Neurosurgery Case Review
Questions and Answers

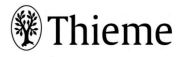

Neurosurgery Case Review
Questions and Answers

Remi Nader, MD, CM, FRCS(C), FACS
Chief, Division of Neurosurgery
Greenwood Leflore Hospital
Greenwood, Mississippi

Clinical Assistant Professor
Department of Neurosurgery
University of Mississippi
Jackson, Mississippi

Abdulrahman J. Sabbagh, MD, FRCS(C)
Director, Neurosurgery Residency Program
Department of Neurosurgery
Neuroscience Center
King Fahd Medical City–Ministry of Health
Riyadh, Saudi Arabia

Thieme
New York • Stuttgart

Thieme Medical Publishers, Inc.
333 Seventh Ave.
New York, NY 10001

Editorial Director: Michael Wachinger
Executive Editor: Kay D. Conerly
Editorial Assistants: Jacquelyn DeSanti, Lauren Henry
International Production Director: Andreas Schabert
Production Editor: Heidi Grauel, Maryland Composition
Vice President, International Sales and Marketing: Cornelia Schulze
Chief Financial Officer: James W. Mitos
President: Brian D. Scanlan
Compositor: MPS Content Services
Printer: Everbest Printing Co.

Library of Congress Cataloging-in-Publication Data

Neurosurgery case review : questions and answers / edited by Remi Nader, Abdulrahman J. Sabbagh.
    p. ; cm.
  Includes bibliographical references and index.
  ISBN 978-1-60406-052-2 (alk. paper)
  1. Nervous system—Surgery—Examinations, questions, etc.   I. Nader, Remi.   II. Sabbagh, Abdulrahman J.
  [DNLM: 1. Nervous System Diseases—surgery—Examination Questions.   2. Neurosurgical Procedures—methods—Examination
Questions.   WL 18.2 C338 2009]
  RD593.C38 2009
  617.4'80076—dc22   2009014543

Important note: Medical knowledge is ever-changing. As new research and clinical experience broaden our knowledge, changes in treatment and drug therapy may be required. The authors and editors of the material herein have consulted sources believed to be reliable in their efforts to provide information that is complete and in accord with the standards accepted at the time of publication. However, in view of the possibility of human error by the authors, editors, or publisher of the work herein or changes in medical knowledge, neither the authors, editors, nor publisher, nor any other party who has been involved in the preparation of this work, warrants that the information contained herein is in every respect accurate or complete, and they are not responsible for any errors or omissions or for the results obtained from use of such information. Readers are encouraged to confirm the information contained herein with other sources. For example, readers are advised to check the product information sheet included in the package of each drug they plan to administer to be certain that the information contained in this publication is accurate and that changes have not been made in the recommended dose or in the contraindications for administration. This recommendation is of particular importance in connection with new or infrequently used drugs.

Some of the product names, patents, and registered designs referred to in this book are in fact registered trademarks or proprietary names even though specific reference to this fact is not always made in the text. Therefore, the appearance of a name without designation as proprietary is not to be construed as a representation by the publisher that it is in the public domain.

All chapters in this book are based on actual cases encountered by the primary or senior authors during the scope of their practices, as are the complications and challenges discussed in each case. Any resemblance with cases or questions presented in formal examinations (such as national board examinations or licensing examinations) or with cases discussed in organized review courses is purely coincidental.

Printed in China

5 4 3 2 1

ISBN 978-1-60406-052-2

Dedication

This book is dedicated to . . .
My lovely wife, Candis, who endured me the past few years during the labor on this project!
My parents, Eleonore and Joseph, and grandmother, Honeine, to whom I owe my life, discipline, and education.
Our pets, Minou and Bibite, who have kept me company and cheered me up during this endeavor.

Remi Nader

To my heroes, my parents, Jafar and Wafa, who selflessly dedicated their lives to their family and country, taught me tolerance and persistence, and told me "never stop before you reach the stars."

To my better half and best friend, my wife, Alaa, without whose true love, altruistic devotion, and unrelenting support I would never have achieved what I have.

To my children, Leen, Jafar, and Omar, and my siblings, Heba, Ahmad, and Mostafa, for making it all worthwhile.

Abdulrahman J. Sabbagh

Contents

Pediatric Cranial Trauma

Developmental Brain Disorders

Stereotactic and Functional Neurosurgery
Neuralgias

Pain Disorders

Other Stereotactic and Functional Procedures

Section II   Spinal and Peripheral Nerve Pathology
Spine
Spinal Trauma

Developmental Spinal Disorders

Peripheral Nerve Pathology
Upper Extremity Peripheral Nerve Disease

Lower Extremity Peripheral Nerve Disease

Section III   Neurology
Epilepsy

Dementias and White Matter Diseases

Foreword

With today's rapid expansion of medical technology and clinical information, it is essential that we are on top of the fundamental knowledge in our field. To this end, Drs. Nader and Sabbagh have compiled a remarkable collection of cases that highlight a variety of clinical entities and syndromes that help in this task.

The cases in this book cover the majority of topics of importance and interest to a junior neurosurgeon. As such, a careful review of all these cases would be particularly helpful in preparing for the in-training written board examination, as well as for the oral board examination. In fact, this comprehensive case book serves as a reminder of all the clinical and diagnostic entities that should be reviewed prior to taking these examinations. Very few publications exist that help accomplish this goal. This book therefore helps fill this void and provides a well thought-out outline of the major neurosurgical topics and a high-quality collection of cases to review and study. The authors should be commended on their efforts.

Raymond Sawaya, MD
Professor and Chairman
Department of Neurosurgery
The University of Texas M. D. Anderson Cancer Center
Houston, Texas

Preface

The amount of material that needs to be reviewed for a national board examination can be very intimidating and formidable. Having taken both the Royal College of Canada examination and the American board examination in neurosurgery, I have noticed that there is a lack of comprehensive texts presenting a case-based approach for the management of neurosurgical problems (such as the cases presented on both of the above-mentioned examinations). This text was written to fill this void.

Furthermore, this book is not only intended for board review (although I do anticipate that this will be one of its primary uses) but it is also meant to bring "the judgment" and "the art" of practicing neurosurgery to the general neurosurgeon. Most published texts provide broad guidelines and indications on how to treat certain conditions. There are very few books that discuss treatment on a case-by-case basis, focusing on the intricacies and nuances of the specific cases, and the complications and outcome.

Also, Abdulrahman and I realize that there are several ways of treating the same condition, or dealing with the same complication or outcome. When deemed appropriate, we will discuss those different ways. However, the main authors typically select and focus on their preferred approach. This does not mean that this is the only correct approach and we do encourage our readers to further discuss these cases and alternatives for treatment with their colleagues. After all, neurosurgery is an ever-evolving field and some cases in this book may be treated by radically different measures even a few years from now.

In 2006, my study partner for the Royal College of Canada examination, Abdulrahman J. Sabbagh, became a good friend and colleague. Together we exchanged multiple cases and discussed their intricacies and details at length. With his great artistic talents, our varied experience, interesting cases I had accumulated, and our network of friends and colleagues in the field, we were able to put together 113 cases covering the whole span of neurosurgery.

This by no means represents an exhaustive review of the field of neurosurgery, but merely a cross-section of each of the main areas in the field. The book consists mainly of common (and some less common) clinical scenarios encountered in a general neurosurgical practice, with pertinent questions on presentation, diagnosis, imaging, management, surgical detail, complications, and outcome. The cases in this book are organized by main sections and subsections. Each case consists of a short clinical presentation followed by a few questions about the case. The answers are kept simple and to the point. Whenever possible, we have tried to use up-to-date, evidence-based reference data to support the management of each case. As you browse through the book, you will notice that certain sections contain more topics than others and certain topics are discussed in more detail. This particular selection of topics was chosen as it reflects the frequency of occurrence of individual components in a general neurosurgical practice, the expertise of the contributors, and the emphasis on the pertinent knowledge needed for examination purposes. Over 380 scans and photographs and about 50 color illustrations contribute to this book's ease of use and richness.

With over 85 contributors from four continents (North America, Europe, Africa, and Asia) and seven countries (United States, Canada, Italy, Saudi Arabia, Egypt, China, and Indonesia), as well as six reviewers from the United States, this book represents a wealth of information that has been distilled to the essentials. Each case has been reviewed by at least three neurosurgeons (the editors and one or two reviewers) and all chapters were tailored to fit U.S. and Canadian general standards of care for practice.

All chapters in this book are based on actual cases encountered by the primary or senior authors during the scope of their practices, as are the complications and challenges discussed in each case. Any resemblance with cases or questions presented in formal examinations (such as national board examinations or licensing examinations) or with cases discussed in organized review courses is purely coincidental.

I hope you enjoy reading this text as much as we enjoyed preparing it.

Remi Nader, MD

Acknowledgments

I would like to acknowledge the help and support of Joseph Nader, PhD, Brent McCaleb, Michele Crescenzo, PhD, and Alain Domkam, MD.

I would like to thank all of our contributors and reviewers who have helped shape this book into a wealth of knowledge and information.

I would like to extend my appreciation to the staff and patients of Greenwood Leflore Hospital and the North Central Mississippi Neurological Surgery Clinic.

I would also like to acknowledge the assistance of Ivy Ip, Birgitta Brandenberg, and Kay D. Conerly from Thieme, who have nursed this book along and without whom this idea would not have become a reality.

Remi Nader

I would like to thank my co-editor, Remi Nader, who inspired me to start this project. I would also thank our Canadian Boards Study Group, Drs. Ahmed Lary, Denis Klironomos, Mohammad Halawani, Pascale Lavoie, Mohamed Bangash, Paul Khuair, Jocelyn Blanchard, Nick Phan, and Anil Kumar for motivating both me and Remi to make this idea a reality. I would like to extend my appreciation to each member of my family away from home at the Montreal Neurological Institute (MNI) and Montreal Children's Hospital. I will never forget the help I got from the MNI librarians. I could not have accomplished this work without the endless support of my patients and family here at our Neuroscience Center, King Fahd Medical City. I thank my new friends at Thieme for being interested in this project. I thank my wife, my parents, and her parents for being my secret to success. Most importantly, I would like to thank the All-Mighty for his guidance and for giving me the fortune of knowing all these people and allowing me to work closely with Remi Nader—despite being oceans apart—to bring this project to life.

Abdulrahman J. Sabbagh

Contributors

Ahmed T. Abdelmoity, MD
Assistant Professor
Departments of Pediatrics and Neurology
Director of Department of Neurophysiology
Director of the Comprehensive Epilepsy Program
University of Missouri at Kansas City
University of Kansas
Children's Mercy Hospitals and Clinics
Kansas City, Missouri

Abdulrazag Ajlan, MD
Neurosurgery Resident
Department of Neurosurgery
McGill University
Montreal Neurological Institute and Hospital
Montreal, Quebec, Canada

Maqsood Ahmad, MMed (RSA)
Consultant Pediatric Neurosurgeon
Pediatric Neurosurgery Section
Consultant Neurosurgeon
Department of Neurosurgery
Neuroscience Center
King Fahd Medical City
Riyadh, Saudi Arabia

Ayman Abdullah Albanyan, MBBS, FRCS(C)
Head
Pediatric Neurosurgery Section
Consultant Pediatric Neurosurgeon
Department of Neurosurgery
Neuroscience Center
King Fahd Medical City
Riyadh, Saudi Arabia

Homoud Aldahash, MBBS
Senior Resident
Section of Neurosurgery
Department of Neurosciences
King Faisal Specialist Hospital and Research Center
Riyadh, Saudi Arabia

Hashem Al Hashemi, MD, FRCPC
Physical Medicine and Rehabilitation Consultant
Division of Physical Medicine and Geriatric
Department of Medicine
King Abdulaziz Medical City
Riyadh, Saudi Arabia

Qasim S. Al-Hinai, BSc, MD, MRCSI
Neurosurgery Resident
Department of Neurosurgery
McGill University
Montreal Neurological Institute and Hospital
Montreal, Quebec, Canada

Hosam Al-Jehani, MD
Neurosurgery Resident
Department of Neurosurgery
McGill University
Montreal Neurological Institute and Hospital
Montreal, Quebec, Canada

Ahmad Al-Jishi, MD
Neurosurgery Resident
Department of Neurosurgery
McGill University
Montreal Neurological Institute and Hospital
Montreal, Quebec, Canada

Ossama Al-Mefty, MD
Professor and Chairman
Department of Neurosurgery
University of Arkansas for Medical Sciences
Little Rock, Arkansas

Khalid N. Almusrea, MD, FRCS(C)
Chairman
Department of Spine Surgery
Consultant Neurosurgeon
Departments of Spine and Neurosurgery
Neuroscience Center
King Fahd Medical City
Riyadh, Saudi Arabia

Fahad Eid Alotaibi, MBBS
Physician
Department of Neurosurgery
Neuroscience Center
King Fahd Medical City
Riyadh, Saudi Arabia

Abdulrahman Yaqub Alturki, MBBS
Neurosurgery Resident
Department of Neurosurgery
Montreal Neurological Institute and Hospital
Montreal, Quebec, Canada

Mahmoud A. Al Yamany, MD, MHA, FRCS(C)
Director, Neuroscience Center
Chairman, Department of Neurosurgery
Consultant Neurosurgeon
Consultant Neurovascular and Skull Base Surgeon
Department of Neurosurgery
Neuroscience Center
King Fahd Medical City
Riyadh, Saudi Arabia

Ahmed Jaman Alzahrani, MD
Senior Resident
Section of Neurosurgery
Department of Neurosciences
King Faisal Specialist Hospital and Research Center
Riyadh, Saudi Arabia

Gmaan Ali M. Al-Zhrani, MBBS
Resident, Neurosurgery Residency Training Program
Department of Neurosurgery
Neuroscience Center
King Fahd Medical City
Riyadh, Saudi Arabia

Carmina M. Angeles, MD
Division of Neurosurgery
University of Texas Medical Branch at Galveston
Galveston, Texas

Jeffrey Atkinson, MD, FRCS(C)
Assistant Professor
Department of Neurosurgery
McGill University
Montreal Children's Hospital
Montreal, Quebec, Canada

Fawziah A. Bamogaddam, MD
Neurology Consultant
Department of Adult Neurology
Neuroscience Center
King Fahd Medical City
Riyadh, Saudia Arabia

Edward Benzel, MD
Chairman
Department of Neurosurgery
Center for Spine Health
The Cleveland Clinic Foundation
Cleveland, Ohio

Michel W. Bojanowski, MD, FRCS(C)
Professor
Department of Neurosurgery
University of Montreal
Hôpital Notre-Dame du CHUM
Montreal, Quebec, Canada

Reem Bunyan, MD
Consultant Neurologist and Neuroimmunologist
Neuroimmunology Program
Departments of Neurology and Neurophysiology
Chair of Neurophysiology
Neurosciences Center
Kind Fahd Medical City
Riyadh, Saudi Arabia

Alwin Camancho, MD
Department of Radiology
University of Texas Medical Branch at Galveston
Galveston, Texas

Ricardo L. Carrau, MD
Department of Otolaryngology
University of Pittsburgh Medical Center
The Eye and Ear Institute Building
Pittsburgh, Pennsylvania

Isaac Chan, MD
Department of Neurological Surgery
Columbia University
College of Physicians and Surgeons
New York, New York

Claude-Edouard Chatillon, MD
Department of Neurosurgery
Montreal Neurological Hospital Institute
Montreal, Quebec, Canada

Deepa Danan, BA
Department of Neurological Surgery
Columbia University
College of Physicians and Surgerons
New York, New York

Rolando Del Maestro, MD, PhD, FRCS(C), FACS
Professor
Department of Neurology and Neurosurgery
Montreal Neurological Institute
Montreal, Quebec, Canada

Samer K. Elbabaa, MD
Assistant Professor
Department of Neurosurgery
University of Arkansas for Medical Sciences
Little Rock, Arkansas

Domenic P. Esposito, MD, FACS
Associate Professor
Department of Neurosurgery
University of Mississippi Medical Center
Jackson, Mississippi

Jean-Pierre Farmer, MD, CM, FRCS(C)
Professor
Department of Neurosurgery
McGill University
Montreal Children's Hospital
Montreal, Quebec, Canada

Paul Gardner, MD
Department of Neurological Surgery
University of Pittsburgh Medical Center
Pittsburgh, Pennsylvania

Cristian Gragnaniello, MD
Chief Resident
Department of Neurosurgery
Second University of Naples
Naples, Italy

Amgad S. Hanna, MD
Assistant Professor
Department of Neurological Surgery
University of Wisconsin, Madison
Madison, Wisconsin

Stephen J. Hentschel, MD
Clinical Assistant Professor
Department of Surgery
University of British Columbia
Victorial General Hospital
Victoria, British Columbia, Canada

Robert Herndon, MD
Professor
Department of Neurology
University of Mississippi Medical Center
Jackson, Mississippi

Melanie Hood, BA
Columbia University
College of Physicians and Surgeons
New York, New York

Glenn C. Hunter, MD
Chief of Vascular Surgery
Southern Arizona VA Health Care System
Tucson, Arizona

Pascal M. Jabbour, MD
Department of Neurological Surgery
Thomas Jefferson University Hospital
Philadelphia, Pennsylvania

Julius July, MD, MHSc
Senior Lecturer
Department of Neurosurgery
Pelita Harapan/Siloam Lippo Karawaci Hospital
Tangerang, Baten, Indonesia

Amin B. Kassam, MD
Professor
Department of Neurological Surgery
University of Pittsburgh Medical Center
Pittsburgh, Pennsylvania

Christopher P. Kellner, MD
Resident
Department of Neurological Surgery
Columbia University
College of Physicians and Surgeons
New York, New York

Dennis Klironomos, MD, FRCS(C)
St. Luke's Neurosurgery Associates
Duluth, Minnesota

William E. Krauss, MD
Associate Professor
Department of Neurological Surgery
Mayo Clinic
Rochester, Minnesota

Michel Lacroix, MD, FRCS(C), FACS
Director of Neurosurgery
Director of Brain and Spine Tumor Institute
Department of Neurosurgery
Geisinger Wyoming Valley
Wilkes-Barre, Pennsylvania

Ahmad I. Lary, MD, FRCS(C)
Director, Neuro-oncology Program
Neurosurgery Department
Neuroscience Center
King Fahd Medical City
Riyadh, Saudi Arabia

Richard Leblanc, MSc, MD, FRCS(C)
Professor
Departments of Neurology and Neurosurgery
McGill University
Montreal Neurological Institute and Hospital
Montreal, Quebec, Canada

Joung H. Lee, MD
Professor
Head of Skull Base Surgery
Brain Tumor and Neuro-oncology Center
Neurological Institute
Cleveland Clinic
Cleveland, Ohio

Jie Ma, MD
Professor
Department of Pediatric Neurosurgery
Xinhua Hospital School of Medicine
Shanghai Jiao Tong University
Shanghai, China

Ramez Malak, MD, MSc
Resident
Department of Neurosurgery
Notre Dame Hospital
Centre Hospitalier de l'Université de Montreal
Montreal, Quebec, Canada

Judith Marcoux, MD, MSc, FRCS(C)
Assistant Professor
Department of Neurosurgery
McGill University
Montreal Neurological Institute and Hospital
Montreal, Quebec, Canada

Nancy McLaughlin, MD
University of Montreal
Department of Neurosurgery
Hôpital Notre-Dame du CHUM
Montreal, Quebec, Canada

Arlan H. Mintz, MD
Department of Neurological Surgery
University of Pittsburgh Medical Center
Pittsburgh, Pennsylvania

Sandeep Mittal, MD, FRCS(C), FACS
Assistant Professor
Department of Neurosurgery
Wayne State University
Detroit, Michigan

Gaetan Moise, MD
Resident
Department of Neurological Surgery
Columbia University
College of Physicians and Surgeons
New York, New York

José Luis Montes, MD, CM
Associate Professor
Department of Neurosurgery, Neurology, and Oncology
McGill University
Montreal, Quebec, Canada

Robert Moumdjian, MD, MSc, FRCS(C)
Associate Professor
Department of Neurosurgery
Notre Dame Hospital
Centre Hospitalier de l'Universite de Montreal
Montreal, Quebec, Canada

Marc-Elie Nader, MD
Department of Otolaryngology
Centre Hospitalier de l'Université de Montreal
Montreal, Quebec, Canada

Maya Nader
Faculty of Medicine
Université de Montréal
Montreal, Quebec, Canada

Remi Nader, MD, CM, FRCS(C), FACS
Chief, Division of Neurosurgery
Greenwood Leflore Hospital
Greenwood, Mississippi
Clinical Assistant Professor
Department of Neurosurgery
University of Mississippi
Jackson, Mississippi

Lissa Marie Ogieglo, MD
Resident
Department of Neurosurgery
University of Saskatchewan
Saskatoow, Saskatchewan, Canada

Yasser I. Orz, MD, PhD
Director, Neurovascular Program
Department of Neurosurgery
King Fahd Medical City
Riyadh, Saudi Arabia

Ravi Pande, MD
Greenwood Neurology Clinic
Greenwood, Mississippi

Kevin Petrecca, MD, PhD
Assistant Professor
Department of Neurology and Neurosurgery
McGill University
Montreal Neurological Institute and Hospital
Montreal, Quebec, Canada

Ian F. Pollack, MD
Chief, Pediatric Neurosurgery
Professor of Neurological Surgery
Department of Neurosurgery
Children's Hospital of Pittsburgh
Pittsburgh, Pennsylvania

Daniel M. Prevedello, MD
Clinical Instructor
Director of the Microsurgical Anatomy Lab
Department of Neurological Surgery
UPMC - Presbyterian - Neurological Surgery
Pittsburgh, Pennsylvania

Nazer H. Qureshi, MD, D. Stat, MSc
Chief, Brain and Spine Tumor Service
Baptist Health Medical Center
North Little Rock, Arkansas

Ali Raja, MD
Assistant Professor
Department of Neurosurgery
University of Arkansas for Medical Sciences
Little Rock, Arkansas

Eric P. Roger, MD, FRCS(C)
Assistant Professor
Department of Neurosurgery
University of Buffalo, State University of New York
Buffalo, New York

Stephen M. Russell, MD
Assistant Professor
Department of Neurosurgery
NYU School of Medicine
New York, New York

Abdulrahman J. Sabbagh, MD, FRCS(C)
Epilepsy and Pediatric Neurosurgeon
Neurosurgery Residency Program Director
Department of Neurosurgery
Neuroscience Center
King Fahd Medical City
Riyadh, Saudi Arabia

Burak Sade, MD
Clinical Associate
Section of Skull Base Surgery
Brain Tumor and Neuro-oncology Center
Cleveland Clinic
Cleveland, Ohio

Brian Seaman, DO
Chief Resident
Department of Neurosurgery
Grant Medical Center
Columbus, Ohio

Bassem Sheikh, MD
Vice Dean for Clinical Affairs
Faculty of Medicine
Taibah University
Al-Madinah, Saudi Arabia

Joseph A. Shehadi, MD, FRCS(C), FACS
Clinical Assistant Professor
Department of Neurosurgery
Ohio University
Grant Medical Center
Columbus, Ohio

Xiaohong Si, MD
Vanderbilt University Medical Center
Children's Hospital
Nashville, Tennessee

Khurram A. Siddiqui, MBBS, FRCP
Consultant Neurologist and Epileptologist
Neurosciences Center
King Fahd Medical City
Riyadh, Saudi Arabia

Allen K. Sills Jr., MD, FACS
Semmes-Murphey Neurologic and Spine Institute
Memphis, Tennessee

David Sinclair, MD, FRCS(C)
Assistant Professor
Department of Neurology and Neurosurgery
Montreal Neurological Institute and Hospital
Montreal, Quebec, Canada

Shobhit Sinha, MBBS
Consultant, Neurology and Epilepsy
Neurosciences Center
King Fahad Medical City
Riyadh, Saudi Arabia

Dennis J. Sirhan, MD, FRCS(C)
Assistant Professor
Department of Neurosurgery
Montreal Neurological Institute and Hospital
Montreal, Quebec, Canada

Carl H. Snyderman, MD
Minimally Invasive Endoneurosurgical Center
Department of Otolaryngology
University of Pittsburgh Medical Center
Pittsburgh, Pennsylvania

Sten Solander, MD
Assistant Professor
Department of Radiology
The University of North Carolina at Chapel Hill
Chapel Hill, North Carolina

Lahbib B. Soualmi, PhD
Director, Neuronavigation Unit and the Intraoperative
   MRI Suite
Neurosurgery Department
Neuroscience Center
King Fahd Medical City
Riyadh, Saudi Arabia
Assistant Professor, Director, Neuronavigation Unit
Montreal Neurological Institute
McGill University
Montreal Quebec, Canada

Robert L. Tiel, MD
Professor
Department of Neurosurgery
University of Mississippi Medical Center
Jackson, Mississippi

Erol Veznedaroglu, MD
Director
Stroke and Cerebrovascular Center of New Jersey Chief
Cerebrovascular and Endovascular Neurosurgery Capital
Health System
Trenton, New Jersey

Rudiger Von Ritschl, MD
Department of Radiology
University of Texas Medical Branch at Galveston
Galveston, Texas

Dennis G. Vollmer, MD
Colorado Brain and Spine Institute
Edgewood, Colorado

Eka Julianta Wahjoepramono, MD
Associate Professor
Department of Neurosurgery
Pelita Harapan/Siloam Lippo Karawaci Hospital
Tangerang, Baten, Indonesia

Adam Sauh Gee Wu, MD
Neurosurgery Resident
University of Saskatchewan
Division of Neurosurgery
Royal University Hospital
Saskatoon, Saskatchewan, Canada

Christopher J. Winfree, MD
Assistant Professor
Department of Neurological Surgery
Columbia University
College of Physicians and Surgeons
New York, New York

John Winestone, MD
Department of Neurosurgery
The University of Tennessee
Memphis, Tennessee

Reviewers

Brain Tumors

Jimmy D. Miller, MD, JD
Attending Neurosurgeon
North Central Mississippi Neurological Surgery
Greenwood Leflore Hospital
Greenwood, Mississippi

Nazer H. Qureshi, MD, D Stat, MSc
Chief, Brain and Spine Tumor Service
Baptist Health Medical Center
North Little Rock, Arkansas

Vascular Neurosurgery

Gustavo D. Luzardo, MD
Assistant Professor of Neurosurgery, Department
  of Neurosurgery
University of Mississippi Medical Center
Jackson, Mississippi

Pediatric and Developmental Disorders

Andrew D. Parent, MD
Professor of Neurosurgery, Department of
  Neurosurgery
University of Mississippi Medical Center
Jackson, Mississippi

Spine

Amgad Hanna, MD
Assistant Professor
Department of Neurological Surgery
University of Wisconsin, Madison
Madison, Wisconsin

Jimmy D. Miller, MD, JD
Attending Neurosurgeon
North Central Mississippi Neurological Surgery
Greenwood Leflore Hospital
Greenwood, Mississippi

Neurology

Jimmy D. Miller, MD, JD
Attending Neurosurgeon
North Central Mississippi Neurological Surgery
Greenwood Leflore Hospital
Greenwood, Mississippi

General and Neuroanatomy

Duane E. Haines, PhD
Chairman and Professor of Anatomy
Department of Anatomy
The University of Mississippi Medical Center
Jackson, Mississippi

Section I Intracranial Pathology

Case 1   Vestibular Schwannoma in Neurofibromatosis Type 2

Burak Sade and Joung H. Lee

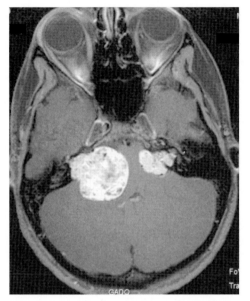

Fig. 1.1 T1-weighted postcontrast axial magnetic resonance image showing bilateral vestibular schwannomas. Note the severe compression of the brainstem.

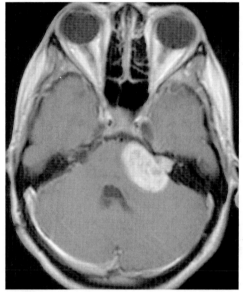

Fig. 1.2 T1-weighted postcontrast axial magnetic resonance image 2 years after surgery showing complete resection of the tumor on the right. At this point, the left-sided tumor was treated with gamma knife radiosurgery.

■ Clinical Presentation

- An 18-year-old left-handed woman with neurofibromatosis type 2 (NF-2) presents with progression of a known vestibular schwannoma (VS).
- Three years ago, she underwent Cyberknife fractionated stereotactic radiosurgery to treat a right-sided VS. Over the last few months, she describes episodes of imbalance and "blackouts" without loss of consciousness.
- Her family history is significant; both her father and sister have NF-2.
- Neurologic evaluation shows bilateral papilledema, decreased hearing on the left side (but still serviceable), and complete loss of hearing on the right side.
- Magnetic resonance imaging (MRI) of the brain is shown in **Fig. 1.1**.

■ Questions

1. What are the diagnostic criteria of NF-2?
2. What additional studies are essential for the decision-making process?
3. What are the main management goals in NF-2 patients?
4. What are the management options?
5. What are the most common surgical approaches?
6. What would be your plan for the right-sided tumor?

She was operated on via a suboccipital retrosigmoid approach, and complete removal of the tumor was achieved with preservation of the facial nerve. During her follow-up, the tumor on the left side showed growth (**Fig. 1.2**), with worsening of her hearing.

7. What would be your plan for the left-sided tumor?
8. What are the outcomes of radiosurgery for VS?

■ Answers

1. *What are the diagnostic criteria for NF-2?*
   - Bilateral vestibular schwannoma
   - Family history of NF-2 (first-degree relative) plus unilateral VS
   - Family history of NF-2 plus two of the following:
     – Meningioma, schwannoma (nonvestibular), glioma, neurofibroma, juvenile posterior subcapsular lenticular cataract, or opacity[1]

2. *What additional studies are essential for the decision-making process?*[2,3]
   - Audiometric evaluation including pure tone (PTA), speech reception threshold (SRT), and speech discrimination score (SDS) values
   - "50/50" rule can be used a cutoff value for serviceable hearing. With PTA showing values <50 dB and speech discrimination with recognition of >50%.
   - Computed tomography (CT) scan of the brain to assess bony landmarks and for surgical planning. Also assess the size of the internal auditory canal (IAC) and whether or not there is any dilatation of the canal.
   - Other tests that may be helpful include brainstem auditory-evoked responses (BSAER) as preoperative baselines, electronystagmography (ENG), stapedial reflex to assess retrocochlear lesion, and cold caloric testing.[2,3]

3. *What are the main management goals in NF-2 patients?*
   - To preserve serviceable hearing as long as possible
   - To decompress the brainstem from the pressure exerted by the right-sided tumor in this case (**Fig. 1.1**)
   - Early counseling about the genetic implications, as well as the need for training in lip reading, and sign language techniques

4. *What are the management options?*
   - Conservative approach with observation is not a good option in this case. This approach is used in cases of small tumor with serviceable hearing. It consists of serial observation with MRI or CT every 6 months for 2 years, then annually.
   - Radiation therapy: External beam radiation or stereotactic radiosurgery (SRS). Gamma knife radiosurgery (a type of SRS) can be used in the following cases:
     – Poor operative candidates because of other medical problems, age, etc.
     – Bilateral VS
     – Tumor progression or tumor residual after surgical resection
     – Usually cases of small tumor and/or tumors with serviceable hearing
   - Surgery is the mainstay of therapy. It is indicated in large- or medium-size tumors with or without serviceable hearing, in signs of brainstem compression, intractable disequilibrium, severe trigeminal symptoms, and hydrocephalus.
   - Note that patients with bilateral VS (as opposed to unilateral) tend to be younger, with larger tumors, worse preoperative hearing, and have greater chances of losing either cranial nerve VII or VIII functions during surgical excision of the tumor.[3,4]

5. *What are the most common surgical approaches?*
   - Suboccipital or retrosigmoid
   - Translabyrinthine
   - Middle fossa
   - Combined approaches[5]

6. *What would be your plan for the right-sided tumor?*
   - Because of the symptomatic increase in size, failure of previous radiation treatment, and absence of hearing, surgery is indicated on the right-sided tumor.

7. *What would be your plan for the left-sided tumor?*
   - Both surgery and radiosurgery are options in this case. Surgery may have the added benefit of removing any mass effect on the brainstem. However, surgery has a significant risk of hearing loss on the only functioning side. Our preferred course of action would be to treat the tumor with SRS. This is to preserve hearing in the only side where it is still present. She was treated with gamma knife radiosurgery.

8. *What are the outcomes of radiosurgery for VS?*
   - This treatment modality has 81% tumor control rate at 15 years with hearing preservation rates of 73% at 1 year and 48% at 5 years.[6] Preservation of hearing in tumors of this size would be very difficult to achieve with microsurgery.[7] Therefore, surgery would not be recommended on this side as the first option, as long as she has serviceable hearing.

■ References

1. Neurofibromatosis, National Institutes of Health Consensus Development Conference. Neurofibromatosis: Conference Statement. Arch Neurol 1988;45:575–578
2. Cheng G, Smith R, Tan AK. Cost comparison of auditory brainstem response versus magnetic resonance imaging screening of acoustic neuroma. J Otolaryngol 2003;32(6):394–399
3. Sahu RN, Mehrotra N, Tyagi I, Banerji D, Jain VK, Behari S. Management strategies for bilateral vestibular schwannomas. J Clin Neurosci 2007;14(8):715–722
4. Nader R, Al-Abdulhadi K, Leblanc R, Zeitouni A. Acoustic neuroma – an outcome study. J Otolaryngol 2002;31(4):207–210
5. Bennett M, Haynes DS. Surgical approaches and complications in the removal of vestibular schwannomas. Otolaryngol Clin North Am 2007;40(3):589–609, ix–x
6. Mathieu D, Kondziolka D, Flickenger JC, et al. Stereotactic radiosurgery for vestibular schwannomas in patients with neurofibromatosis type 2: an analysis of tumor control, complications, and hearing preservation rates. Neurosurgery 2007;60:460–470
7. Mohr G, Sade B, Dufour JJ, Rappaport JM. Preservation of hearing in patients with vestibular schwannoma: degree of meatal filling. J Neurosurg 2005;102:1–5

Case 2 Subependymal Giant Cell Astrocytoma

Remi Nader

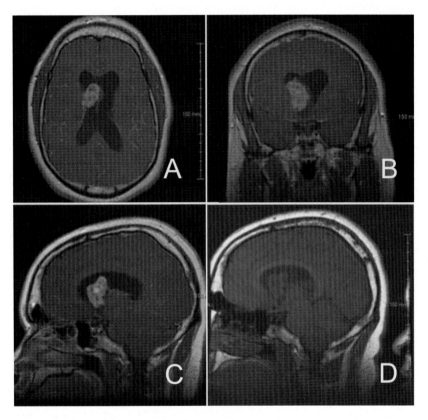

Fig. 2.1 Magnetic resonance imaging (MRI) scan of the brain **(A–C)** with gadolinium intravenous contrast and **(D)** without contrast showing **(A)** pertinent axial, **(B)** coronal, and **(C,D)** sagittal sections.

■ Clinical Presentation

- A 21-year-old man presents with 2-year history of headaches, exacerbated over the past 3 to 4 months.
- He also complains of blurred vision intermittently and some episodes of nausea and vomiting.
- Neurologic examination reveals bilateral papilledema; otherwise, no focal deficits are seen.

- Upon further questioning, he claims he had a history of seizures as a child, but this resolved by the time he was 12 years old.
- Magnetic resonance imaging (MRI) scan of the brain is ordered (**Fig. 2.1**).

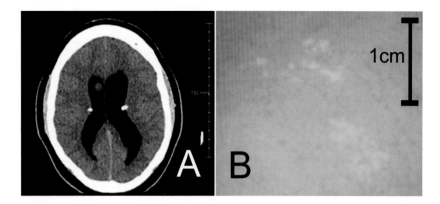

Fig. 2.2   (A) Axial computed tomography (CT) scan without contrast at the level of the ventricles showing hyperdense lesions along the lateral walls of both ventricles. **(B)** Photograph of macular skin lesion with loss of pigmentation.

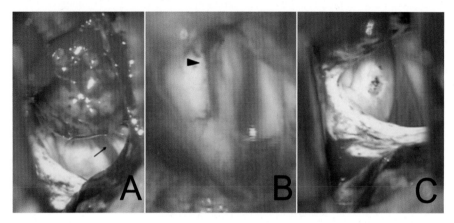

Fig. 2.3   Intraoperative pictures taken with microscope magnification (300×) showing the inside of the right lateral ventricle **(A)** with large fleshy mass superiorly representing the tumor. A small draining vein within the ventricle is pointed out (*arrow*). Following tumor resection, the picture is taken while inside the lateral ventricle showing the slitlike opening (*arrowhead*) into the third ventricle via the foramen of Monro **(B)**. Picture taken while retracting with a self-retaining retractor and exposing the medial wall of the lateral ventricle **(C)**.

■ Questions

1. Interpret the lesion on the MRI.
2. Give a differential diagnosis.
3. What further studies should you obtain?

A computed tomography (CT) scan of the brain is done and upon further examination, you observe the following skin lesions (multiple on his trunk and lower extremities) (**Fig. 2.2**).

4. Name the lesions seen on the CT and on the skin.
5. What is the diagnosis?
6. What other lesions are associated with the presenting diagnosis?
7. What are the operative options in this case?
8. Which option do you choose and why?
9. What preoperative studies would you like to obtain?

10. You elect to perform a right transcallosal approach. As you enter the right ventricle, you see the tumor anterior to your corpus callosal opening and the falx laterally. Identify the following vessel (**Fig. 2.3A**, *arrow*) and name the parent or immediate tributary vessel.
11. As you start dissecting the tumor, cerebrospinal fluid (CSF) is let out and the septum pellucidum bulges out and obstructs your view. What is your course of action?
12. You perform a complete resection. The tumor was seen to extend in the 3rd ventricle, shown in **Fig. 2.3B**. It was attached on the structure inside the lateral ventricle as shown in **Fig. 2.3B** (*arrowhead*). Identify this structure and give the function of this structure.

■ Answers

1. *Interpret the lesion on the MRI.*
   - MRI shows a lesion in the right lateral ventricle at the level of the foramen of Monroe.
   - The lesion is ~2.5 × 3 cm in size, well circumscribed, heterogeneous with enhancement. It is hypointense on T1-weighted sequences.
   - There is evidence of obstructive hydrocephalus and ventriculomegaly.

2. *Give a differential diagnosis.[1]*
   The mnemonic is "CENTRAL MS" for intraventricular lesion:
   - C – Choroid plexus papilloma or carcinoma, colloid cyst, central neurocytoma, cavernoma
   - E – Ependymoma, epidermoid/dermoid
   - N – Neurocytoma
   - T – Teratoma, tuber
   - R – "Rule out" infection
   - A – Astrocytoma, arteriovenous malformation (AVM), aneurysm, abscess
   - L – Lipoma, lymphoma
   - M – Metastases, meningioma
   - S – Subependymoma, subependymal giant cell astrocytoma

3. *What further imaging studies and pertinent laboratory studies should you obtain?[1]*
   - CT scan of the brain
   - MRI neuraxis to rule out drop metastases
   - Angiogram and venogram, especially if you plan to perform an operative resection
   - Tumor markers: carcinoembryonic antigen, α-fetoprotein, beta human chorionic gonadotropin
   - Basic laboratory panel: complete blood count, electrolytes, prothrombin time, partial thromboplastin time, type and screen

4. *A CT scan of the brain is done and upon further examination, you observe the following skin lesion. Name the lesions seen on the CT and on the skin.*
   - CT scan shows subependymal nodules that are hyperdense in both ventricles (lateral walls).
   - Skin lesion is a patchy macular discoloration or loss of pigmentation consistent with an ash-leaf spot

5. *What is the diagnosis?*
   - Tuberous sclerosis with subependymal giant cell astrocytoma in the right ventricle

6. *What other lesions are associated with the presenting diagnosis?[1,2]*
   - Facial angiofibromas, multiple ungual fibromas, tubers, multiple calcified subependymal nodules, multiple retinal astrocytomas, cardiac rhabdomyoma, retinal hamartomas or achromic patch, shagreen patch, forehead plaque, pulmonary lymphangiomyomatosis, renal angiomyolipoma, renal cysts

7. *What are the operative options in this case?[3,4]*
   - Transcallosal approach
     - Preferred over transcortical, in general
     - Advantages
       - Short trajectory to 3rd ventricle
       - No cortical transgression
       - Can visualize both foramina of Monro
     - Complications
       - Weakness
       - Akinetic mutism
       - Memory deficits
   - Transcortical, transventricular approach
     - Good for anterosuperior 3rd ventricle lesions
     - Especially if lesion extends into frontal horns
     - Passage through the right middle frontal gyrus (F2)
     - Disadvantages
       - Higher risk of seizures (11%)
       - Need larger ventricles
   - Ventriculoperitoneal (VP) shunt
     - Does not get rid of the mass effect caused by the tumor
     - Reserve for palliative cases
   - Endoscopic resection
     - May be a better option with smaller tumor sizes
     - Is associated with a potential risk of hemorrhage
     - Requires extensive operator's experience

8. *Which one do you choose and why?[3,4]*
   - The transcallosal approach is preferred in this case because of the advantages listed above.

9. *What preoperative studies would you like to obtain?*
   - Cerebral arteriogram and venogram
     - To better define the arterial supply to the tumor
     - For possible embolization
     - To define the cortical venous anatomy, especially on the right side at the site of entry in the lateral ventricle
   - Frameless stereotactic MRI study for navigation
   - Other studies as per question 3

10. *You elect to perform a right transcallosal approach. As you enter the right ventricle, you see the tumor anterior to your corpus callosal opening and the falx laterally. Identify the following vessel (arrow) and name the parent or immediate tributary vessel.[5]*
    - Thalamostriate vein
    - Empties into the internal cerebral vein

11. *As you start dissecting the tumor, CSF is let out and the septum pellucidum bulges out and obstructs your view. What is your course of action?[5,6]*
    - Perform a septostomy to let out CSF from the contralateral lateral ventricle (**Fig. 2.3C**)

■ Answers *(continued)*

12. *You perform a complete resection. The tumor was seen to extend in the 3rd ventricle, shown below. It was attached on the following structure inside the lateral ventricle (arrowhead). Identify this structure and give the function of this structure.*[5]	• Fornix • Location: From hippocampus to hypothalamus, the body of fornix is under the corpus callosum. • Function: memory, emotion, part of the limbic system and hippocampal formation

■ References

1. Koeller KK, Sandberg GD. Armed Forces Institute of Pathology. From the archives of the AFIP. Cerebral intraventricular neoplasms: radiologic-pathologic correlation. Radiographics 2002;22(6):1473–1505

2. Hurst JS, Wilcoski S. Recognizing an index case of tuberous sclerosis. Am Fam Physician 2000;61(3):703–710

3. D'Angelo VA, Galarza M, Catapano D, Monte V, Bisceglia M, Carosi I. Lateral ventricle tumors: surgical strategies according to tumor origin and development – a series of 72 cases. Neurosurgery 2005; 56(1, Suppl)36–45

4. Cuccia V, Zuccaro G, Sosa F, Monges J, Lubienieky F, Taratuto AL. Subependymal giant cell astrocytoma in children with tuberous sclerosis. Childs Nerv Syst 2003;19(4):232–243

5. Rhoton A. Microsurgical anatomy of the lateral ventricles. In: Rengashary SS, Wilkins RH, eds. Neurosurgery. 2nd ed. New York: McGraw-Hill; 1996:1419–1434

6. Schneider JH, Chandrasoma P, Nedzi L, Apuzzo ML. Neoplasms of the pineal and third ventricular region. In: Youman JR. Neurological Surgery. 4th ed. Philadelphia, PA: WB Saunders Co; 1996: 2715–2747

Case 3   Sturge–Weber Syndrome

Remi Nader

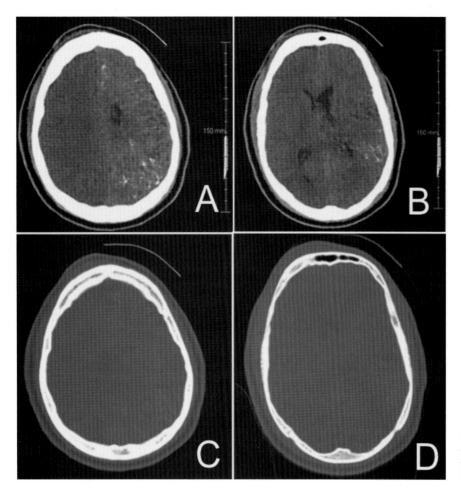

Fig. 3.1   (A,B) Computed tomography scan without contrast, brain windows, and bone windows **(C,D)**, showing lesion in the left hemisphere.

■ **Clinical Presentation**

- A 31-year-old man had a grand mal seizure episode at home while eating.
- He is brought to the emergency room at an outside hospital, where he obtains a computed tomography (CT) scan, which is read as "suspicious subarachnoid hemorrhage." He is then transferred to your hospital for further care. On arrival, the patient was in status epilepticus, intubated, and receiving diazepam and phenytoin.
- Initial CT scan is shown in **Fig. 3.1**.
- The family arrives shortly after patient is stabilized and further history is obtained.

- The patient is known to have a seizure disorder, and the first seizure was 6 years ago. He also has a longstanding expressive speech deficit. He has had a left-sided hemiparesis for the past 6 years with joint contractures.
- The family was told by his primary care physician that he has a "brain condition" for which they did not know the name.
- He recovers back to his baseline neurologic status the next day.

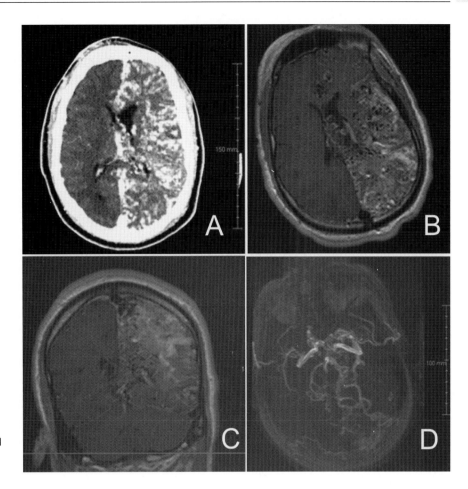

Fig. 3.2 **(A,B)** Magnetic resonance images with contrast, **(C)** magnetic resonance angiography coronal, and **(D)** axial reconstructed images showing abnormality in the left hemisphere.

■ Questions

1. Interpret the initial computed tomography (CT) scan.
2. What is the differential diagnosis?
3. What is the most likely diagnosis based on the history given by the family?
4. What other findings do you expect on general and neurologic examination?
5. How do you manage status epilepticus?
6. What other investigations would you like to obtain?

7. CT with contrast, magnetic resonance imaging (MRI) and magnetic resonance angiography (MRA) are obtained and shown in **Fig. 3.2**. Interpret the studies.
8. What is the treatment of this condition?
9. Describe some surgical options of managing seizures for this condition.
10. What are the indications for hemispherectomy?

■ Answers

1. *Interpret the initial CT.*
   - On brain windows: Hyperdensities are seen involving the left hemisphere only. These findings could represent acute blood, calcifications, tumor cells, or an abnormal vascular pattern (which is the most likely possibility).
   - On bone windows: Calcifications are seen involving the left temporal and parietal region. The calcifications are most likely cortical in nature and are not representing acute hemorrhage.

   - There is mild mass effect with a mild amount of left-to-right shift.
2. *What is the differential diagnosis?*
   - Congenital: neurocutaneous disorder (Sturge–Weber syndrome)
   - Infectious: encephalitis (viral, bacterial), purulent meningitis
   - Traumatic: contusion, subarachnoid hemorrhage
   - Tumor: gliomatosis, metastatic disease, lymphoma

■ Answers (*continued*)

- Inflammatory: progressive multifocal leukoenceph-alopathy, viral encephalitis, ossifying meningoen-cephalopathy
- Vascular: arteriovenous malformation, venous an-giomas[1]

3. *What is the most likely diagnosis based on the history given by the family?*
   - Sturge–Weber syndrome[1]

4. *What other findings do you expect on general and neu-rologic examination?*
   - Port-wine stain (facial angiomas): usually unilateral involvement of the skin supplied by the ophthalmic division of the trigeminal nerve.[2,3] Rarely can be bilateral.
   - Leptomeningeal angiomas: usually occipital and posterior parietal
   - Seizures (by age 3 years: 75–90%).[2,3]
   - Hemiparesis (25–60%) and hemiatrophy (possibly from chronic cerebral hypoxia)[1]
   - Mental retardation or learning disability (50–75%)[2]
   - Glaucoma (30–70%) and vascular eye abnormalities
   - Hemianopsia (40–45%)
   - Vascular headaches (40–60%)[2]
   - Developmental delay and mental retardation (50–75%)
   - Moya moya disease
   - Arteriovenous malformations of the lung and liver

5. *How do you manage status epilepticus?*
   - Intravenous (i.v.) glucose 50% 50 mL, i.v. thiamine 100 mg (folate/multivitamin), intubate, i.v. access
   - Laboratory: complete blood count (CBC), electro-lytes, serum glucose, serum calcium levels, arterial blood gas
   - Neurologic examination
   - Pharmacologic treatment (as follows, in order given):
     – Lorazepam 1–2 mg every 5 minutes, up to 9 mg (0.1 mg/kg) or diazepam 5 mg every 5 minutes, up to 20 mg (0.2 mg/kg)
     – Phenytoin – loading dose 20 mg/kg
     – Phenobarbital – drip load 20 mg/kg
     – Pentobarbital – drip 20 mg/kg if seizure did not arrest in 30 minutes
   - General anesthesia[4,5]

6. *What other investigations would you like to obtain?*
   - CT of the brain with contrast
   - MRI/magnetic resonance angiography (MRA) of the brain
   - 4-vessel cerebral angiogram

- Electroencephalogram
- Laboratory tests: CBC, electrolytes, prothrombin time, partial thromboplastin time, type and screen[3]

7. *CT with contrast, MRI, and MRA are obtained and described below. Interpret the studies.*
   - CT with contrast: There is extensive serpentine leptomeningeal enhancement involving the left temporal and parietal region.
   - MRI: Extensive cortical parenchymal calcification in the left cerebral hemisphere predominantly in the parietal and occipital region with some extension into the frontal and temporal lobes is demonstrated with decreased signal. Postcontrast examination again demonstrated serpentine enhancement of almost the entire cerebral hemisphere with enhance-ment also within the brain parenchyma. Minimal mass effect with slight midline shift is seen.
   - MRA: Extensive abnormal cerebral arteries are demonstrated in the left cerebral hemisphere con-sistent with leptomeningeal venous abnormalities.

8. *What is the treatment of this condition?*
   - Aggressive treatment of seizures with antiepileptics (carbamazepine is the usual first-line medication)
   - Stroke prevention (aspirin, good hydration, etc.)
   - Aggressive treatment of fever
   - Treat iron deficiency with anemia vitamin supple-mentation
   - Flu shot
   - Treat headaches symptomatically

9. *Describe some surgical options of managing seizures for this condition.*
   - Hemispherectomy (functional or anatomic)
   - Corpus callosum interruption
   - Localized cortical resection[6]

10. *What are the indications for hemispherectomy?*
    - Indications: intractable epilepsy with unilateral hemisphere damage, congenital hemiplegia, chronic encephalitis, hemimegalencephaly, or Sturge–Weber syndrome
    - It is performed only on patients who have a dense hemianopsia and are already hemiplegic with no fine motor activity on the affected side.
    - The acute surgical risk is that some crude move-ment or sensation on the opposite side of the body would be adversely affected.
    - Chronic risks include superficial cerebral hemosid-erosis.[7,8]

■ References

1. Akpinar E. The tram-track sign: cortical calcifications. Radiology 2004;231(2):515–516
2. Nathan N, Thaller SR. Sturge-Weber syndrome and associated congenital vascular disorders: a review. J Craniofac Surg 2006;17(4):724–728
3. Thomas-Sohl KA, Vaslow DF, Maria BL. Sturge-Weber syndrome: a review. Pediatr Neurol 2004;30:303–310
4. Treiman DM. Treatment of convulsive status epilepticus. Int Rev Neurobiol 2007;81:273–285
5. Nandhagopal R. Generalised convulsive status epilepticus: an overview. Postgrad Med J 2006;82(973):723–732
6. Comi AM. Advances in Sturge-Weber syndrome. Curr Opin Neurol 2006;19(2):124–128
7. McClelland S III, Maxwell RE. Hemispherectomy for intractable epilepsy in adults: the first reported series. Ann Neurol 2007;61(4):372–376
8. Morino M, Shimizu H, Uda T, et al. Transventricular hemispherotomy for surgical treatment of intractable epilepsy. J Clin Neurosci 2007;14(2):171–175

Case 4   Von Hippel–Lindau Disease—Hemangioblastoma

Ramez Malak and Robert Moumdjian

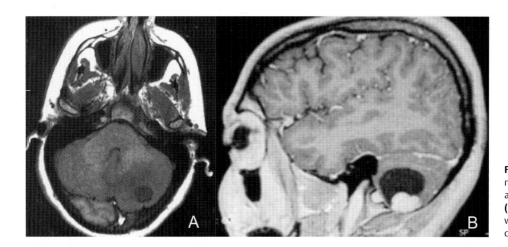

Fig. 4.1   (A) T1-weighted magnetic resonance image (MRI) of the brain, axial cut through the posterior fossa. **(B)** T1-weighted MRI of the brain with contrast enhancement, sagittal cut.

■ Clinical Presentation

- A 32-year-old man presents with nausea, vomiting, and headache for the last week.
- He is otherwise neurologically intact.

- Magnetic resonance imaging (MRI) scan of his brain is shown in **Fig. 4.1**.

■ Questions

1. Interpret the MRI scan (**Fig. 4.1**).
2. What is your initial management?
3. Give a differential diagnosis of cerebellar lesions. Which is the most likely?
4. Provide diagnostic criteria of Von Hippel–Lindau disease (VHL), associated systemic lesions, and chromosomal abnormalities.
5. Name other phakomatoses and their main features.
6. Describe the preoperative evaluation for this hemangioblastoma.
7. What are the treatment options?
8. Describe your postoperative follow-up.
9. A spinal MRI demonstrates hemangioblastoma at the T5 level. What is your management (**Fig. 4.2**)?

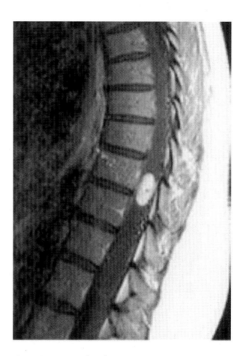

Fig. 4.2   T1-weighted magnetic resonance image of the thoracic spine with contrast enhancement, midsagittal cut.

■ Answers

1. *Interpret the computed tomography (CT) scan.*
   - Nonenhanced MRI T1-weighted scan (**Fig. 4.1A**) shows a cystic lesion in the left cerebellar hemisphere, ~1 cm in diameter with associated edema and no mass effect on the 4th ventricle. There is no hydrocephalus.
   - Sagittal view T1-weighted with contrast (**Fig. 4.1B**) shows a cystic cerebellar lesion with densely enhancing nodule. The cyst wall does not enhance.

2. *What is your initial management?*
   - Admission to intensive care unit
   - Symptomatic treatment: analgesics, antiemetics, hydration with i.v. fluids
   - Dexamethasone could be indicated in the presence of vasogenic edema.
   - Initial blood workup: complete blood count, electrolytes, coagulation profile, type and screen
   - Be prepared to place a ventriculostomy if patient decompensates.
   - If an urgent shunt is indicated for acute hydrocephalus (rare), keep draining at a low rate (10–15 mL/h) to avoid overdrainage and upward herniation.

3. *Given a differential diagnosis of cerebellar lesions, which is the most likely?*
   - Hemangioblastoma (the most likely), metastasis, medulloblastoma, pilocytic astrocytoma, ependymoma, choroid plexus papilloma, brainstem glioma, abscess, cavernous angioma, hemorrhage, infarction

4. *Provide diagnostic criteria of VHL and associated systemic lesions.*
   - The hallmark features of the condition include[1,2]
     - Retinal angiomas
     - Hemangioblastomas of the cerebellum and spinal cord
     - Renal cell carcinomas (RCCs)
   - Additionally, this condition can cause
     - Angiomatous or cystic lesions in the kidneys, pancreas, and epididymis
     - Adrenal pheochromocytomas, polycythemia
   - Minimal diagnostic criteria
     - If positive family history of VHL, one of the following: retinal or cerebellar hemangioblastoma, RCC, or pheochromocytoma
     - In an isolated case: Two or more retinal or central nervous system hemangioblastomas or a single hemangioblastoma and a characteristic visceral tumor

5. *Name other phakomatoses and their main features.*
   - See **Table 4.1**.[3]
   - Other, less common: incontinentia pigmenti, ataxia, telangiectasia, Peutz–Jeghers syndrome, Osler–Weber–Rendu syndrome

6. *Describe the preoperative evaluation for this hemangioblastoma.*
   - Craniospinal MRI
   - Ophthalmologic examination
   - Abdominal CT scan
   - Laboratory work (to rule out polycythemia)
   - 24-Hour urine metanephrine vanillylmandelic acid, homovanillic acid, and catecholamine determinations
   - Genetic screening for VHL gene
   - Cerebral angiography and embolization (especially for solid highly enhancing nodules) to decrease preoperative bleeding

7. *What are the treatment options?*
   - The aim of surgical treatment remains the complete removal of the hemangioblastoma.
   - However, multiplicity of lesions and their frequent proximity to vital structures can preclude complete excision. Only symptomatic lesions should be operated.
   - Surgical technique
     - Suboccipital craniotomy
     - Cervicospinal fluid draining via cisterna magna
     - Aspiration of the cyst content
     - En bloc removal of the nodule to avoid profuse bleeding by dissecting along the gliotic margin and by dividing vascular supply.
     - The cyst wall should not be removed because it does not contain tumor.
     - Careful closure is critical because of frequent recurrences and need for reexploration.[4]
   - Radiosurgery for hemangioblastomas
     - Radiosurgery controls the majority of primary and recurrent hemangioblastomas less than 3 cm in size. Radiosurgery also offers the ability to treat multiple lesions in a single treatment session. With cystic tumors, radiosurgery does not reduce the cyst size, and additional surgical removal or repeated evacuations of the cyst may be necessary.[5]

8. *Describe your postoperative follow-up.*
   - Hemangioblastomas are slow-growing tumors, but a risk of rapidly enlarging cysts is still present and a striking tendency for multiple occurrences is habitual in VHL disease.

Table 4.1   Summary of Findings in Neurocutaneous Disorders

Disorder	Prevalence	Tumors	Other Features	Genetic Mutation
NF1	1:4000	Neurofibroma, glioma, leukemia	Cafe-au-lait macules, skin-fold freckling, Lisch nodules, skeletal dysplasia, learning disability, vascular disorder	NF1 gene mutation on chr 17
NF2	1:40,000	Schwannoma, meningioma, ependymoma, glioma, neurofibroma	Cataract	NF2 gene mutation on chr 22
Tuberous sclerosis	1:6,000	Subependymal nodule, giant cell astrocytoma	Seizures, cardiac rhabdomyoma, renal angiomyolipoma, hypopigmented macules, angiofibroma, collagenous plaque, pulmonary lymphangiomyomatosis, retinal hamartoma	TSC1 and TSC2 gene mutation on chr 9 and 16
Sturge–Weber	1:3000		Facial port-wine birthmark, vascular eye abnormalities, ipsilateral occipital leptomeningeal angioma, subcortical calcifications, glaucoma, seizures, hemiparesis, developmental delays, and mental retardation	?
VHL	1:30,000	Hemangioblastoma, renal cell carcinoma, pheochromocytoma	Pancreatic, hepatic, and epididymal cysts	VHL gene mutation on chromosome 3P

Abbreviations: chr, chromosome; NF, neurofibromatosis; TSC, tuberous sclerosis; VHL, Von Hippel–Lindau disease.

Source: Adapted from Korf BR. The phakomatoses. Clinics in Dermatology 2005;23(1):78–84. Adapted with permission.

■ **Answers (*continued*)**

- Pregnancy can be accompanied by the enlargement of a cyst within a few months, sometimes leading to dramatic complications for both mother and fetus.
- Regular surveillance includes periodic craniospinal gadolinium-enhanced MRI, abdominal CT scan or ultrasonography, urinary metanephrins, and ophthalmoscopy, for both early diagnosis and follow-up of different manifestations. Rising hematocrit may mean progression or recurrence. The periodicity of specific examinations depends on age, number, and type of manifestations in each patient. We generally repeat craniospinal MRI every 6 months in the presence of lesions and later yearly if stable.

9. *A spinal MRI demonstrates hemangioblastoma at the T5 level. What is your management (**Fig. 4.2**)?*
   - Symptomatic or growing lesions should be treated surgically.
   - Microneurosurgery has improved outcome and safe tumor removal in patients with intramedullary tumors.
   - Preoperative embolization may be considered.
   - Because of its well-defined margins, careful surgical removal of this benign lesion provides a cure.
   - It is important to stay just outside the lesion to avoid uncontrollable bleeding, and draining veins must be preserved until the arterial supply has been interrupted.[6]

References

1. Couch V, Lindor NM, Karnes PS, Michels VV. von Hippel-Lindau disease. Mayo Clin Proc 2000;75(3):265–272
2. Lin DD, Barker PB. Neuroimaging of phakomatoses. Semin Pediatr Neurol 2006;13(1):48–62
3. Korf BR. The phakomatoses. Clin Dermatol 2005;23(1):78–84
4. Winn RH. Neurological Surgery. 5th ed. Philadelphia: WB Saunders; 2004
5. Richard S, David P, Marsot-Dupuch K, Giraud S, Beroud C, Resche F. Central nervous system hemangioblastomas, endolymphatic sac tumors, and von Hippel-Lindau disease. Neurosurg Rev 2000;23(1):1–22
6. Miller DJ, McCutcheon IE. Hemangioblastomas and other uncommon intramedullary tumors. J Neurooncol 2000;47(3):253–270

Case 5 Parasagittal Meningioma

Remi Nader

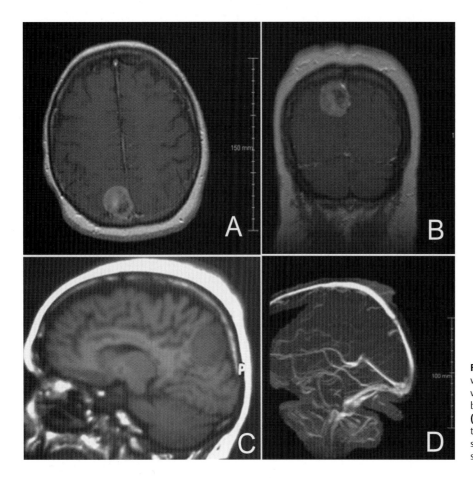

Fig. 5.1 **(A)** Axial and **(B)** coronal T1-weighted magnetic resonance images (MRIs) with contrast showing parafalcine dural-based lesion in the parietooccipital lobe. **(C)** Sagittal T1-weighted MRI showing the tumor. **(D)** Magnetic resonance venography showing patency of the superior sagittal sinus at the site of the tumor.

■ Clinical Presentation

- A 69-year-old healthy woman presents with episodic headaches and dizziness.
- There is no deficit on examination, and there are no other symptoms.
- Her family physician obtained the following study (magnetic resonance imaging [MRI] scan shown in **Fig. 5.1**).

- She has seen a neurosurgeon who told her that she had nothing to worry about and the mass seen in the MRI scan can be observed.
- She comes to see you for a second opinion.

■ Questions

1. Outline a management plan for this particular patient. She asks you, "Is the other neurosurgeon right?" What do you tell her?
2. What are your indications for surgery?
3. If the patient is demanding to have surgery, how do you approach this situation?

4. What is the most serious potential surgical complication specific to this case, and how do you avoid it and manage it if it were to occur?
5. If you decide to operate and have a residual mass postoperatively, how do you manage it?
6. What are some adjuvant treatments for meningioma?
7. What are the outcomes of these treatments?

■ Answers

1. *Outline a management plan for this particular patient.*
   - This is likely an incidental meningioma. You may get magnetic resonance angiography (MRA)/MR venography (MRV) and MR spectroscopy to evaluate vasculature and tumor type. Then you need to have a discussion with the patient about the different options: observation, surgery, and radiosurgery. A discussion about potential risks of surgery and radiosurgery and benefits of each option is in order.
   - You may mention that the other neurosurgeon's view is a valid option.[1]
   - This may not be the only option available to manage this condition.[1–3]
2. *What are your indications for surgery?*
   - Uncertain diagnosis
   - Increase in size more than 1 cm in a year or any other change in radiologic features such as extensive edema
   - Symptomatic patient
   - Location of tumor (operative difficulty)
   - Patient's wishes (controversial)[2]
3. *If the patient is demanding to have surgery, how do you approach this situation?*
   - Patient autonomy is important and should be respected.
   - However, one must take into account any other potential prohibitive factors such as age, other medical problems (none in this case), psychosocial situation, etc.
   - If there are some doubts about the benefits of surgery, then these should be clearly explained to the patient.[1]
   - If the patient seems to have an unreasonable behavior or expectations, a psychological evaluation may help.
4. *What is the most serious potential surgical complication specific to this case, and how do you avoid and manage it?*
   - The risk of venous sinus injury, which may lead to profuse hemorrhage, air embolism, or venous infarction

   - Avoidance is achieved by
     - Obtaining detailed preoperative venous imaging (MRV or venogram)
     - Assistance with neuronavigation
     - Attention during opening not to injure the sinus while drilling the skull
   - Attention during tumor resection not to apply any extensive retraction on the sinus or large draining veins and to avoid sinus occlusion
   - Be prepared and have a strategy to repair the sinus and to treat a potential air embolus (have graft ready, precordial Doppler probe, warn anesthesia to monitor P_{CO_2}, etc.).[3,4]
5. *If you decide to operate and have a residual mass postoperatively, how do you manage it?*
   - Observation with serial MRI is an option with an increase in size warranting further treatment.
   - Stereotactic radiosurgery is another option, depending on the size of the residual mass and pathology.[5,6]
6. *What are some adjuvant treatments for meningioma?*
   - Radiation therapy
     - Shown to arrest the growth of some tumors
     - Good for residual or recurrent tumors
     - Good for malignant pathologies
   - Other nonsurgical therapies
     - Restricted to recurrence or incomplete resections
     - Tamoxifen
     - Mifepristone (RU-486)
     - Trapidil — platelet-derived growth factor antagonist[6,7]
7. *What are the outcomes of these treatments?*
   - Radiosurgery shows tumor control rates of 84–100%.
   - Complications of radiosurgery are mainly related to edema and include seizure, cranial nerve deficits (trigeminal symptoms, oculomotor palsy, dysphasia, hearing loss), hemiparesis, headache, mental status changes, and imbalance.
   - Permanent morbidity secondary to gamma knife surgery occurs in 5.7% of cases.[6,8]

■ References

1. Yano S, Kuratsu J, Kumamoto Brain Tumor Research Group. Indications for surgery in patients with asymptomatic meningiomas based on an extensive experience. J Neurosurg 2006;105:538–543
2. Nabika S, Kiya K, Satoh H, Mizoue T, Oshita J, Kondo H. Strategy for the treatment of incidental meningiomas. [Japanese] No Shinkei Geka 2007;35(1):27–32
3. Sindou MP, Alvernia JE. Results of attempted radical tumor removal and venous repair in 100 consecutive meningiomas involving the major dural sinuses. J Neurosurg 2006;105:514–525
4. Czepko R, Pietraszko W, Turski T, Kamieniecka B, Kwinta B, Adamek D. Direct surgical outcome of meningiomas obliterating the superior sagittal sinus. [Polish] Przegl Lek 2006;63(8):610–615
5. Goldsmith B, McDermott M. Meningioma. Neurosurg Clin N Am 2006;17(2):111–120, vi
6. Pamir MN, Peker S, Kilic T, Sengoz M. Efficacy of gamma-knife surgery for treating meningiomas that involve the superior sagittal sinus. Zentralbl Neurochir 2007;68(2):73–78
7. Haddad G, Al-Mefty O. Meningioma – An Overview. In: Rengashary SS, Wilkins RH. Neurosurgery. 2nd ed. New York: McGraw-Hill; 1996:833–841
8. Kollova A, Liscak R, Novotny J Jr, Vladyka V, Simonova G, Janouskova L. Gamma knife surgery for benign meningioma. J Neurosurg 2007;107(2):325–336

Case 6   Olfactory Groove Meningioma

Stephen J. Hentschel and Lissa Marie Ogieglo

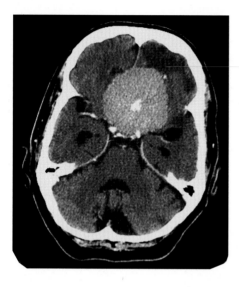

Fig. 6.1   Axial computed tomography (CT) scan of the brain plus contrast.

■ Clinical Presentation

- A 78-year-old woman presented with increasing difficulties with ambulation and memory deficits. The patient also complained of progressive visual loss for an unspecified period.
- Medical history is significant for atrial fibrillation and hypothyroidism treated with Eltroxin (GlaxoSmithKline, Brentford, London, UK), digoxin, and warfarin.

- On examination, the patient was confused and agitated. She had a right temporal visual field cut and decreased acuity in the left eye. Her examination was otherwise unremarkable but difficult to assess because of her confusion.
- A computed tomography (CT) scan of the head was performed (**Fig. 6.1**). The patient was then admitted for further management.

■ Questions

1. What is your differential diagnosis?
2. What is your initial management?
3. What is Foster–Kennedy syndrome?
4. What further imaging studies, if any, would you request?
5. Magnetic resonance imaging (MRI) scan is obtained; please describe the findings (**Fig. 6.2**).
6. What are the main features differentiating an olfactory groove meningioma and a tuberculum sellae meningioma?

7. Describe the pros and cons of the most common potential operative approaches for olfactory groove meningiomas.
8. Describe the general operative technique including management for the arterial supply and plan for resection.
9. What is the expected prognosis of this lesion following your treatment? What intraoperative steps can you take to minimize recurrence of the lesion?

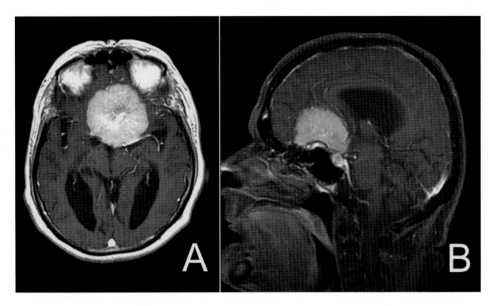

Fig. 6.2 **(A)** Axial T1-weighted magnetic resonance image (MRI) plus gadolinium of the brain. **(B)** Sagittal T1-weighted MRI plus gadolinium of the brain.

■ Answers

1. *What is your differential diagnosis?*
   - Skull-base meningiomas (olfactory groove meningioma, tuberculum sellae meningioma)
   - Pituitary adenoma
   - Craniopharyngioma
2. *What is your initial management?*
   - Reversal of warfarin in preparation for operation with vitamin K and fresh frozen plasma
   - Corticosteroid: dexamethasone – loading dose of 10 mg intravenously (i.v.) followed by 4 mg i.v./p.o. (by mouth) every 6 hours
   - Preoperative assessment for fitness of surgery
3. *What is Foster–Kennedy syndrome?*
   - Foster–Kennedy syndrome has been described with olfactory groove meningiomas. The components of this syndrome include
     - Anosmia
     - Unilateral optic atrophy
     - Contralateral papilledema
4. *What further imaging studies, if any, would you request?*
   - Further imaging studies should include an MRI scan with MR angiography.
   - There is no need for conventional catheter angiography because the relationship of the vessels of the lesion should be well defined in noninvasive angiography.

5. *An MRI scan is obtained; please describe the findings.*
   - The T1-weighted MRI sequence with gadolinium demonstrates a large diffusely enhancing tumor arising from the anterior skull base with the anterior cerebral arteries located posterior to the lesion and the optic chiasm located inferior to the lesion.
6. *What are the main features differentiating an olfactory groove meningioma and a tuberculum sellae meningioma?*
   - The main feature distinguishing olfactory groove meningiomas and tuberculum sellae meningiomas is the location of the chiasm. The optic nerves and chiasm are located inferolateral to the tumor in olfactory groove meningiomas but are located superolateral to the tumor in tuberculum sellae meningiomas.[1]
7. *Describe the pros and cons of the most common potential operative approaches for olfactory groove meningiomas.*
   - The most common operative approaches for olfactory groove meningiomas are described below.

■ Answers (*continued*)

- Subfrontal approach ± orbital osteotomies
  - For larger tumors (>3 cm), a bicoronal flap is turned.
  - For smaller tumors (<3 cm), a unicoronal flap is turned.[1]
  - Advantages
    - Early devascularization along the skull base with division of feeding vessels[2]
    - Allows for access into orbits to coagulate the ethmoidal arteries that supply the majority of the tumor[3]
    - Orbital osteotomies minimize frontal lobe retraction.[1]
    - Allows for harvesting of vascularized pericranium for skull base reconstruction
  - Disadvantages
    - Opens frontal sinus, the increasing risk of postoperative cerebrospinal fluid (CSF) leak and infection[2]
    - Sacrifice of anterosuperior sagittal sinus
- Pterional
  - Advantages
    - Early exposure of optic apparatus and carotid artery prior to tumor manipulation[1,2,4]
    - Early access to basal cisterns for CSF drainage for brain relaxation[4]
    - Shorter distance to tumor[4]
    - Avoids entry into frontal sinus[1]
    - Spares venous structures[2,4]
    - Less frontal lobe retraction unless orbital osteotomies are preformed with subfrontal approach[1]
  - Disadvantages
    - Narrow working angle[4]
    - May be blinded in upper portion of tumor, which may require extensive frontal lobe retraction[4]
    - Difficult to access ethmoid arteries[2]
    - Difficult to repair basal skull defects[2]
- Interhemispheric (2)
  - Advantages
    - Preserves superior sagittal sinus
    - Frontal sinus not opened
  - Disadvantages
    - Higher risk of contusion to frontal lobes
    - Operative route is long and narrow.
    - Risk to bridging veins
    - Difficult to access vascular supply

8. *Describe the general operative technique including management for the arterial supply and plan for resection.*
   - Craniotomy ± orbital osteotomies
   - Early interruption of the blood supply
     - If using a subfrontal approach, isolate and cauterize the anterior and posterior ethmoidal arteries within the orbit to reduce the risk of intraoperative hemorrhage.
   - Gentle retraction of the frontal lobes with exposure of tumor[1,2]
   - The tumor capsule must be dissected, cauterized, and opened. The tumor is then debulked using an ultrasonic aspirator.
   - At the posterior aspect of the tumor, an intact arachnoid plane should be identified separating the tumor from the anterior cerebral arteries, chiasm, and optic nerves.
   - Excellent visualization of the anterior cranial fossa floor to permit tumor resection and repair of defects[1]

9. *What is the expected prognosis of this lesion following your treatment? What intraoperative steps can you take to minimize recurrence of the lesion?*
   - Prognosis
     - Clinically, this patient has a high likelihood of returning to normal mental status with a reversal of her visual changes.[1,5]
     - It has been shown that these tumors have a high predilection for late recurrence at the cranial base and sinuses with a rate approximated at 30% at 5 years and 41% at 10 years.[6]
     - Due to the increased difficulty and risks associated with reoperations, reducing the chance of recurrence following the primary resection should be a goal of this surgery[4,7]
     - Aggressive primary resection including drilling of hyperostotic bone, removal of dura as well as resection of sinus extension is recommended.[1] In these circumstances, reconstruction of the skull base is a necessity to prevent postoperative CSF leaks and meningitis.

■ References

1. Hentschel SJ, DeMonte F. Olfactory groove meningiomas. Neurosurg Focus 2003;14:1–6
2. Mayfrank L, Gilsbach JM. Interhemispheric approach for microsurgical removal of olfactory groove meningiomas. Br J Neurosurg 1996;10:541–545
3. McDermott MW, Rootman J, Durity FA. Subperiosteal, subperiorbital dissection and division of the anterior and posterior ethmoid arteries for meningiomas of the cribiform plate and planum sphenoidale: technical note. Neurosurgery 1995;36:1215–1219
4. Spektor S, Valarezo J, Fliss DM, et al. Operative groove meningiomas from neurosurgical and ear, nose and throat perspectives: approaches, techniques, and outcomes. Neurosurgery 2005;57:268–280
5. Turazzi S, Cristofori L, Gambin R, Bricolo A. The pterional approach for the microsurgical removal of olfactory groove meningiomas. Neurosurgery 1999;45:821–826
6. Mirimanoff RO, Dosoretz DE, Lingood RM, Ojemann RG, Martuza RL. Meningioma: analysis of recurrence and progression following neurosurgical resection. J Neurosurg 1985;62:18–24
7. Obeid F, Al-Mefty O. Recurrence of olfactory groove meningiomas. Neurosurgery 2003;53:534–543

Case 7 Sphenoid Wing Meningioma

Remi Nader

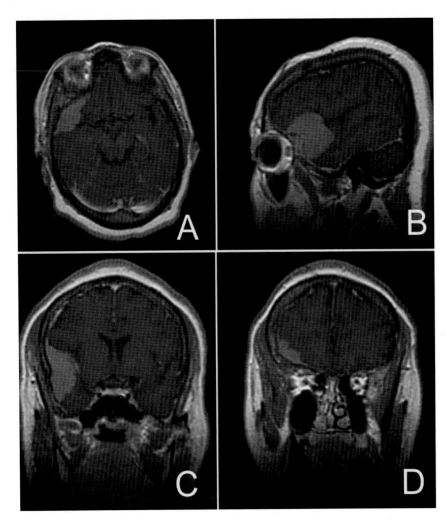

Fig. 7.1 T1-weighted magnetic resonance imaging sequences with contrast illustrating sphenoid wing meningioma. **(A)** Axial, **(B)** sagittal, and **(C,D)** coronal sections of interest are shown.

■ Clinical Presentation

- A 53-year-old woman presents with a history of chronic headaches on the right side for several years with more recent exacerbation.
- She reports a history of partial seizures for the past 9 months.
- The patient has a long history of left-sided decreased sensation along her face, arm, and lower extremity, as well as some subjective weakness along her left side. She claims that these symptoms have been present since she sustained a stroke about a year ago.

- She also complains of some right-sided blurred vision and decreased visual acuity along the right eye.
- She has some gait disturbances.
- She is referred with magnetic resonance imaging (MRI) (**Fig. 7.1**). You are told that the lesion observed was present 5 years ago but was about half its current size.

■ Questions

1. Interpret the MRI scan.
2. Give a differential diagnosis and the most likely diagnosis.
3. Give a classification of the most likely diagnosis.
4. What is your initial management?
5. How would you approach the lesion surgically?
6. You decide to resect the lesion via a pterional approach. After the lesion is completely removed, you have a large dural defect. How do you address this defect?
7. You are able to remove the lesion in its entirety and a surrounding rim of dura up to the level of the sphenoid wing, where you can only cauterize the adherent dural edge, but are unable to resect it. How would you grade your resection and based on what classification?
8. What are the clinical implications to this grading?
9. How do you manage her seizures postoperatively?

■ Answers

1. *Interpret the MRI scan.*
   - A 4 × 4 × 2-cm right frontotemporal dural-based tumor is seen.
   - The mass is abutting the sylvian fissure.
   - There also appeared to be an attachment along the lateral aspect of the right sphenoid wing.
   - There is some mild mass effect; however, there is no midline shift and no hydrocephalus.
2. *Give a differential diagnosis and the most likely diagnosis.*
   - Most likely diagnosis is meningioma.
   - Differential diagnosis
     - Tumor
       - Primary: hemangiopericytoma, primary bony lesion
       - Metastatic lesion
   - Less likely diagnoses include
     - Infection: brain abscess, subdural empyema, meningitis
     - Vascular lesion: arteriovenous malformation
     - Inflammatory condition: sarcoidosis
     - Traumatic: subdural or epidural hematoma
3. *Give a classification based on this location of the most likely diagnosis.*
   - Sphenoid wing meningioma[1]
     - Lateral
     - Intermediate
     - Medial
4. *What is your initial management?*
   - Admit the patient to the hospital.
   - Obtain preoperative laboratory studies: complete blood count, electrolytes, prothrombin time/partial thromboplastin time, type and cross match 2 to 4 units.
   - Start dexamethasone (6 mg every 6 hours recommended) if vasogenic edema is suspected.
   - Seizure prophylaxis: continue her home regimen or if uncontrolled, change regimen (phenytoin, phenobarbital, or valproate are the recommended options; levetiracetam [Keppra, U.C.B. S.A., Brussels, Belgium] may be used as an adjunct)
   - Obtain preoperative angiogram with possibility of embolization.
   - Obtain medical clearance because of her history of stroke.
   - May also get other imaging studies such as a computed tomography (CT) scan to assess hyperostosis, and magnetic resonance angiography (MRA) if an angiogram is unobtainable.[1,2]
5. *How would you approach the lesion surgically?*
   - Preoperative steps in surgical management
     - Priority is to preserve and improve function.
     - Steroids preoperatively for 48 hours
     - Control blood pressure during anesthesia.
     - Furosemide, mannitol, intravenous antibiotics
     - Head positioning (Mayfield 3-point fixation)
       - Elevate the head above heart level.
       - Head rotation: 30 to 40 degrees
       - Supine, elevated shoulder ipsilateral to tumor
     - Preoperative frameless navigation scan to mark incision and location of the tumor
   - Intraoperative considerations
     - Minimize brain retraction.
     - Plan skin incision to allow full exposure of the tumor.
     - Preserve pericranial tissue attachment to scalp for dural repair.
     - Right pterional or cranio-orbito-zygomatic craniotomy
     - Exposure of lateral sphenoid wing extradurally via bone drilling of the sphenoid
     - Intraoperative ultrasound may be used as an adjunct.
     - Expose as little normal brain as possible.
     - Extensive internal decompression prior to capsule resection
     - Use Cavitron ultrasonic surgical aspirator or cautery loop.
     - Use intraoperative microscope for magnification.
     - Have a self-retaining retractor such as the Budde halo (Integra, Plainsboro, NJ) or Greenberg halo (Codman, Raynham, MA) available.
     - Debulk tumor internally prior to resecting the outer capsule.
     - Remove en block if possible with rim of dura surrounding the tumor.
     - Spare vessels "en passage" especially at the sylvian fissure.
     - Drill hyperostotic bone.

■ Answers (*continued*)

- Postoperative considerations
  - Postoperative steroids
  - Monitor neurologic status in the intensive care unit.
  - Taper steroid schedule over 1 to 2 weeks.[1–4]
6. *You decide to resect the lesion via a pterional approach. After the lesion is completely removed, you have a large dural defect. How do you address this defect?*
   - The defect needs to be closed; several options are available.
     - Bovine pericardium
     - Fascia lata (requires preparing a harvesting site)
     - Pericranium (also requires harvesting and potentially expanding the incision)
     - Synthetic dural substitute
   - Closure of the defect may be further optimized by using fibrin glue around the suture line to prevent cerebrospinal fluid seepage.[1,2]
7. *You are able to remove the lesion in its entirety and a surrounding rim of dura up to the level of the sphenoid wing, where you can only cauterize the adherent dural edge but are unable to resect it. How would you grade your resection and based on what classification?*
   - Simpson grade 2 resection

- Note the Simpson grading scale for meningioma resection[5,6]:
  - Grade 1 – Resection complete with the dural attachment
  - Grade 2 – Coagulation of dural attachment
  - Grade 3 – Resection of tumor only with dural attachment left behind
  - Grade 4 – Subtotal resection
  - Grade 5 – Decompression
8. *What are the clinical implications to this grading?*
   - There is a 20% rate of recurrence at 5 years with Simpson grade 2 resections.[5,6]
9. *How do you manage her seizures postoperatively?*
   - Keep her on her preoperative antiepileptic regimen if this was controlling seizures before the surgery.
   - Do not discontinue for at least 6 months to 1 year until you are sure she is seizure free.
   - Frequent follow-ups (monthly) to check antiepileptic levels
   - May elect to get the neurology service involved
   - Seizure control can be achieved in up to 88% of patients undergoing complete resection of meningioma.[7]

■ References

1. Ojemann RG. Supratentorial meningiomas, clinical features and surgical management. In: Rengashary SS, Wilkins RH. Neurosurgery. 2nd ed. New York: McGraw-Hill;1996:873–890
2. Basso A, Carrizo A. Sphenoid ridge meningiomas. In: Schmidek H. Operative Neurosurgical Techniques – Indications, Methods and Results. Philadelphia: WB Saunders Co; 2006:226–237
3. Schick U, Bleyen J, Bani A, Hassler W. Management of meningiomas en plaque of the sphenoid wing. J Neurosurg 2006;104(2):208–214
4. Carrizo A, Basso A. Current surgical treatment for sphenoorbital meningiomas. Surg Neurol 1998;50:574–578
5. Rockhill J, Mrugala M, Chamberlain MC. Intracranial meningiomas: an overview of diagnosis and treatment. Neurosurg Focus 2007;23(4):E1
6. Simpson D. The recurrence of intracranial meningiomas after surgical treatment. J Neurol Neurosurg Psychiatry 1957;20:22–39
7. Chozick BS, Reinert SE, Greenblatt SH. Incidence of seizures after surgery for supratentorial meningiomas: a modern analysis. J Neurosurg 1996;84(3):382–386

Case 8   Hemangiopericytoma

Burak Sade and Joung H. Lee

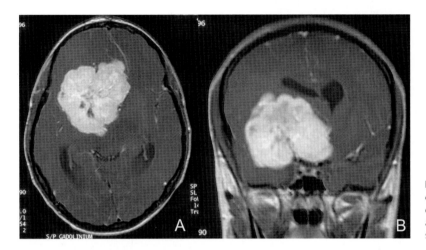

Fig. 8.1   (A) T1-weighted postcontrast axial and **(B)** coronal magnetic resonance images showing a diffusely enhancing 8-cm perisellar mass originating from the anterior clinoid process. Note the significant midline shift and ventricular dilatation.

■ Clinical Presentation

• A 17-year-old right-handed boy presents with a few months' history of behavioral changes and worsening school performance.

• His neurologic evaluation is significant for severe visual deterioration at the level of light perception and central-type facial weakness on the left side.
• Magnetic resonance imaging (MRI) scan of the brain is presented in **Fig. 8.1**.

■ Questions

1. What are the significant findings in the MRI?
2. What is your differential diagnosis?
3. What would be your initial management?

The patient was operated through a right frontotemporal craniotomy. The surgery had to be staged because of extensive bleeding. Gross total resection was achieved after the second stage (**Fig. 8.2**). The tumor histology confirmed the diagnosis of hemangiopericytoma.

4. How is hemangiopericytoma classified in the most recent World Health Organization (WHO) classification in 2007, and how does it differ from meningioma in this classification?
5. Is there any role for adjuvant treatment?

Following surgery, the patient received intensity modulated radiotherapy (IMRT).

Seven years after his initial surgery and radiotherapy, he had a recurrence to the left ventral petrous region, which was treated with surgery and IMRT. Nine years after his initial surgery, he developed recurrence to his original tumor bed, which was resected.

At the time of his second recurrence, a metastasis was detected in his pancreas, which was treated with radiotherapy. Currently, he is 11 years out of his first surgery, with no intracranial detectable disease and stable pancreatic metastasis.

6. What is the prognosis for hemangiopericytoma?

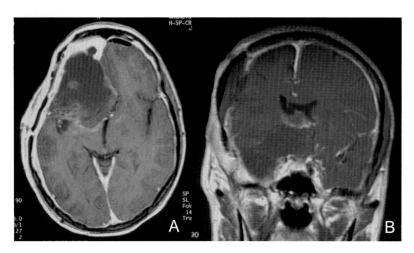

Fig. 8.2 Postoperative T1-weighted postcontrast **(A)** axial and **(B)** coronal magnetic resonance images following the second stage of the resection showing gross total resection.

■ Answers

1. *What are the significant findings in the MRI?*
   - Tumor size and location
   - Site of origin: parasellar or clinoidal
   - Severe midline shift, edema, dilatation of both lateral ventricles
   - Hypointense areas within the diffusely enhancing tumor suggesting hypervascularity.
2. *What is your differential diagnosis?*
   - Meningioma
   - Hemangiopericytoma
   - Less likely: metastases, glioma, lymphoma, brain abscess
3. *What would be your initial management?*
   - Admit to the ward or intensive care unit.
   - Obtain laboratory studies (complete blood count, electrolytes, prothrombin time, partial thromboplastin time, type and screen or cross-match 4 units of packed red blood cells if surgery is anticipated.
   - Steroids (dexamethasone). Note though that the impact may be subtle due the multifactorial nature of the raised intracranial pressure in this case (huge tumor size, hydrocephalus, edema).
   - Seizure prophylaxis
   - Preoperative angiography with possible embolization
   - Obtain further imaging to plan surgery, if necessary: computed tomography scan to determine bony landmarks, magnetic resonance angiography if unable to get an angiogram.
   - Schedule surgery on a semiurgent basis – it may need to be a staged procedure.
4. *How is hemangiopericytoma classified in the most recent WHO classification in 2007, and how does it differ from meningioma in this classification?*
   - Both tumors are under the main group of "Tumors of the Meninges."
   - However, hemangiopericytoma is classified under the subgroup of "Mesenchymal (Nonmeningothelial) Tumors" along with tumors such as solitary fibrous tumor, malignant fibrous histiocytoma, and chondrosarcoma
   - Meningioma is classified under the subgroup of "Tumors of Meningothelial Cells."[1,2]
5. *Is there any role for adjuvant treatment?*
   - Hemangiopericytoma is considered a sarcoma; therefore, it should be treated as such. The role and efficacy of radiation treatment and chemotherapy are controversial.[3,4]
   - However, the often dramatic radiographic regression with radiation continues to support its use both in primary and recurrent disease.[3]
   - It can be administered either in the form of fractionated radiotherapy or stereotactic radiosurgery.
   - Chemotherapy, on the other hand is usually administered as a salvage treatment. Most commonly used agents include doxorubicin, ifosfamide, etoposide, methotrexate, cyclophosphamide, cisplatin, mitomycin, and vincristine.[4]
6. *What is the prognosis for hemangiopericytoma?*
   - In a recent surgical series, 5-year survival and disease-free survival rates are reported as 93% and 89%, respectively.[3]
   - Recurrence can be seen in up to 80% and metastasis in up to 30% of the patients.[3,4]
   - Spine, long bones, liver, lung, and abdominal cavity are the most common sites of metastasis.[4]

■ References

1. Kleihues P, Louis DN, Scheithauer BW, et al. The WHO classification of tumors of the nervous system. J Neuropathol Exp Neurol 2002;61(3):215–225
2. Louis DN, Ohgaki H, Wiestler OD, et al. The 2007 WHO Classification of Tumours of the Central Nervous System. Acta Neuropathol 2007;114:97–109
3. Ecker RD, Marsh R, Pollock BE, et al. Hemangiopericytoma in the central nervous system: treatment, pathological features, and long-term follow up in 38 patients. J Neurosurg 2003;98:1182–1187
4. Mena H, Ribas JL, Pezeshkpour GH, Cowan DN, Parisi JE. Hemangiopericytoma of the central nervous system: a review of 94 cases. Hum Pathol 1991;22:84–91

Case 9   Clinoidal Meningioma

Burak Sade and Joung H. Lee

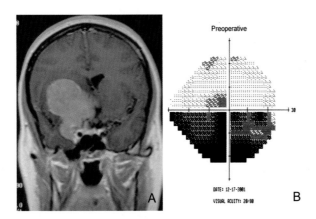

Fig. 9.1 **(A)** T1-weighted postcontrast coronal magnetic resonance image showing a 7 cm enhancing mass arising from the anterior clinoid process and compressing the chiasm laterally and superiorly. **(B)** Visual field examination is shown on the right and reveals an inferior arcuate visual field defect.

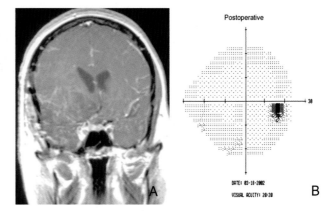

Fig. 9.2 **(A)** Postoperative T1-weighted postcontrast coronal magnetic resonance image showing gross total resection of the tumor with minimal residual within the cavernous sinus. **(B)** Postoperative visual field examination is shown on the right and reveals resolution of the defect.

■ Clinical Presentation

• A 44-year-old right-handed woman presents with a 1-month history of right-sided blurred vision and retroorbital pressure headache. Over the last 8 months, she describes episodes of "funny smell," each lasting ~45 seconds.

• Her neurologic evaluation is significant for papilledema, visual acuity of 20/80, and an inferior arcuate visual field defect on the right side. A magnetic resonance imaging (MRI) scan is obtained (**Fig. 9.1**).

■ Questions

1. What is your differential diagnosis?
2. How would you classify clinoidal meningiomas?
3. How would you initially manage this patient?
4. What are your treatment goals and options?
5. What other evaluations would you like to have before the surgery?

Management: The patient was operated on through a right frontotemporal craniotomy using a skull-base approach, which enables early decompression of the optic nerve and enhanced exposure and resectability of the tumor.[1–3] Gross total resection was achieved with small residual in the cavernous sinus (**Fig. 9.2**). The histology was grade I meningothelial meningioma. Her retroorbital headache, visual acuity loss, and field defect resolved completely following surgery (**Fig. 9.2**).

6. What are the critical structures in the vicinity of clinoidal meningiomas?
7. What is your follow-up plan?

■ Answers

1. *What is your differential diagnosis?*
   - Based on the location and imaging characteristics of the lesion, differential diagnoses include meningioma and hemangiopericytoma.
   - Other less likely diagnoses include glioma, lymphoma, metastases, or abscess.

2. *How would you classify clinoidal meningiomas?*
   - Grade I: Tumor with origin proximal to the end of the cistern, attachment on the lower part of the clinoid, encase the carotid artery within its cistern, and adhere to the adventitia in the absence of an arachnoidal membrane.
   - Grade II tumors originate from the superior or lateral aspect of the anterior clinoid process, come into contact with the carotid artery, with presence of an arachnoid membrane in between, deriving from carotid and sylvian cisterns.
   - Grade III tumors originate from the optic foramen in which the arachnoid membrane is present between vessels and tumor but may be absent between tumor and the optic nerve.[4,5]

3. *How would you initially manage this patient?*
   - Admit to the ward or intensive care unit.
   - Obtain laboratory studies (complete blood count, electrolytes, prothrombin time, partial thromboplastin time, type and screen)
   - Steroids (dexamethasone). This might provide some relief with her pressure headache and some improvement of her visual deficits.
   - Seizure prophylaxis. The history of "funny smell" is suspicious for temporal lobe seizures. Therefore, seizure prophylaxis would be reasonable.

4. *What are your treatment goals and options?*
   - The patient presents with a 7-cm lesion causing significant mass effect and visual deterioration. Therefore, surgery is indicated.
   - The main goals of the surgery would be to decompress the optic nerve and achieve as maximum resection as possible.[1] Because of the age of the patient, extent of resection is important as a significant residual will likely result in tumor regrowth in her lifetime.

   - A tumor of this size cannot be treated with gamma-knife stereotactic radiosurgery. However, if she were to have significant medical comorbidities, which would make surgery not feasible, fractionated radiotherapy could be an option.[4–6]
   - Conservative management is not advisable in her case.

5. *What other evaluations would you like to have before the surgery?*
   - Neuroophthalmologic consultation. In this location, even in patients who do not present with visual symptoms, this assessment is warranted because of the proximity of the tumor to the optic nerve and the frequent involvement of the optic canal by the tumor.
   - Computed tomography (CT) scan of the head to evaluate for bone remodeling and possible hyperostosis[4]
   - Angiography. The role of angiography is controversial. In selected cases, it may be helpful in demonstrating the critical vascular structures, and it may be used to embolize the tumor preoperatively in some cases.[4]

6. *What are the critical structures in the vicinity of clinoidal meningiomas?*
   - Critical neurovascular structures include the optic and oculomotor nerves, internal carotid, middle cerebral, anterior cerebral arteries and their branches, pituitary stalk, and contents of the cavernous sinus (especially in tumors with cavernous sinus extension).[2,3]

7. *What is your follow-up plan?*
   - The histology of the tumor and extent of resection are the main factors that dictate the follow-up plan.
   - Simpson grading can be helpful in evaluating likelihood of recurrence (see Case 7, Sphenoid Wing Meningioma).
   - In this case, because of the grade I histology and gross total resection, no further treatment is necessary at this point. The patient can be followed up by imaging periodically.
   - In the case of a recurrence, the recurrent portion's proximity to the optic nerve will dictate the management strategy.[4,5]

■ References

1. Lee JH, Sade B, Park BJ. A surgical technique for the removal of clinoidal meningiomas. Neurosurgery 2006; 59(1, Supp 1)ONS108–ONS114
2. Evans JJ, Hwang YS, Lee JH. Pre- versus post-anterior clinoidectomy measurements of the optic nerve, internal carotid artery, and opticocarotid triangle: a cadaveric morphometric study. Neurosurgery 2000;46(4):1018–1023
3. Sade B, Kweon CY, Evans JJ, Lee JH. Enhanced exposure of caroticooculomotor triangle following extradural anterior clinoidectomy: a comparative anatomical study. Skull Base 2005;15:157–162

4. Puzzilli F, Ruggeri A, Mastronardi L, Agrillo A, Ferrante L. Anterior clinoidal meningiomas: report of a series of 33 patients operated on through the pterional approach. Neuro-oncol 1999;1(3):188–195
5. Al-Mefty O. Clinoidal meningiomas. J Neurosurg 1990;73:840–849
6. Kondziolka D, Lunsford LD, Coffey RJ, Flickinger JC. Gamma knife radiosurgery of meningiomas. Stereotact Funct Neurosurg 1991;57:11–21

Case 10   Velum Interpositum Meningioma

Michel W. Bojanowski and Denis Klironomos

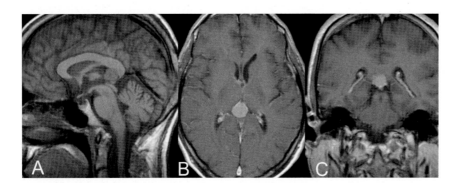

Fig. 10.1   **(A)** Sagittal, **(B)** axial, and **(C)** coronal T1-weighted magnetic resonance images with gadolinium.

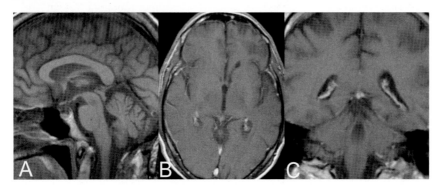

Fig. 10.2   Postoperative **(A)** sagittal, **(B)** axial, and **(C)** coronal T1-weighted magnetic resonance images with gadolinium.

■ Clinical Presentation

• A 40-year-old man previously in good health presented with a history of a nonprogressive headache ongoing for 1 year. There was no nausea, vomiting, or visual disturbance.

• The magnetic resonance imaging (MRI) scan is shown in **Fig. 10.1**.

■ Questions

1. Interpret the MRI.
2. What is the differential diagnosis?
3. What additional studies would you like to order?

You decide to obtain tissue for histopathologic analysis.

4. What are the possible surgical approaches?
5. What are the anatomic relationships of the pineal region?

6. What are the potential surgical complications?

The postoperative MRI (**Fig. 10.2**) reveals complete resection of the tumor. The histopathological study is diagnostic for a World Health Organization grade I transitional meningioma.

7. Explain the presumed origin of this tumor.
8. What are the reported locations of meningiomas without dural attachment?

■ Answers

1. *Interpret the MRI.*
   - There is a well-circumscribed, round mass in the pineal region, isointense to cortex with homogeneous enhancement after gadolinium injection. This lesion does not seem to originate from the pineal gland, which is compressed by the tumor.
   - There is no mass effect on the tectal plate or on the aqueduct of Sylvius and no hydrocephalus. The internal cerebral veins are pushed downward and consequently are beneath the tumor. The mass does not have any relation or attachment to the falco–tentorial junction.

2. *What is the differential diagnosis?*
   - Meningioma: In the pineal region, meningiomas usually arise from tentorium cerebelli and falx. Few cases described without dural attachment are located in the velum interpositum.[1,2]
   - Pineoblastoma: Most are large, greater than 3 cm with peripheral calcifications. Usually associated with obstructive hydrocephalus.
   - Pineocytoma: An enhancing, well-circumscribed pineal tumor with calcifications that rarely extends into the third ventricle.
   - Germ cell tumors: Engulf the pineal gland. Hyperintense to gray matter
   - Astrocytoma: Arises from midbrain tectum or thalamus; rarely from the pineal gland
   - Ependymoma: Mild to moderate heterogenous enhancement
   - Metastases

3. *What additional studies would you like to order?*
   - Because neuroimaging alone is not consistently diagnostic for third ventricular meningioma, these lesions are usually evaluated according to standard algorithms for pineal masses.
   - Alfa-fetoprotein and beta human chorionic gonadotropin are markers of germ cell malignancy and should be measured in serum and cerebrospinal fluid if possible because patients with elevated markers suggestive of germinomas can be treated with chemotherapy and radiation without histologic diagnosis.
   - For patients with a previous history of malignancy, a complete metastatic workup should be done.
   - Also consider a spinal survey MRI.

4. *What are the possible surgical approaches?*
   - Stereotactic-guided biopsy
     - Ideally suited for patients with contraindications to open surgery and general anesthesia. Also for tumors that clearly invade the brainstem.[3]
     - However, it provides limited amount of tissue from lesions that may be histologically diverse.
     - The potential of hemorrhage is increased in the pineal region compared with other locations.[4]
   - Open surgical resection

   - The selection of surgical approaches is determined according to
     - The relationship of the tumor to the deep venous system and other surrounding structures
     - Particular characteristics of the tumor (size, spread, etc.)
     - Degree of surgeon's familiarity
   - Approaches include **(Fig. 10.3)**
     - Infratentorial supracerebellar approach
       - For tumors that displace the internal cerebral veins dorsally
       - Tumor is reached through the midline, below the deep cerebral veins
       - Avoids violation of normal tissues
     - Occipital transtentorial
       - For lesion above the deep venous system, midline, or above the tentorial edge
       - With this approach, it is difficult to dissect the tumor from the tela choroidea of the third ventricle
       - Necessitates retraction of the visual cortex
     - Posterior transcallosal
       - For lesions anterior to the confluence of the deep cerebral veins
       - For lesions that displace the internal cerebral veins ventrally
   - Because of its relatively small size, the tumor was approached through an infratentorial supracerebellar corridor, avoiding violation of normal tissues.

5. *What are the anatomic relationships of the pineal region?*
   - The pineal gland is attached to the posterior wall of the third ventricle and projects posteriorly in the quadrigeminal cistern.
   - The splenium of the corpus callosum lies above this region and the thalamus is located on each side.
   - The roof of the third ventricle is formed by the body and crura of the fornices, the dorsal and ventral layers of the tela choroidea. The space between these two layers is the velum interpositum. The internal cerebral veins and the medial posterior choroidal arteries course through this space.
   - The vein of Galen is located behind the posterior wall of the third ventricle.[5]

6. *What are the potential surgical complications?*
   - Oculomotor deficits including Parinaud syndrome
   - Injury of the deep venous system
     - Venous sinus tear
     - Venous infarction
     - Venous air embolism
   - Infratentorial–supracerebellar approach: related to the sitting position
   - Transcallosal approach: hemisensory or motor deficit (brain retraction), venous cortical infarction, disconnection syndrome

■ Answers (*continued*)

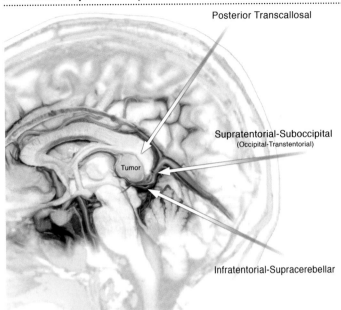

Fig. 10.3 Surgical approaches to the pineal region.

- Transtentorial approach: Visual-fields deficit, venous cortical infarction
7. *Explain the presumed origin of this tumor.*
   - This case represents a meningioma of the third ventricle without dural attachment.
   - Meningothelial cells are normally found in the arachnoid and choroidal tela. During embryologic development, arachnoid tissue migrates together with the choroid plexus as the ventricular system invaginates, and thus meningocytes are found in the stroma of the choroid plexus.[6]
   - Ventricular meningiomas arise from choroid plexus or from the tela choroidea.[6]

- The velum interpositum is the potential space between the dorsal and ventral layers of the tela choroidea. In the present case, it is presumed that the meningioma originated from arachnoid cap cells of the dorsal tela choroidea of the third ventricle with ventral displacement of the internal cerebral veins.[2]
8. *What are the reported locations of meningiomas without dural attachment?*
   - Meningiomas rarely occur in cerebral ventricles.
   - They are more commonly seen in the atrium of the lateral ventricle and for unknown reasons more frequently on the left side.[6] They have also been found in the third ventricle, and only few cases have been reported in the fourth ventricle.[6]

■ References

1. Osborn AG, Blaser SI, Salzman KL, et al. Diagnostic Imaging Brain. Salt Lake City: Amirsys; 2004
2. Lozier AP, Bruce JN. Meningiomas of the velum interpositum: surgical considerations. Neurosurg Focus 2003;15(1):E11
3. Bruce JN. Pineal region masses: clinical features and management. 55(1):786–797
4. Field M, Witham TF, Flickinger JC, et al. Comprehensive assessment of hemorrhage risks and outcomes after stereotactic brain biopsy. J Neurosurg 2001;94:545–551
5. Rhoton AL Jr. The lateral and third ventricles. Neurosurgery 2002; 51(4, Suppl)S207–S271
6. Bhatoe HS, Singh P, Dutta V. Intraventricular meningiomas: a clinicopathological study and review of the literature. Neurosurg Focus 2006;20(3):1–6

Case 11   **Pituitary Apoplexy**

Michel W. Bojanowski and Denis Klironomos

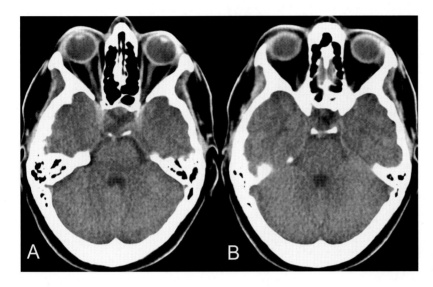

Fig. 11.1   (A,B) Head computed tomography (CT) scan showing axial cuts through the sella turcica.

■ Clinical Presentation

- A 46-year-old woman with no previous medical history presents to you after awakening from a sudden headache associated with nausea and vomiting. She also has temporary visual loss, which subsides spontaneously after 1 hour. She currently has a persistent severe headache.

- On examination, she is slightly obese. Blood pressure is 110/80 mm Hg. The neurologic and neuro-ophthalmic examinations are within normal limits.
- **Fig. 11.1** shows the computed tomography (CT) scan of the head.

■ Questions

1. Interpret the CT scan.
2. What is your initial diagnosis and why?
3. What are important questions to ask when obtaining the history and points to look for on the physical examination?
4. What is your initial management?

The headaches have gradually decreased over the next few hours. A magnetic resonance imaging (MRI) scan of the brain is obtained (**Fig. 11.2**).

5. Describe the MRI. What is your management now?
6. What are the indications for surgery?

An MRI is obtained a few weeks later (**Fig. 11.3**).

7. Discuss the findings.
8. What is the pathophysiology of this condition?
9. What are the precipitating factors?
10. What is the expected outcome after appropriate management?

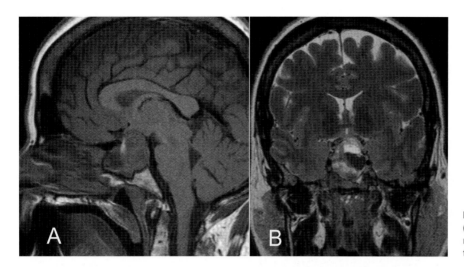

Fig. 11.2 **(A)** Sagittal T1-weighted and **(B)** coronal T2-weighted weighted magnetic resonance imaging of the brain at the level of the sella.

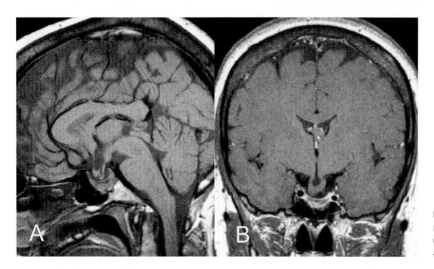

Fig. 11.3 **(A)** Sagittal T1-weighted magnetic resonance imaging (MRI) scan without gadolinium and **(B)** coronal T1-weighted MRI scan with gadolinium at the level of the sella.

■ Answers

1. *Interpret the CT scan.*
   - The CT scan reveals significant enlargement of the pituitary fossa suggestive of an intrasellar tumor. There is no evidence of subarachnoid blood.

2. *What is your initial diagnosis and describe why.*
   - Pituitary apoplexy
   - This condition typically presents with sudden onset, evolving within hours to 1 or 2 days. It includes severe headaches associated with nausea, vomiting, and/or decreased level of consciousness. It may be accompanied by impairment of visual acuity, restriction of visual fields, ophthalmoplegia, and endocrinologic deficits.[1–3]
   - Although some authors describe pituitary apoplexy as having a more subtle onset or even occurring as clinically silent,[4] for the majority pituitary apoplexy is characterized by acute symptoms with patients seeking emergent medical attention.[1–3]

3. *What are the important questions to ask when obtaining the history and points to look for on the physical examination?*

- The history should include questions regarding symptoms and signs resulting from sudden and fulminant expansion of the pituitary tumor (which may be due to hemorrhage, infarction, or hemorrhagic infarction).
- Hypocortisolism resulting from destruction or compression of the pituitary gland
- Impairment of visual acuity or fields and ophthalmoplegia resulting from compression of neural structures when the sudden enlargement is superior or lateral
- Meningismus due to leakage of blood and necrotic tissue in the subarachnoid space
- Look for precipitating factors (*refer to Question 9*).
- Symptoms and signs related to the presence of a secreting or nonsecreting (hypopituitarism) pituitary tumor
- Differential diagnosis involves most commonly subarachnoid hemorrhage, followed by meningitis.[1,5]

4. *What is your initial management?*
   - Hypopituitarism is present in the majority of patients who present with apoplexy[1,2] and requires rapid initiation of steroid replacement to avoid an adrenal crisis.

■ Answers (*continued*)

- Urgent surgical decompression is not necessary if the patient is neurologically intact with no visual impairment.
- MRI should be obtained to confirm the suspected diagnosis and visualize the underlying pathology.
- Send endocrine laboratory panel including prolactin, luteinizing hormone, follicle-stimulating hormone, thyroid-stimulating hormone, T_3, T_4, AM cortisol, and insulin-like growth factor-1. Also obtain endocrinology consultation to assist in management.
- Obtain ophthalmologic consultation to document visual-field deficit.
- Magnetic resonance angiography may also be obtained if subarachnoid hemorrhage is suspected to rule out the possibility of aneurysm.

5. *Describe the MRI. What is your management now?*
- The MRI (**Fig. 11.2**) reveals a pituitary tumor with a suprasellar extension containing mixed intensities suggestive of an acute intratumoral hemorrhage.
- Neurologic and neuro-ophthalmologic examinations are normal, and a large part of the tumor appears necrotic. Hence, conservative management is justified: obtain follow-up MRI in a few weeks provided the patient remains stable.

6. *What are the indications for surgery?*
- Opinions may vary among different authors.
- Urgent decompression is required for sudden onset of blindness, for progressive deterioration of vision, or for neurologic deterioration due to hydrocephalus.
- Surgery is indicated for decreased level of consciousness and for hypothalamic dysfunction. It is also required for impairment of visual acuity, constriction of visual fields, or progressive deterioration of oculomotricity. For visual impairment, surgery is recommended within the first week.[3]
- Ventricular drainage may be necessary in the presence of hydrocephalus.

7. *Discuss the findings.*
- The MRI (**Fig. 11.3**) reveals a complete disappearance of the tumor. Sporadic cases of pituitary apoplexy cured by isolated medical treatment have been reported.[6]

8. *What is the pathophysiology of this condition?*
- This is controversial. For the majority of cases, it results from hemorrhage, infarction, or hemorrhagic infarction of a pituitary tumor secondary to its rapid growth.[1] This may be due to a discrepancy between the rate of neoplastic progression and the availability of circulatory input. However, although pituitary apoplexy typically occurs in pituitary macroadenomas, small tumors also hemorrhage.[7] One theory suggests intrinsic vasculopathy of the pituitary adenoma with secondary susceptibility to infarction and hemorrhage.[8]

- Most patients had an undiagnosed pituitary adenoma at the time of apoplexy presentation.[9] Although pituitary apoplexy occurs most of the time in pituitary adenomas, it may also occur in[1,2]
  - Healthy pituitary gland
  - Pituitary abscess
  - Metastatic tumor
  - Lymphocytic hypophysitis
  - Craniopharyngioma

9. *What are the precipitating factors?*
- Precipitating factors are identified in ~50% of cases.[4] There is no preponderance of tumor type.[10] Precipitating factors that have been involved include[10]
  - Treatment with bromocriptine
  - Treatment with anticoagulants
  - Stimulation tests of hormonal therapy with gonadotrophin-releasing hormone agonists
  - Thrombocytopenia
  - Reduced blood flow in the gland: head trauma, recent surgery
  - Pregnancy

10. *What is the expected outcome after appropriate management?*
- Pituitary apoplexy is a potentially life-threatening condition, but the overall outcome with appropriate management is good.[5,9]
  - Visual acuity: Outcome is related to duration, severity of the initial defect, appearance of the optic disk, and timing of decompression.[1,11] However, even complete blindness may have remarkable improvement if surgical decompression is undertaken early.[12]
  - Ophthalmoparesis is reported to have good outcome whether treated conservatively or with surgical decompression.[8]
  - Endocrine function: The majority of patients require endocrine replacement therapy.[1,3,8,9]
- Thickening of the sphenoid sinus mucosa during acute pituitary apoplexy may represent an indirect measure of increased intrasellar pressure. This finding has been associated with higher grades of apoplexy, larger tumors with compression of parasellar structures, and worse endocrinologic and neurologic outcomes.[13]
- Recurrent apoplexy has been documented in patients managed conservatively after their first apoplectic event but rarely after surgical treatment of the initial episode.[3]

■ References

1. Semple PL, Webb MK, de Villiers JC, Laws ER Jr. Pituitary apoplexy. Neurosurgery 2005;56(1):65–72

2. Dubuisson AS, Beckers A, Stevenaert A. Classical pituitary tumour apoplexy: clinical features, management and outcomes in a series of 24 patients. Clin Neurol Neurosurg 2007;109:63–70

3. Randeva HS, Schoebel J, Byrne J, Esiri M, Adams CBT, Wass JAH. Classical pituitary apoplexy: clinical features, management and outcome. Clin Endocrinol (Oxf) 1999;51(2):181–188

4. Verrees M, Arafah BM, Selman WR. Pituitary tumor apoplexy: characteristics, treatment, and outcomes. Neurosurg Focus 2004;16(4):E6

5. Maccagnan P, Macedo CLD, Kayath MJ, Nogueira RG, Abucham J. Conservative management of pituitary apoplexy: a prospective study. J Clin Endocrinol Metab 1995;80(7):2190–2197

6. Schatz NJ, Job OM, Glaser JS. Spontaneous resolution of pituitary adenoma after apoplexy. J Neuroophthalmol 2000;20(1):42–44

7. Cardoso ER, Petersen EW. Pituitary apoplexy: A review. Neurosurgery 1984;14:363–373

8. Bills DC, Meyer FB, Laws ER Jr, et al. A retrospective analysis of pituitary apoplexy. Neurosurgery 1993;33:602–609

9. Lubina A, Olchovsky D, Berezin M, Ram Z, Hadani M, Shimon I. Management of pituitary apoplexy: clinical experience with 40 patients. Acta Neurochir (Wien) 2005;147:151–157

10. Biousse V, Newman NJ, Oyesiku NM. Precipitating factors in pituitary apoplexy. J Neurol Neurosurg Psychiatry 2001;71(4):542–545

11. Chuang CC, Chang CN, Wei KC, et al. Surgical treatment for severe visual compromised patients after pituitary apoplexy. J Neurooncol 2006;80:39–47

12. Agrawal D, Mahapatra AK. Visual outcome of blind eyes in pituitary apoplexy after transsphenoidal surgery: a series of 14 eyes. Surg Neurol 2005;63:42–46

13. Liu JK, Couldwell WT. Pituitary apoplexy in the magnetic resonance imaging era: clinical significance of sphenoid sinus mucosal thickening. J Neurosurg 2006;104:892–898

Case 12   **Pituitary Adenoma**

Remi Nader and Marc-Elie Nader

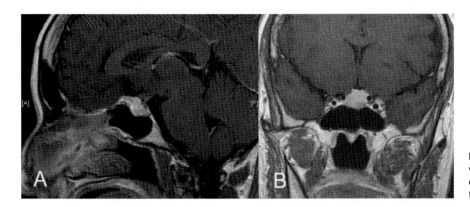

Fig. 12.1   (A) Sagittal and **(B)** coronal T1-weighted magnetic resonance images with contrast demonstrating lesion at the level of the sella.

■ Clinical Presentation

- A 40-year-old woman presents with headaches and blurred vision ongoing for several years. Recently, her headaches were getting worse and she went to see a neurologist, who ordered a magnetic resonance imaging (MRI) scan (**Fig. 12.1**).

- Upon examination, you find that she has a right temporal hemianopsia and decreased visual acuity of 20/50 in both eyes. The remainder of her neurologic exam is normal.

■ Questions

1. Interpret the MRI.
2. What other symptoms/signs do you suspect in this patient, and what other investigative measures would you like to obtain?
3. What is your differential diagnosis?

You obtain a computed tomography (CT) scan (**Fig. 12.2**) after having referred your patient to your otolaryngology colleague. The endocrinology workup reveals no abnormalities. The ophthalmologist confirms your examination findings. The patient wants to have this lesion treated.

4. What are the indications for surgical intervention in this case?
5. What approach would you use and why?

You elect to proceed with a transnasal transsphenoidal approach to resect this tumor. Your otolaryngology colleague helps with the exposure. After opening the dura, you notice that the mass behind the dura appears firm and yellowish. You send a small biopsy piece to pathology for a frozen section and you are told that this may be meningioma, normal pituitary, or adenoma. The pathologist is not able to give you an exact diagnosis based on frozen section.

You then elect to remove whatever portion can be safely removed, without applying any tension on the carotid arteries or the diaphragm sella. However, you notice a small opening in the right cavernous sinus that you pack with fibrin glue at the end of the case. You also do notice a cerebrospinal fluid (CSF) fistula at the end of your resection.

You were able to achieve ~80–90% resection. You were also able to remove the suprasellar portion of the mass. You left behind a part that abuts the carotid arteries directly.

6. How do you manage CSF fistulas in transsphenoidal surgery?
7. What will be your next course of action in the event that the pathology reveals meningioma?

The patient develops transient diabetes insipidus (DI) postoperatively that lasts ~4 days. After having received desmopressin acetate (DDAVP; 3 doses), her sodium levels drop from 150 meq/L to the upper 120s mEq/L within 72 hours. However, her mental status remains stable. You watch her another few days and the sodium and urine output normalize.

■ Questions (*continued*)

She develops a partial oculomotor nerve palsy on the right side, 2 weeks postoperatively. You obtain a CT scan (**Fig. 12.3**). You are unable to obtain an MRI as the patient had a pacemaker placed prior to her surgery. She has an elevated white blood cell (WBC) count (20,000–25,000) and no fever. A lumbar puncture (LP) reveals 0 WBC and no organisms.

After discharge, she presents 4 days later with headaches, nausea, increasing urine output, hypotension, and sodium level of 143 mEq/L.

8. Explain the fluctuations in her sodium and urine output and your management of this disorder now.
9. Explain the potential causes of the delayed oculomotor palsy and your management.

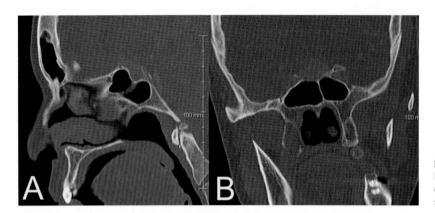

Fig. 12.2 **(A)** A computed tomography scan of the head with sagittal and **(B)** coronal reconstructions demonstrating the same lesion in the sella and the sphenoid sinus anatomy at that level.

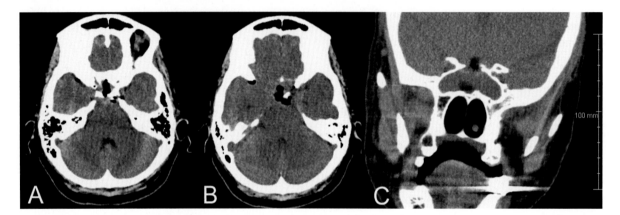

Fig. 12.3 **(A)** A computed tomography scan of the head with axial images through the sella, **(B)** suprasellar, and **(C)** coronal reconstruction. Intrasellar and suprasellar air and fat graft are visualized. No intracranial hematoma or hydrocephalus is seen.

■ **Answers**

1. *Interpret the MRI.*
   - MRI sagittal and coronal cuts through the sella demonstrate a pituitary neoplasm that enhances brightly with contrast. It is displacing the optic chiasm superiorly and the pituitary stalk posteriorly.
   - There is a small suprasellar extension of the mass.
   - Laterally, the mass seems to abut on both carotid arteries.

2. *What other symptoms/signs do you suspect in this patient, and what other investigative measures would you like to obtain?*
   - Endocrinologic signs and symptoms need to be evaluated as the tumor may cause compression of the stalk or may be actively secreting a certain pituitary hormone, most commonly prolactin. Ask for weight gain or loss, lacrimation, changes in menstrual cycle, peripheral edema, mood swings, temperature fluctuations, sweats, chills, etc. Look for signs of acromegaly, edema, etc.
   - An endocrine laboratory panel consisting of serum prolactin, luteinizing hormone, follicle-stimulating hormone, thyroid-stimulating hormone, adrenocorticotropic hormone, AM cortisol, growth hormone, and insulin-like growth factor-1.[1,2]
   - Evaluate thoroughly all cranial nerves, particularly the optic, oculomotor, trigeminal, trochlear, and abducens as they are in proximity to the mass.
   - Endocrine and ophthalmology consultations should be sought.

3. *What is your differential diagnosis?*
   - Pituitary adenoma
   - Meningioma (tuberculum sella, diaphragma sella)
   - Other (less likely) diagnoses: Mnemonic is "SATCHMO."[1]
     - Sarcoid, sarcoma
     - Aneurysms
     - Teratoma
     - Craniopharyngioma, cyst (Rathke), carcinoma
     - Hamartoma
     - Metastases
     - Optic glioma

4. *What are the indications for surgical intervention in this case?*
   - Documented tumor growth
   - Symptomatic mass: visual or endocrinologic symptoms
   - Compression of the optic chiasm

5. *What approach would you use and why?*
   - Transsphenoidal approach is preferred in this case as the tumor is accessible via this route. The suprasellar portion of the mass appears to be small and easily resectable. If it does not displace inferiorly during the initial approach, a staged procedure may be done. Alternatively, an extended transsphenoidal approach may be attempted with unroofing of the sphenoid sinus.[3]
   - Other approaches also include
     - Craniotomy with pterional or subfrontal approach[3]
     - Endoscopic endonasal approach[4]

6. *How do you manage CSF fistulas in transsphenoidal surgery?*
   - Preoperative preparation[5]
     - Place a lumbar drain preoperatively.
     - Harvest a fat graft from the abdomen or right thigh.
     - Have some fibrin glue available intraoperatively.
   - Intraoperative care
     - Avoid excessive pulling on the diaphragm sella during resection.
     - Use intraoperative C-arm radiographic guidance and possibly stereotactic frameless navigation to evaluate the anatomy of the sella and its posterior and superior borders.
     - Microscope magnification
     - May also use an endoscope
     - Pack the sella with layered fat graft and fibrin glue; you may also place a small piece of cartilage of bone harvested during the approach to close the posterior wall of the sphenoid sinus.[5]
   - Postoperatively
     - Keep the lumbar drain at 10–15 mL/h drainage for ~72 hours.
     - Keep the head of bed elevated at ~30 degrees at all times.
     - Caution the patient to avoid nose blowing, sucking through a straw, sneezing, or straining.
     - Frequently monitor for CSF rhinorrhea postoperatively.
     - If the leak persists, the patient may need further packing via intranasal approach with otolaryngologic assistance. Alternatively, you may elect to proceed with a bicoronal craniotomy with laying a vascularized periosteal flap over the sella.[6]

7. *What will be your next course of action in the event that the pathology reveals meningioma?*
   - As 80–90% resection was achieved, one may elect to observe the mass with serial scans and monitor for recurrence.
   - An alternative is to treat the residual or recurrence with stereotactic radiosurgery.[7] However, there may be a significant risk of radiation injury to the optic nerves or chiasm by using this modality.

8. *Explain the fluctuations in her sodium and urine output and your management of this disorder now.*
   - The patient most likely sustained a triphasic response of DI.[8] Initially, the vasopressin releasing is halted due to the direct trauma of surgery. After a few days, the vasopressin-releasing cells that were traumatized die off, causing a surge of serum arginine vasopressin and a clinical picture of syndrome of inappropriate antidiuretic hormone. After a few

■ Answers (*continued*)

days to weeks, once the surge subsides, the patient will then be in permanent DI requiring vasopressin replacement.

- Of note is that the diagnosis of DI does not necessarily require an elevated serum sodium level. In this case, the level was normal; however, the diagnosis was made based on the elevated urine output of >300 mL/h, low urine specific gravity (<1.005) and urine osmolality (150), in the face of normal serum osmolality (280).[9]
- Initially, give DDAVP intravenously 1–2 µg every day until the DI resolves and her condition is stabilized. Then you may switch to an intranasal route.

9. *Explain the potential causes of the delayed oculomotor palsy and your management.*
   - Possible causes include[10]
     - Inflammatory response: This is the most likely cause, as the cavernous sinus was entered intraoperatively on the right side.
     - Infection such as meningitis (less likely given the normal LP findings and no other systemic symptoms – the elevated WBC count may be due to steroid replacement or postoperative response).
     - Local trauma (fracture of surrounding orbital bone, direct trauma to the nerve, excessive packing of the sella): also less likely due to the delay in presentation.
     - Vascular/hemorrhagic: The CT scan does not show any intracranial hemorrhage. Nevertheless, there might still be a small hematoma within the cavernous sinus that is too small to be visualized with CT. Alternatively, there may be an arteriovenous fistula that formed at the level of the intracavernous carotid artery.

- Management[10]
  - Start steroids (high dose initially, then taper) for suspected inflammatory response.
  - May continue with antibiotic coverage if infection is not completely ruled out. Use antibiotics with good CSF penetration such as a third- or fourth-generation cephalosporin and vancomycin.
  - May further investigate with computed tomographic angiography (CTA) or angiography if the condition does not improve after a few days, to rule out other vascular causes.[10]
  - Obtain ophthalmology consultation to document deficit and progress accurately.

■ References

1. Thapar K, Kovaks K, Horvath E, Asa S. Classification and pathology of pituitary tumors. In: Rengashary SS, Wilkins RH. Neurosurgery. 2nd ed. New York: McGraw-Hill, 1996:1273–1289
2. Zervas NT, Biller BMK. Endocrine diagnosis in neurosurgery. In: Rengashary SS, Wilkins RH. Neurosurgery. 2nd ed. New York: McGraw-Hill; 1996:1291–1298
3. Kitano M, Taneda M, Nakao Y. Postoperative improvement in visual function in patients with tuberculum sellae meningiomas: results of the extended transsphenoidal and transcranial approaches. J Neurosurg 2007;107(2):337–346
4. Charalampaki P, Reisch R, Ayad A, et al. Endoscopic endonasal pituitary surgery: surgical and outcome analysis of 50 cases. J Clin Neurosci 2007;14(5):410–415
5. Esposito F, Dusick JR, Fatemi N, Kelly DF. Graded repair of cranial base defects and cerebrospinal fluid leaks in transsphenoidal surgery. Neurosurgery 2007;60(4, Suppl 2)295–303

6. Yoon JH, Lee JG, Kim SH, Park IY. Microscopical surgical management of cerebrospinal fluid rhinorrhoea with free grafts. Rhinology 1995;33(4):208–211
7. Zachenhofer I, Wolfsberger S, Aichholzer M, et al. Gamma-knife radiosurgery for cranial base meningiomas: experience of tumor control, clinical course, and morbidity in a follow-up of more than 8 years. Neurosurgery 2006;58(1):28–36
8. Ultmann MC, Hoffman GE, Nelson PG, Robinson AG. Transient hyponatremia after damage to the neurohypophyseal tracts. Neuroendocrinology 1992;56(6):803–811
9. Sheehan JM, Sheehan JP, Douds GL, Page RB. DDAVP use in patients undergoing transsphenoidal surgery for pituitary adenomas. Acta Neurochir (Wien) 2006;148(3):287–291
10. Foroozan R, Bhatti MT, Rhoton AL. Transsphenoidal diplopia. Surv Ophthalmol 2004;49(3):349–358

Case 13   Craniopharyngioma: Endoscopic Approach

Daniel M. Prevedello, Amin B. Kassam, Paul Gardner, Arlan H. Mintz, Carl H. Snyderman, and Ricardo L. Carrau

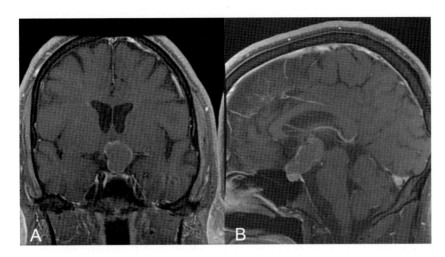

Fig. 13.1   (A) Coronal and **(B)** sagittal T1-weighted magnetic resonance images of the brain with contrast showing a suprasellar mass.

■ Clinical Presentation

• A 44-year-old woman presents with mild decreased peripheral vision, increased thirst, and fatigue.
• A recent diagnosis of hypothyroidism was given by her primary care physician.

• Magnetic resonance imaging (MRI) scan is shown (**Fig. 13.1**).
• The patient also underwent a computed tomography (CT) scan of the brain, which does demonstrate calcifications at the level of the lesion (*not shown here*).

■ Questions

1. What is the diagnosis?
2. What is the differential diagnosis?
3. What are the treatment options?
4. What are the classic surgical approaches for craniopharyngiomas and their main limitations?
5. How are craniopharyngiomas classified in relation to the infundibulum? Which type is demonstrated in this case?

You decide to approach the tumor via an endoscopic endonasal route.

6. Describe the advantages of an endoscopic endonasal approach (EEA) over the standard transcranial approaches.
7. What are the limitations for EEAs for the treatment of craniopharyngiomas?
8. What are the prognostic factors for risks of recurrence or regrowth?

■ Answers

1. *What is the diagnosis?*
   - Craniopharyngioma is most likely – The diagnosis is made based on both radiologic and clinical findings.
   - The contrast-enhanced MRI demonstrates a heterogeneous enhancing sellar and suprasellar lesion with solid and cystic components.
   - In addition, CT images confirm the presence of calcifications in the lesion, which are present in ~80% of craniopharyngioma cases.
   - Clinically, the presentation of panhypopituitarism and occasionally diabetes insipidus combined with these imaging studies is diagnostic for craniopharyngioma.

2. *What is the differential diagnosis?*
   - The differential diagnosis for suprasellar enhancing lesions includes (see Case 12, Pituitary Adenoma)[1] craniopharyngioma, Rathke cleft cyst, gliomas, germinoma, pituitary adenoma, meningioma, metastases, brain abscess, aneurysm, sarcoid, teratoma

3. *What are the treatment options?*
   - The main treatment modality for craniopharyngiomas is surgical resection. A total surgical resection decreases the possibility of a tumor recurrence. The first surgical attempt is the most important in determining the outcome because reoperation on a recurrent or residual craniopharyngioma is less likely to result in a complete resection due to scar tissue formation caused by the previous surgery or radiation.[2]
   - Other modalities of treatment, in general reserved for recurrent tumors, include
     - Radiation (radiosurgery, intensity modulated radiation therapy, or fractionated radiotherapy)[2,3]
     - Stereotactic cystic drainage (with or without Ommaya reservoir placement)
     - Stereotactic intracystic delivery of radioactive or immunoactive substances
       - Bleomycin[4]
       - Radioactive substances
         - Phosphorous-32 (P32)[5]
         - Yttrium-90 (Y90)[6]
         - Rhenium-186 (Re186)[7]
       - Interferon-α[8]

4. *What are the classic surgical approaches for craniopharyngiomas?*

   - Frontal interhemispheric and pterional transsylvian approaches[9]:
     - May include orbitozygomatic osteotomies and other variations
     - The cranial–caudal angle of approach has a substantial limitation with the optic apparatus positioned between the surgeon and the target.
     - To improve corridors around the parachiasmatic space, critical positioning of the chiasm needs to be considered via these approaches, specifically whether the chiasm is positioned anteriorly (prefixed) or posteriorly (postfixed).
     - Anterior interhemispheric approach with subsequent opening of the lamina terminalis
       - This is an option for tumors eroding the floor of the 3rd ventricle. It is a midline approach well indicated to resect a midline lesion; however, it is very limited in the exposure of the undersurface of the optic apparatus and is usually indicated only for intraventricular craniopharyngiomas.
   - Lateral presigmoid combined with a transtentorial subtemporal approach
     - Option to minimize optic apparatus manipulation is a caudal–cranial angle of attack.
     - Allows for exposure of the pre-pontine and interpeduncular cisterns.
     - Nevertheless, any dissection through this lateral view is divided into many small corridors in between the cranial nerves (II to XII) that are present in the midline cisterns' lateral walls.

5. *How are craniopharyngiomas classified in relation to the infundibulum? Which type is demonstrated in this case?*
   - The classification is summarized in **Fig. 13.2**.[10]
     - Type I is preinfundibular.
     - Type II is transinfundibular (extending into the stalk) – This case illustration.
     - Type III is retroinfundibular (extends behind the gland and stalk).[11]
     - Type IV is isolated to the 3rd ventricle and/or optic recess and may not be accessible via an endonasal approach.

6. *Describe the advantages of an EEA over the standard transcranial approaches.*
   - The main advantage of an endonasal corridor to approach craniopharyngiomas is the fact it is a midline

■ Answers (*continued*)

approach for a midline lesion. In contrast to the lateral approaches for the interpeduncular fossa, it offers a direct visualization of the midline without the need for cranial nerve dissection.

- At the same time, it offers a caudal–cranial angle of attack, allowing for better visualization of the inferior aspect of the optic apparatus, which is essential for preservation of chiasmatic perforators during tumor dissection.
- When compared with standard transsphenoidal approach, which uses the same corridor with microscopic visualization, the endoscopic technique is proven to be superior by offering a wider visualization of the ventral skull base.[12]

7. *What are the limitations for EEA for the treatment of craniopharyngiomas?*
- Lack of space and/or three-dimensional perception
  — Freedom of movements is improved by using two surgeons synergistically performing the surgery through both nostrils coupled with better depth perception generated by continuous movements of the camera.
- Any extension of the lesion laterally beyond the optic nerves formally determines a limitation for an endoscopic endonasal resection of craniopharyngiomas. Lesions located in those territories have to be accessed through paramedian corridors (craniotomies) either as a complementary or an exclusive approach for resection of specific lesions.
- Lack of surgeon's experience with the endoscope.[12]

8. *What are the prognostic factors for risks of recurrence or regrowth?*
- Favorable prognostic factors for risk of recurrence/regrowth in craniopharyngioma include[2]
  – Size (<4 cm)
  – Favorable location
  – Complete surgical removal
  – Age (>5 years carries favorable prognosis)
  – Absence of severe hypothalamic involvement

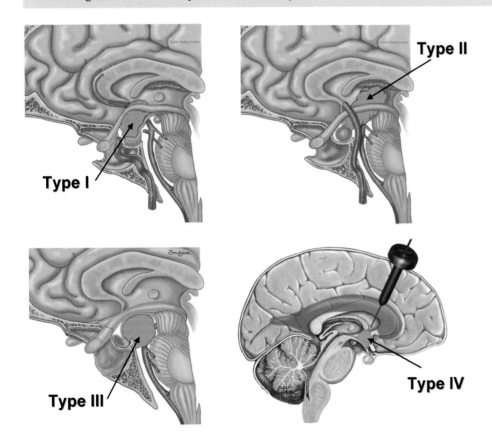

Fig. 13.2 Artist's rendering of anatomic classification of craniopharyngioma based on location with respect to the optic chiasm. See text for details (*Question 5*). Endoscopic endonasal approaches may not be ideal for resection of type IV craniopharyngiomas. However, these pure third-ventricular lesions can be approached through a minimally invasive transcortical endoscopic approach. An Endoport (Carl Zeiss A.G., Oberkochen/Wuerttenberg, Germany), a transparent cylinder with 11.5 mm of diameter, is inserted through the frontal cortex after dilatation of the cerebral tissue by an introducer. The dissection is performed under pure endoscopic visualization of the ventricles and the lesion.[10,12] (From Kassam AB, Gardner PA, Snyderman CH, et al. Expanded endonasal approach, a fully endoscopic transnasal approach for the resection of midline suprasellar craniopharyngiomas: a new classification based upon the infundibulum. J Neurosurg 2008;108(4):715–728, Figures 3 and 5. Modified with permission. From Kassam AB, Prevedello DM, Thomas A, et al. Endoscopic endonasal pituitary transposition for transdorsum sellae approach to the interpeduncular cistern. Neurosurgery 2008;62(ONS Suppl 1):ONS57–74, Figure 1. Reprinted with permission.)

References

1. Osborn AG. *Diagnostic Neuroradiology*. St Louis, MO: Mosby; 1994
2. Garre ML, Cama A. Craniopharyngioma: modern concepts in pathogenesis and treatment. Curr Opin Pediatr 2007;19(4):471–479
3. Mansur DB, Klein EE, Maserang BP. Measured peripheral dose in pediatric radiation therapy: a comparison of intensity-modulated and conformal techniques. Radiother Oncol 2007;82(2):179–184
4. Hukin J, Steinbok P, Lafay-Cousin L, et al. Intracystic bleomycin therapy for craniopharyngioma in children: the Canadian experience. Cancer 2007;109(10):2124–2131
5. Sadeghi M, Moradi S, Shahzadi S, Pourbeigi H. Dosimetry of (32)P radiocolloid for treatment of cystic craniopharyngioma. Appl Radiat Isot 2007;65(5):519–523
6. Julow J, Backlund EO, Lanyi F, et al. Long-term results and late complications after intracavitary yttrium-90 colloid irradiation of recurrent cystic craniopharyngiomas. Neurosurgery 2007;61(2):288–295
7. Voges J, Sturm V, Lehrke R, Treuer H, Gauss C, Berthold F. Cystic craniopharyngioma: long-term results after intracavitary irradiation with stereotactically applied colloidal beta-emitting radioactive sources. Neurosurgery 1997;40(2):263–269
8. Cavalheiro S, Dastoli PA, Silva NS, Toledo S, Lederman H, da Silva MC. Use of interferon alpha in intratumoral chemotherapy for cystic craniopharyngioma. Childs Nerv Syst 2005;21(8–9):719–724
9. Shi XE, Wu B, Zhou ZQ, Fan T, Zhang YL. Microsurgical treatment of craniopharyngiomas: report of 284 patients. Chin Med J (Engl) 2006;119(19):1653–1663
10. Kassam AB, Gardner PA, Snyderman CH, Carrau RL, Mintz AH, Prevedello DM. Expanded endonasal approach, a fully endoscopic transnasal approach for the resection of midline suprasellar craniopharyngiomas: a new classification based on the infundibulum. J Neurosurg 2008;108(4):715–728
11. Kassam AB, Prevedello DM, Thomas A, et al. Endoscopic endonasal pituitary transposition for a trans dorsum sellae approach to the interpeduncular cistern. Neurosurgery 2008; 62(3, Suppl 1)57–72 discussion 72–4
12. Laufer I, Anand VK, Schwartz TH. Endoscopic, endonasal extended transsphenoidal, transplanum transtuberculum approach for resection of suprasellar lesions. J Neurosurg 2007;106(3):400–406

Case 14   High-grade Glioma: Surgical Treatment

Ramaz Malak and Robert Moumdjian

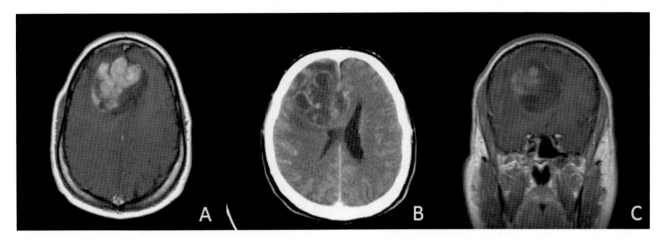

Fig. 14.1   T1-weighted magnetic resonance images (MRIs) of the head with contrast enhancement, axial **(A)** and coronal **(C)** sections. **(B)** Computed tomography (CT) scan of the head with contrast enhancement.

■ Clinical Presentation

• A 52-year-old woman presents with a de novo tonic–clonic seizure.

• She is otherwise neurologically intact.

• Computed tomography (CT) and magnetic resonance imaging (MRI) scans of her brain are obtained (**Fig. 14.1**).

■ Questions

1. Describe the CT and MRI scans.
2. Provide a differential diagnosis of this ring-enhancing lesion.
3. What are the prognostic factors for glioblastoma multiforme (GBM)?
4. Describe perioperative technologies that enhance the rate of total resection.
5. Describe the relation between extent of resection and survival.
6. What factors hinder a complete resection?

The patient has a recurrence of symptoms after 10 months. An MRI shows an enhancing lesion at the site of resection (**Fig. 14.2**).

7. What are your differential diagnoses and investigations?
8. Provide indications for reoperation and describe complications of a reoperation.

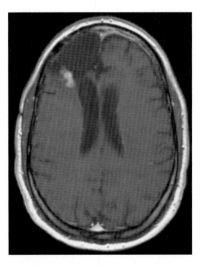

Fig. 14.2   T1-weighted magnetic resonance image (MRI) of the head with contrast enhancement, axial section, 10 months postresection.

■ Answers

1. *Describe the CT and MRI scans.*
   - The scans show a nonhomogeneously enhancing lesion with a necrotic center in the right frontal lobe invading the corpus callosum.
2. *Provide a differential diagnosis of this ring-enhancing lesion.*
   - Malignant astrocytoma, metastases, abscess including toxoplasmosis, lymphomas, resolving hematoma, cysticercosis cyst, trauma, infarction
3. *What are the prognostic factors for GBM?*
   - Age (the younger the better)
   - Karnofsky performance score (KPS; >70 associated with better survival)
   - General and medical conditions
   - Cystic component (suggestive of necrosis)
   - Completeness of the resection (>90% resection associated with better survival)

- Adjuvant therapy (standard of care conferring best survival rates remains a combination of surgery, radiation, and chemotherapy)[1]
4. *Describe perioperative technologies that enhance the rate of total resection.*
   - Table 14.1[2-5]
   - Other modalities include
     - Cortical mapping
     - Awake craniotomy[6]
     - Robotics
5. *Describe the relation between extent of resection and survival.*
   - Table 14.2[7-9]
6. *What factors hinder a complete resection?*
   - Tumor location in a functionally eloquent brain region
   - Deep structures and brainstem invasion of the tumor
   - Invasion of vascular structures

Table 14.1   Perioperative Technologies Used in Resection of Glioblastoma Multiforme

Method	Advantages	Disadvantages
CT/MRI localization Frameless stereotaxy[5]	No special equipment necessary High degree of accuracy Helps with incision and bone flap planning	Requires an additional imaging study No real-time imaging capability Requires special equipment Requires an additional imaging study
Intraoperative ultrasound	Real-time imaging	Requires special equipment Does not help design incision/bone flap planning
Intraoperative imaging (CT or MRI)	Real-time imaging High degree of accuracy	Requires special equipment in the OR Intraoperative MRI requires special surgical instruments.
Fluorescence-guided tumor resection[6,7]	The tumor is stained yellow and intense enough to be readily perceived for resection.	Surgical microscope must be modified to include a special illumination source and filters.

Source: Data from Hou LC, Veeravagu A, Hsu AR, Tse VC. Recurrent glioblastoma multiforme: a review of natural history and management options. Neurosurgical Focus 2006;20(4):E5.

Abbreviations: CT, computed tomography; MRI, magnetic resonance imaging; OR, operating room.

Table 14.2   Relation between Extent of Resection and Survival in Glioblastoma Multiforme Patients

Reference	Extent of Resection	No. of Patients	Median Survival (Weeks)
Lacroix et al., 2001[7]	<98%	219	40
	>98%	197	52
Laws et al., 2003[8]	Biopsy	84	21
	Resection	329	45
Ushio et al., 2005[9]	Biopsy	13	33
	Partial	57	57
	Total	35	80

Source: Data from Lacroix M, Abi-Said D, Fourney DR, et al. A multivariate analysis of 416 patients with glioblastoma multiforme: prognosis, extent of resection, and survival. J Neurosurg 2001;95(2):190–198; Laws ER, Parney IF, Huang W, et al., Glioma Outcomes Investigators. Survival following surgery and prognostic factors for recently diagnosed malignant glioma: data from the Glioma Outcomes Project. J Neurosurg 2003;99(3):467–473; Ushio Y, Kochi M, Hamada J, Kai Y, Nakamura H. Effect of surgical removal on survival and quality of life in patients with supratentorial glioblastoma. Neurol Med Chir (Tokyo) 2005;45(9):454–460, discussion 460–461.

■ Answers (*continued*)

• Multiloculated GBM
7. *What are your differential diagnoses and investigations?*
   • Differential diagnosis
     – Tumor recurrence
     – Distinct tumor de novo (genetic predisposition)
     – Nonneoplastic lesion: abscess, radiation necrosis, inflammation, pseudotumor
   • Investigation
     – In addition to basic imaging (CT/ MRI with and without contrast) and basic laboratory panel. Investigations also include those described below.
     – The main two diagnoses to differentiate remaining tumor recurrence versus radiation necrosis
     – See **Table 14.3**[10] for comparison of some studies
     – MRI with gadolinium: Both tumor recurrence and radiation necrosis show enhancement.
     – MR spectroscopy: In specimens with mixed necrosis and neoplasm, the spectral patterns are less definitive.
     – Cerebral blood volume (CBV) mapping: Lesions with relative CBV greater than 2.6 mL blood/g of tissue were indicative of tumor recurrence, and relative CBV of less than 0.6 was consistent with radiation necrosis. However, there was significant overlap between the groups.
     – Positron emission tomography (PET) scan: Metabolic activity (glucose uptake) is increased in tumor and decreased in radiation necrosis.
     – Biopsy: may ultimately be necessary to distinguish tumor recurrence, radiation necrosis, and abscess.

8. *Provide indications for reoperation and describe complications of a reoperation.*
   • Indications for reoperation
     – Favorable location: possibility of total or subtotal resection (≥90%)
     – KPS more than 70
     – Long disease-free interval
     – Good general condition: hematologic reserve, immunity, coagulation profile
     – Variable depending on previous treatment: surgery, irradiation, chemotherapy, steroids
     – In highly selected patients with GBM recurrence, average overall survival after maximal tumor resection is 30 weeks.[11]
     – **Table 14.4**[11]
   • Complications of reoperation
     – Death in 17%, edema, infection, bleeding, seizure, neurologic deterioration, cerebrospinal fluid fistula, functional deterioration (decreased KPS), wound dehiscence

Table 14.3   Comparison of Imaging Characteristics: Tumor Recurrence versus Radiation Necrosis

	MR Spectroscopy	Perfusion MRI	PET
Tumor	↑↑ Cho/NAA ↑↑ Ch/Cr ↓↓ NAA/Cr ↓ NAA and Cr ↑ Cho and Lac	↑ Relative CBV (>2.6 mL blood/g of tissue)	↑ Metabolic activity
Radiation necrosis	↑ Cho/NAA ↑ Ch/Cr ↑ NAA/Cr ↑ Cho	↓ Relative CBV (<0.6 mL blood/g of tissue)	↓ Metabolic activity

Source: Adapted from Hou LC, Veeravagu A, Hsu AR, Tse VC. Recurrent glioblastoma multiforme: a review of natural history and management options. Neurosurgical Focus 2006, 20(4):E5.

Abbreviations: NAA, N-acetylaspartate, a neuronal marker that decreases with neuronal disease or loss of integrity; Cr, creatine plus phosphocreatine, a measure of energy stores; Lac, lactate, a product of anaerobic metabolism; Cho, choline, a cell membrane marker that is elevated in tumors and inflammatory processes; MR, magnetic resonance; MRI, magnetic resonance imaging; PET, positron emission tomography; CBV, cerebral blood volume.

Table 14.4   Survival after Treatment of Glioblastoma Multiforme Recurrence

Reference	Treatment	No. of Patients	Survival (Weeks)
Brem et al., 1995	Resection	112	23
	Resection plus BCNU polymer	110	31
Subach et al., 1999	Resection	45	50
	Resection plus BCNU polymer	17	14
Muehling et al., 1999	Resection	35	29
Barker et al., 1998	Resection	46	36
Ammirati et al., 1987	Resection	55	36
Sipos and Afra, 1997	Resection	60	19
Harsh et al., 1987	Resection	39	36
Total		519	30

Source: Adapted from Nieder C, Grosu AL, Molls M. A comparison of treatment results for recurrent malignant gliomas. Cancer Treat Rev 2000;26:397–409.

Abbreviations: BCNU, bis chloroethyl nitrosourea

■ **References**

1. Ashby LS, Ryken TC. Management of malignant glioma: steady progress with multimodal approaches. Neurosurg Focus 2006;20(4):E3
2. Modha A, Shepard SR, Gutin PH. Surgery of brain metastases—is there still a place for it? J Neurooncol 2005;75(1):21–29
3. Willems PW, Taphoorn MJ, Burger H, Berkelbach van der Sprenkel JW, Tulleken CA. Effectiveness of neuronavigation in resecting solitary intracerebral contrast-enhancing tumors: a randomized controlled trial. J Neurosurg 2006;104(3):360–368
4. Stummer W, Novotny A, Stepp H, Goetz C, Bise K, Reulen HJ. Fluorescence-guided resection of glioblastoma multiforme by using 5-aminolevulinic acid-induced porphyrins: a prospective study in 52 consecutive patients. J Neurosurg 2000;93(6):1003–1013
5. Shinoda J, Yano H, Yoshimura S, et al. Fluorescence-guided resection of glioblastoma multiforme by using high-dose fluorescein sodium. Technical note. J Neurosurg 2003;99(3):597–603
6. Kurimoto M, Asahi T, Shibata T, et al. Safe removal of glioblastoma near the angular gyrus by awake surgery preserving calculation ability—case report. Neurol Med Chir (Tokyo) 2006;46(1):46–50
7. Lacroix M, Abi-Said D, Fourney DR, et al. A multivariate analysis of 416 patients with glioblastoma multiforme: prognosis, extent of resection, and survival. J Neurosurg 2001;95(2):190–198
8. Laws ER, Parney IF, Huang W, et al; Glioma Outcomes Investigators. Survival following surgery and prognostic factors for recently diagnosed malignant glioma: data from the Glioma Outcomes Project. J Neurosurg 2003;99(3):467–473
9. Ushio Y, Kochi M, Hamada J, Kai Y, Nakamura H. Effect of surgical removal on survival and quality of life in patients with supraten-
torial glioblastoma. Neurol Med Chir (Tokyo) 2005;45(9):454–460, discussion 460–461
10. Hou LC, Veeravagu A, Hsu AR, Tse VC. Recurrent glioblastoma multiforme: a review of natural history and management options. Neurosurg Focus 2006;20(4):E5
11. Nieder C, Grosu AL, Molls M. A comparison of treatment results for recurrent malignant gliomas. Cancer Treat Rev 2000;26(6):397–409
12. Brem H, Piantadosi S, Burger PC, et al. Placebo-controlled trial of safety and efficacy of intraoperative controlled delivery by biodegradable polymers of chemotherapy for recurrent gliomas. Lancet 1995;345:1008–1012
13. Subach BR, Witham TF, Kondziolka D, Lunsford LD, Bozik M, Schiff D. Morbidity and survival after 1,3-bis(2-chloroethyl)-1-nitrosurea wafer implantation for recurrent glioblastoma: a retrospective case-matched cohort series. Neurosurgery 1999;45:17–22
14. Muehling M, Krage S, Hussein S, Samii M. Indication for repeat surgery of glioblastoma: influence of progress of disease. Front Radiat Ther Oncol 1999;33:192–201
15. Barker FG, Chang SM, Gutin PH, et al. Survival and functional status after resection of recurrent glioblastoma multiforme. Neurosurgery 1998;42:709–720
16. Ammirati M, Galicich JC, Arbit E, Liao Y. Reoperation in the treatment of recurrent intracranial malignant gliomas. Neurosurgery 1987;21:607–614
17. Sipos L, Afra D. Re-operations of supratentorial anaplastic astrocytomas. Acta Neurochir 1997;139:99–104
18. Harsh GR, Levin VA, Gutin PH, Seager M, Silver P, Wilson CB. Reoperation for recurrent glioblastoma and anaplastic astrocytoma. Neurosurgery 1987;21:615–621

Case 15   **High-grade Glioma**

Remi Nader and Abdulrahman J. Sabbagh

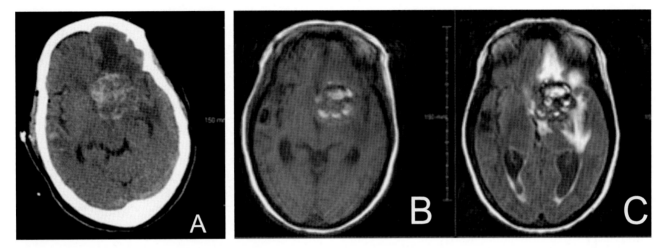

Fig. 15.1   (A) Initial computed tomography (CT) brain without contrast obtained in the emergency room (ER). **(B)** T1-weighted and **(C)** fluid-attenuated inversion-recovery (FLAIR) magnetic resonance images of the brain obtained during initial workup. Note that the lesion does extend down to the hypothalamus (not shown in these images).

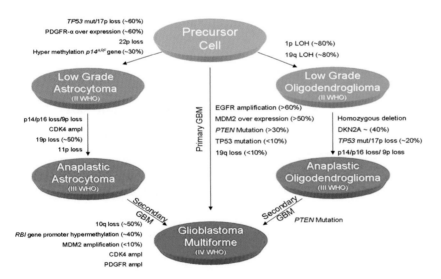

Fig. 15.2   Summary of glioma progression pathways and genetic alterations. CDK4, cyclin-dependent kinase 4; EGFR, epidermal growth factor receptor; GBM, glioblastoma multiforme; LOH, loss of heterozygosity; MDM2, murine double minute 2; PDGFR, platelet-derived growth factor receptor; PTEN, phosphatase and tensin homologue gene; WHO, World Health Organization.

■ Clinical Presentation

- A 62-year-old women presents with gradual deterioration in mental status over the course of 2 weeks.
- Now she is unable to walk. She also suffers from a right-sided hemiparesis and profound expressive aphasia for 2 weeks.

- She presents to the emergency room (ER) dehydrated and malnourished with a serum sodium (Na^+) of 166 mEq/L
- A computed tomography (CT) scan of the brain is obtained in the ER (**Fig. 15.1A**).

■ Questions

1. Interpret the CT scan.
2. Give a differential diagnosis.
3. What is your initial management?
4. What studies do you order?
5. Magnetic resonance imaging (MRI) scans of the brain are obtained (**Fig. 15.1B and Fig. 15.1C**), interpret the images.

You decide to biopsy the small lesion in the right temporal lobe. The pathologist tells you that he or she sees some astrocytosis and possibly a low-grade glioma, but he or she is unable to confirm the diagnosis.

6. Outline your next plan of care.

During your initial management, the patient responds at first to fluids, resuscitation, and electrolyte corrections and gets better. However, she starts to deteriorate over the next few hours; she becomes more lethargic and harder to arouse.

7. What are the possible causes of her deterioration?
8. How will you manage her now?
9. What adjuvant treatment protocol would you give according to the latest evidence from the literature (therapeutic agent(s) and doses required)?
10. What is the expected prognosis with your treatment?
11. Discuss genetic pathways as it relates to glioma progression.
12. What is the epigenetic mechanism that is related to glioblastoma multiforme (GBM) and alkylating agents? What are the implications of this mechanism?

■ Answers

1. *Interpret the CT scan.*
   - There are two lesions: a large left frontal lesion measuring ~4 × 4 cm, heterogeneous with mixed intensity, and well circumscribed.
   - It is involving the lentiform nuclei as well as the caudate and is abutting on the lateral ventricle, causing close to 1 cm of midline shift and mass effect.
   - There appears to be a significant amount of edema anterior and lateral to the lesion.
   - The second lesion is a smaller right temporal lesion, rather superficial, near the tip of the temporal lobe, mostly hyperdense with some areas of increased density.
   - The hyperdensity in the larger lesion may be consistent with hemorrhage, hypercellularity, or vascular markings.
2. *Give a differential diagnosis.*
   - Differential diagnosis includes multifocal GBM, lymphoma, metastasis, and optic chiasm glioma with hypothalamic extension.
   - The other less likely diagnosis includes multiple hemorrhage from vasculitis, embolic hemorrhage, or abscess.

3. *What is your initial management?*
   - Admission to the intensive care unit or at least a step-down unit
   - Fluid resuscitation
   - Correction of metabolic disorder
   - Intravenous Dexamethasone 10 mg bolus followed by 6 mg daily with histamine 2 (H_2) blockers
   - Phenytoin (Dilantin; Pfizer Pharmaceuticals, New York, NY), bolus 1 g followed by 100 mg every 8 hours
   - Endocrine assessment, serum and urine osmolality
   - Other specific laboratories include complete blood cell count, electrolytes, coagulation profile, type and screen
   - Seizure prophylaxis with phenytoin
4. *What studies do you order?*
   - MRI of the brain with and without contrast
   - MR angiography
5. *An MRI of the brain is obtained (**Fig. 15.1B and Fig. 15.1C**); interpret the images.*
   - The MRI shows again the two lesions described above in the CT findings.

■ Answers (*continued*)

- Of note is that the large mass appears to have a "popcorn-like" appearance with old and new hemorrhage within the lesion as well as a hypointense rim on fluid-attenuated inversion-recovery (FLAIR) sequences.

6. *Outline your next plan of care.*
   - Present all options to the patient, including[1-3]
     - Observation/no treatment
     - Stereotactic biopsy of the left frontal lesion
     - Open biopsy or resection of the left frontal lesion
     - Stereotaxic biopsy of the nondominant right-sided lesion appears to be the least risky procedure and is the authors' preferred choice.
   - Consider obtaining an angiogram.
   - Also consider obtaining MR spectroscopy, cultures (blood, urine).

7. *What are the possible causes of her deterioration?*
   - Differential diagnosis of further deterioration
     - Hemorrhage into the mass
     - Diffuse worsening of edema
     - Trapped ventricle with hydrocephalus
     - Deteriorating hypothalamic function

8. *How will you manage her now?*
   - Given that the diagnosis remains unclear, the patient needs further treatment and investigations for causes of deterioration. Consider
     - Urgent CT of the head
     - Continuing steroids
     - Repeating electrolytes, coagulation profile, and other laboratories
   - In this case, the deterioration was due to a trapped ventricle from increasing edema and the patient was treated with a ventriculostomy. She did improve postprocedure and remained more awake for about a week, at which point a stereotactic biopsy of the larger lesion was considered.
   - This final diagnosis was of GBM. The sequence of steps outlined above in her management is important, however, even though the final outcome is still dismal in retrospect.

9. *What adjuvant treatment protocol would you give according to the latest evidence from the literature (therapeutic agent (s) and doses required)?*

- According to the Stupp protocol[4]: Temozolomide (Temodal; Schering-Plough, Kenilworth, NJ) – a methylating agent is administered concomitantly and sequentially with radiotherapy (RT) as follows:
  - RT: 2 Gy given 5 days per week for 6 weeks, for a total of 60 Gy
  - Concomitantly administer daily temozolomide 75 mg/m^2, 7 days a week from the first to the last day of RT
  - Sequentially, beginning 4 weeks after the end of concomitant administration:
    - Six cycles of temozolomide 150 to 200 mg/m^2 once daily on days 1 to 5 of a 28-day cycle

10. *What is the expected prognosis with your treatment?*
    - In this case, due to the poor Karnofsky performance score and the underlying metabolic disorder, the survival will be less than the expected median survival generally quoted for GBM[5,6]:
    - Concomitant RT + temozolomide:
      - Median survival: 14.6 months
      - Two-year survival rate: 26.5%
    - RT alone:
      - Median survival: 12.1 months
      - Two-year survival rate: 10.4%

11. *Discuss genetic pathways as related to glioma progression.*
    - Glioma progression pathway[6] (**Fig. 15.2**)
      - Precursor cells may progress to
        - Diffuse (grade II) astrocytoma
        - Then to anaplastic (grade III) astrocytoma
        - Then to secondary GBM (grade IV)
        - They are associated with *TP53* mutation in 60% of cases, which present as primary (de novo GBM).
      - GBM is associated with epidermal growth factor receptor amplification or overexpression.
      - Oligodendroglioma development is associated with chromosome 1p and 19q loss of heterozygosity.

12. *What is the epigenetic mechanism that is related to GBM and alkylating agents? What are the implications of these mechanisms?*

■ **Answers (continued)**

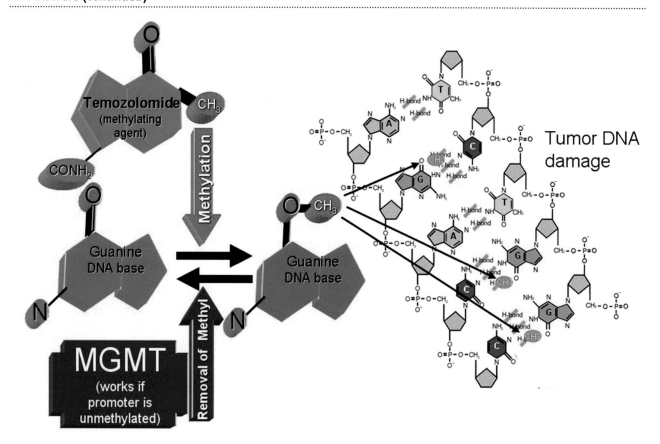

Fig. 15.3 Epigenetic mechanisms of action of temozolomide on malignant glial tumor DNA and opposing O^6-methylguanine-DNA methyltransferase gene (MGMT) repair.

- Epigenetic mechanisms of action of temozolomide on malignant glial tumor DNA and opposing MGMT (O^6-methylguanine–DNA methyltransferase) repair is summarized below (**Fig. 15.3**)[4,7,8]:
  - Temozolomide (Temodal) is an alkylating agent that adds a methyl group to guanine (one of the four DNA bases). The product is O^6-methylguanine DNA.
  - This initiates a futile recycling of the mismatch repair pathway causing DNA strand breaks and apoptotic tumor cell death.
  - MGMT is a DNA repair enzyme that repairs the damaged tumor DNA through a stoichiometric reaction by removing the methyl group.
  - If the MGMT promoter gene is methylated, then MGMT is inactive and the tumor cells are not protected from temozolomide.
  - MGMT is a suicide enzyme because it protects tumor cells from temozolomide.

■ **References**

1. Lacroix M, Abi-Said D, Fourney DR, et al. A multivariate analysis of 416 patients with glioblastoma multiforme: prognosis, extent of resection, and survival. J Neurosurg 2001;95(2):190–198
2. Shastri-Hurst N, Tsegaye M, Robson DK, Lowe JS, Macarthur DC. Stereotactic brain biopsy: an audit of sampling reliability in a clinical case series. Br J Neurosurg 2006;20(4):222–226
3. McGirt MJ, Villavicencio AT, Bulsara KR, Friedman AH. MRI-guided stereotactic biopsy in the diagnosis of glioma: comparison of biopsy and surgical resection specimen. Surg Neurol 2003;59(4):277–281
4. Stupp R, Mason WP, van den Bent MJ, et al. Radiotherapy plus concomitant and adjuvant temozolomide for glioblastoma. N Engl J Med 2005;352(10):987–996

5. Ellison D, Love S, Chimell L, Harding B, Lowe JS, Vinters HV. Neuropathology – A Reference Text to CNS Pathology. St Louis, MO: Mosby; 2004
6. Kleihues P, Cavanee WK. Pathology and Genetics of Tumors of the Nervous System. Lyon, France: World Health Organization;2000
7. Esteller M, Garcia-Foncillas J, Andion E, et al. Inactivation of the DNA-repair gene MGMT and the clinical response of gliomas to alkylating agents. N Engl J Med 2000;343:1350–1354
8. Hegi ME, Diserens AC, Gorlia T, et al. MGMT gene silencing and benefit from temozolomide in glioblastoma. N Engl J Med 2005;352:997–1003

Case 16 Eloquent Cortex Low-grade Glioma

John Winestone and Allen K. Sills Jr.

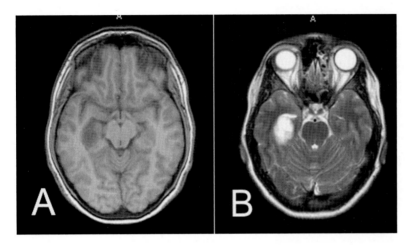

Fig. 16.1 (A) T1- and **(B)** T2-weighted axial magnetic resonance images of the brain at the level of the temporal lobe.

■ Clinical Presentation

- A 22-year-old woman presents with a 2-month history of seizures: she loses concentration, stares, but does not lose consciousness.
- Seizures were controlled on carbamazepine, but now have progressed to tremors in the left hand and are refractory to medications.

- She is right-handed and has no significant past medical history.
- Neurologic examination is unremarkable.
- A magnetic resonance imaging (MRI) scan is obtained (**Fig. 16.1**).

■ Questions

1. Describe the images. (Note: The lesion is nonenhancing on contrasted images – not shown here.)
2. What is the differential diagnosis?
3. What is it about the nature of her seizures that can help to localize them?
4. Which hemisphere would you expect to be dominant and how may it be determined?
5. What is a Wada test and how would it assist in planning treatment?
6. Describe any further investigation and how it would guide you in your treatment plans.
7. What is the treatment for diffuse low-grade glioma in eloquent cortex?

8. Describe some adjuncts used in surgical resection.

The patient underwent surgical resection of the mass via a right temporal approach. The sylvian fissure was split, and a corridor to the lesion was opened via a corticotomy in the mesial temporal lobe. Abnormal tissue was identified and confirmed by a pathologist. Tumor was removed until clear margins were reached in all planes. The pathology was consistent with low-grade oligodendroglioma.

9. What should the follow-up of this patient include?
10. What does the 1p 19q genetic mutation imply?
11. What is the prognosis?

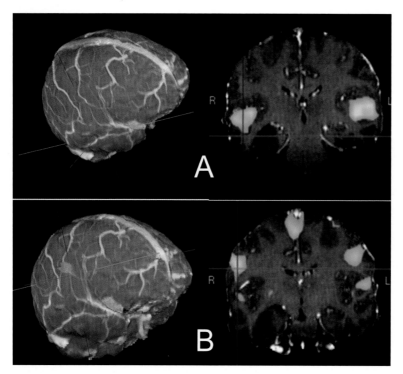

Fig. 16.2 Functional magnetic resonance imaging (fMRI) demonstrating bilaterality of **(A)** listening and **(B)** speech areas in the brain.

■ Answers

1. *Describe the images.*
   - There is a 3 × 2-cm temporal mass on the right side, located in the mesial temporal lobe.
   - The mass is hypointense on T1- and hyperintense on T2-weighted images.
   - There is no significant mass effect or midline shift.
2. *What is the differential diagnosis?*
   - The differential diagnosis includes[1]
     - Low-grade glioma
     - Lymphoma
     - Demyelinating lesion
     - Infectious pathologies (such as herpes encephalitis)
     - Other less likely possibilities include metastases, infarction, arachnoid cyst, epidermoid.
3. *What is it about the nature of her seizures that can help to localize them?*
   - Her neurologic symptoms describe a partial complex seizure, which may be traced to the temporal lobe.
4. *Which hemisphere would you expect to be dominant and how may it be determined?*
   - The presence of a right-sided lesion causing language-related problems is suggestive of bihemispheric language input.
5. *What is a Wada test and how would it assist in planning treatment?*
   - A Wada test (intracarotid sodium amobarbital procedure) consists of a selective intracarotid amobarbital injection while performing an angiogram.[2]
   - Neuropsychological testing is performed on an awake patient, and deficits are observed in speech and memory as hemiplegia occurs on the side of injection of amobarbital.
   - A Wada test can help localize speech when there is concern for bihemispheric input.
   - It is also used to assess temporal lobe dominance in terms of memory.
6. *Describe any further investigation and how it would guide you in your treatment plans.*
   - Functional MRI (fMRI), electroencephalogram, positron emission tomography, or single photon emitted computed tomography scan[2,3]
   - The fMRI (**Fig. 16.2**) clearly demonstrates speech areas away from the lesion, even on the ipsilateral side.
   - This finding enables planning of surgical resection with the possibility of sparing of eloquent cortex.
7. *What is the treatment for diffuse low-grade glioma in eloquent cortex?*
   - There is no class I evidence guiding the timing and extent of treatment of low-grade gliomas. Treatment options include[4]
     - Observation with serial imaging
     - Chemotherapy ± biopsy
     - Radiation therapy ± biopsy
     - Chemotherapy and radiation ± biopsy
     - Surgical resection

■ Answers (*continued*)

- The risks of early gross total resection depend on location of the lesion and its relation to surrounding structures. The best outcomes occur with a gross total resection, and this must be weighed with the possibility of causing deficits in the area of resection.[5]
- Other factors favoring early and aggressive intervention include management of medically intractable seizures, prevention of progression to a more malignant lesion, and surgery before the tumor further spreads into eloquent structures.[5]
- Aggressive resection of a tumor is beneficial for many reasons: seizure control, avoiding misdiagnosis, reducing mass effect, and in most cases improving neurologic defect. However, there must be clear understanding between the surgeon and the patient of the tradeoffs involved with a potential cure and permanent iatrogenic deficit, where relevant.[3]

8. *Describe some adjuncts used in surgical resection.*
   - Image guidance is a useful instrument in resection. Its reliability must be tempered with the inherent limitations of most guidance systems.
   - Intraoperative imaging
   - Frameless navigation
   - Ultrasound, mapping
   - Awake craniotomy
   - Direct cortical electrocorticography[3]

9. *What should the follow-up of this patient consist of?*
   - National Comprehensive Cancer Network (NCCN) guidelines recommend maximal resection where possible, followed by observation in younger patients. In those older than 45, external-beam radiation and/or chemotherapy in tumors with 1p/19q deletions are recommended. Patients should be followed with annual MRIs indefinitely.[6]

10. *What does the 1p 19q genetic mutation imply?*
    - More likely to be of oligodendroglial origin[7]
    - Better prognosis[8]
    - More responsive to chemotherapy[8]
    - Longer tumor-free survival after chemotherapy[8]
    - Chemotherapy used for treatment may include PCV (procarbazine, CCNU, vincristine) with 50% complete resolution versus non 1p-19q → only 25% response.[7]
    - Temozolomide may be used for recurrent tumors.[8]

11. *What is the prognosis?*
    - Mean survival = 4.4–9.8 years (after operative treatment)[5,7]
    - 5-year survival = 38–75%
    - 10-year survival = 19–59%

■ References

1. Osborn AG. Diagnostic Neuroradiology. St Louis, MO: Mosby;1994
2. Abou-Khalil B. An update on determination of language dominance in screening for epilepsy surgery: the Wada test and newer noninvasive alternatives. Epilepsia 2007;48(3):442–455
3. Duffau H. New concepts in surgery of WHO grade II gliomas: functional brain mapping, connectionism and plasticity–a review. J Neurooncol 2006;79(1):77–115
4. Schiff D, Brown PD, Giannini C. Outcome in adult low-grade glioma: the impact of prognostic factors and treatment. Neurology 2007;69(13):1366–1373
5. Morantz RA. Low grade astrocytoma. In: Rengashary SS, Wilkins RH, eds. Neurosurgery. 2nd ed. New York: McGraw-Hill;1996:789–797
6. Brem S, Bierman P, Black P, et al. NCCN Clinical Practice Guidelines in Oncology – Central Nervous System Cancers [Online] 2007. Available at: http://www.nccn.org/professionals/physician_gls/PDF/cns.pdf. Accessed December 8, 2007
7. Kleihues P, Cavanee WK. Pathology and Genetics of Tumors of the Nervous System. Lyon, France: World Health Organization; 2000
8. Kaloshi G, Benouaich-Amiel A, Diakite F, et al. Temozolomide for low-grade gliomas: predictive impact of 1p/19q loss on response and outcome. Neurology 2007;68(21):1831–1836

Case 17   Single Brain Metastasis

Joseph A. Shehadi and Brian Seaman

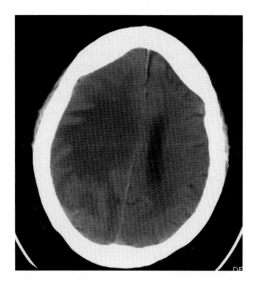

Fig. 17.1   Computed tomography (CT) scan of the brain without contrast.

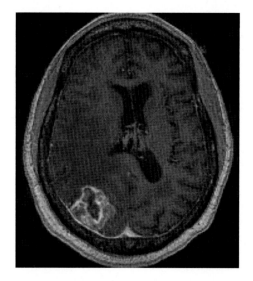

Fig. 17.2   T1-weighted magnetic resonance image (MRI) of the brain, axial cut with contrast.

■ Clinical Presentation

• A 55-year-old right-handed man with a 20-year history of tobacco abuse presents to the emergency room (ER) with severe headaches and left-sided weakness.
• On neurologic examination, the patient was lethargic with dysarthria. Motor exam was significant for left hemiparesis. Sensory exam revealed decreased light touch in the left upper and lower extremities.

• Computed tomography (CT) scan of the brain was obtained in the ER (**Fig. 17.1**).

■ Questions

1. Interpret the CT of the brain.
2. A magnetic resonance imaging (MRI) scan of the brain with contrast was then obtained (**Fig. 17.2**). Interpret the images.
3. What is the differential diagnosis for a solitary enhancing mass lesion with cerebral edema?
4. What is your initial management for this patient?
5. Name the common primary sources for brain metastases.

The patient's left-sided weakness improved significantly with steroids. CT of the chest, abdomen, and pelvis was unremarkable. The bone scan failed to reveal evidence

of skeletal lesions. Surgical intervention was sought to establish a histologic diagnosis and alleviate mass effect for symptom relief and improvement in quality of life.

6. Describe a treatment plan for this patient.
7. What is the efficacy of surgical resection for the treatment of metastatic brain lesions?
8. What are the benefits and limitations of stereotactic radiosurgery (SRS) for metastatic brain lesions?
9. How does the addition of whole brain radiation therapy (WBRT) to surgical resection affect tumor recurrence?

■ Questions (*continued*)

10. What is the role for surgical intervention with recurrent brain metastasis?
11. Because this lesion is in close proximity to the sensory–motor strip, describe how you might delineate eloquent brain areas both preoperatively and intraoperatively.

The patient underwent a right parietal craniotomy utilizing Stealth MRI guidance, two-dimensional ultrasonography, and intraoperative electrocortical mapping. A gross total resection was achieved. Pathology revealed metastatic squamous cell carcinoma. Postoperatively he was treated with hyperfractionated WBRT. Further investiga-

tion revealed the primary to be esophageal carcinoma. Chemotherapy was initiated consisting of 5-fluorouracil and cisplatin. The patient died 7 months later secondary to extracranial disease progression.

12. What are the potential long-term complications of WBRT?
13. Discuss the role of brachytherapy for the treatment of brain metastasis.
14. Do patients with a known primary lesion have a better chance of survival than do individuals with an undiagnosed primary tumor?

■ Answers

1. *Interpret the CT of the brain (**Fig. 17.1**).*
   - A 4 × 4-cm right parietal lobe mass with significant vasogenic edema
   - This lesion exerts mass effect on the right lateral ventricle and right to left midline shift of 7 mm.
2. *MRI scan of the brain with contrast was then obtained (**Fig. 17.2**). Interpret the images.*
   - There is a solitary 4.4 × 4-cm ring-enhancing lesion in the right posterior parietal region near the postcentral sulcus.
   - There is a significant amount of vasogenic edema subcortically, throughout the right centrum semiovale.
3. *What is the differential diagnosis for a solitary enhancing mass lesion with cerebral edema?*
   - Primary brain tumor (astrocytoma/glioblastoma multiforme)
   - Metastasis
   - Cerebral abscess
   - Other: resolving hematoma, lymphoma, infarction, and demyelination
4. *What is your initial management for this patient?*
   - Admission to the intensive care unit for close neurologic observation
   - Because the patient is highly symptomatic from significant cerebral edema, the patient should be given steroids immediately: dexamethasone 10 mg intravenous (i.v.) bolus followed by 6 mg i.v. every 6 hours with gastrointestinal prophylaxis.
   - Consideration should be given to the use of prophylactic antiepileptic drugs, although controversial because the patient has not had a seizure.
   - Expeditiously, a metastatic workup can be performed, consisting of a CT scan of the chest, abdomen, and pelvis; a radiograph of the chest; a bone scan; stool guaiac test; and tests using appropriate laboratory tumor markers.

5. *Name the common primary sources for brain metastases.*
   - Lung, breast, renal cell, colon cancer, and melanoma.[1] Lung, colon, and renal cancers account for 80% of metastatic brain tumors in men.
   - However, breast, lung, colon, and melanoma cancers account for 80% of metastatic brain tumors in women.
6. *Describe a treatment plan for this patient.*
   - Surgical intervention is necessary to obtain a histologic diagnosis and alleviate mass effect. Differentiating between neoplastic and infectious etiology is critical. If neoplastic, the tissue type has significant prognostic value and treatment implications.
   - Metastatic tumors typically require adjuvant postoperative WBRT.
   - However, if the lesion is of infectious etiology, the treatment options are radically different (i.e., i.v. antibiotics).
7. *What is the efficacy of surgical resection for the treatment of metastatic brain lesions?*
   - In a randomized trial of surgery in the treatment of single metastases to the brain,[2] patients were randomly assigned to surgical removal of the brain tumor followed by RT (surgical group) or needle biopsy and RT (radiation group).
   - The overall length of survival was significantly longer in the surgical group (median, 40 weeks versus 15 weeks in the radiation group; *P* <0.01).
   - Patients treated with surgery remained functionally independent longer (median, 38 weeks versus 8 weeks in the radiation group; *P* <0.005).
   - This study demonstrated increases survival with a lower recurrence rate in those individuals with surgical resection of their single metastasis.
8. *What are the benefits and limitations of SRS for metastatic brain lesions?*

■ Answers (*continued*)

- Advantages of SRS
  - Noninvasive, general anesthesia is avoided.
  - Radiation doses to normal brain tissue are minimized.
  - Treatable lesions include those that are surgically inaccessible.
  - SRS can sometimes be effective for typically radio-resistant tumors such as melanoma, renal cell carcinoma, and sarcoma.[3]
  - The addition of SRS to WBRT may improve neurologic outcomes in selected patients who are candidates for SRS.[4,5]
- Disadvantages of SRS include a treatment restriction to lesions under 4 cm. Also symptomatic radionecrosis may occur, which at times requires treatment with steroids or surgical resection.[6]

9. *How does the addition of WBRT to surgical resection affect tumor recurrence?*
   - Patchell et al.[7] randomly assigned patients to treatment with postoperative WBRT or no further treatment after complete surgical resections for their brain metastasis.
   - Tumor recurrence was less frequent in the RT group than in the observation group (18 vs. 70%).
   - Postoperative RT prevented local recurrence (10 vs. 46%).
   - Patients in the RT group were less likely to die of neurologic causes than were patients in the observation group (14% of whom died vs. 44%).

10. *What is the role for surgical intervention with recurrent brain metastasis?*
    - Initial and second reoperation was shown to improve survival and quality of life in patients with recurrent disease.[8]
    - Factors shown to negatively influence survival
      - Presence of systemic disease
      - Lower Karnofsky performance score (KPS; <70)
      - Short time to recurrence (<4 months), age (>40)
      - Specific types of primary tumor (breast or melanoma)[8]

11. *Because this lesion is in close proximity to the sensory–motor strip, describe how you might delineate eloquent brain areas both preoperatively and intraoperatively.*
    - Preoperatively, functional MRI (fMRI) can be matched with high-resolution MR or CT navigation to aid in delineating eloquent areas in the brain.[9]

- Intraoperatively, cortical mapping is most commonly used when resecting lesions near the sensorimotor cortex.
- Direct bipolar electrical stimulation of exposed cortex for motor cortex mapping is favored over monitoring of cortical somatosensory evoked potentials and phase reversal phenomena.[10]
- Furthermore, an awake craniotomy technique is used for lesions in or around the speech center.

12. *What are the potential long-term complications of WBRT?*
    - Long-term complications include radiation-induced neurotoxicity, symptoms of which include dementia, gait ataxia, and incontinence.[11]
    - Elderly patients are at particular risk for this complication.
    - Symptomatic radionecrosis may also occur, which at times requires treatment with steroids or surgical resection.

13. *Discuss the role of brachytherapy for the treatment of brain metastasis.*
    - Emerging technology includes Iodine-125 brachytherapy. Dagnew et al.[6] researched placement of permanent brachytherapy with ^{125}I seeds, after the gross total resection of single brain metastasis.
    - At median follow-up evaluation of 12 months, the local tumor control rate was 96%. Median survival was 17.8 months.
    - The author states that 92% never required WBRT, avoiding potential radiation-induced neurotoxicity.[6]
    - Results of the Phase II GliaSite Trial revealed local tumor control rate and survival to be similar to individuals who underwent surgical resection of a single metastasis + WBRT[12] (implantable inflatable balloon catheter and liquid ^{125}I radiation source.[12])

14. *Do patients with a known primary lesion have a better chance of survival than do individuals with an undiagnosed primary tumor?*
    - In a retrospective study of 342 patients, survival was not statistically different between patients with an undiagnosed primary lesion versus those with a diagnosed primary tumor.[13]
    - The authors conclude that delaying treatment in pursuit of a primary diagnosis may not be appropriate.[13]

■ References

1. Schouten LJ, Rutten J, Huveneers HA, Twijnstra A. Incidence of brain metastases in a cohort of patients with carcinoma of the breast, colon, kidney, lung and melanoma. Cancer 2002;94:2698–2705

2. Patchell RA, Tibbs PA, Walsh JW, et al. A randomized trial of surgery in the treatment of single metastases to the brain. N Engl J Med 1990;322:494–500

3. Brown PD, Brown CA, Pollock BE, Gorman DA, Foote RL. Stereotactic radiosurgery for patients with "radioresistant" brain metastases. Neurosurgery 2002;51(3):656–665

4. Baisden JM, Benedict SH, Sheng K, Read PE, Larner JM. Helical TomoTherapy in the treatment of central nervous system metastasis. Neurosurg Focus 2007;22(3):E8

5. Andrews DW, Scott CB, Sperduto PW, et al. Whole brain radiation therapy with or without stereotactic radiosurgery boost for patients with one to three brain metastases: phase III results of the RTOG 9508 randomized trial. Lancet 2004;363:1665–1672

6. Dagnew E, Kanski J, McDermott MW, et al. Management of newly diagnosed single brain metastasis using resection and permanent iodine-125 seeds without initial whole-brain radiotherapy: a two institution experience. Neurosurg Focus 2007;22(3):E3

7. Patchell RA, Tibbs PA, Regine WF, et al. Postoperative radiotherapy on the treatment of single metastases to the brain: a randomized trial. JAMA 1998;280:1485–1489

8. Bindal RK, Sawaya R, Leavens ME, Hess KR, Taylor SH. Reoperation for recurrent metastatic brain tumors. J Neurosurg 1995;83:600–604

9. Vlieger EJ, Majoie CB, Leenstra S, Den Heeten GJ. Functional magnetic resonance imaging for neurosurgical planning in neurooncology. Eur Radiol 2004;14:1143–1153

10. Ranasinghe MG, Sheehan JM. Surgical management of brain metastases. Neurosurg Focus 2007;22(3):E2

11. Smith ML, Lee JYK. Stereotactic radiosurgery in the management of brain metastasis. Neurosurg Focus 2007;22(3):E5

12. Rogers LR, Rock JP, Sills AK, et al. Results of a phase II trial of the GliaSite Radiation Therapy System for the treatment of newly diagnosed, resected single brain metastases. J Neurosurg 2006;105:375–384

13. D'Ambrosio AL, Agazzi S. Prognosis in patients presenting with brain metastasis from an undiagnosed primary tumor. Neurosurg Focus 2007;22(3):E7

Case 18   Multiple Brain Metastases

Ramez Malak and Robert Moumdjian

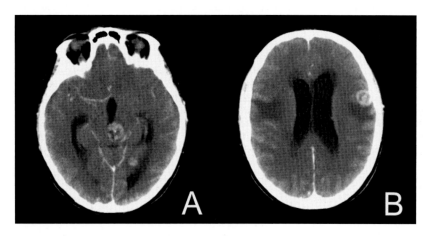

Fig. 18.1   (A,B) Computed tomography (CT) scans of the head with contrast brain windows.

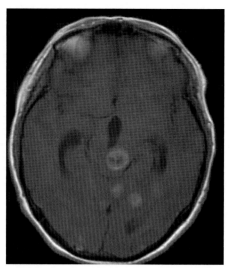

Fig. 18.2   T1-weighted magnetic resonance image (MRI) of the brain with contrast, axial section.

■ Clinical Presentation

• A 63-year-old woman presents with history of breast cancer treated successfully a year ago.
• She presents with progressive fatigue, drowsiness, and downward gaze for the last 3 weeks.

• Neurologic examination reveals no lateralization or localization.

■ Questions

1. Describe the computed tomography (CT) scan (**Fig. 18.1**).
2. What is your initial workup?
3. A magnetic resonance imaging (MRI) scan was ordered and revealed more than 10 lesions. Give the differential diagnosis of multiple cerebral lesions (**Fig. 18.2**).
4. What are the indications for biopsy?
5. What are the indications for aggressive treatment with surgery or radiosurgery?
6. What are the factors in favor of surgery over radiosurgery?
7. Describe some adjuvant therapies.
8. What is the prognosis?

■ Answers

1. *Describe the CT scan (**Fig. 18.1**).*
   - Multiple lesions in the brain parenchyma are visualized (at least four lesions)
     - Left frontal precoronal cortico-subcortical round enhancing lesion with associated edema
     - Right frontal edema, no lesion seen
     - Left thalamic enhancing lesion with compression of the 3rd ventricle and moderate hydrocephalus with cerebrospinal transependymal transudation
     - Left occipital periventricular enhancing lesion
2. *What is your initial workup?*
   - Metastatic workup
     - If primary is unknown or controlled for a long time
     - CT scan of the chest, abdomen, and pelvis
     - Radionuclide bone scan
     - Tumor markers (serum, cerebrospinal fluid)
   - Brain MRI with contrast and spectroscopy
   - Total body positron emission tomography scan
3. *An MRI was ordered and revealed more than 10 lesions. Give the differential diagnosis of multiple cerebral lesions (**Fig. 18.2**).*
   - **Table 18.1**[1]
4. *What are the indications for biopsy?*
   - Unknown primary (10% of brain metastasis have no primary)
   - Remote history of systemic cancer
   - To rule out radiation necrosis in patients previously treated with radiation to the brain
   - Unusual appearing lesions, or unusual clinical presentation such as fever in a patient with known cancer[2]
5. *What are the indications for aggressive treatment with surgery or radiosurgery?*
   - Primary control
   - Expected relatively long disease-free interval
   - Karnofsky performance score (KPS) of 70 or greater
   - Young age (age is a predictor of survival length)
   - Absence of leptomeningeal involvement
   - Fewer than four brain metastases (the probability of tumor control is 64% for one tumor, 51% for two, and 41% for three lesions).[3]
6. *What are the factors in favor of surgery over radiosurgery?*
   - Factors favoring surgery[2,4]
     - Surgical accessibility
     - Undiagnosed primary
     - Need for immediate tumor debulking (rapid deterioration due to mass effect)
     - A lesion that is causing hydrocephalus
     - Rapid weaning of steroids
     - Lesions unlikely to respond to radiation
     - Radiation resistant tumors (thyroid carcinoma, renal cell carcinoma, and melanoma)
     - Highly cystic tumors
     - Very large tumors (>3 cm)
   - Factors favoring radiosurgery[2]
     - To avoid the need for multiple craniotomies
     - Associated morbidities (prior general status)
     - Surgery is usually not indicated for the following brain metastases
       - Small cell cancer of the lung
       - Germ cell tumors
       - Multiple myeloma
       - Leukemia and lymphoma
7. *Describe some adjuvant therapies.*
   - Patients with poor (low) KPS scores and progressive systemic disease often receive WBRT alone.
   - Current radiation doses are either 20 Gy in five fractions or 30 Gy in 10 fractions.
   - In patients with longer life expectancy (i.e., 1 year or more), a prolonged fractionation regimen of 40 Gy in 2-Gy fractions may decrease radiation-induced morbidity.
   - The combination of WBRT and surgery or stereotactic radiosurgery for the treatment of patients with two to four tumors significantly improves the control of brain disease.[5]
8. *What is the prognosis?*
   - If no treatment is given, survival can be as little as 4 weeks.
   - When the patient is taking high-dose glucocorticoids survival increases to 8 weeks.
   - WBRT can improve survival to 3 to 6 months.[2]
   - The addition of either tumor resection or SRS in a subset of these patients is associated with improved outcome.[3,6-9] Survival was similar to a matched control group of patients with single metastases (average 14-month).[6]
   - Patients with four or more brain metastases continue to have a particularly poor prognosis and are usually not treated surgically.[4]

Table 18.1 Differential Diagnosis for Multiple Brain Lesions

Primary tumor	Multifocal glioma, tuberous sclerosis (giant cell astrocytoma), multiple meningiomas, lymphoma, primitive neuroectodermal tumor, multiple neuromas (neurofibromatosis)
Metastasis	Lung, breast, melanoma, leukemia
Infection	Bacterial, toxoplasmosis, *Cryptococcus*, aspergillosis, herpes simplex encephalitis
Inflammation	Multiple sclerosis, tuberculosis gummas, granuloma, amyloidosis, sarcoidosis, vasculitis
Vascular	Multiple hemorrhages, venous infarct, moyamoya disease, multiple strokes
Other	Intracerebral calcifications, radiation necrosis

Source: Greenberg, MS. Handbook of Neurosurgery. 6th ed. New York: Thieme Medical Publishing; 2006.

■ References

1. Greenberg MS. Handbook of Neurosurgery. 6th ed. New York: Thieme Medical Publishing; 2006
2. Modha A, Shepard SR, Gutin PH. Surgery of brain metastases–is there still a place for it? J Neurooncol 2005;75(1):21–29
3. Chang SD, Adler JR Jr. Current treatment of patients with multiple brain metastases. Neurosurg Focus 2000;9(2):e5
4. Sills AK. Current treatment approaches to surgery for brain metastases. Neurosurgery 2005; 57(5, Suppl)S24–S32
5. Kondziolka D, Patel A, Lunsford LD, Flickinger JC. Decision making for patients with multiple brain metastases: radiosurgery, radiotherapy, or resection? Neurosurg Focus 2000;9(2):e4
6. Bindal RK, Sawaya R, Leavens ME, et al. Surgical treatment of multiple brain metastases. J Neurosurg 1993;79:210–216
7. Joseph J, Adler JR, Cox RS, et al. Linear accelerator-based stereotactic radiosurgery for brain metastases: the influence of number of lesions on survival. J Clin Oncol 1996;14:1085–1092
8. Kondziolka D, Patel A, Lunsford LD, et al. Stereotactic radiosurgery plus whole brain radiotherapy versus radiotherapy alone for patients with multiple brain metastases. Int J Radiat Oncol Biol Phys 1999;45:427–434
9. Loeffler JS, Alexander E III. Radiosurgery for the treatment of intracranial metastasis. In Loeffler JS, Lunsford LD, Alexander E III, eds. Stereotactic Radiosurgery. New York: McGraw-Hill; 1993:197–206

Case 19   Meningeal Carcinomatosis

Ramez Malak and Robert Moumdjian

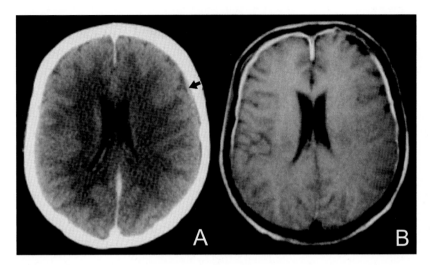

Fig. 19.1   (A) Computed tomography scan of the brain and **(B)** T1-weighted axial magnetic resonance image of the brain, both with contrast. *Arrow* in **(A)** points to contrast enhancement of the meninges.

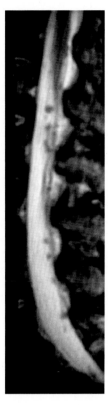

Fig. 19.2   T2-weighted magnetic resonance image of the lumbar spine, midsagittal section.

■ Clinical Presentation

• A 45-year-old woman presents with headache, nuchal rigidity, diplopia, and weakness in the left leg.

• A computed tomography (CT) scan shows contrast enhancement of the leptomeninges (**Fig. 19.1**)

■ Questions

1. Provide a differential diagnosis of meningeal enhancement.
2. What are the most common causes of meningeal carcinomatosis (MC)?
3. What investigations would you obtain?
4. What is the yield of lumbar puncture (LP) in MC and how can you improve this yield?
5. What is the mechanism of invasion?
6. What are the characteristics of meningeal carcinomatosis on craniospinal magnetic resonance imaging (MRI)?

MRI of the lumbar spine (**Fig. 19.2**) shows multiple metastases along the cauda equina.

7. Describe symptomatic treatment.
8. Describe the advantage and complications of Ommaya reservoir placement.
9. Outline the treatment of meningeal carcinomatosis.
10. What is the prognosis?

■ Answers

1. *Provide a differential diagnosis of meningeal enhancement.*
   - Neurogenic: increased cerebrospinal fluid (CSF) pressure, intracranial hypotension
   - Inflammatory: sarcoidosis
   - Infectious: subacute and chronic meningitis including tuberculosis, fungal infection, granulomatous cell infiltration
   - Vascular: local ischemia, venous thrombosis, hypoxia, subarachnoid hemorrhage
   - Traumatic
   - Drug induced: chemotherapeutic agents, heavy metals
   - Neoplastic: local tumor infiltration, primary meningeal glioma, primitive neuroectodermal tumor, isolated primary meningeal melanomas, rhabdomyosarcoma of the leptomeninges[1,2]
   - Other: ionizing radiation, metabolic disturbances, reaction to hyperventilation

2. *What are the most common causes of MC?*
   - MC is estimated to occur in ~5% of all patients with cancer. There is a greater prevalence of solid tumors compared with hematologic malignancies[3]
   - Hematologic malignancies presenting mostly with spinal or radicular symptoms
     - Breast and lung cancers
     - Head and neck cancers
     - Melanoma
     - Gastric cancer
   - Hematologic malignancy presenting more frequently with cranial nerve dysfunction or multifocal neurologic symptoms
     - Leukemia
     - Lymphoma
     - Adenocarcinoma of unknown primary

3. *What investigations would you obtain?*
   - CSF cytology
   - Radiologic studies
     - Cranial CT
     - Brain and spine MRI
     - CT myelography (rarely used)
   - Radionuclide CSF flow studies
   - Meningeal biopsy from an enhancing region on MRI, in cases where CSF exams remain inconclusive

4. *What is the yield of LP in MC and how can you improve this yield?*
   - The initial cytology is falsely negative in up to 40–50% of patients with pathologically proven leptomeningeal carcinomatosis. Diagnostic yield improves with[2]
     - Repeated sampling (50% for the first to 90% for the third spinal tap)
     - CSF sample volume (10 mL at least)
     - Avoiding delays in (i.e., immediate) processing and cytospin of the samples in the laboratory
     - Sampling site (LP provides a higher yield than ventricular CSF)

5. *What is the mechanism of invasion?*
   - Hematogenous spread via the arterial circulation or retrograde venous pathways along the valveless Batson venous plexus
   - Perineural and perivascular lymphatics route
   - Direct spread from central nervous system (CNS) tumors into the subarachnoid or ventricular spaces
   - Iatrogenic spread during invasive procedures or neurosurgery through an ependymal or dural breach
   - Common pathway: Once malignant cells enter the CSF, they disseminate to distant parts of the CNS, where they form secondary leptomeningeal deposits. The areas of predilection are basilar cisterns, posterior fossa, and cauda equina.[2]

6. *What are the characteristic aspects of meningeal carcinomatosis on craniospinal MRI?*
   - Enhancement and enlargement of cranial nerves
   - Superficial linear sulcal, cisternal, or dural enhancement
   - Irregular tentorial or ependymal enhancement
   - Cisternal or sulcal obliteration
   - Communicating hydrocephalus
   - Subarachnoid or intraventricular enhancing nodules
   - Multiple small nodular superficial brain nodules
   - Spinal linear enhancement
   - Spinal cord enlargement
   - Asymmetry of the roots with clumping of the roots of the cauda equina[1,2]

7. *Describe symptomatic treatment.*
   - Symptomatic treatment includes
     - Pain relief using analgesics: acetaminophen, opioids
     - Neuropathic pain often requires amitriptyline, clonazepam, or antiepileptic drugs (AEDs) such as egabalin (Lyrica; Pfizer Pharmaceuticals, New York, NY) or gabapentin (Neurontin; Pfizer Pharmaceuticals, New York, NY).
     - Focal irradiation of symptomatic sites is often quite efficient in relieving pain.
   - Seizures are managed with anti-epileptic drugs (AEDS), but prophylactic administration of AEDs is not recommended in patients who have never had seizures.
   - Headaches related to edema or increased intracranial pressure can sometimes be treated with steroids.
   - In cases of hydrocephalus secondary to CSF blockade, a course of steroids during whole brain or skull-base radiotherapy (RT) is sometimes appropriate, but shunting is often required.
   - Repeated LPs in the absence of cerebral edema or mass effect are often a good way to relieve headache.

8. *Describe the advantages and complications of Ommaya reservoir placement.*

■ Answers (*continued*)

- Advantages over repeated LP[4]:
  - Drug administration is painless and easier to perform.
  - Better drug distribution in the entire subarachnoid ventricular spaces
  - Possibility of delivering frequent small doses of drug to reduce neurotoxicity
  - Can be used when the platelet count is around 20,000 cell/mm[3]
  - Provides a certainty that the drug has not been given in the epidural space (which is the case in 10% of LPs)
  - Avoids some complications of LPs such as
    - Local obstruction of CSF circulation secondary to arachnoiditis
    - Brain herniation in the presence of brain mass effect
- Complications[5]
  - If there is a concern due to risks for general anesthesia, it can be performed with local anesthesia.
  - Infections
  - Epilepsy by extravasation of the drug into the brain
  - Failure to puncture slit ventricles
  - Hemorrhages are rare complications occurring especially with repeated puncture attempts.
  - Reservoir or catheter obstruction or dysfunction

9. *Outline the treatment of meningeal carcinomatosis.*
  - The treatment of meningeal carcinomatosis today is palliative and rarely curative with a median patient survival of 2 months. However, palliative therapy often affords the patient protection from further neurologic deterioration and consequently an improved neurologic quality of life.[3]
  - Radiotherapy
    - Although it may stabilize or delay progression of neurologic symptoms, it does not prolong survival.[3]
    - RT is also indicated to relieve CSF blocks, which reduce the efficacy and increase the toxicity of intrathecal chemotherapy.
    - RT is administered at a dose of 30 Gy delivered in 10 fractions over 2 weeks. It provides effective relief of pain and stabilizes neurologic symptoms but rarely leads to significant recovery[2]
    - Irradiation of the entire neuraxis is too toxic in patients who have generally already received multiagent chemotherapy and are prone to severe bone marrow toxicity.

- Chemotherapy
  - Chemotherapy can be administered intrathecally and/or systemically. Methotrexate is usually the first-line agent followed by cytarabine and thiotepa.
  - Following the placement of an intraventricular catheter, methotrexate may be administered as 2 mg per day for 5 consecutive days every other week for four treatment cycles[2-4]
- Prophylactic treatment in lymphoma and leukemia
  - Prevention of CNS relapse is increasingly a goal of primary therapy for patients with either non-Hodgkin's lymphoma or acute lymphocytic leukemia, high-dose systemic and/or intrathecal chemotherapy are used depending on the presence of risk factors for CNS involvement. These risk factors include
  - Lymphoma grade and stage
    - Extent of extranodal disease
    - Young age
    - Elevated serum lactate dehydrogenase levels
    - Presence of human immunodeficiency virus-(HIV)-related NHL
    - Presence of a primary CNS lymphoma[3]

10. *What is the prognosis?*
  - Despite therapy, median survival for meningeal carcinomatosis is about 4 months from diagnosis. This is particularly true of patients with leptomeningeal metastasis from solid tumors. Patients with breast cancer have a relatively better prognosis with median survival of 6 months from the time of diagnosis of meningeal carcinomatosis.
  - Patients with leukemia and lymphoma have the best prognosis with meningeal carcinomatosis. Such patients may respond rapidly and remain in a sustained remission for months to years.[4]

■ References

1. Schumacher M, Orszagh M. Imaging techniques in neoplastic meningosis. J Neurooncol 1998;38(2–3):111–120
2. Taillibert S, Laigle-Donadey F, Chodkiewicz C. Leptomeningeal metastases from solid malignancy: a review. J Neurooncol 2005;75:85–99
3. Chamberlain MC, Nolan C, Abrey LE. Leukemic and lymphomatous meningitis: incidence, prognosis and treatment. J Neurooncol 2005;75:71–83
4. DeAngelis LM. Current diagnosis and treatment of leptomeningeal metastasis. J Neurooncol 1998;38(2–3):245–252
5. Berweiler U, Krone A, Tonn JC. Reservoir systems for intraventricular chemotherapy. J Neurooncol 1998;38(2–3):141–143

Case 20   Primary Central Nervous System Lymphoma

John Winestone and Allen K. Sills Jr.

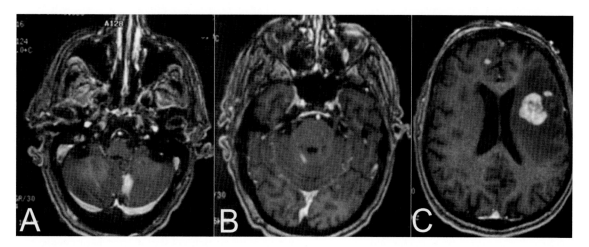

Fig. 20.1   (A–C) Enhanced T1-weighted magnetic resonance images showing multiple lesions, **(C)** the largest one being in the left frontal lobe.

■ Clinical Presentation

- An 81-year-old man presents with several days of confusion and a medical history significant for hypertension and hyperlipidemia.
- On examination, there are no focal neurologic deficits other than confusion.

- Computed tomography (CT) scan shows multiple intraparenchymal brain lesions.
- A magnetic resonance imaging (MRI) scan is obtained (**Fig. 20.1**).

■ Questions

1. Describe the MRI.
2. What is the differential diagnosis for the imaging findings in this scenario?
3. What is an appropriate workup to help narrow the differential diagnosis?
4. If a tissue sample was needed, which would be the best lesion to biopsy?

After a metastatic and immunodeficiency workup was negative, we elected to biopsy the left frontal lobe lesion.

Care was taken to have the patient off of steroids for 2 weeks before the biopsy. The pathology results confirmed central nervous system (CNS) lymphoma.

5. Name the different ways to diagnose CNS lymphoma.
6. Describe the treatment course.
7. What is the role of surgery?
8. What is the outcome with and without treatment?

■ Answers

1. *Describe the MRI.*
   - The MRI shows multiple enhancing lesions. They are dispersed throughout the brain with some lesions abutting the ventricular system.
   - The largest lesion is in the left frontal lobe, measuring ~2 × 2.5 cm with some local edema.
   - The lesions are bilateral.

2. *What is the differential diagnosis for the imaging findings in this scenario?*
   - Periventricular solid enhancing lesions may represent[1]
     - Primary CNS lymphoma (PCNSL)
     - Ependymoma
     - Metastatic lesions
     - Glioblastoma multiforme (multifocal)
     - Toxoplasmosis
     - Other less likely diagnoses include brain abscess, multiple sclerosis, and vasculopathy

3. *What is an appropriate workup to help narrow the differential diagnosis?*
   - An aggressive medical workup searching for neoplastic disease is in order. CT scans of the viscera as well as basic screening tests for common malignancies such as breast, lung, prostate, and colon cancer would help define a metastatic source.
   - Blood work for neoplastic markers as well as immunodeficiency (prostate-specific antigen, human immunodeficiency virus, carcinoembryonic antigen) may aid in the workup.
   - Cerebrospinal fluid (CSF) sampling may be helpful in determining demyelinating disease as well as detecting cells from a lymphoma process including tumor markers such as lactate dehydrogenase.
   - Beta-glucuronidase and beta 2-microglobulin may also be sought out in the CSF.[2,3]

4. *If a tissue sample were needed, which would be the best lesion to biopsy?*
   - The left frontal lesion is the most easily accessible for tissue diagnosis. If there were complications from the surgery, this location would be the most tolerant in terms of subsequent deficits.

5. *Name the different ways to diagnose CNS lymphoma.*
   - National Comprehensive Cancer Network (NCCN) guidelines recommend holding steroids when lymphoma is suspected by history, physical examination, and imaging.
   - The diagnosis can be made with CSF cytology and flow cytometry, a biopsy of the lesion, and/or ophthalmologic examination.
   - The lesion having dissipated with prior steroids is suggestive of PCNSL and a trial of steroids followed by biopsy of any growing lesion is the treatment of choice. Almost all patients will develop resistance after prolonged exposure to steroids. Consequently, steroids should be avoided in suspected but undiagnosed PCNSL. Steroid-induced remission may impact biopsy results[2]
   - Systemic workup for the hematologic or solid organ source of the lymphoma is suggested.[3]

6. *Describe the treatment course.*
   - High-dose methotrexate is the treatment of choice. Intrathecal methotrexate should be used when there is evidence of disease in the CSF by lumbar puncture or on a MRI of the spine.[2,3]
   - Radiation therapy is currently not recommended for PCNSL when the patient is older than 60 years.[2,3]
   - Low-dose whole brain radiation treatment may be used as an adjunct to chemotherapy in selective elderly patients.[2,4]

7. *What is the role of surgery?*
   - Surgery does not improve survival and has a limited role.[2]
     - Masses large enough to cause impending herniation
     - For diagnostic purposes

8. *What is the outcome with and without treatment?*
   - Survival
     - Median survival less than 3 months without treatment (supportive care only)[5]
     - Median overall survival is 37 months with treatment.[6]
     - Median survival in elderly patients is 7 months (including partial or limited treatment).[4]
   - Predictors of poor survival include increased age, low Karnofsky performance score, hemiparesis, altered mental status, and decreased creatinine clearance.[6]

■ References

1. Osborn AG. Diagnostic Neuroradiology. St Louis, MO: Mosby, 1994
2. Mohile NA, Abrey LE. Primary central nervous system lymphoma. Semin Radiat Oncol 2007;17(3):223–229
3. Brem S, Bierman P, Black P, et al. NCCN Clinical Practice Guidelines in Oncology - Central Nervous System Cancers [Online] 2007. Available at: http://www.nccn.org/professionals/physician_gls/PDF/cns.pdf. Accessed December 11, 2007
4. Panageas KS, Elkin EB, Ben-Porat L, Deangelis LM, Abrey LE. Patterns of treatment in older adults with primary central nervous system lymphoma. Cancer 2007;110(6):1338–1344
5. Ferreri AJ, Reni M. Primary central nervous system lymphoma. Crit Rev Oncol Hematol 2007;63(3):257–268
6. Abrey LE, Ben-Porat L, Panageas KS, et al. Primary central nervous system lymphoma: The Memorial Sloan-Kettering Cancer Center prognostic model. J Clin Oncol 2006;24:5711–5715

Case 21   Posterior Fossa Tumor

Julius July and Eka Julianta Wahjoepramono

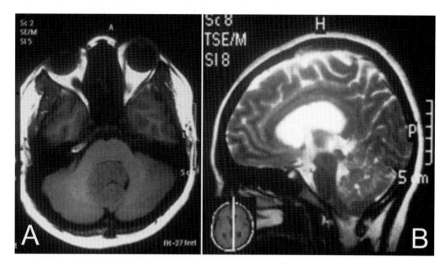

Fig. 21.1   (A) T1-weighted magnetic resonance image (MRI), axial plane at the level of the posterior fossa, and **(B)** T2-weighted MRI midsagittal section.

■ Clinical Presentation

• A 28-year-old woman presents with balance problems for the past 2 months.
• She is also experiencing progressing headache and blurred vision for 3 weeks.

• Physical examination reveals mild ataxia, altered tandem gait, and bilateral papilledema.
• A magnetic resonance imaging (MRI) scan without contrast is obtained (**Fig. 21.1**).

■ Questions

1. Interpret the MRI.
2. What is your differential diagnosis?
3. What is your treatment plan?
4. What adjuvant therapy is recommended based on your differential diagnosis?

The histopathology reveals medulloblastoma.

5. What are the differences between medulloblastoma in childhood and adulthood?
6. List familial cancer syndrome associated with medulloblastoma.
7. What is the prognosis for this tumor?
8. What is the current staging for medulloblastoma?

■ Answers

1. *Interpret the MRI.*
   - The T1-weighted axial MRI (**Fig. 21.1A**) shows a lesion involving the midline posterior fossa and compression of the 4th ventricle (vermis lesion).
   - The T2-weighted sagittal MRI (**Fig. 21.1B**) demonstrates the same lesion in the vermis and hydrocephalus.

2. *What is your differential diagnosis?*
   - Differential diagnosis for a single posterior fossa lesion in a young adult includes[1,2]
     - Metastasis (most common brain lesion in an adult)
     - Hemangioblastoma (accounts for 7–12% of posterior fossa tumors)
     - Pilocytic astrocytoma (could be solid or cystic form)
     - Medulloblastoma (more common in childhood. There is a second peak between 20–40 years. It accounts for 5% of all adult posterior fossa tumors and 1% of all adult brain tumors. Medulloblastoma in adulthood is more likely laterally located; in childhood, it tends to be in the midline.)
     - Other less likely lesions include tuberculoma, cavernous hemangioma, brain abscess, high-grade glioma, lymphoma, dermoid, infarction, hemorrhage, etc.

3. *What is your treatment plan?*
   - The tumor is located in the vermis, just posterior to the 4th ventricle with signs of hydrocephalus (both radiographically and clinically).
   - Initial management[3]
     - The patient should be admitted to the intensive care unit.
     - Place the patient on steroids (dexamethasone 10 mg intravenous (i.v.) once, the 6 mg i.v. every 6 hours) with histamine blockers for gastric ulcer prevention.
     - Obtain a basic preoperative laboratory panel: complete blood count, electrolytes, prothrombin time/partial thromboplastin time, type and cross-match 2 units of packed red blood cells.
     - Due to the presence of hydrocephalus, surgical intervention should be performed urgently (within a few hours).
     - If possible, also obtain preoperative brain and spine MRIs with contrast to better delineate the tumor and its vasculature and to rule out drop metastases

   - Definitive treatment should include surgical removal of the lesion with likely temporary external ventricular drain to control the intracranial pressure and anticipate postoperative cerebellum swelling.[3]
     - Posterior fossa craniotomy with prone positioning (Concorde) and midline incision
     - May place Frazier burr hole for ventricular catheter (3 to 4 cm from the midline and 6 cm above the inion)
     - Adjuncts to surgery should include
       - Microscope
       - Intraoperative ultrasound
       - If available – frameless navigation
   - The histopathology of the tumor will guide further treatment plan.

4. *What adjuvant therapy is recommended based on your differential diagnosis?*
   - Metastatic disease: whole brain radiation 45–50 Gy plus a boost to the tumor bed to bring the total treatment up to 55 Gy, all with low fractions of 1.80–2.0 Gy. Possible combination with chemotherapy for certain entities such as small cell lung carcinoma, adenocarcinoma of colorectal, etc. A workup for the primary tumor is also recommended (such as CT thorax, abdomen and pelvis, mammogram, and serum tumor markers).[3]
   - Medulloblastoma: often spreads through the subarachnoid space and the tumors are radiosensitive. Radiotherapy of the entire neuraxis is considered standard, even if no obvious lesions are present on postoperative imaging. Best survival rates are obtained with 3600 to 4000 cGy to the whole craniospinal axis, supplemented to 5400 – 5600 cGy at the primary site.[3]
   - Hemangioblastoma, cavernoma, and pilocytic astrocytoma should be completely removed as a definitive treatment. Adjuvant therapy remains controversial with this diagnosis.[3]
   - Tuberculoma: It is not necessary to remove completely. It requires postoperative antituberculosis treatment: rifampicin 450–600 mg/day (10 mg/kg), isoniazid 300–450 mg/day (3–10 mg/kg), ethambutol 15 mg/kg/day, pyrazinamide 20–30 mg/kg/day. All these medications are given orally every day for the initial 3–4 months. Then the first two medications are continued (rifampicin and isoniazid) for 16–18 months. Pyridoxine (10 mg/day) is invariably added to prevent peripheral neuropathy due to isoniazid. Streptomycin could be added for the initial treatment, given intramuscularly 1 g/day (20–25 mg/kg).

■ **Answers (*continued*)**

5. *What are the differences between medulloblastoma in childhood and adulthood?*
   - **Table 21.1** summarizes the differences between medulloblastoma in childhood and adulthood.[4,5]
6. *List familial cancer syndrome associated with medulloblastoma.*
   Syndrome associated with medulloblastoma[4,5]
   - Gorlin syndrome (multiple nevoid basal cell carcinomas)
   - Rubinstein–Taybi syndrome
   - Ataxia-telangiectasia
   - Turcot's syndrome (polyposis-glioma)
   - Li–Fraumeni syndrome (germ line TP53)
   - Neurofibromatosis
   - Tuberous sclerosis
7. *What is the prognosis for this tumor?*
   - The prognosis for patients with medulloblastoma is related to[5]
     - Tumor size: Large tumors have been shown to have a lower 5-year disease-free survival rate.
     - Invasiveness of the tumor to surrounding structure such as brainstem could prevent complete removal of the tumor.
     - Dissemination of the tumor through the neuraxis correlates with poor outcome.
     - Age of patients: younger age is much more likely to have dissemination.
     - Postoperative residual tumor correlates with poor outcome.

   - Overall, with surgery and radiation, the 5-year disease-free survival rate could approach 80%.[5]
8. *What is the current staging for medulloblastoma?*
   - Current staging for medulloblastoma divides the risk into standard and poor risk based on several factors, such as extent of tumor, resection, age, and histology.[5,6]
   - **Table 21.2** summarizes the factors affecting survival in medulloblastoma.[5]

Table 21.1 Differences between Medulloblastoma in Childhood and Adulthood

	Children	Adult
Peak incidence	3–5 Years	20–40 Years
Location	Midline	Hemispheric/lateral
CT / MRI	Contrast enhancement	Less contrast enhancement
Macroscopic appearance	Mostly solid	Cystic & necrotic
Margins	Well-defined margins	Poorly defined margins

Sources: Data from Kleihues P, Cavanee WK. Pathology and Genetics of Tumors of the Nervous System. Lyon: World Health Organization; 2000; and Kunschner LJ, Lang FF. Medulloblastoma. In Winn HR, ed. Youmans Neurological Surgery. 5th ed. Philadelphia, PA: Saunders Elsevier, 2004:1031–1042.

Abbreviations: CT, computed tomography; MRI, magnetic resonance imaging.

Table 21.2 Factors Affecting Survival in Medulloblastoma

Factors	Standard Risk	Poor Risk
Extent of tumor	Posterior fossa, no brainstem involvement, no metastasis	Disseminated to intracranial and/or spinal, extraneural lump
Extent of resection	Near total, <1.5 cm² residual tumor	Subtotal, >1.5 cm² residual tumor
Age	Older than 3 years	Younger than 3 years
Histology	Undifferentiated	Differentiated

Source: Adapted from Kunschner LJ, Lang FF. Medulloblastoma. In Winn HR, ed. Youmans Neurological Surgery. 5th ed. Philadelphia, PA: Saunders Elsevier, 2004:1031–1042. Adapted with permission.

■ References

1. Osborn AG. Diagnostic Neuroradiology. St. Louis, MO: Mosby, 1994:465
2. Greenberg MS. Handbook of Neurosurgery. 6th ed. New York: Thieme Medical Publishers, 2006:923–924
3. Miller JP, Cohen AR. Surgical management of tumors of the fourth ventricle. In: Roberts DW, Schmideck HH, eds., Schmidek & Sweet's Operative Neurosurgical Techniques. Indication, Methods, and Results. 5th ed. Philadelphia, PA: Saunders Elsevier; 2006:881–913
4. Kleihues P, Cavanee WK. Pathology and Genetics of Tumors of the Nervous System. Lyon: World Health Organization; 2000
5. Kunschner LJ, Lang FF. Medulloblastoma. In Winn HR, ed., Youmans Neurological Surgery. 5th ed. Philadelphia, PA: Saunders Elsevier, 2004:1031–1042
6. Rodriguez FJ, Eberhart C, O'Neill BP, et al. Histopathologic grading of adult medulloblastomas. Cancer 2007;109(12):2557–2565

Case 22   Fibrous Dysplasia of the Skull

Burak Sade and Joung H. Lee

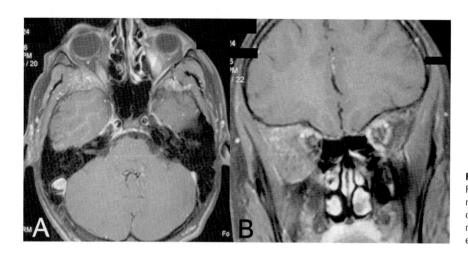

Fig. 22.1 **(A)** T1-weighted postcontrast FatSat (fat saturation) axial and **(B)** coronal magnetic resonance images. Note the hyperostotic abnormal bone involving the orbital roof, the posterolateral wall of the orbit, and extending into the infratemporal fossa.

■ Clinical Presentation

• A 15-year-old right-handed boy is referred by a pediatric neurologist because of a right frontal, retroorbital headache not responding to aggressive medical treatment.

• Neurologic evaluation is within normal limits.
• Magnetic resonance imaging (MRI) scan of the brain is obtained (**Fig. 22.1**).

■ Questions

1. Interpret the MRI scan.
2. What is your differential diagnosis?
3. What additional studies would you obtain?
4. What would be the indications for surgery based on your preoperative diagnosis?

Because of the intractable nature of his headaches, the patient was offered surgery. A right frontotemporal craniotomy was performed with a skull-base approach consisting of extensive extradural removal of the lesion involving the orbital roof and the posterolateral wall of the orbit. The resection was further extended to the inferior orbital fissure inferiorly and foramen ovale posteriorly until normal bone texture was seen at all margins.

Postoperative MRI confirming complete resection of the tumor is shown in **Fig. 22.2**.

The histology of the tumor was reported as "benign bone and fibrous tissue," consistent with fibrous dysplasia. At 6-week follow-up, his headaches were significantly improved.

5. What would be your management goals?
6. What is the role of radiation therapy in the treatment of fibrous dysplasia?
7. What is the McCune–Albright syndrome?

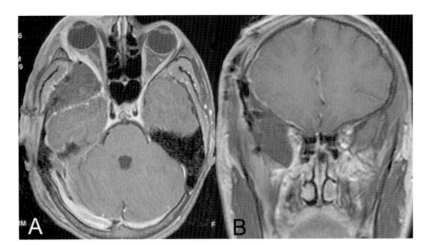

Fig. 22.2 Postoperative T1-weighted postcontrast **(A)** axial and **(B)** coronal magnetic resonance images, confirming complete removal of the dysplastic bone.

■ Answers

1. *Interpret the MRI scan.*
   - There is an enhancing hyperostotic lesion of the sphenoid bone on the right involving the orbital roof and posterolateral orbital wall.
   - It is extending into the infratemporal fossa to the level of the inferior orbital fissure.
2. *What is your differential diagnosis?*
   - The differential diagnosis includes
     - Fibrous dysplasia
     - Fibro-osseous tumors (i.e., ossifying fibroma)
     - Primary bone tumors
     - Intradural process causing hyperostosis of the adjacent bone (i.e., sphenoid wing meningioma)
     - Metastasis
     - Other less likely diagnoses include lymphoma, rhabdomyosarcoma, Paget disease, Langerhans cell histiocytosis, infection (osteomyelitis, soft tissue infection, etc.)
3. *What additional studies would you obtain?*
   - Computed tomography scan: to better identify the osseous structures, and assess the extent of the pathologic bone[1]
   - Neuroophthalmologic examination: because of the proximity of the lesion to the optic nerve[2]
   - Laboratory studies including serum alkaline phosphatase, calcium[3]
   - Possibly preoperative angiography or magnetic resonance angiography with or without embolization, if surgery is planned
4. *What would be the indications for surgery based on your preoperative diagnosis?*
   - Indications for surgery include[2,4]
     - Cosmetic concerns such as ocular proptosis or skull deformity
     - Compromise of the vision or ocular motility
     - Intractable headache or local pain
     - Rapid or aggressive growth
5. *What would be your management goals?*
   - Rather than being a true neoplasm, fibrous dysplasia is a result of the arrest of the bone maturation in the lamellar/woven stage.
   - Because of its polyostotic occurrence and poor demarcation from the normal bone, complete resection may be difficult at times, or not possible. In one series, gross total resection was possible in only 25% of the patients.[5] Although subtotal resection may carry a risk for future regrowth of the residual lesion, its growth usually slows down after puberty.
   - Calcitonin or bisphosphonates have been used in multifocal or nonoperable cases.[2]
6. *What is the role of radiation therapy in the treatment of fibrous dysplasia?*
   - The role of radiotherapy is unproven.[4]
   - There may be a 44% of malignant transformation of fibrous dysplasia with radiation and it is therefore relatively contraindicated.[2]
7. *What is the McCune–Albright syndrome?*
   - The McCune–Albright syndrome is characterized by the following features[2,6]:
     - Fibrous dysplasia (usually polyostotic)
     - Precocious puberty and endocrinopathies
     - Areas of cutaneous pigmentation (café-au-lait spots)

■ **References**

1. Osborn AG. Diagnostic Neuroradiology. St. Louis, MO: Mosby; 1994:465
2. Dumont AS, Boulos PT, Jane JA, Ellegala DB, Newman SA, Jane JA. Cranioorbital fibrous dysplasia: with emphasis on visual impairment and current surgical management. Neurosurg Focus 2001;10(5):e6
3. Greenberg MS. Handbook of Neurosurgery. 6th ed. New York: Thieme Medical Publishers; 2006:923–924
4. Ozek C, Gundogan H, Bilkay U, Tokat C, Gurler T, Songur E. Craniomaxillofacial fibrous dysplasia. J Craniofac Surg 2002;13(3):382–389
5. Maher CO, Friedman JA, Meyer FB, Lynch JJ, Unni K, Raffel C. Surgical treatment of the fibrous dysplasia of the skull in children. Pediatr Neurosurg 2002;37:87–92
6. Albright F, Butler AM, Hampton AO, et al. Syndrome characterized by osteitis fibrosa disseminata, areas of pigmentation and endocrine dysfunction with precocious puberty in females, report of five cases. N Engl J Med 1937;216:727–746

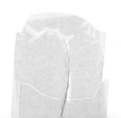

Case 23   **Orbital Tumor**

Michel Lacroix

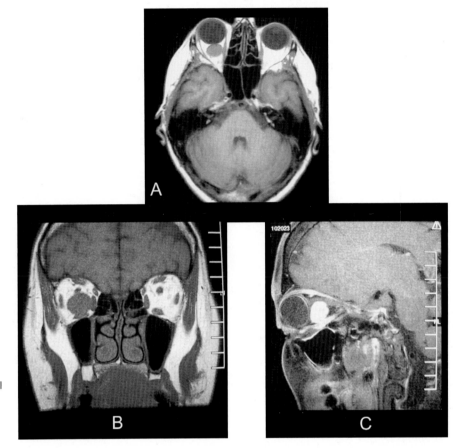

Fig. 23.1   (A) Axial T1-weighted, **(B)** coronal T1-weighted, and **(C)** sagittal T1-weighted magnetic resonance images (MRIs) of the brain with gadolinium contrast brought by the patient during the initial visit.

■ Clinical Presentation

- A 52-year-old woman presents with gradual proptosis.
- Examination reveals no diplopia, loss of vision, or other neurologic deficits.
- A magnetic resonance imaging (MRI) scan is shown in **Fig. 23.1**.

■ Questions

1. Interpret the MRI.
2. Give a general classification of orbital tumors.
3. What structures are contained in the annulus of Zinn?
4. Give a differential diagnosis.
5. What is your initial management?
6. Describe the surgical approach and choose the one you consider best.

You proceed with a lateral microsurgical approach, achieve a complete macroscopic resection, and the diagnosis is hemangioma.

7. What is the prognosis and what will be your follow-up?

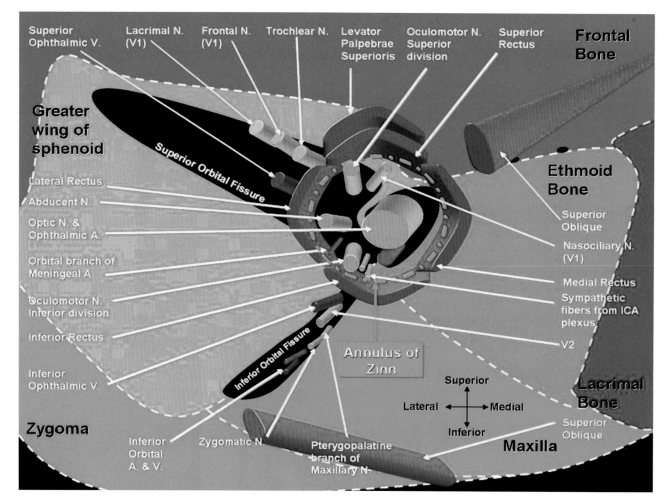

Fig. 23.2 Artist's rendering of the content of the annulus of Zinn.

■ Answers

1. *Interpret the MRI.*
   - In the right orbit there is a round lesion 1.3 cm in diameter. The lesion is homogeneous and is enhanced strongly after gadolinium injection.
   - The lesion lies inferiorly to the optic nerve to which it may or may not be attached, pushing it upward. There is a significant mass effect with displacement and/or invasion of the inferior rectus muscle and significant secondary proptosis.

2. *Give a general classification of orbital tumors.*
   - Based on their location and presentation with some specific symptoms, there are three categories of orbital tumors[1] excluding the primary ocular tumors.
     – Within the muscle cone (intraconal): visual loss and/or impaired orbital motility by mass effect; potential axial proptosis
     – Outside the muscle cone (extraconal): proptosis and orbital displacement; visual loss and impaired mobility by compression of individual muscles and deformity of the eye globe
     – Within the optic canal (intracanalicular): loss of vision and optic disk swelling; rare proptosis

3. *What structures are contained in the annulus of Zinn?*
   - Cranial nerve (CN) II, ophthalmic artery, CN III (superior and inferior divisions), CN V1 (nasociliary), CN VI (abducens)
   - **Figure 23.2**

4. *Give a differential diagnosis.*
   - The lesion appears to be extraaxial and intraconal and does not involve the eye globe. Considering the appearance of the lesion and the broad differential diagnosis of orbital lesions,[2] one should probably list these pathologies in this sequence:
     – Hemangioma: the most common benign lesion of this location
     – Meningioma of the optic nerve sheath
     – Neurofibroma
     – Melanoma: the most frequent primary malignancy in adults in this location or other metastatic tumor
     – Lymphoma: a frequent cause of painless proptosis
     – Vascular, endocrine, infectious, and inflammatory diseases are unlikely. It is not a congenital malformation.

■ Answers (*continued*)

5. *What is your initial management?*
   - Present all options to the patient including
     - Observation/no treatment
     - Surgical resection for diagnosis and treatment
   - Present all the potential surgical complications including
     - General (infection, hematoma, systemic complications, coma, death)
     - Specific (loss of vision, diplopia, xerophthalmia, hypoesthesia)
   - Consult ophthalmology for visual fields, extraocular movements' assessment, and surgical assistance
   - Computed tomography scan is moderately helpful in this circumstance. The MRI is providing all required imaging information. Consider selective angiogram.[3]
   - A metastatic workup will not change the initial management.

6. *Describe the surgical approach and choose the one you consider best.*
   - Relying on the MRI, the lesion can be located inferior to the optic nerve and lateral to the optic apex.

   - A lateral microsurgical approach is a viable surgical option[4,5]: the skin incision is made superolateral to the eyebrow and is carried posteriorly ~4 cm.
   - A lateral orbito-zygomatectomy allows exposure of the periorbital fascia. A traction suture can be placed to identify the lateral rectus muscle and follows it. The incision in the periorbita is inferior to the lateral rectus muscle.
   - A medial rotation of the globe is performed by light traction. Access is then achieved to the intraconal lesion.
   - For lesions with intracranial extension, lesions involving the optic canal and lesions medial to the optic apex, a transcranial fronto-orbital temporal approach is essential.
   - A medial orbitotomy is preferred for a tumor located anteriorly to the orbit and medial to the optic nerve.

7. *What is the prognosis and what will be your follow-up?*
   - A complete resection of a hemangioma is curative. No other treatment or long-term follow-up is required.[6]

■ References

1. Winn RH. Neurological Surgery. 5th ed. Philadelphia, PA: Saunders, 2004:1371–1387
2. Greenberg MS. Handbook of Neurosurgery. 6th ed. New York: Thieme Medical Publishers; 2006:923–924
3. Kennedy RE. Arterial embolization of orbital hemangiomas. Trans Am Ophthalmol Soc 1978;76:266–277
4. Czirjak S, Szeifert GT. The role of the superciliary approach in the surgical management of intracranial neoplasms. Neurol Res 2006;28(2):131–137
5. Maus M, Goldman HW. Removal of orbital apex hemangioma using new transorbital craniotomy through suprabrow approach. Ophthal Plast Reconstr Surg 1999;15(3):166–170
6. Hamilton HB, Voorhies RM. Tumors of the Skull. In: Wilkins RH, Rengashary SS. Neurosurgery. 2nd ed. New York: McGraw-Hill; 1996:1503–1528

Case 24   Multiple Ring-enhancing Cerebral Lesions

Kevin Petrecca and Rolando Del Maestro

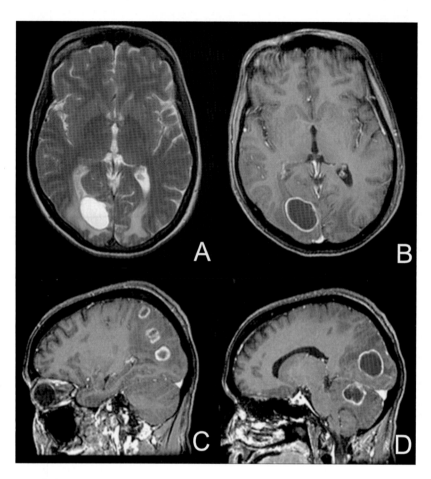

Fig. 24.1 **(A)** T2-weighted axial magnetic resonance image (MRI), **(B)** T1-weighted axial MRI with contrast, and **(C,D)** T1-weighted sagittal MRI showing intraparenchymal lesions.

■ Clinical Presentation

- A 44-year-old woman presents with sudden onset right ear pain 2 months ago associated with headache, dizziness, and difficulty getting out of bed while vacationing in the Dominican Republic.

- Patient is a smoker.
- She was given a 1-week course of antibiotics for a presumed otitis media.
- She developed a progressive unsteady gait.

■ Questions

1. Describe the magnetic resonance imaging (MRI) findings (**Fig. 24.1**).
2. What information should be obtained on history?
3. What is the differential diagnosis?
4. What are your initial investigations and how would you manage this patient?
5. Are there any MRI findings that can distinguish a bacterial abscess from a neoplasm?
6. What are the histologic stages of bacterial abscess formation and what are their radiologic correlates?
7. What are the sources of bacterial abscesses?

A stereotactic biopsy for diagnosis was performed and was nondiagnostic and the lesions are not decreasing in size on broad spectrum antibiotics.

8. What is the next step in your management?

A right parietal craniotomy was performed and one of the lesions was resected. Pathology was consistent with an adenocarcinoma. A computed tomography (CT) scan of the chest and abdomen revealed a small mass adjacent to the right main stem bronchus.

■ Answers

1. *Describe the MRI findings (**Fig. 24.1**).*
   - The T2-weighted MRI shows a right occipital cystic lesion with surrounding edema. There is also edema in the contralateral occipital lobe. The lesion exhibits a small amount of mass effect, evident as a loss of sulcation in the area of the lesion.
   - The contrast-infused images reveal multiple lesions, a larger lesion in the cerebellar vermis, and two other lesions in the right parieto-occipital region. Each lesion has similar characteristics including a well-formed enhancing capsule surrounding a cystic center. A developmental venous anomaly is present in the left frontal lobe.

2. *What information should be obtained in the history?*
   - It is important to identify risk factors for cerebral abscess formation and for metastatic disease: smoking, weight loss, night sweats, fatigue, cough, intravenous drug use, cardiac or pulmonary abnormalities, human immunodeficiency virus status, other high-risk behaviors, etc.

3. *What is the differential diagnosis?*
   - The differential diagnosis includes multiple bacterial abscesses, neurocysticercosis, toxoplasmosis, tuberculomas, metastases, and multifocal glioblastoma.

4. *What are your initial investigations and how would you manage this patient?*
   - Markers of infections include an elevated white blood cell count, erythrocyte sedimentation rate, and C-reactive protein.
   - A chest radiograph to rule out pneumonia, tuberculosis, and a neoplasm
   - Metastatic workup may be initiated with CT of the chest, abdomen, and pelvis.
   - Gram stain, blood and urine cultures to identify a hematogenous origin to an abscess as well as serum antitoxoplasma titers
   - Radiographs of the arms and legs to identify subcutaneous or muscular calcifications that can be present in cysticercosis
   - Western blot tests to detect *Taenium solium* antigens from serum
   - An electrocardiogram to assess cardiac rhythm and an abdominal ultrasound to identify a mass

5. *Are there any MRI findings that can distinguish a bacterial abscess from a neoplasm?*
   - Cerebral abscesses can mimic necrotic tumors and cystic metastases on conventional MRI. These lesions can often, however, be differentiated on diffusion-weighted imaging (DWI).
   - Cerebral abscesses typically demonstrate restricted diffusion on DWI, whereas tumors and cystic metastases usually do not.[1]

6. *What are the histologic stages of bacterial abscess formation and what are their radiologic correlates?*
   - There are four histologic stages in cerebral abscess formation[2,3]:
     - Early suppurative cerebritis (days 1–2) defined by endothelial cell swelling, perivascular neutrophil infiltration. CT findings include an area of hypodensity that may exhibit patchy enhancement.
     - Late suppurative cerebritis with confluent central necrosis (days 3–7) defined by adjacent foci of necrosis, which enlarge and become confluent. The infiltrate now includes macrophages, lymphocytes, and plasma cells. CT findings include a more pronounced central hypodensity with a thick enhancing ring surrounded by a hypodensity.
     - Early encapsulation (days 8–14) defined by capsular neovascularity, fibroblast infiltration, collagen deposition, and perilesional edema. CT findings include a well-developed central core with a thinner well-formed enhancing ring.
     - Late encapsulation (days >14) defined by central necrosis, a thin collagen capsule and lymphocytes. Note: Capsule is thinner along the ventricular wall, increasing the susceptibility of rupture into ventricular system. CT findings include a very thin enhancing ring surrounded by a hypodensity.

7. *What are the sources of bacterial abscesses?*
   - There are three sources of cerebral bacterial abscesses.
   - The most common route is hematogenous, which accounts for 25% of abscesses. The most common pathogen is *Streptococcus viridans*.
   - A second etiology is from a contiguous source such as a paranasal sinus, middle ear, dental root, osteomyelitis, or emissary vein. The most common pathogen is *Streptococcus milleri*.
   - The third route is direct from a trauma or postsurgical, especially postsinus breach. The common pathogens are *Staphylococcus aureus* and *epidermidis*.[3]

8. *What is the next step in your management?*
   - Because the stereotactic biopsy was nondiagnostic and the lesions are not decreasing in size on broad-spectrum antibiotics, a more invasive approach to make a diagnosis is necessary.
   - Treatment options include steroid therapy for symptom relief, resection of one or more lesions followed by whole brain radiotherapy (WBRT), radiosurgery for each lesion with or without WBRT, or WBRT alone.

■ References

1. Chang SC, Lai PH, Chen WL, et al. Diffusion-weighted MRI features of brain abscess and cystic or necrotic brain tumors. Comparison with conventional MRI. Clin Imaging 2002;26(4):227–236

2. Lu CH, Chang WN, Lui CC. Strategies for the management of bacterial brain abscess. J Clin Neurosci 2006;13(10):979–985

3. Ellison D, Love S, Chimell L, Harding B, Lowe JS, Vinters HV. Neuropathology – A Reference Text to CNS Pathology. St. Louis, MO: Mosby; 2004

Case 25   **Paraganglioma**

Nazer H. Qureshi and Ossama Al-Mefty

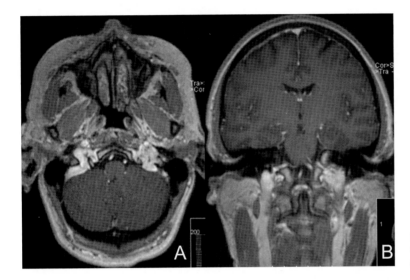

Fig. 25.1 T1-weighted magnetic resonance image with contrast injection. **(A)** Axial cut taken at the level of the skull base and **(B)** coronal cut.

■ Clinical Presentation

- A 44-year-old hypertensive woman with type 2 diabetes mellitus presented with a concussion. She had a history of speech difficulty and tongue wasting.
- The patient was noted to have ipsilateral tongue fasciculations, atrophy, and deviation. She also had slight ipsilateral sternocleidomastoid weakness with normal gag reflex and mild ipsilateral high-frequency sensorineural hearing loss.
- Magnetic resonance imaging (MRI) scan with contrast is shown in **Fig. 25.1**.

■ Questions

1. Describe the MRI findings and explain what the computed tomography (CT) scan would have shown.
2. What is the most probable diagnosis and what is the differential diagnosis?
3. What other studies would you order for this patient?
4. The serum epinephrine-level test that you ordered was reported 5 times above normal level. What is the significance of this and what would you do next?
5. Interpret the angiogram (**Fig. 25.2**).
6. How would you describe the treatment options to the patient?
7. The patient chooses surgery. What preoperative and intraoperative measures would you take to avoid complications?
8. What would you do if the patient were also noted to have (a) an ipsilateral carotid body lesion or (b) a bilateral jugular fossa lesion?

At the first follow-up visit you discuss the pathology report with the patient, which reads as follows, "… sustentacular cell density and the immunohistochemical staining with S-100 and chromogranin of the chief cells in this tumor was very low."

9. How would you interpret these pathologic findings?
10. The patient asks about the risk of her two sons getting this tumor. How would you address this issue with her?
11. Describe a classification system for glomus tympanicum tumors.
12. Describe the syndromes of the jugular foramen.

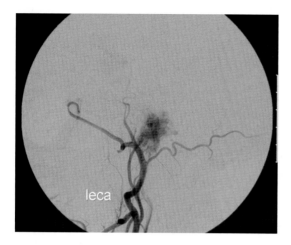

Fig. 25.2 Left external carotid artery injection angiogram.

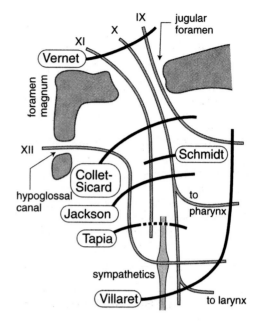

Fig. 25.3 Schematic diagram of jugular foramen syndromes. (From Greenberg MS. Handbook of Neurosurgery. 6th ed. New York: Thieme Medical Publishers; 2006:86. Adapted with permission.)

■ Answers

1. *Describe the MRI findings and explain what the CT scan would have shown.*
   - T1-weighted MRI with gadolinium enhancement shows a left-sided jugular foramen lesion in the petrous bone that takes up contrast brightly and is noted to have "speckled pattern" suggestive of flow voids depicting high vascularity. Intracranial extension is not clearly evident in this slice but could be expected.
   - A CT scan would have shown an enlarged jugular foramen indicating the presence of a lesion in the petrous bone.

2. *What is the most probable diagnosis and what is the differential diagnosis?*
   - Tumors arising from the jugular foramen are most likely glomus jugulare (paraganglioma).
   - Other common possible lesions in the differential diagnosis include schwannoma and meningioma.
   - Other surrounding tumors may invade into the jugular foramen. These constitute chordoma, chondrosarcoma, giant-cell tumor, cholesterol granuloma, endolymphatic sac tumor, temporal bone carcinomas, metastases, etc.[1]

3. *What other studies would you order for this patient?*
   - Other relevant studies would include an angiogram; CT scan of the head; and CT scans of the chest, abdomen, and pelvis.
   - Serum and urine catecholamine levels and urine vanillylmandelic acid levels.
   - Glomus jugulare belongs to the neuroendocrine tumor family that includes other paragangliomas including pheochromocytoma.[2]

4. *The serum epinephrine-level test that you ordered was reported 5 times above normal level. What is the significance of this and what would you do next?*
   - Conversion of norepinephrine to epinephrine requires phenylethanolamine-N-methyl transferase (PNMT) that is present in the adrenal medulla. A very high serum epinephrine level raises the suspicion for pheochromocytoma. Glomus jugulare, when chemically active, generally produces norepinephrine.[3]
   - The patient should undergo both α- and β-adrenergic blockade (e.g., phenoxybenzamine and propranolol) prior to embolization or surgery. Note: Do not initiate β-adrenergic blockade until α- blockage is partially established.[2]

5. *Interpret the angiogram* (**Fig. 25.2**).
   - A left-sided external carotid angiogram showing tumor blush fed via the ascending pharyngeal artery. Other arteries that may feed the glomus tumor are the occipital artery, internal maxillary artery, and the vertebrobasilar system.

6. *How would you describe the treatment options to the patient?*
   - Surgery, radiation therapy (RT), as well as radiosurgery have all been used for the treatment of glomus tumor.
   - A 20-year actuarial survival of 94% and a 20-year actuarial disease-free survival of 77% are reported with RT.[4]

■ Answers (*continued*)

- The aim of radiosurgery is tumor control. It has no reported mortality and 2.1% recurrence rate, but the regression in tumor size is reported in a little less than one-third of the patients. It can be used for smaller recurrences and residuals. In comparison, surgical resection is reported to have 1.3% mortality, 3.1% recurrence rate along with 92.1% surgical control, and a gross total resection of tumor in 88.2%.[5]
- Similar surgical success is also reported for complex glomus jugulare tumors.[6]

7. *The patient chooses surgery. What preoperative and intraoperative measures would you take to avoid complications?*
- Because glomus tumor is a highly vascular tumor, preoperative embolization performed 3–5 days prior to the surgery prevents excessive bleeding in the operating room.
- Similarly, the patient should be started on α– and β-blockers for blood pressure control if the tumor is hormonally active.
- Intraoperative monitoring of cranial nerves (CNs) VII, IX, X, XI, and XII is recommended along with brainstem auditory-evoked response and somatosensory-evoked potentials.
- The relationship of the CNs to the jugular foramen and hence, the tumor, are vital to the risk of damage to these nerves. Generally the lower CNs are pushed medially by the tumor and are at less risk than CNs VII and IX that may be in the path of the approach to resection of the tumor.[7]

8. *What would you do if the patient were also noted to have (a) an ipsilateral carotid body lesion, or (b) a bilateral jugular fossa lesion?*
- An ipsilateral carotid body tumor can be addressed at the same setting with the neck dissection that is performed with the tumor resection from the temporal bone.
- If the patient has bilateral glomus tumors as is seen in ~10% of sporadic cases and as high as 25–55% or more in familial cases, the resection on the opposite site should be performed only if the surgical resection on one side did not cause lower CN deficit.[6]

9. *How would you interpret these pathologic findings?*
- Sustentacular cell density and the intensity of immunohistochemical staining of the chief and sustentacular cells are inversely proportional to the tumor aggressiveness.[8]
- Anaplastic or metastasizing paragangliomas are either devoid or very depleted of sustentacular cells.[9]

10. *The patient asks about the risk of her two sons getting this tumor. How would you address this issue with her?*
- Embryologically, glomus jugulare tumor is of neuroectodermal origin. Genes for this tumor are located on chromosome 11q[23.1] and 11q[13.1]. The germline mutation is in succinate dehydrogenase subunits of mitochondrial enzyme system transmitted in an autosomal dominant inheritance pattern with variable penetrance only from the father.
- The responsible gene from an affected mother is inactivated but may become active in the subsequent generations if one of her sons gets the gene in question.[3]

11. *Describe a classification system for glomus tympanicum tumors.*
- There are two well-recognized classification systems, summarized in **Table 25.1**.[2]

12. *Describe the syndromes of the jugular foramen.*
- Vernet syndrome affects CNs IX, X, and XI and is due to an intracranial lesion.
- Collet–Sicard syndrome affects CNs IX, X, XI, and XII and is usually due to an extracranial lesion.
- Villaret syndrome affects CNs IX, X, XI, XII, and the sympathetic nervous system and is usually due to a posterior retropharyngeal lesion.
- Jackson syndrome affects CNs X, XI, and XII and is usually due to a vascular infarction of the medullary tegmentum.
- Tapia syndrome affects CNs X, XII, and possibly IX and is usually due to a high cervical lesion.
- See **Fig. 25.3** for further illustration.[10,11]

Table 25.1   Classification of Glomus Tympanicum Tumors

Type	Fisch Classification	Glasscock–Jackson Classification
A or I	Limited to middle ear cleft	Small; involves jugular bulb, middle ear, and mastoid
B or II	Limited to tympanomastoid without destruction of bone in the infralabyrinthine area	Extends to internal auditory canal with possible intracanalicular extension
C or III	Involvement of infralabyrinthine compartment & extending into the petrous apex along the carotid canal (subdivided into C1, C2, & C3)	Extends to petrous apex; possible intracranial extension
D or IV	Intracranial extension of tumor of <2 cm in diameter (D1) and >2 cm in diameter (D2)	Beyond petrous apex to clivus and infratemporal fossa; possible intracranial extension

Source: Adapted from Sampson JH, Wilkins RH. Paraganglioma of the carotid body and temporal bone. In: Wilkins RH, Rengashary SS, eds. Neurosurgery. 2nd ed. New York: McGraw-Hill; 1996:1559–1571.

■ References

1. Osborn AG. Diagnostic Neuroradiology. St. Louis, MO: Mosby; 1994:465
2. Sampson JH, Wilkins RH. Paraganglioma of the carotid body and temporal bone. In: Wilkins RH. Rengashary SS, eds. Neurosurgery. 2nd ed. New York: McGraw-Hill; 1996:1559–1571
3. Heth J. The basic science of glomus jugulare tumors. Neurosurg Focus 2004;17(2):E2
4. Dawes PJ, Filippou M, Welch AR, Dawes JD. Management of glomus jugulare tumors. Clin Otolaryngol Allied Sci 1987;12(1):15–24
5. Gottfried ON, Liu JK, Couldwell WT. Comparison of radiosurgery and conventional surgery for the treatment of glomus jugulare tumors. Neurosurg Focus 2004;17(2):E4
6. Al-Mefty O, Teixeira A. Complex tumors of the glomus jugulare: criteria, treatment, and outcome. J Neurosurg 2002;97(6):1356–1366
7. Inserra MM, Pfister M, Jackler RK. Anatomy involved in the jugular foramen approach for jugulotympanic paraganglioma resection. Neurosurg Focus 2004;17(2):E6
8. Kliewer KE, Wen DR, Cancilla PA, Cochran AJ. Paragangliomas: assessment of prognosis by histologic, immunohistochemical, and ultrastructural techniques. Hum Pathol 1989;20(1):29–39
9. Kleihues P, Cavanee WK. Pathology and Genetics of Tumors of the Nervous System. Lyon: World Health Organization; 2000
10. Greenberg MS. Handbook of Neurosurgery. 6th ed. New York: Thieme Medical Publishers; 2006.
11. Rengashary SS. Cranial nerve examination. In Rengashary SS, Wilkins RH, eds. Neurosurgery. 2nd ed. New York: McGraw Hill; 1996:67–86

Case 26   Colloid Cyst of the Third Ventricle

Remi Nader

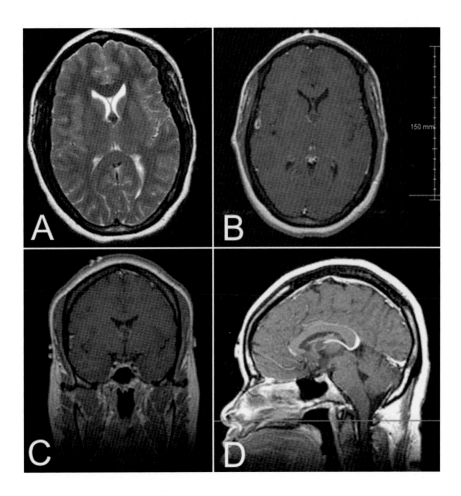

Fig. 26.1 **(A)** T2-weighted axial magnetic resonance image (MRI) at the level of the foramen of Monroe. **(B)** Corresponding T1-weighted MRI with contrast. **(C)** Coronal and **(D)** midsagittal MRI with contrast.

■ Clinical Presentation

- A 37-year-old woman presents with history of headaches and head pain for 3 months.
- Previous history of migraines over several years.
- She also has some dizziness and gait ataxia by history that started 3 months ago.

- Neurologic examination shows no deficits.
- Magnetic resonance imaging (MRI) scan of the brain with contrast is shown in **Fig. 26.1**.

■ Questions

1. Interpret the MRI.
2. Give a differential diagnosis of the lesion observed.
3. What is your initial management?
4. Would you resect the mass? Why or why not?
5. What are the different approaches for surgical treatment and which one is the preferred option in this case?

6. Describe your approach to resection of the lesion. Given a skull, show the landmarks for the skin incision, burr holes, and craniotomy flap. Describe all important structures encountered along the way.
7. What are the important potential complications and what do you do to avoid them?

■ Answers

1. *Interpret the MRI.*
   - MRI shows a lesion in the anterior 3rd ventricle at the level of the foramen of Monroe.
   - The lesion is ~1 cm in size, circular, homogeneous with thin rim enhancement. It is hypointense on both T1- and T2-weighted sequences. It appears to be abutting on both fornices and the internal cerebral veins (see sagittal view). It is in the midline.
   - There is no evidence of hydrocephalus or ventriculomegaly.

2. *Give a differential diagnosis of the lesion observed.*
   - Anterior 3rd ventricle lesion (mnemonic is "SACHMO")[1,2]
     - Colloid cyst is the most likely diagnosis.
     - Sellar mass
     - Metastases
     - Other less likely lesions: aneurysm, abscess, hypothalamic glioma, histiocytosis, meningioma, optic glioma, sarcoidosis

3. *What is your initial management?*
   - Discuss treatment options with the patient
   - If she elects to have surgery then obtain:
     - Imaging: MRI frameless stereotaxy protocol
     - Laboratory studies: complete blood count, electrolytes, prothrombin time/partial thromboplastin time, type and cross match 2 units of packed red blood cells
   - Ventriculostomy placement is not needed as there is no evidence of hydrocephalus.

4. *Would you resect the mass? Why or why not?*
   - The patient is symptomatic from the mass (headaches, gait ataxia, etc.).
   - There is no medical treatment for colloid cysts.
   - It is therefore reasonable to offer her surgical treatment.
   - Best approach would be to present to her the options of observation versus surgical intervention, explain the risks and benefits of both, and let the patient decide.[2]

5. *What are the different approaches for surgical treatment and which one is the preferred option in this case?*
   - Transcallosal approach[3]
     - Preferred over transcortical, in general
     - Good if ventricles are small
     - Advantages:
       - Short trajectory to 3rd ventricle
       - No cortical transgression
       - Can see both foramina of Monro
     - Complication
       - Weakness
       - Akinetic mutism
       - Memory deficits
     - Preferred approach in this case, given small size of ventricles. Note: This is the approach of choice if surgeon has limited experience with the endoscope.

- Endoscopic approach[4,5]
  - Less invasive than open craniotomy
  - Direct vision
  - Good decompression using endoscopic rongeurs
  - Shorter operation and hospitalization
  - Lower incidence of postoperative seizures than transcortical approach
  - Disadvantages
    - Better if ventricles are dilated
    - Poor control of bleeding
    - Cortex/brain matter may be too thick for penetration
- Transcortical, transventricular approach[5]
  - Good for anterior superior 3rd ventricle lesions
  - Especially if lesion extends into frontal horns
  - Trajectory through the right middle frontal gyrus (F2)
  - Disadvantages
    - Higher risk of seizures (11%)
    - Need larger ventricles
- Subfrontal approach[5]
  - Best for lesions in the anterior-inferior 3rd ventricle such as craniopharyngiomas
  - Four different corridors to enter
    - Subchiasmal
    - Opticocarotid
    - Lamina terminalis (if there is a prefixed chiasm)
    - Transfrontal–transsphenoidal (if there is a prefixed chiasm)
- Stereotactic aspiration (± endoscopic guidance)[5]
  - Good if patient is not a candidate for craniotomy
  - Good for cysts >1 cm and not very viscous
  - Enter just anterior to right coronal suture
- Ventriculoperitoneal shunt placement[5]

6. *Describe your approach to resection of the lesion. Given a skull, show the landmarks for the skin incision, burr holes, and craniotomy flap. Describe all important structures encountered along the way.*
   - Interhemispheric transcallosal approach[3,6,7]
   - Preparation
     - Frameless stereotaxy
     - Review venous anatomy on MRI/magnetic resonance venography to check for cortical vein locations as they enter the superior sagittal sinus.
     - Position the patient supine with the head in neutral position.
     - Head of bed slightly elevated
     - Medicate with preoperative antibiotics, dexamethasone, and mannitol.

■ Answers (*continued*)

- Opening
  - ¾ suttar incision (i.e., bicoronal)
  - Open more on the right side than on the left; preserve temporalis fascia and pericranium tissues
  - Expose coronal, sagittal sutures, and bregma.
  - Lateral exposure up to the temporalis muscle insertion
  - Burr holes: Two behind and two in front of the coronal suture, 6 cm apart. Straddling the superior sagittal sinus (SSS), ⅔ in front, and ⅓ behind the coronal suture
  - Trapezoid bone flap – cut last the part that is straddling the SSS.
- Dissection
  - Open dura in "C"-shaped fashion based on the SSS.
  - Visualize bridging veins; avoid or dissect with microdissectors to create room for interhemispheric approach.
  - Gently place retractors on the right frontal lobe and the falx toward the left side. Be careful not to occlude the SSS.
  - Dissect your way down the interhemispheric fissure. You will identify the cingulate gyrus, callosomarginal and pericallosal arteries, corpus callosum (white structure).
  - Open the corpus callosum just distal to the genu, ~2 × 1 cm, as close to the midline as possible.
- 3rd ventricle approaches (**Fig. 26.2**)[8]
  - Identify which lateral ventricle has been entered.
  - Choroid plexus goes forward in the choroidal fissure to the foramen of Monro (which is medial), where it converges with the thalamostriate vein.
  - The septal and caudate veins approach the foramen from anterior.
  - With colloid cysts, the foramen of Monro may be hard to recognize initially as it will be plugged with the cyst, which is slightly grayer than the ependymal lining of the ventricle.
  - Interforniceal approach
    - Danger of permanent short-term memory loss if both fornices damaged
- Lateral ventricular approach through the foramen of Monro
  - May enlarge the foramen of Monro by opening the foramen laterally or posteriorly (sacrificing the thalamostriate vein), which is supposedly well tolerated

- Closure
  - Consider leaving ventricular catheter in place, tunneled through one of the burr holes.

7. *What are the important potential complications and what do you do to avoid them?*
Complications include[3,6,7]
- Venous infarction
  - Sacrifice of critical cortical draining veins
    - Avoid through preoperative planning and imaging review
  - Sagittal sinus thrombosis leading to venous infarction
    - Retraction injury: avoid excessive retraction; keep moist
    - Injury during opening of the bone flap above the sinus
    - Overuse of coagulation in the region of the sinus
    - Hypercoagulable state of the patient, including dehydration
- Bilateral cingulate gyrus retraction or thalamic injury
  - Transient mutism
  - Care must be taken when retracting deeper structures
- Injury to the fornices
  - Injury to both fornices may result in short-term memory deficits and inability to learn new knowledge.
  - Avoid taking both fornices
- Other potential complications
  - Hemiparesis from injury to the motor cortex
  - Seizure
  - Arterial injury to pericallosal or callosomarginal arteries with infarction of the regions supplied by these vessels
  - Disconnection syndrome from wider opening of the corpus callosum
  - Internal cerebral vein injury via coagulation
  - Intraventricular hemorrhage from inadequate hemostasis
  - Other systemic problems: infection, myocardial infarction, deep vein thrombosis, pulmonary embolism, etc.

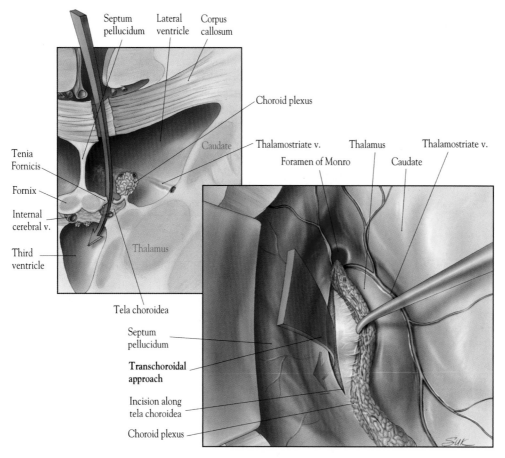

Fig. 26.2 The transchoroidal approach into the 3rd ventricle. A corridor into the 3rd ventricle can be achieved via a transchoroidal approach when the foramen of Monro is small. Upper left shows a coronal view of interhemispheric transcallosal entry into lateral ventricle. The safest passage to the 3rd ventricle is on the medial side of the choroid plexus (along the tenia fornicis). (*Lower right*) An incision is made along the tenia fornicis through the tela choroidea. The surgeon can then dissect between both internal cerebral veins to be free of any vessels. By beginning at the foramen of Monro exposure of the entire 3rd ventricle can be achieved. (From Yao KC, Lang FF. Surgical approach to tumors of the third ventricle. In: Badie B, ed. Neurosurgical Operative Atlas – Neuro-Oncology. 2nd ed. New York: Thieme Medical Publishers; 2006:50. Reprinted with permission).

■ References

1. Osborn AG. Diagnostic Neuroradiology. St. Louis, MO: Mosby; 1994:465
2. Greenberg MS. Handbook of Neurosurgery. 6th ed. New York: Thieme Medical Publishers; 2006
3. Hernesniemi J, Leivo S. Management outcome in third ventricular colloid cysts in a defined population: a series of 40 patients treated mainly by transcallosal microsurgery. Surg Neurol 1996;45(1):2–14
4. Grondin RT, Hader W, MacRae ME, Hamilton MG. Endoscopic versus microsurgical resection of third ventricle colloid cysts. Can J Neurol Sci 2007;34(2):197–207
5. Horn EM, Feiz-Erfan I, Bristol RE, et al. Treatment options for third ventricular colloid cysts: comparison of open microsurgical versus endoscopic resection. Neurosurgery 2007;60(4):613–618
6. Villani RM, Tomei G. Transcallosal approach to tumors of the third ventricle. In: Schmideck HH, Roberts DW, eds. Schmidek & Sweet's Operative Neurosurgical Techniques. Indication, Methods, and Results. 5th ed. Philadelphia, PA: Elsevier; 2006:772–785
7. Connelly ES, McKhann GM, Huang J, Choudhri TF. Fundamentals of Operative Techniques in Neurosurgery. New York: Thieme Medical Publishers; 2002
8. Yao KC, Lang FF. Surgical approach to tumors of the third ventricle. In: Badie B, ed. Neurosurgical Operative Atlas—Neuro-Oncology. 2nd ed. New York: Thieme Medical Publishers; 2006:50

Case 27   **Dural Arteriovenous Fistula**

Nancy McLaughlin and Michel W. Bojanowski

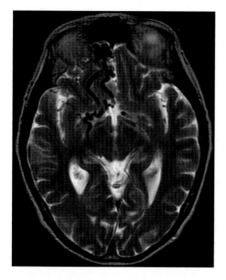

Fig. 27.1   Axial T2-weighted magnetic resonance image of the head.

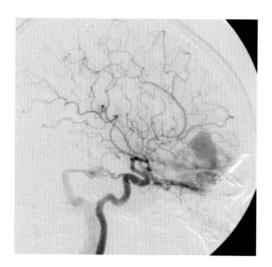

Fig. 27.2   Digital subtraction angiography lateral view, right carotid injection.

■ Clinical Presentation

- A 68-year-old woman was referred for evaluation of a pulsatile tinnitus ongoing for the past 7 years and a more recent headache of variable intensity occurring daily for one year. The patient is in otherwise excellent health. No other symptoms were reported.

- Neurologic examination was normal; specifically, no bruit was auscultated over the skull and no pulsatile tinnitus was documented.

■ Questions

1. What is your differential diagnosis for pulsatile tinnitus?
2. What are the indications to investigate a pulsatile tinnitus?

Findings on the magnetic resonance imaging (MRI) scan (**Fig. 27.1**) revealed a vascular anomaly and required an angiography (**Fig. 27.2**).

3. Describe the angiography.
4. What is your management? Justify.

You decided to treat the anterior cranial fossa dural arteriovenous fistula (DAVF) surgically.

5. What is the main step during surgery to eliminate the fistula?
6. What are the possible complications of surgical treatment?

The postoperative angiography shows a complete exclusion of the anterior cranial fossa DAVF. However, there is now a retrograde venous drainage from the sigmoid sinus fistula (**Fig. 27.3**).

7. What is your management?
8. What are the causes of DAVFs?
9. How are DAVFs classified?

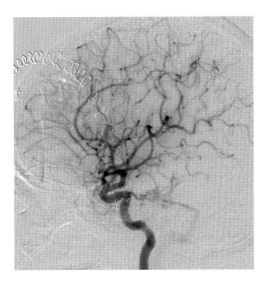

Fig. 27.3   Digital subtraction angiography postoperative lateral view, right carotid injection.

■ Answers

1. *What is your differential diagnosis for pulsatile tinnitus?*
   - See **Table 27.1** for details.[1,2]
2. *What are the indications to investigate a pulsatile tinnitus?*
   - In the absence of an audible bruit, MRI–magnetic resonance angiography (MRA) is an appropriate initial diagnostic step for subjective pulsatile tinnitus.
   - In the presence of an objective pulsatile tinnitus, the clinician may proceed initially with an MRI–MRA. However, in patients with an audible bruit and those with a history of trauma accompanied with de novo pulsatile tinnitus, an angiography is warranted.[1]
3. *Describe the angiography.*
   - The angiography showed a right anterior cranial fossa DAVF supplied by branches of the right and left ophthalmic arteries, right and left internal maxillary arteries, and right middle meningeal artery.
   - A large venous pouch located in the right anterior fossa was identified. Retrograde venous drainage to cortical veins toward the basal vein of Rosenthal and great cerebral vein of Galen was present.
   - Other cortical veins refluxed toward the longitudinal superior sagittal sinus.
   - The angiography also revealed a right sigmoid sinus fistula nourished by the right tentorial artery. No retrograde venous reflux was noted (**Fig. 27.2**).
4. *What is your management? Justify.*
   - Treatment is indicated to eliminate the risk of hemorrhages and neurologic deficits. The overall morbidity and mortality rate of patients harboring a DAVF with cortical venous retrograde drainage (CVR) are 15% and 10%, respectively.[3]
   - Anterior cranial fossa DAVFs always drain via cortical venous drainage and therefore mandate an aggressive treatment.[4]

- Transarterial embolization is limited to branches of the external carotid artery. Embolization of ophthalmic arteries is avoided due to the inherent risk of central retinal artery occlusion.
- Transvenous embolization is not feasible for most of these fistulas because of the lack of venous access.
- Surgery is the best treatment option for anterior cranial fossa dural arteriovenous fistulas.[5,6]
- Lesions without CVR such as the sigmoid sinus fistula do not require treatment except if symptoms are intolerable. In such situations, a palliative treatment may be indicated.[4]

5. *What is the main step during surgery to eliminate the fistula?*
   - The goal is to interrupt the draining veins at their dural origin.
6. *What are the possible complications of surgical treatment?*
   - Possible complications of anterior fossa DAVFs treated by surgical means include excessive blood loss, venous hypertension, venous infarct, cerebral edema, and seizures.
7. *What is your management?*
   - Prior to surgery of the anterior fossa DAVF, the sigmoid fistula was initially considered for conservative treatment.
   - However, after the surgery of the anterior fossa DAVF, the sigmoid fistula developed a retrograde venous drainage and a curative treatment for this fistula should be sought.
   - Transvenous embolization should be considered initially.
   - If endovascular treatment fails, surgery should be performed for patients with CVR.
   - Whenever possible, transarterial embolization should be attempted to reduce intraoperative bleeding.[4]

■ Answers (*continued*)

8. *What are the causes of DAVFs?*
- The etiology of DAVFs remains poorly understood. Some conditions have been associated with DAVF such as head injury, prior craniotomy, infection, arterial dysplasia, dural venous sinus thrombosis.
- Most of these etiologies have a sinus occlusion in common.

9. *How are DAVFs classified?*
- The most commonly used classifications are those of Borden and colleagues[7] and Cognard and colleagues.[8] These classifications are based on the pattern of venous drainage of the arteriovenous fistulas (**Fig. 27.4** and **Table 27.2**).

Table 27.1   Causes of Pulsatile Tinnitus

Causes of Pulsatile Tinnitus Reported in the Literature

Type of lesion	Etiology
Arterial lesion	Arteriovenous malformation
	Dural arteriovenous fistula
	Carotid cavernous fistula
	Aneurysm of the ICA
	Fibromuscular dysplasias of the ICA
	Dissection of ICA
	Aberrant carotid artery
	Atherosclerosis
	Vascular anomaly of the ear
	Vascular compression of the eighth nerve
Venous lesion	Jugular bulb anomalies (high-riding jugular bulb, dehiscent jugular vein, jugular diverticulum)
	Dominant or attenuated transverse sinus
	Benign intracranial hypertension
	Abnormal condylar or mastoid emissary veins
Neoplasm	Glomus jugular tumors
	Facial nerve hemangiomas
	Cavernous hemangioma
	Histiocytosis X
	Paget disease
Miscellaneous	Anemia
	High cardiac outflow
	Thyrotoxicoses
	Otosclerosis

Source: From Shin EJ, Lalwani AK, Dowd CF. Role of angiography in the evaluation of patients with pulsatile tinnitus. Laryngoscope 2000;110:1916–1920; Weissman JL, Hirsch BE. Imaging of tinnitus: a review. Radiology 2000;216:342–349.

Abbreviations: AVM, arteriovenous malformation; ICA, internal carotid artery.

■ **Answers (*continued*)**

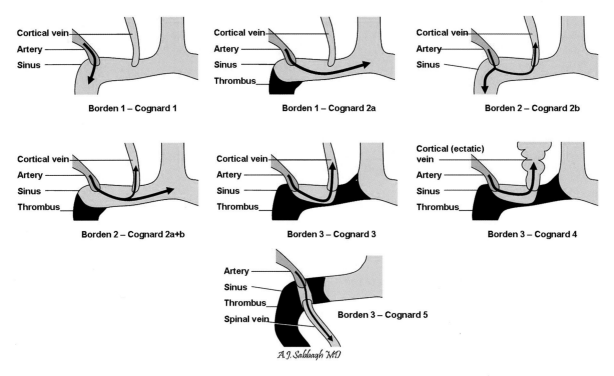

Dural Arteriovenous Fistula Classification

Fig. 27.4 Artist's rendering of venous drainage pattern of dural arteriovenous fistulas according to Borden and Cognard classification schemes. (From Borden JA, Wu JK, Shucart WA, Proposed A. Classification for spinal and cranial dural arteriovenous fistulous malformations and implications for treatment. J Neurosurg 1995;82:166–179; Cognard C, Gobin YP, Pierot L, et al. Cerebral dural arteriovenous fistulas: clinical and angiographic correlation with a revised classification of venous drainage. Radiology 1995;194:671–680.)

Table 27.2   Venous Drainage Pattern of Dural Arteriovenous Fistulas According to Borden and Cognard Classification Schemes

Borden Classification[7]	Cognard Classification[8]
Type I: Drainage into dural venous sinus or meningeal vein only	Type I: Drainage into dural venous sinus only, normal anterograde flow
Type II: Drainage into dural venous sinus or meningeal vein + cortical venous reflux	Type IIa: Drainage into dural venous sinus only, with retrograde flow
Type III: Cortical venous reflux only	Type IIb: Drainage into dural venous sinus (anterograde flow) + CVR
	Type III: CVR only without venous ectasia
	Type IV: CVR only with venous ectasia
	Type V: Drainage into spinal perimedullary veins

Source: From Borden JA, Wu JK, Shucart WA, Proposed A. Classification for spinal and cranial dural arteriovenous fistulous malformations and implications for treatment. J Neurosurg 1995;82:166–179; Cognard C, Gobin YP, Pierot L, et al. Cerebral dural arteriovenous fistulas: clinical and angiographic correlation with a revised classification of venous drainage. Radiology 1995;194:671–680.

Note: All three types of dural arteriovenous fistulous malformation (AVFM) are subclassified as subtype a: simple fistula, and subtype b: multiple fistulas with multiple dural-based AVFMs fed by multiple arteries.

Abbreviation: CVR, cortical venous retrograde.

■ References

1. Shin EJ, Lalwani AK, Dowd CF. Role of angiography in the evaluation of patients with pulsatile tinnitus. Laryngoscope 2000;110:1916–1920

2. Weissman JL, Hirsch BE. Imaging of tinnitus: a review. Radiology 2000;216:342–349

3. Van Dijk JM, terBrugge KG, Willinsky RA, et al. Clinical course of cranial dural arteriovenous fistulas with long term persistent cortical venous reflux. Stroke 2002;33:1233–1236

4. Javadpour M, Wallace CM. Surgical management of cranial dural arteriovenous fistulas. In: Roberts DW, Schmidek HH, eds. Operative Neurosurgical Techniques–Indications, Methods and Results. Philadelphia: Saunders Elsevier; 2006:1287–1305

5. Van Rooij WJ, Sluzewski M, Beute GN. Dural arteriovenous fistulas with cortical venous drainage: incidence, clinical presentation, and treatment. AJNR Am J Neuroradiol 2007;28:651–655

6. Lawton MT, Chun J, Wilson CB, Halbach VV. Ethmoidal dural arteriovenous fistulae: an assessment of surgical and endovascular management. Neurosurgery 1999;45:805–811

7. Borden JA, Wu JK, Shucart WA, Proposed A. Classification for spinal and cranial dural arteriovenous fistulous malformations and implications for treatment. J Neurosurg 1995;82:166–179

8. Cognard C, Gobin YP, Pierot L, et al. Cerebral dural arteriovenous fistulas: clinical and angiographic correlation with a revised classification of venous drainage. Radiology 1995;194:671–680

Case 28   Cerebral Arteriovenous Malformation

Pascal M. Jabbour and Erol Veznedaroglu

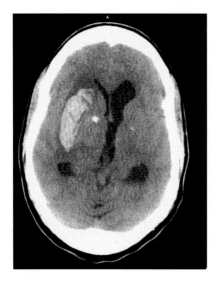

Fig. 28.1   Computed tomography scan of the head showing a right basal ganglia bleed.

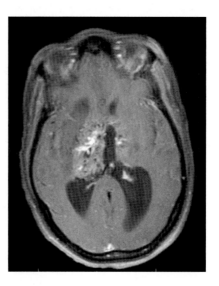

Fig. 28.2   Magnetic resonance imaging scan of the head showing a basal ganglia arteriovenous malformation.

■ Clinical Presentation

- A 36-year-old woman presented to the emergency room for sudden onset of headaches and right hemiplegia.
- Her medical and familial history was noncontributory.
- Neurologic evaluation showed that the patient was awake, alert, and strength was 5/5 on the right; she was hemiplegic on the left, with right-sided gaze preference, anosognosia, and hemiasomatognosia.
- Computed tomography (CT) scan is shown in **Fig. 28.1**; magnetic resonance imaging (MRI) scan of the head is shown in **Fig. 28.2**.

■ Questions

1. Considering the age of the patient, what is the most likely etiology of the bleed?
2. What is the next test to order?
3. What is the most common arteriovenous malformation (AVM) grading system used? And what is the patient's grade?
4. What is the risk of rupture of an AVM and the lifetime cumulative risk for this patient?
5. What are the different treatment options for this patient?
6. What are some important steps of AVM surgery?
7. What is normal perfusion pressure breakthrough and how is it treated?

Answers

1. *Considering the age of the patient, what is the most likely etiology of the bleed?*
   - Any intracerebral hemorrhage in a young patient without any past medical history should raise the suspicion of a vascular malformation.
2. *What is the next test to order?*
   - The CT of the head showed a basal ganglia bleed in a young patient; the next test to be ordered should be an imaging modality that is able to demonstrate any vascular abnormality, like a CT angiogram, MRI, or magnetic resonance angiography.
3. *What is the most common AVM grading system used? And what is the patient's grade?*
   - The Spetzler–Martin grading system (**Table 28.1**).[1]
   - The patient's grade is 2 (size) + 1 (eloquence) + 1 (venous drainage) = 4
4. *What is the risk of rupture of an AVM and the lifetime cumulative risk for this patient?*
   - The risk of rupture of this AVM is ~4% per year.[2]
   - Risk is 1 (risk of not hemorrhaging) raised to the power of years left to live.
   - In a 36-year-old patient, at an average life expectancy of 79 years, the years left to live can be calculated to be 43 years.
   - Risk = $1 - (1 - \text{risk of hemorrhage})^{43}$
   - Risk = $1 - (0.96)^{43} = 83$
   - The patient has a lifetime risk of hemorrhage of 83%.
5. *What are the different treatment options for this patient?*
   - The different options are[1,3,4]
     - No intervention if the risk of intervening is higher than the natural history risk of the AVM rupturing.
     - Embolization in preparation for surgical resection
     - Embolization with the goal of reducing the volume of the AVM in preparation for radiosurgery
     - Surgery alone
     - Radiosurgery alone with possible volume fractionation

6. *What are some important steps of AVM surgery?*
   - Furosemide + mannitol prior to dural opening
   - Proximal temporary occlusion can be performed with aneurysm clips.
   - Smaller vessels are occluded with AVM mini-clips.
   - Large draining veins are clipped with large aneurysm clips.
   - Do not commit on vessel occlusion until the vessel is seen to enter the AVM.
   - "If it looks like it may be AVM, it probably is."
   - Difficult-to-control bleeding during this dissection is commonly an indication that the AVM–brain interface has been breached on the side of the AVM.
   - As a safety measure, before taking the major draining vein, an aneurysm clip is placed across it for 10–15 minutes and dissect out in a different area.
   - Always obtain a postoperative angiogram and CT scan.[5]
7. *What is normal perfusion pressure breakthrough and how is it treated?*
   - It is a disorder of autoregulation of the brain vasculature.
   - May present with sudden onset of brain swelling and bleeding from multiple sites
   - May be due to draining vein that was taken too soon
   - Also occurs from raw normal brain surfaces, that have lost autoregulatory capacity
   - Close inspection of the operative field will identify any residual AVM.
   - Treatment
     - Elevation of the patient's head
     - Administration of mannitol and furosemide
     - Barbiturate- or etomidate-induced coma
     - Hypotension may be beneficial.
     - Focal hypotension by means of proximal vessel occlusion with temporary clip[5]

Table 28.1 The Spetzler–Martin Grading System

Size of AVM		Eloquence of Adjacent Brain		Pattern of Venous Drainage	
Small (<3 cm)	1	Noneloquent	0	Superficial only	0
Medium (3–6 cm)	2	Eloquent	1	Deep component	1
Large (>6 cm)	3	—		—	

Source: Data from Spetzler RF, Martin NA. A proposed grading system for arteriovenous malformations. J Neurosurg 1986;65(4):476–483.

Abbreviation: AVM, arteriovenous malformation.

■ References

1. Spetzler RF, Martin NA. A proposed grading system for arteriovenous malformations. J Neurosurg 1986;65(4):476–483
2. Ondra SL, Troupp H, George ED, Schwab K. The natural history of symptomatic arteriovenous malformations of the brain: a 24-year follow-up assessment. J Neurosurg 1990;73(3):387–391
3. Veznedaroglu E, Andrews DW, Benitez RP, et al. Fractionated stereotactic radiotherapy for the treatment of large arteriovenous malformations with or without previous partial embolization. Neurosurgery 2004;55(3):519–530
4. Heros RC, Korosue K, Diebold PM. Surgical excision of cerebral arteriovenous malformations: late results. Neurosurgery 1990;26(4):570–577
5. Fisher WS. Surgical treatment of arteriovenous malformations of the cerebral convexity. In: Wilkins RH, Rengachary SS, eds. Neurosurgical Operative Atlas. Vol. 3. Chicago, IL: The American Association of Neurological Surgeons; 1993:283–291

Case 29   Cavernous Angioma

Julius July and Eka Julianta Wahjoepramono

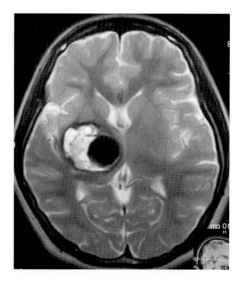

Fig. 29.1   T2-weighted magnetic resonance image showing a lesion involving the right basal ganglia and thalamus.

■ Clinical Presentation

- A 19-year-old woman presents with chronic headache since early childhood. For the last 6 months her headaches have become progressively worse. She also felt that her left side was becoming weaker.
- Her left upper and lower extremities were weak since early childhood.

- There is no history of seizure.
- On initial assessment, she has left-side weakness and left hemi-hypesthesia.
- She was referred from other hospital with the magnetic resonance imaging (MRI) study shown. (**Fig. 29.1**)

■ Questions

1. Describe the MRI feature and provide a differential diagnosis.
2. What are the treatment options?
3. What treatment would you recommend for this case?
4. What is your argument between a surgical and non-surgical option?
5. If you decide to do the surgery, what is your approach to remove the lesion?
6. What are the potential complications of surgery?

■ Answers

1. *Describe the MRI feature and provide a differential diagnosis.*
   - Considering the clinical presentation and based on the T2-weighted MRI, the lesion most likely represents a longstanding condition with repeated acute onset of bleeding.
   - The reticulated core of decreased and increased intensity with prominent surrounding rim of reduced intensity may represent hemosiderin-laden macrophages from previous hemorrhage.
   - This might represent an intracranial vascular malformation. Although unlikely, spontaneous hemorrhage and intratumoral bleeding still should be on the differential diagnosis.
   - Intracranial vascular malformation are divided into
     - Arteriovenous malformation (AVM)
     - Venous malformation
     - Capillary malformation
     - Cavernous malformation (cavernoma = cavernous angioma = cavernous hemangioma)[1,2]

2. *What are the treatment options?*
   - Conservative treatment
     - Asymptomatic or minimally symptomatic lesions because they may remain quiescent and if they rebleed, this tends to be mild and not catastrophic.
     - Multiple lesions with familial history
     - Deep or eloquent area when the surgical risks exceed the benefit, especially in elderly patients
   - Radiosurgery
     - In cases of surgically inaccessible lesions with at least one prior hemorrhage
     - Several studies show that radiosurgery could reduce the risk of hemorrhage to one-third of initial risk.
     - However, because of the high complication rate of radiosurgery, its routine use for cavernoma fell out of favor. The benefits of radiosurgery are difficult to assess because of the unclear natural history of cavernomas, the inability to evaluate the status of the malformation vessels, and the lack of completeness of obliteration of the malformation.
   - Surgery
     - Recurrent hemorrhage, especially at a young age
     - Progressive neurologic deficits
     - Intractable epilepsy when the benefit outweighs the risk
     - Lesion located in the cerebellum or the cerebral cortex
     - Lesions that do not respond to radiosurgery
     - In special circumstances (e.g., a young woman who wants to become pregnant with an accessible lesion)
     - To prevent future bleeding[2,3]

3. *What treatment would you recommend for this case?*
   - Considering the patient's young age and history of repeated hemorrhage with progressive neurologic deterioration, surgical treatment should be recommended.

4. *What is your argument between a surgical and nonsurgical option?*
   - Kondziolka et al.'s[4] prospective study of 122 cavernomas has shown that the annual bleeding rate for symptomatic lesions is 4.5%.
   - The patient has a 93.6% chance of sustaining another hemorrhage in her lifetime (with life expectancy of 79 years, based on formula from Case 28). The hemorrhage could be catastrophic.[1]
   - Although the lesion is located in eloquent brain (thalamus-basal ganglia), surgical resection still provides significant benefits that are greater than the above risk.
   - Based on the MRI (**Fig. 29.1**), the sylvian fissure appears to be quite relaxed. Resection can be achieved with image-guided surgery by performing a sylvian fissure dissection. A corticotomy along the insular gyrus of ~1–2 cm is enough to remove the cavernoma (**Fig. 29.2** and **Fig. 29.3**).
   - Alternatively, a parietal transcortical-transventricular approach may also be used.

5. *What are the potential complications of surgery?*
   - The complications of surgery consist of general risk that might happen during any neurosurgical cases (such as infection, cerebrospinal fluid leak leak, seizure, stroke, deep vein thrombosis, pneumonia, coma, death, etc.).
   - They also include neurologic worsening related to lesion location (such as paraesthesia, hemiparesis or hemiplegia, visual field deficits, etc.).[3,4]

■ Answers (*continued*)

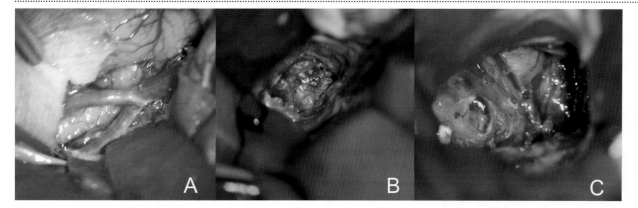

Fig. 29.2 (A) Intraoperative photograph (300×) showing a sylvian fissure dissection, exposing the M2 segment of the right middle cerebral artery. Further dissection of the M2 segment provides maximal exposure of the long insular gyrus. **(B)** Intraoperative photograph (300×) taken after corticotomy completed at the long insular gyrus.

The typical appearance of a cavernoma is situ is visualized. Very often, there is a good cleavage plane between the lesion and the surrounding brain. The surrounding brain has also undergone gliotic changes, which facilitates complete resection. **(C)** Intraoperative photograph taken after complete removal of the lesion.

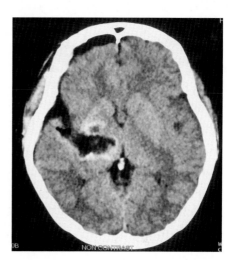

Fig. 29.3   Postoperative computed tomography scan showing the surgical track through the sylvian fissure.

■ References

1. Greenberg MS. Handbook of Neurosurgery. 6th ed. New York: Thieme Medical Publishers; 2006
2. Tew JM, Sathi S. Cavernous malformations. In Caplan LR, Reis DJ, Siesjo BK, Weir B, Welch KMA, eds. Primer on Cerebrovascular Disease. San Diego: Academic Press; 1997:549–556
3. Amin-Hanjani S, Ojemann RG, Ogilvy CS. Surgical management of cavernous malformations of the nervous system. In: Roberts DW, Schmidek HH, eds. Schmidek & Sweet's Operative Neurosurgical Techniques. Indications, Methods, and Results. 5th ed. Philadelphia: Saunders Elsevier; 2006:1307–1324
4. Kondziolka D, Lunsford LD, Kestle JRW. The natural history of cerebral cavernous malformations. J Neurosurg 1995;83:820–824

Case 30   Subarachnoid Hemorrhage and Vasospasm

Qasim Al Hinai, Claude-Edouard Chatillon, David Sinclair, and Dennis J. Sirhan

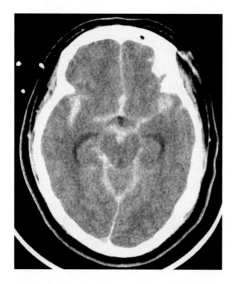

Fig. 30.1 Computed tomography of the head axial cut through basal cisterns.

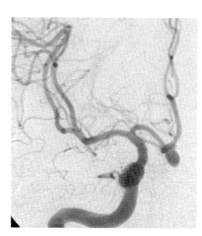

Fig. 30.2 Cerebral angiogram, anteroposterior view, right carotid injection.

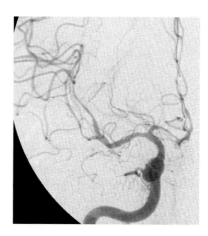

Fig. 30.3 Cerebral angiogram, antero-posterior view, right carotid injection, performed 6 days later, after a therapeutic intervention.

■ Clinical Presentation

• A 55-year-old woman presents to the emergency room with sudden-onset severe headache, vomiting and photophobia.

• On examination, she is confused and drowsy. There are no focal neurologic deficits. She opens her eyes spontaneously and obeys commands.

• Computed tomography (CT) scan of the head is obtained in the ER (**Fig. 30.1**).

■ Questions

1. Interpret the CT (**Fig. 30.1**).
2. What is the diagnosis?
3. Describe two clinical grading systems of your diagnosis. What is the grade in this case?
4. Give one radiologic grading system of your diagnosis and its prognostic significance. What is the grade in this case?
5. What is your management?
6. Describe the cerebral angiogram shown in **Fig. 30.2**.

The patient was admitted to the intensive care unit (ICU) and underwent a therapeutic procedure for the finding on the previous angiogram. Six days later, the patient de-veloped dysphasia and right-sided hemiparesis (right leg is weaker than right arm). A CT of the head reveals a right frontal hypodensity with surrounding mild edema.

7. What is the most likely diagnosis and what studies do you obtain?
8. Describe the cerebral angiogram shown in **Fig. 30.3**.
9. What is the pathophysiology of this condition?
10. What additional investigations can you obtain at this stage?
11. What intervention can be done during the angiography?
12. How will you treat this condition medically?

■ Answers

1. *Interpret the CT (Fig. 30.1)*
   - There is extensive subarachnoid hemorrhage (SAH) involving anterior interhemispheric fissure and bilateral sylvian fissures.
2. *What is the diagnosis?*
   - SAH, likely secondary to aneurysmal rupture
3. *Describe two clinical grading systems of your diagnosis. What is the grade in this case?*
   - Hunt & Hess (H&H) and World Federation of Neurosurgical Societies (WFNS)
   - H & H grading[1]:
     - 1: Asymptomatic, or mild headache (H/A) and slight nuchal rigidity
     - 2: Cranial nerve palsy, moderate to severe H/A, nuchal rigidity
     - 3: Mild focal deficit, lethargy, or confusion
     - 4: Stupor, moderate to severe hemiparesis, early decerebrate rigidity
     - 5: Deep coma, decerebrate rigidity, moribund appearance
   - WFNS grading[2]:
     - 1: Glasgow Coma Score (GCS) 15 with no major focal deficit
     - 2: GCS 13–14 with no major focal deficit
     - 3: GCS 13–14 with major focal deficit
     - 4: GCS 7–12 with or without major focal deficit
     - 5: GCS 3–6 with or without major focal deficit
   - This patient has an H&H grade 3 and WFNS grade 2.
4. *Give one radiologic grading system of your diagnosis and its prognostic significance. What is the grade in this case?*
   - Fisher grading system[3]:
     - 1: No SAH
     - 2: Diffuse or vertical layer <1 mm thick
     - 3: Localized clot and/or vertical layer >1 mm
     - 4: Intracerebral hemorrhage or intravenous hemorrhage with minimal diffuse or no SAH
   - This patient has Fisher grade 3.
   - The amount of subarachnoid blood correlates with the risk of vasospasm.
   - Grade 3 carries the worst prognosis.
5. *What is your management?*
   - Management includes the steps here[4]:
     - ICU admission
     - Arterial and central lines
     - Monitor systolic blood pressure (SBP), mean arterial pressure (MAP), and central venous pressure (CVP) closely
     - Phenytoin (dilantin™) loading (18 mg/kg) and maintenance doses (100 mg tid × 1 week unless seizures)

     - Nimodipine (60 mg by mouth every 4 hours × 21 days)
     - Analgesics
     - In cases of hydrocephalus or H&H grade >3, an external ventricular drain (EVD) should be inserted.
     - Cerebral angiography ± coiling (if the cause of SAH is aneurysm). If the aneurysm is not coilable, then craniotomy and aneurysm clipping.
     - In cases of poor H&H grade (V) at presentation, prognosis is very poor unless the comatose state is partly due to hydrocephalus or to a postictal state. Initial management usually consists of an EVD insertion and observation for a few hours. The decision to initiate aggressive management depends on the patient's clinical improvement.
6. *Describe the cerebral angiogram shown in Fig. 30.2.*
   - The right anteroposterior projection internal carotid artery angiogram reveals an aneurysm at the level of the anterior communicating artery (ACOM) pointing inferiorly.
7. *What is the most likely diagnosis and what studies do you obtain?*
   - The likely diagnosis is vasospasm affecting the right anterior cerebral artery (ACA).
   - Vasospasm is a major complication of SAH.
   - Clinical vasospasm occurs in 30% of SAH.
   - Infarction occurs in about half of these cases if vasospasm remains untreated.
   - 7% of attributed deaths are due to vasospasm.[5]
   - Very few preventive and therapeutic measures have reproducible benefits in randomized trials.
   - A cerebral angiogram may be done to confirm the presence of radiographic vasospasm, which may correlate with the clinical picture.
8. *Describe the cerebral angiogram shown in Fig. 30.3.*
   - As suspected clinically and based on the CT scan findings, the angiogram reveals severe stenosis suggesting cerebral vasospasm affecting the right A2 segment of the ACA.
   - Note the occluded right ACOM aneurysm, which has been treated by endovascular coiling.
9. *What is the pathophysiology of this condition?*
   - The exact pathophysiology is unknown. However, there are two theories that might explain the pathophysiology[6]:
   - Theories of "spasmogens"
     - Components of erythrocytes
     - Oxyhemoglobin
     - Plasma and buffy coat (white blood cells) do not induce vasospasm.

■ Answers (*continued*)

- Structural theories
  - Proliferative vasculopathy
  - Immune vasculopathy
  - Vessel wall inflammation
  - Extracellular lattice contraction
- Vasoconstriction theories
  - Free-radical lipid peroxidation
  - Derangement in eicosanoid production
  - Nitric oxide deficit
  - Endothelin excess[4]

10. *What additional investigations can you obtain at this stage?*
  - Transcranial Doppler
  - Electroencephalogram
  - Cerebral blood flow studies using positron emission tomography and single photon emitted computed tomography scans

11. *What intervention can be done during the angiography?*
  - Vasodilation by angioplasty or intraarterial verapamil or papaverine

12. *How will you treat this condition medically?*
  - Start "triple H" therapy, which traditionally comprises hypervolemia, hypertension, and hemodilution[7]
    - Hypertension: Keep systolic blood pressure at 160 mm Hg, or mean arterial pressure at 120 mm Hg or above
    - Hemodilution: Hematocrit 30–35%
  - Alternatively, normovolemia may be used as hypervolemia can increase the risk of cardiorespiratory complications (central venous pressure is kept around 6 mm Hg).
  - Normonatremia: $[Na^+] > 140$ mEq/L
  - Normoglycemia: [glucose] < 8 mmol/L
  - Normothermia
  - Norepinephrine bitartrate (Levophed; Abbott Laboratories, Abbott Park, IL) may be used to maintain blood pressure at pretreatment levels on an as needed basis.
  - Induced hypertension and/or angioplasty may be performed if the patient is refractory to other treatments.
  - Milrinone: a phosphodiesterase III inhibitor reducing the incidence of vasospasm may also be used in an intravenous infusion form

■ References

1. Hunt WE, Hess RM. Surgical risk as related to time of intervention in the repair of intracranial aneurysms. J Neurosurg 1968;28:14–20

2. Drake CG. Report of World Federation of Neurological Surgeons Committee on a Universal Subarachnoid Hemorrhage Grading Scale. J Neurosurg 1988;68:985–986

3. Fisher CM, Kistler JP, Davis JM. Relation of cerebral vasospasm to subarachnoid hemorrhage visualized by CT scanning. Neurosurgery 1980;6:1–9

4. Greenberg MS. Handbook of Neurosurgery. 6th ed. New York: Thieme Medical Publishers; 2006

5. Brant-Zawadzki M, Barnwell S, Dowd C, Hieshima GB. Transluminal angioplasty for treatment of intracranial arterial vasospasm. J Neurosurg 1989;71:648–653

6. Winn RH. Neurological Surgery. 5th ed. Philadelphia: Saunders; 2004:1371–1387

7. Origitano TC, Wascher TM, Reichman OH, Anderson DE. Sustained increased cerebral blood flow with prophylactic hypertensive hypervolemic hemodilution ('Triple-H" Therapy) after subarachnoid hemorrhage. Neurosurgery 1990;27:729–740

Case 31   Unruptured Anterior Communicating Artery Aneurysm

Yasser I. Orz

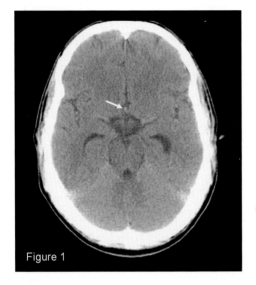

Figure 1

Fig. 31.1 Computed tomography scan of the head showing hyperdensity in the interhemispheric fissure (*arrow*).

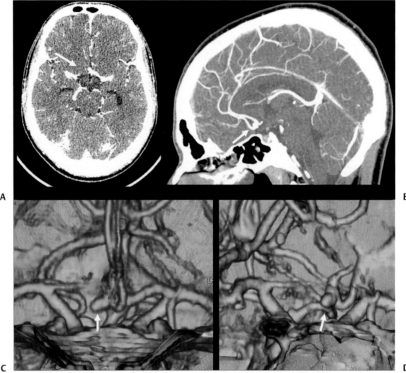

Fig. 31.2 **(A)** Axial and **(B)** sagittal contrast-enhanced T1-weighted magnetic resonance angiography images, with three-dimensional reconstructions **(C)** anteroposterior and **(D)** oblique views.

■ Clinical Presentation

- A 42-year-old man presents with a 2-year history of recurrent bouts of headache.
- On examination, he had no neurologic deficit.

- A computed tomography (CT) scan of the brain is done (**Fig. 31.1**).

■ Questions

1. Interpret the CT findings.
2. What is the most probable diagnosis?
3. What other investigations would you order?
4. What are the options and associated risks for management of the lesion?
5. What is the natural history of unruptured aneurysms?
6. Name factors favoring treatment of unruptured cerebral aneurysms.
7. How would you classify anterior communicating artery (ACOM) aneurysms?
8. If you chose to manage the lesion surgically, what approaches may be utilized?
9. In the case of a pterional approach, what side would you choose?
10. In the case of surgery of nonruptured aneurysms, what are less-favorable outcome factors?

■ Answers

1. *Interpret the CT findings.*
   - CT of the brain showed a small hyperdense lesion in the suprasellar interhemispheric cistern at the site of the ACOM.
2. *What is the most probable diagnosis?*
   - The most probable diagnosis is a nonruptured ACOM aneurysm.
3. *What other investigations would you order?*
   - Other investigations (see Case 36 for a detailed comparison of the different treatment measures)
   - Three-dimensional CT angiography (CTA) (**Fig. 31.2**)
     - It is a noninvasive reliable method for diagnosis of cerebral aneurysms with sensitivity of 95%.
     - In some centers, CTA has become the only diagnostic and pretreatment planning study for patients with ruptured and unruptured cerebral aneurysms.
   - Conventional cerebral angiography
     - The gold standard for evaluation of cerebral aneurysms
     - Four-vessel digital subtraction angiography (DSA) should be done to exclude the presence of multiple aneurysms.
   - Magnetic resonance angiography (MRA)
     - There are several parameters that affect the MRA's ability to detect the intracranial aneurysms including
       - Aneurysm size
       - Rate and direction of blood flow in the aneurysm relative to the magnetic field
     - Currently MRA may be useful as a screening test in high-risk patients.
4. *What are the options and associated risks for management of the lesion?*
   - Occlusion of this aneurysm can be done either by microsurgical clipping (see **Fig. 31.3** for a postclipping DSA) or by endovascular coiling.[1-4]
   - Alternatively, observation may be an option if the patient so chooses.
- **Table 31.1** summarizes surgical morbidity rates based on size and location.[2]
- **Table 31.2** summarizes overall risks of coiling of unruptured aneurysms.[3-5]

5. *What is the natural history of unruptured aneurysms?*
   - According to the International Study of Unruptured Intracranial Aneurysms (ISUIA),[2] risk of bleeding from unruptured cerebral aneurysms differs from aneurysms that have ruptured.
   - The natural history and treatment results are affected by the following factors[1-4]:
     - Patients' factors
       - Smoking[6]
       - Age of the patient
       - Associated medical conditions
       - History of previous subarachnoid hemorrhage (SAH)
     - Aneurysm characteristics
       - Size
         - The most important predictor for future rupture[2] as the estimated annual risk of rupture for aneurysms less than 10 mm in diameter is 0.05% and ~1% or more for aneurysms with diameter more than 10 mm, based on initial ISUIA study results of 1998.[2]
         - ISUIA follow-up study from 2003[7] stated that 5-year cumulative rupture rates for patients with unruptured aneurysm at internal carotid artery (ICA), ACOM, anterior cerebral artery (ACA), and middle cerebral artery (MCA) are 0%, 2.6%, 14.5%, and 40% for aneurysms less than 7 mm, 7–12 mm, 13–24 mm, and 25 mm or greater, respectively, compared with rates of 2.5%, 14.5%, 18.4%, and 50%, respectively, for the same size categories involving posterior circulation and posterior communicating artery (PCOM) aneurysms.
       - The relative risk is 1.11/mm in diameter.[6]

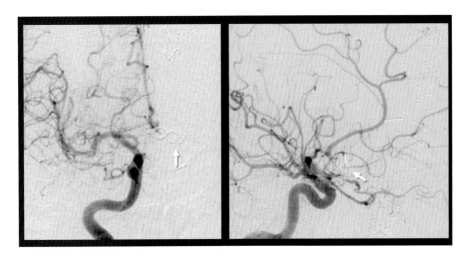

Fig. 31.3 Digital subtraction angiogram with **(A)** anteroposterior and **(B)** lateral views showing aneurysm clip (*arrow*) in place.

■ **Answers (*continued*)**

Table 31.1 Surgical Morbidity in Operated Cases of Unruptured Aneurysms Based on Location and Size

Criteria		Rate (%)
Size	<5 mm	2.3
	6–15 mm	6.8
	16–25 mm	14
Location	PCOM	4.8
	MCA	8.1
	Ophthalmic	11.8
	ACOM	15.5
	Carotid bifurcation	16.8

Source: Adapted from Unruptured intracranial aneurysms-risk of rupture and risks of surgical intervention. International Study of Unruptured Intracranial Aneurysms Investigators. N Engl J Med 1998;339(24):1725–1733. Reprinted with permission.

Abbreviations: ACOM, anterior communicating artery; MCA, middle cerebral artery; PCOM, posterior communicating artery.

Table 31.2 Risks and Results of Endovascular Coiling in Cases of Unruptured Aneurysms

Aneurysm perforation	2.4%
Ischemic complication	8–16%
Permanent complications	3–12%
Decrease in functional score	1–3%
Mortality rate	1.4%
Complete aneurysm occlusion	47%
Near-complete occlusion (90–99%)	43%
Incomplete occlusion	9%
Recurrences	20%
Rebleeding rate	0.9%

Source: Data from Chen PR, Frerichs K, Spetzler R. Current treatment options for unruptured intracranial aneurysms. Neurosurg Focus 2004;17(5):E5; Johnston SC, Higashida RT, Barrow DL, et al. Recommendations for the Endovascular Treatment of Intracranial Aneurysms: A Statement for Healthcare Professionals from the Committee on Cerebrovascular Imaging of the American Heart Association Council on Cardiovascular Radiology. Stroke 2002;33(10):2536–2544; Brilstra EH, Rinkel GJ, van der Graaf Y, van Rooij WJ, Algra A. Treatment of intracranial aneurysms by embolization with coils: a systematic review. Stroke 1999;30:470–476.

- Location
  - PCOM, vertebrobasilar, and basilar termination unruptured aneurysms are more likely to rupture.
  - Aneurysm morphology: The irregular and multilobular aneurysms are more likely to rupture.
- **Table 31.3** summarizes rupture rates based on aneurysm size.[2]
6. *Name factors favoring treatment of unruptured cerebral aneurysms.*
   - These factors include
     - Young age
     - Previous SAH
     - Larger aneurysm size
     - Aneurysm location and configuration

- Juvela et al.[6] stated that the cumulative rate of unruptured aneurysm rupture is 10.5% at 10 years, 23% at 20 years, and 30.3% at 30 years after diagnosis.
7. *How would you classify ACOM aneurysms?*
   - There are two classification schemes of ACOM aneurysms (**Fig. 31.4**).
   - Yasargil classified the ACOM aneurysms into[8]
     - Superior
     - Inferior
     - Anterior
     - Posterior

Table 31.3 Rates of Rupture in Unruptured Aneurysm Cases Based on Size and Location

Size of Unruptured Aneurysm (mm)	5-Year Rate of Hemorrhage for Anterior Circulation Aneurysm (%)	5-Year Rate of Hemorrhage for Posterior Circulation Aneurysm Including PCOM (%)
<7	<0.01	2.5
7–12	2.5	14
13–24	14	18
>24	40	50

Source: Adapted from Unruptured intracranial aneurysms—risk of rupture and risks of surgical intervention. International Study of Unruptured Intracranial Aneurysms Investigators. N Engl J Med 1998;339(24):1725–1733.

Abbreviation: PCOM, posterior communicating artery.

■ **Answers** (*continued*)

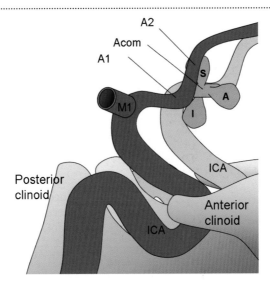

Fig. 31.4 Classification of anterior communicating artery aneurysms. ICA, internal carotid artery; A, anterior; S, superior; I, inferior; A1, first segment of the anterior cerebral artery; A2, second segment of the anterior cerebral artery; ACOM, anterior communicating artery; M1, first segment of the middle cerebral artery.

- Kobayashi classified ACOM aneurysms in terms of approach selection.[9]
  - Anterior type: (Between 1 and 5 o'clock) The aneurysm lies away from the brain and in relation to the arachnoid membrane. Therefore, wide dissection of the arachnoid lessens the degree of frontal lobe retraction.
  - Inferior type: (Between 5 and 9 o'clock) The aneurysm is likely to be adherent to the chiasm. Therefore, frontal lobe retraction can be dangerous and should be done very carefully.
  - Superior (posterior) type: (Between 9 and 1 o'clock) The aneurysm is usually hidden behind the parent arteries or the gyrus rectus. Therefore, it is difficult to clip via the pterional approach and it may be more suitable to coil them.

8. *If you chose to manage the lesion surgically, what approaches may be used?*
   - Surgical approaches that can be used to clip ACOM aneurysms include
     - Pterional approach: This is the most commonly used approach for ACOM aneurysms. It may be supplemented by the cranio-orbital approach in more diffcult to reach or larger aneurysms.
     - Interhemispheric approach: It is infrequently used and indicated if the aneurysm is large or giant and when the aneurysm is in high position (13 mm or more above the anterior clinoid process.[8,9]

9. *In the case of a pterional approach, what side would you choose?*
   - The right pterional approach is the most commonly used approach for the ACOM aneurysms. The left pterional approach is indicated in the following situations:
     - The left A1 is dominant.
     - When the origin of the right A2 is located anterior to that of the left A2, so the neck of the aneurysm is hidden by the right A2 if the right pterional approach is taken.
     - In cases of multiple aneurysms with other aneurysms are located on the left side.

10. *In the case of surgery of unruptured aneurysms, what are less favorable outcome factors?*
    - Factors for less favorable outcome post-surgery[10]:
      - Aneurysm size larger than 15 mm
      - Location: Posterior circulation
      - Number: Multiple aneurysms
      - Associated medical conditions

References

1. Brisman JL, SongJK, Newell DW. Cerebral aneurysms. N Engl J Med 2006;355:928–939
2. Unruptured intracranial aneurysms-risk of rupture and risks of surgical intervention. International Study of Unruptured Intracranial Aneurysms Investigators. N Engl J Med 1998;339(24):1725–1733
3. Chen PR, Frerichs K, Spetzler R. Current treatment options for unruptured intracranial aneurysms. Neurosurg Focus 2004;17(5):E5
4. Johnston SC, Higashida RT, Barrow DL, et al. Recommendations for the Endovascular Treatment of Intracranial Aneurysms: A Statement for Healthcare Professionals from the Committee on Cerebrovascular Imaging of the American Heart Association Council on Cardiovascular Radiology. Stroke 2002;33(10):2536–2544
5. Brilstra EH, Rinkel GJ, van der Graaf Y, van Rooij WJ, Algra A. Treatment of intracranial aneurysms by embolization with coils: a systematic review. Stroke 1999;30:470–476
6. Juvela S, Porras M, Poussa K. Natural history of unruptured intracranial aneurysms: probability of and risk factors for aneurysm rupture. J Neurosurg 2008;108(5):1052–1060
7. Wiebers DO, Whisnant JP, Huston J III, et al. International Study of Unruptured Intracranial Aneurysms Investigators. Unruptured intracranial aneurysms: natural history, clinical outcome, and risks of surgical and endovascular treatment. Lancet 2003;362(9378):103–110
8. Yasargil MG. Microneurosurgery II. New York: Thieme Medical Publishers; 1984
9. Kobayashi S, Nitta J, Hongo K, Goel A. Anterior communicating artery aneurysms. In: Goel A, Hongo K, Kobayashi S, eds. Neurosurgery of Complex Tumors & Vascular Lesions. New York: Churchill Livingstone; 1997:47–62
10. Orz YI, Hongo K, Tanaka Y, et al. Risks of surgery for patients with unruptured intracranial aneurysms. Surg Neurol 2000;53(1):21–27

Case 32   Posterior Communicating Artery Aneurysm

Pascal M. Jabbour and Erol Veznedaroglu

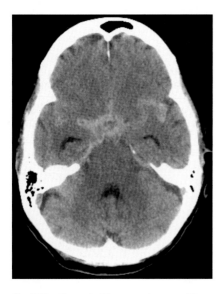

Fig. 32.1   Computed tomography scan of the head showing diffuse subarachnoid hemorrhage.

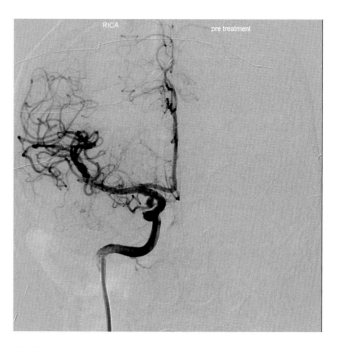

Fig. 32.2   Cerebral angiogram, right carotid injection showing a cerebral aneurysm.

■ Clinical Presentation

- A 64-year-old right-handed woman with a history of high blood pressure and smoking presents to the emergency room after experiencing the worst headache of her life while she was driving her car.
- She does not have a history of migraine headaches and never complained of headaches before this episode.
- Her familial history is significant—a maternal aunt died 10 years ago from a ruptured brain aneurysm.

- Neurologic evaluation showed that the patient was alert, awake-oriented, with a dilated nonreactive pupil on the right side, with decreased ocular motility upward, inward and downward.
- A computed tomography (CT) scan of the head is shown in **Fig. 32.1** and a cerebral angiogram is shown in **Fig. 32.2**.

■ Questions

1. What is the most likely diagnosis based on clinical history?
2. What are this patient's Hunt & Hess and Fisher grades?
3. What are the risk factors for subarachnoid hemorrhage (SAH) in this patient?
4. How are the findings on the clinical examination of this patient relevant; and where is most likely the anatomical location of the lesion based on the imaging studies provided?

5. What are the treatment options available for this patient?
6. You opt to proceed with surgical repair. Describe the details of the operation including positioning, opening, details of dissection and repair, closure, and other assistive measures.

■ **Answers**

1. *What is the most likely diagnosis of this patient?*
   - The patient experienced the worst headache of her life, with no previous history of headaches. This is highly suspicious of SAH.
2. *What are this patient's Hunt & Hess and Fisher grades?*
   - The patient has a Hunt & Hess grade 2 and a Fisher grade 3.[1,2]
3. *What are the risk factors for SAH in this patient?*
   - Female, high blood pressure, smoker, and familial history of aneurysms.[3]
4. *How are the findings on the clinical examination of this patient relevant and where is the most likely anatomic location of the lesion based on the imaging studies provided?*
   - The patient has a partial third nerve palsy involving the pupil.
   - Most probably the patient has a right posterior communicating artery (PCOM) aneurysm because of the proximity of the third nerve to the PCOM.
5. *What are the treatment options available for this patient?*
   - The patient's treatment options are either open surgery and clip ligation of the aneurysm or endovascular treatment with coils, depending on the patient's comorbidities, the shape of the aneurysm and the neck, and the preference of the surgeon. The literature is not clear about whether any of the modalities are better for the third nerve recovery.[4–6]
6. *You opt to proceed with surgical repair. Describe the details of the operation including positioning, opening, details of dissection and repair, closure and other assistive measures.*
   - Positioning and preoperative preparation
     - Supine, shoulder roll, head rotated 45 degrees, Mayfield 3-point fixation
     - Preoperative antibiotics, mannitol, furosemide available
     - Phenobarbital or etomidate available
     - Ventriculostomy ready to be placed
     - Assistive devices: microscope, loops, headlight, ultrasound; if have intraoperative angiography, have it ready
     - Retractors: Greenberg, Fukushima; Lela bar or Budde halo
     - Consider somatosensory evoked potential, electroencephalogram intraoperatively if feasible.
     - Anesthetize the pin sites before pinning.
     - Prepare the neck for possible early proximal control.

- Opening and dissection
  - Curvilinear incision, pterional craniotomy
  - Take down sphenoid wing extradurally down to the meningo-orbital artery.
  - Clinoid may have to be partially removed to obtain adequate exposure and proximal control of the internal carotid artery.
  - Wax all bone edges to prevent air embolism.
  - Place tack-up sutures.
  - Open the dura based on sphenoid wing.
  - Split the fissure under the microscope from proximal to distal.
  - Open between the veins and frontal cortex.
  - May place retractors on frontal lobe and gently start sharp dissection.
  - Identify the optic nerve and carotid artery and dissect the carotid to be able to place a proximal clip.
  - Work your way back to identify the carotid bifurcation.
  - Wide opening of the sylvian fissure greatly facilitates the safety of clipping.
  - Dissection done with caution in laterally projecting aneurysms to avoid avulsion of the fundus from the temporal lobe attachments.
  - Approach directed more frontal is preferred until the aneurysm neck is visualized.
- Clipping and precautions
  - May then place temporary clips and work on dissecting the neck and dome
  - Note: Can temporarily clip internal carotid artery up to 15 minutes before opening and reperfusing the brain.
  - Use systemic hypertension, phenobarbital or etomidate, mild hypothermia, mannitol during temporary clip.
  - Dissect neck before the dome, then place clip, then dissect dome and check for perforators
  - Advance the clip just beyond the course of the PCOM, without compromising the patency of that artery or that of the anterior thalamoperforators, internal carotid perforators, or anterior choroidal artery.
  - Use ultrasound to the dome to verify that there is no flow.
  - If no flow and no perforators, open the dome.
  - Open the membrane of Liliequist widely to visualize and release any tethering or compromise of the PCOM and its thalamoperforating vessels.
  - Obtain intraoperative angiogram if possible to confirm patency.
- Closure
  - Close and transfer to intensive care unit.
  - Obtain immediate postoperative CT and angiogram as well as neurologic exam.[7,8]

■ References

1. Hunt WE, Hess RM. Surgical risk as related to time of intervention in the repair of intracranial aneurysms. J Neurosurg 1968;28:14–20

2. Fisher CM, Kistler JP, Davis JM. Relation of cerebral vasospasm to subarachnoid hemorrhage visualized by CT scanning. Neurosurgery 1980;6:1–9

3. Wiebers DO, Whisnant JP, Huston J III, et al. Unruptured intracranial aneurysms: actual history, clinical outcome, and risks of surgical and endovascular treatment. Lancet 2003;362:103–110

4. Molyneux A, Kerr R, Stratton I, et al. International Subarachnoid Aneurysm Trial (ISAT) of neurosurgical clipping versus endovascular coiling in 2143 patients with ruptured intracranial aneurysms: a randomised trial. Lancet 2002;360:1267–1274

5. Ahn JY, Han IB, Yoon PH, et al. Clipping vs coiling of posterior communicating artery aneurysms with third nerve palsy. Neurology 2006;66:121–123

6. Stiebel-Kalish H, Maimon S, Amsalem J, Erlich R, Kalish Y, Rappaport HZ. Evolution of oculomotor nerve paresis after endovascular coiling of posterior communicating artery aneurysms: a neuro-ophthalmological perspective. Neurosurgery 2003;53:1268–1273

7. Greenberg MS. Handbook of Neurosurgery. 6th ed. New York: Thieme MedicalPublishers; 2006

8. Winn RH. Neurological Surgery. 5th ed. Philadelphia: Saunders; 2004:1371–1387

Case 33   Familial Cerebral Aneurysms

Hosam Al-Jehani and Richard Leblanc

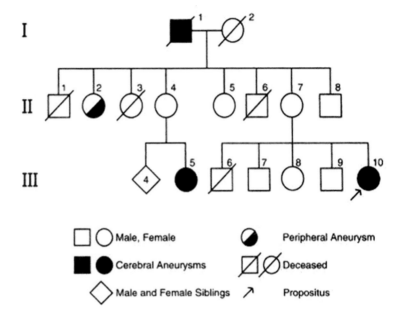

Fig. 33.1   Pedigree demonstrating familial history of cerebral and peripheral aneurysms. (From Leblanc R. *De novo* formation of familial cerebral aneurysms. Neurosurgery 1999;44:871–877. Reprinted with permission.)

■ **Clinical Presentation**

• A 24-year old white female was admitted to the hospital because of an episode of transient global amnesia, headache, nausea, and neck pain.
• The patient gave a family history of intracranial and peripheral aneurysms (**Fig. 33.1**),[1] but the review of systems was unremarkable.
• She was normotensive and the remainder of the general and neurologic examinations were normal.
• A complete blood count, serum electrolytes, liver function tests, and urinalysis were normal. A chest x-ray, electrocardiogram, and ultrasound examination of the kidneys were unremarkable.
• A contrast-enhanced computed tomographic (CT) scan demonstrated a right internal carotid artery aneurysm, which was confirmed by four-vessel intraarterial cerebral angiography (**Fig. 33.2**).[1] No other aneurysms were seen, but both posterior communicating arteries (PCOMs) had an infundibular origin.
• The patient underwent a right pterional craniotomy and uneventful clipping of the aneurysm.
• The patient remained well until 10 years later when, at the age of 34 years, she was readmitted to the hospital because of severe headache. Cerebral angiography showed

the presence of de novo aneurysms of the right internal carotid artery between the posterior communicating and anterior choroidal arteries, of the right middle cerebral artery at its bifurcation, of the anterior communicating artery, and on the left middle cerebral artery at the distal aspect of its first segment (M1) and at the bifurcation of its second segment (M2). The previously clipped aneurysm did not fill (**Fig. 33.3**).[1]
• The anterior communicating artery (ACOM) aneurysm was clipped, and the right internal carotid artery aneurysm was treated with detachable coils. The patient made an uneventful recovery. She was discharged home and returned to her previous occupation.
• The patient remained well for another 10 years when, at the age of 44 years, she underwent CT scanning for investigation of chronic, nonspecific facial pain. The CT scan showed that the previously untreated aneurysm of the second segment of the left middle cerebral artery had enlarged, a finding confirmed by intraarterial angiography. Angiography also demonstrated new aneurysms of the proximal and distal right middle cerebral artery, of the right ACOM and of the distal right superior cerebellar artery.

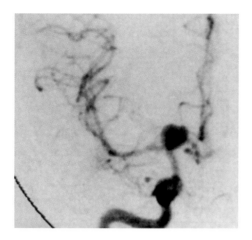

Fig. 33.2   Right carotid artery angiogram demonstrating the presence of a 1 × 1.5 cm aneurysm of the right internal carotid artery at the level of its bifurcation into anterior and middle cerebral arteries. (From Leblanc R. *De novo* formation of familial cerebral aneurysms. Neurosurgery 1999;44:871–877. Reprinted with permission.)

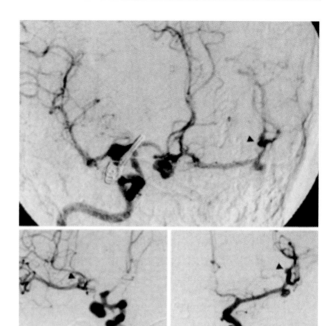

Fig. 33.3   Right internal carotid artery angiogram performed during compression of the left internal carotid artery (top) demonstrating the anterior communicating artery aneurysm and the aneurysms of the left middle cerebral artery at its bifurcation and at the origin of its second segment (*arrowheads*). The later two aneurysms are further illustrated at the bottom right image after the performance of a left internal carotid artery angiogram. The aneurysm at the origin of the right middle cerebral artery is illustrated at the bottom left of the figure. (From Leblanc R. *De novo* formation of familial cerebral aneurysms. Neurosurgery 1999; 44:871–877. Reprinted with permission.)

■ Questions

1. What are the risk factors of subarachnoid hemorrhage (SAH)?
2. What is the prognosis of aneurysmal SAH?
3. What are some of the common genetically determined conditions associated with intracranial aneurysms?
4. What is the incidence of familial aneurysms that are not associated with other genetically determined conditions?
5. What are the features of familial aneurysms compared with sporadic ones?
6. What have been the results of genetic studies of familial cerebral aneurysms?
7. What are the limitations to the genetic studies of familial intracranial aneurysm?
8. How can genetic factors interact with other risk factors in familial aneurysms?
9. What are your recommendations for screening for familial intracranial aneurysms?

■ Answers

1. *What are the risk factors of SAH?*
   - Risk factors for aneurysmal SAH include[2-4]
     - Cigarette smoking (odds ratio of 3.1)
     - Arterial hypertension (odds ratio of 2.6)
     - Excessive use of alcohol
     - A family history of aneurysmal SAH
     - Advancing age
     - The use of cocaine

2. *What is the prognosis of aneurysmal SAH?*
   - Subarachnoid hemorrhage from a ruptured intracranial aneurysm has a poor prognosis: In population-based studies mortality is of the order of 50% and 20% of survivors remain severely disabled.[5]

3. *What are some of the common genetically determined conditions associated with intracranial aneurysms?*
   - Syndromes associated with intracranial aneurysms include[6,7]
     - Autosomal dominant polycystic kidney disease
     - Ehlers–Danlos syndrome type I and IV
     - Marfan syndrome
     - Fibromuscular dysplasia
     - Neurofibromatosis type 1
     - Tuberous sclerosis
     - Osteogenesis imperfecta type 1
     - Achondroplasia
     - α1-Antitrypsin deficiency

4. *What is the incidence of familial aneurysms that are not associated with other genetically determined conditions?*
   - Up to 15% of individuals with a ruptured aneurysm in the absence of other familial conditions associated with cerebral aneurysms will have a first-degree relative who also has a cerebral aneurysm compared with ~5% for age-matched controls.[8]
   - The risk of harboring intracranial aneurysm is proportional to the number of affected first-degree relatives.[9-12]

5. *What are the features of familial aneurysms compared with sporadic ones?*
   - In initial studies comparing familial cerebral aneurysms and sporadic cerebral aneurysms, it was found that familial aneurysms rupture at a younger age, especially in women, and at a smaller size than sporadic aneurysms. Familial aneurysms tend to rupture within the same decade in families, and within 5 years of each other in identical twins.[11,13,14]
   - Others have suggested that familial aneurysms may be diagnose when they are a larger size than sporadic ones, that they more often occur on the middle cerebral artery and that patients that harbor them are more likely to have multiple aneurysms than individuals with sporadic aneurysms. Familial aneurysms have been shown to have a worse outcome following rupture than sporadic aneurysms.[11,15]

6. *What have been the results of genetic studies of familial cerebral aneurysms?*
   - Initial studies aimed at identifying genetic factors associated with cerebral aneurysms not associated with other well-defined genetic conditions have been largely negative. We were unable to identify a link to the human leucocyte antigen (HLA) system in our cases, and sequencing of the type III collagen gene showed that it is was preserved in our patients.[16,17]
   - Others have suggested a linkage to the 7q11 locus near the elastin gene, to the collagen type 1A2 gene,[18] and to 19q12–13 and 9p21, which contain several loci related to cerebrovascular disease that may be important for aneurysm formation. The loci 1p34.3–p36.13 and Xp22 were found to be associated with familial intracranial aneurysms across different populations.[19,20]

7. *What are the limitations to the genetic studies of familial intracranial aneurysm?*
   - The limitations to genetic studies are multiple. Varying definitions of what constitutes a familial incidence of aneurysms are in use. This implies a different genetic load in the families studied that may lead to different findings.
   - The mode of inheritance is unknown and is most likely heterogeneous. It is difficult to determine whether a sibling is not affected because aneurysms may develop after a negative screening examination.
   - Finally, large cooperative international studies probably are not applicable because different populations and different ethnic groups have different risks for SAH and thus probably also have different genetic determinants for intracranial aneurysms.[19,21-23]

8. *How can genetics factors interact with other risk factors in familial aneurysms?*
   - The interaction between genetic and other risk factors such as atherosclerosis, arterial hypertension, and cigarette smoking may predispose to weakening of the arterial wall. This would be expected to result in a higher risk of developing large and multiple aneurysms in familial cases, or more fragile aneurysms that might rupture at a smaller size.
   - The possibility of such interactions is supported by the findings that cerebral aneurysms are associated with several loci related to cerebrovascular disease that could predispose to atherosclerosis, hypertension, and aneurysm formation[20] and by the observation that polymorphic variants of the eNOS allele, which are associated with cigarette smoking, are more frequent in patients with SAH than in patients with unruptured aneurysms.[18,24-26]

9. *What are your recommendations for screening for familial intracranial aneurysms?*

◼ Answers (*continued*)

- The possible usefulness of elective screening of asymptomatic relatives of individuals with familial intracranial aneurysms is controversial and is best evaluated by decision analysis.
- However, most of the studies fail to support a role for systematic screening of individuals felt to be at risk of harboring a cerebral aneurysm because of their family history or at best suggest a very limited role for this practice, which may benefit only the young.[10,27–29]
- More recently, some have suggested that screening may be of benefit for first-degree relatives who are in their fourth decade or older and who have a history of cigarette smoking or of arterial hypertension, especially if they are female; and others have suggested that magnetic resonance angiography (MRA) screening is cost-effective, especially for patients 50 years and older.[30,31]
- One of the factors that militate against elective screening of asymptomatic individuals with a family history of cerebral aneurysms is the risk attendant to intraarterial angiography.
- However, less invasive diagnostic procedures, such as CT or MRA are becoming well established in the non-invasive diagnosis of individuals suspected of having even a small aneurysm.[32,33]
- Thus, we currently recommend MRA to our patients with a family history of cerebral aneurysms who desire screening, but we usually wait until the patient is 20 years old or older.
- This is followed by conventional angiography if the results are equivocal or if an aneurysm that warrants treatment is found.
- A negative examination, however, does not rule out that an aneurysm may develop in the future.
- There are currently no firm guidelines to suggest that screening should be repeated if an initial examination is negative. We have previously suggested that periodic reexamination should be considered for individuals with a treated aneurysm who have a family history of cerebral aneurysms because, as illustrated by the case of the patient described here, new aneurysms can develop decades later.[1,34]

◼ References

1. Leblanc R. De novo formation of familial cerebral aneurysms: case report. Neurosurgery 1999;44(4):871–876
2. Kissela BM, Sauerbeck L, Woo D, et al. Subarachnoid hemorrhage: a preventable disease with a heritable component. Stroke 2002;33(5):1321–1326
3. Johnston SC, Selvin S, Gress DR. The burden, trends, and demographics of mortality from subarachnoid hemorrhage. Neurology 1998;50(5):1413–1418
4. Leblanc R. Intracranial hemorrhage from coagulopathies and vasculopathies. In: Cooper PR, Barrow DL, Tindall GT, eds. The Practice of Neurosurgery. Baltimore: Williams & Wilkins; 1996:2311–2343
5. Hop JW, Rinkel GJ, Algra A, van Gijn J. Case-fatality rates and functional outcome after subarachnoid hemorrhage: a systematic review. Stroke 1997;28(3):660–664
6. Schievink WI. Genetics of intracranial aneurysms. Neurosurgery 1997;40(4):651–662
7. Lozano AM, Leblanc R. Cerebral aneurysms and polycystic kidney disease: a critical review. Can J Neurol Sci 1992;19(2):222–227
8. Bromberg JE, Rinkel GJ, Algra A, et al. Familial subarachnoid hemorrhage: distinctive features and patterns of inheritance. Ann Neurol 1995;38(6):929–934
9. Rinkel GJ. Intracranial aneurysm screening: indications and advice for practice. Lancet Neurol 2005;4(2):122–128
10. Leblanc R, Melanson D, Tampieri D, Guttmann RD. Familial cerebral aneurysms: a study of 13 families. Neurosurgery 1995;37(4):633–638
11. Leblanc R. Familial cerebral aneurysms. Can J Neurol Sci 1997;24(3):191–199
12. Mathieu J, Hébert G, Pérusse L, et al. Familial intracranial aneurysms: recurrence risk and accidental aggregation study. Can J Neurol Sci 1997;24(4):326–331
13. Lozano AM, Leblanc R. Familial intracranial aneurysms. J Neurosurg 1987;66(4):522–528
14. Leblanc R. Familial cerebral aneurysms. A bias for women. Stroke 1996;27(6):1050–1054
15. Ruigrok YM, Rinkel GJ, Algra A, Raaymakers TW, Van Gijn J. Characteristics of intracranial aneurysms in patients with familial subarachnoid hemorrhage. Neurology 2004;62(6):891–894
16. Leblanc R, Lozano AM, van der Rest M, Guttmann RD. Absence of collagen deficiency in familial cerebral aneurysms. J Neurosurg 1989;70(6):837–840
17. Kuivaniemi H, Prockop DJ, Wu Y, et al. Exclusion of mutations in the gene for type III collagen (COL3A1) as a common cause of intracranial aneurysms or cervical artery dissections: results from sequence analysis of the coding sequences of type III collagen from 55 unrelated patients. Neurology 1993;43(12):2652–2658
18. Khurana VG, Meissner I, Sohni YR, et al. The presence of tandem endothelial nitric oxide synthase gene polymorphisms identifying brain aneurysms more prone to rupture. J Neurosurg 2005;102(3):526–531
19. Ruigrok YM, Rinkel GJ. Genetics of intracranial aneurysms. Stroke 2008;39(3):1049–1055
20. Helgadottir A, Thorleifsson G, Magnusson KP, et al. The same sequence variant on 9p21 associates with myocardial infarction, abdominal aortic aneurysm and intracranial aneurysm. Nat Genet 2008;40(2):217–224
21. Ruigrok YM, Rinkel GJ, Wijmenga C. Familial intracranial aneurysms. Stroke 2004;35(3):e59–e60
22. Wermer MJ, Rinkel GJ, van Gijn J. Repeated screening for intracranial aneurysms in familial subarachnoid hemorrhage. Stroke 2003;34(12):2788–2791

■ References (*continued*)

23. Feigin VL, Rinkel GJ, Lawes CM, et al. Risk factors for subarachnoid hemorrhage: an updated systematic review of epidemiological studies. Stroke 2005;36(12):2773–2780

24. Onda H, Kasuya H, Yoneyama T, et al. Genomewide-linkage and haplotype-association studies map intracranial aneurysm to chromosome 7q11. Am J Hum Genet 2001;69(4):804–819

25. Olson JM, Vongpunsawad S, Kuivaniemi H, et al. Search for intracranial aneurysm susceptibility gene(s) using Finnish families. BMC Med Genet 2002;3:7

26. Foroud T, Sauerbeck L, Brown R, et al. Genome screen to detect linkage to intracranial aneurysm susceptibility genes: the Familial Intracranial Aneurysm (FIA) study. Stroke 2008;39(5):1434–1440

27. Leblanc R, Worsley KJ, Melanson D, Tampieri D. Angiographic screening and elective surgery of familial cerebral aneurysms: a decision analysis. Neurosurgery 1994;35(1):9–18

28. Kirkpatrick PJ, McConnell RS. Screening for familial intracranial aneurysms. BMJ 1999;319(7224):1512–1513

29. Magnetic Resonance Angiography in Relatives of Patients with Subarachnoid Hemorrhage Study Group. Risks and benefits of screening for intracranial aneurysms in first-degree relatives of patients with sporadic subarachnoid hemorrhage. N Engl J Med 1999;341(18):1344–1350

30. Brown RD Jr, Huston J, Hornung R, et al. Screening for brain aneurysm in the Familial Intracranial Aneurysm study: frequency and predictors of lesion detection. J Neurosurg 2008;108(6):1132–1138

31. Takao H, Nojo T, Ohtomo K. Screening for familial intracranial aneurysms: decision and cost-effectiveness analysis. Acad Radiol 2008;15(4):462–471

32. Gibbs GF, Huston J III, Bernstein MA, Riederer SJ, Brown RD Jr. 3.0-Tesla MR angiography of intracranial aneurysms: comparison of time-of-flight and contrast-enhanced techniques. J Magn Reson Imaging 2005;21(2):97–102

33. Tampieri D, Leblanc R, Oleszek J, Pokrupa R, Melançon D. Three-dimensional computed tomographic angiography of cerebral aneurysms. Neurosurgery 1995;36(4):749–754

34. Leblanc R. Incidental aneurysms, multiple aneurysms, familial aneurysms and aneurysms in pregnancy. In: Awad I, ed. Cerebral Aneurysms. Rolling Meadows, IL: American Association of Neurological Surgeons; 1993:277–295

Case 34   Blister Carotid Aneurysm

Nancy McLaughlin and Michel W. Bojanowski

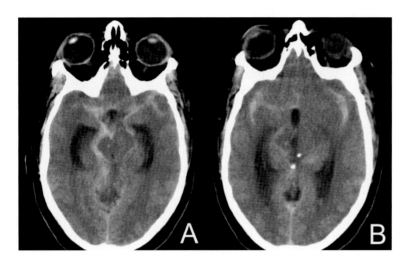

Fig. 34.1 **(A,B)** Computed tomography scan of the head showing a subarachnoid hemorrhage.

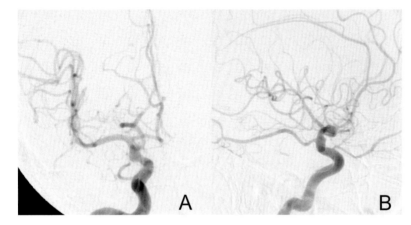

Fig. 34.2 Cerebral angiography. **(A)** Anteroposterior and **(B)** lateral views of a right internal carotid.

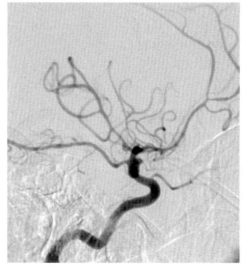

Fig. 34.3 Cerebral angiography: Lateral view, right internal carotid done 3 days later.

■ Clinical Presentation

• A 42-year-old woman presents with a sudden-onset headache. Her past medical history is unremarkable and she is on no medications.

• Her vital signs are stable and the physical examination is normal. Blood pressure is 125/80 mmHg.

• Except for drowsiness, her neurologic examination is unremarkable.

• A computed tomography (CT) scan of the head is performed (**Fig. 34.1**) and subsequently a four-vessels cerebral angiography (**Fig. 34.2**) reveals ectatic appearance of the supraclinoidal segment of the right internal carotid artery with possibly a faint bulge at the level of the posterior communicating artery. The angiogram is otherwise normal.

■ Questions

1. What are the possible causes of subarachnoid hemorrhage (SAH) with a negative angiogram?
2. What are the CT criteria for pretruncal nonaneurysmal SAH?
3. What is your initial management?

You decide to repeat the angiogram 3 days later (**Fig. 34.3**).

4. Interpret the angiogram.
5. What are the definition of and the various nomenclatures for this lesion?

6. What are the pathologic features?

After discussion with the neurointerventional team, you recommend a direct surgical approach of the lesion.

7. What are the pitfalls regarding the surgical treatment?
8. What surgical strategies should be taken into consideration?
9. What is the prognosis?

■ Answers

1. *What are the possible causes of SAH with a negative angiogram?*
   - Aneurysm not visualized on initial angiogram
     – Incomplete or suboptimal quality images
     – Very small micro-aneurysms
     – Thrombosis of an aneurysm after SAH
     – Lack of filling due to vasospasm
     – Nonaneurysmal SAH
   - Pretruncal nonaneurysmal SAH
     – Angiographically occult vascular malformations including cavernous malformations
     – Coagulation disorders
     – Drug abuse (e.g., cocaine)
     – Cerebral artery dissection (e.g., vertebral intracranial)
     – Pituitary apoplexy
2. *What are the CT criteria for pretruncal nonaneurysmal SAH?*
   - Epicenter of hemorrhage anterior to the brainstem (interpeduncular and/or prepontine)
   - There may be extension into the anterior part of the ambient cistern or the basal part of the sylvian fissure
   - Absence of complete filling of the anterior interhemispheric fissure
   - No more than minute amounts of blood in the lateral portion of the sylvian fissure
   - Absence of frank intraventricular hemorrhage: Small amounts of blood sedimenting in the occipital horns of the lateral ventricle are permissible.[1]
3. *What is your initial management?*

- The CT has shown an aneurysmal SAH distribution and does not satisfy the criteria of pretruncal SAH mainly because of the filling of the sylvian and interhemispheric fissures. Accordingly, a ruptured intracranial aneurysm is not entirely excluded. Note the presence of moderate hydrocephalus. The initial management includes
  – Admission to intensive care unit
  – External ventricular drain (EVD) if there is progression of hydrocephalus or clinical deterioration
  – Bed rest and symptomatic treatment (e.g., analgesic, antiemetic)
  – Control of the blood pressure
  – Cardiac monitoring
  – Intravenous (IV) fluids: mild volume expansion and slight hemodilution
  – Calcium channel blockers: nimodipine
  – Laboratories: arterial blood gas (ABG), electrolytes, complete blood count (CBC), international normalized ratio (INR), partial thromboplastin time (PTT)
  – Seizure prophylaxis
4. *Interpret the angiogram.*
   - The right internal carotid injection reveals a small bulbous, broad-based dilatation at the anterior wall of the right internal carotid artery.
   - This finding is compatible with the diagnosis of a ruptured blister-like internal carotid aneurysm. These aneurysms reportedly exhibit rapid growth and changes in shape as in this case.[2]
5. *What are the definition of and the various nomenclatures for this lesion?*

■ Answers (*continued*)

- Blister-like aneurysms are small sessile, hemispherical expansions at a nonbranching site of the anterior aspect of supraclinoid segment of the internal carotid artery (ICA).
- They are characterized by a very fragile wall and a poorly defined neck and are histologically distinct from saccular aneurysms.
- In relation to the ICA, they have been referred as
  - Dorsal
  - Distal-medial
  - Superior
  - Anterior wall[1-4]

6. *What are the pathologic features?*
   - These aneurysms are associated with arteriosclerosis of the neighboring carotid wall.[5]
   - Abrupt termination of the internal elastic lamina is seen at the border between the normal and sclerotic carotid wall.
   - The dome is composed of fibrinous tissue and adventitia whereas the usual collagenous layer of saccular aneurysm is absent.
   - Dissection and infiltration of the arterial wall by inflammatory cells is absent.
   - Because of their very fragile walls and poorly defined necks, surgical exploration and clipping are very hazardous with a high rate of intraoperative or postoperative rupture.[6]

7. *What are the pitfalls regarding the surgical treatment?*
   - Blister-like aneurysms have a high risk of intraoperative rupture with large lacerations of the ICA during clipping. These aneurysms require special consideration.

8. *What surgical strategies should be taken into consideration?*
   - Surgical strategies include[2,6-10]
     - Opening of the sylvian fissure before accessing the carotid and chiasmatic cisterns
     - Frontal lobe retraction should be minimized and performed as late as possible because of adhesion of the frontal lobe to the aneurysm dome.
     - Clips should be applied while pressure within the ICA is low with temporary clipping of the ICA.
     - Clips' blade should be applied parallel to the parent artery and should catch the arterial wall beyond the lesion.
     - Confirming the stability of clips is essential and is done with induced blood pressure elevation and repeated irrigation before closing the dura mater.
   - Other potential surgical treatments
     - Wrapping the full circumference of the ICA and applying an encircling clip. Sundt clips can be used for wrapping because they allow encircling of the vessel with Dacron (Invista, Inc., Wichita, KS).
     - ICA trapping with or without bypass
     - Direct suturing
     - Stent placement, alone or with coiling, is increasingly being used or tested as a modality of treatment. It is based on the rationale of redirecting flow away from the dome. Long-term results are not available at present.
     - Bipolar coagulation has been used by some without documented long-term results.

9. *What is the prognosis?*
   - The prognosis is related to the clinical status on admission, evaluated by the Hunt and Hess clinical classification.
   - However, because of the high incidence of intraoperative or postoperative bleeding, the prognosis is markedly worse than for those patients with saccular-type aneurysm.[6]

■ References

1. Rinkel GJ, Wijdicks EF, Vermeulen M, et al. Nonaneurysmal perimesencephalic subarachnoid hemorrhage: CT and MR patterns that differ from aneurysmal rupture. AJNR Am J Neuroradiol 1991;12(5):829–834
2. Sim SY, Shin YS, Cho KG, et al. Blood blister-like aneurysms at nonbranching sites of the internal carotid artery. J Neurosurg 2006;105:400–405
3. Abe M, Tabuchi K, Yokoyama H, Uchino A. Blood blisterlike aneurysm of the internal carotid artery. J Neurosurg 1998;89:419–424
4. Nakagawa F, Kobayashi S, Takemae T, Sugita K. Aneurysms protruding from the dorsal wall of the internal carotid artery. J Neurosurg 1986;65:303–308
5. Ishikawa T, Nakamura N, Houkin K, Nomura M. Pathological consideration of a «blister-like» aneurysm at the superior wall of the internal carotid artery: case report. Neurosurgery 1997;40(2):403–406
6. Ogawa A, Suzuki M, Ogasawara K. Aneurysms at nonbranching sites in the supraclinoid portion of the internal carotid artery: internal carotid artery trunk aneurysms. Neurosurgery 2000;47(3):578–583
7. Yanaka K, Meguro K, Nose T. Repair of a tear at the base of a blister-like aneurysm with suturing and an encircling clip: technical note. Neurosurgery 2002;50(1):218–221
8. Pelz DM, Ferguson GG, Lownie SP, Kachur E. Combined endovascular/neurosurgical therapy of blister-like distal internal carotid aneurysms. Can J Neurol Sci 2003;30:49–53
9. Sekula RF Jr, Cohen DB, Quigley MR, Jannetta PJ. Primary treatment of a blister-like aneurysm with an encircling clip graft: technical case report. Neurosurgery 2006; 59(Suppl 1)ONS-E168
10. Park JH, Park IS, Han DH, et al. Endovascular treatment of blood blister-like aneurysms of the internal carotid artery. J Neurosurg 2007;106:812–819

Case 35   Concomitant Arteriovenous Malformation and Aneurysm

Julius July and Eka Julianta Wahjoepramono

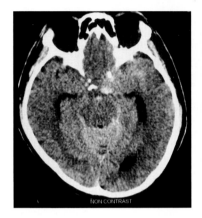

Fig. 35.1   Plain axial computed tomography scan of the head.

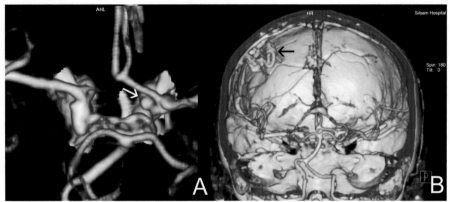

Fig. 35.2   Three-dimensional reconstructed computed tomography angiogram showing **(A)** aneurysm (*white arrow*) and **(B)** arteriovenous malformation (*black arrow*).

■ Clinical Presentation

- A 50-year-old man with past medical history of hypertension and heavy smoking presented to the ER with sudden onset left partial ptosis.
- Ten days prior, he had a very severe headache and was admitted to another hospital for 3 days and was sent home without imaging studies of his head or lumbar puncture.

- Physical examination reveals that he is fully oriented with moderate headache. He has a left partial ptosis and a left dilated pupil (5 mm, compare with the right, 3 mm) and is less reactive to the light. The remainder of the neurologic examination is normal.
- Initial plain computed tomography (CT) scan is shown in **Fig. 35.1**.

■ Questions

1. What is the most probable diagnosis in this case? Explain.
2. What further imaging studies should you obtain on this patient? What is their diagnostic yield?
3. Please describe the three-dimensional (3D) reconstructed computed tomography angiogram (CTA) shown in **Fig. 35.2**.
4. What are some relations between concomitant arteriovenous malformations (AVMs) and aneurysms?
5. You elect to proceed with surgical intervention. Describe the important steps of the surgery.

After the surgery, the patient had an excellent recovery. The partial left third nerve palsy did not resolve, however, no new neurologic deficits were noted. He was observed one night in the intensive care unit then moved to the ward. On the third day after the surgery, he developed slurred speech and a mild right-sided hemiparesis (power 4+/5). A CT scan was done (**Fig. 35.3**).

6. Describe the CT scan findings.
7. What are the possible causes of this condition and how do you want to treat the patient?

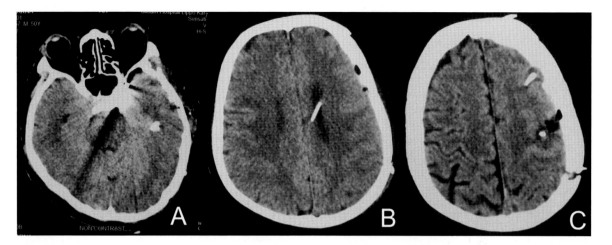

Fig. 35.3   Postoperative computed tomography scan of the head performed after neurologic deterioration. Sequential images showing **(A)** basilar cisterns, **(B)** course of ventriculostomy, and **(C)** site of resection of arteriovenous malformation.

■ Answers

1. *What is the most probable diagnosis in this case? Explain.*
   - According to the clinical history, it seems that the patient had a "warning headache," also known as "sentinel hemorrhage" from an aneurysm rupture. These types of headache occur in 30–60% of patients presenting with subarachnoid hemorrhage (SAH).
   - The SAH may then clear and the patient may not seek medical attention.
   - Unfortunately, in this case, the patient was not investigated properly initially. A plain CT head should have been performed at the outside hospital.
   - Newer generation CT scans will detect SAH in more than 95% of cases if scanned within 48 hours of the SAH. The blood will appears as high-density (white) streaks within the subarachnoid spaces.
   - If the CT turns out to be normal, then a lumbar puncture (LP) is indicated. LP is the most sensitive test for detecting SAH. However, a false-positive may occur such as traumatic taps. Caution must be exerted while performing an LP as intracranial pressure changes may occur and may trigger further bleeding from the rupture site.
   - The development of ptosis points to specific aneurysm location: this is more common with posterior communicating artery (PCOM) aneurysm, or less commonly basilar apex aneurysm. This is an imminent rupture sign that should be considered seriously and treated as soon as possible.
   - A CT scan done upon presentation to our ER (not shown here) showed a hyperdensity in the left supraclinoid region. Also, the temporal horns were dilated, which is suggestive of hydrocephalus. Delayed hydrocephalus is one of SAH's main complications

and may be caused by pia-arachnoid adhesions or permanent impairment of the arachnoid granulation function.[1,2]

2. *What further imaging studies should you obtain for this patient? What is their diagnostic yield?*
   - Cerebral angiography is the gold standard for evaluation of SAH and aneurysms. It is an invasive procedure and has inherent risks (e.g., stroke) and may cause delays in treatment.
   - CTA has a sensitivity of 95% and specificity of 83% in detecting aneurysm as small as 2.2 mm. It is not an invasive procedure and can be done within minutes. The 3D reconstruction of the CTA is very helpful for surgical planning and the head positioning. Even if the endovascular treatment with coiling is considered, CTA can provide further information to determine whether an aneurysm can be treated by coiling.
   - Magnetic resonance arteriography (MRA) provides the ability to detect aneurysms and determine the size, rate, and direction of flow in an aneurysm relative to the magnetic field. It also helps visualize thrombosis and calcifications within an aneurysm. Its sensitivity to detect aneurysms greater than 3 mm is around 86%, and the false-positive rate is 16%. As the false-positive rate is elevated, this modality may be useful for screening high-risk patients, including first-degree relatives of aneurysm patients.
   - Magnetic resonance imaging (MRI) alone is not sensitive within the first 24–48 hours. After 4–7 days, MRI is excellent for detecting subacute to remote SAH. It may be helpful to determine which aneurysm bled in cases of multiple aneurysms.[1,2]

3. *Please describe the 3D reconstructed CTA shown in* **Fig. 35.2**.

■ Answers (*continued*)

- 3D CTA shows the presence of a left internal carotid artery (ICA) aneurysm (**Fig. 35.2A**), most probably at the level of the PCOM segment. The dome of the aneurysm is pointing posteriorly and inferiorly. The left A1 segment is hypoplastic. The aneurysm itself has a wide neck, almost fusiform-like.
- There is also a coincidental finding of an arteriovenous malformation (AVM) in the left frontal area (**Fig. 35.2B**). The major feeders of the AVM appear to be originating from branches of the middle cerebral artery. The drainage of the AVM appears to be via the superior sagittal sinus.

4. *What are some relations between concomitant AVMs and aneurysms?*
   - Aneurysms are present in 2.7–23% of patients with an AVM.
   - Aneurysm occurring in the presence of AVMs may be flow related, intranidal, or unrelated to the AVM.
   - In flow-related cases, hemodynamic stress of the increased flow traveling toward the AVM may contribute to the formation of proximal arterial aneurysms. These are more common in males. They arise along the course of arteries that eventually supply the AVM.
   - Proximal flow-related aneurysms are typically located at these sites:
     - Supraclinoid internal carotid artery
     - Circle of Willis
     - Middle cerebral artery up to bifurcation
     - Anterior cerebral artery up to anterior communicating artery
     - Vertebrobasilar trunk
   - All flow-related aneurysms beyond these locations are distal flow-related aneurysms.
   - Intranidal aneurysms lie within the AVM nidus and are also more common in males.
   - Unrelated aneurysms are remote to the AVM and more common in females.
   - The pathogenesis of AVM and concomitant aneurysms may relate to a combination of factors such as underlying vascular defect, hemodynamic stress, vasoactive substances, and locally generated growth factors.
   - Distal flow-related aneurysms are the most likely to regress with definitive AVM treatment, but the proximal flow-related aneurysms are unlikely to change.
   - The treatment plan in this case will involve repair of the imminently ruptured internal carotid-posterior communicating artery (IC-PC) aneurysm and then continue with the AVM resection, if safely achievable in the same sitting. The wide neck of the aneurysm excludes the endovascular treatment option in this case.[3]

5. *You elect to proceed with surgical intervention. Describe the important steps of the surgery.*
   - Extended pterional approach is used.
   - Image guidance may aid in planning the incision and the bone flap.
   - Ventriculostomy insertion may be performed as a first step.
   - Sylvian fissure dissection from proximal to distal is performed to visualize parent vessels and the aneurysm neck (see Case 32).
   - It may be necessary to put temporary clips on parent vessels and the aneurysm's major branches to reconstruct the aneurysm.
   - After the clipping, always confirm the flow of all surrounding vessels with intraoperative Doppler; also confirm that there is no flow in the aneurysm dome.
   - Then, if safely feasible, one may continue with the resection of the AVM.
   - Note that this step can be done in a separate sitting if difficulties are encountered during aneurysm clipping.
   - Follow the general principles of AVM surgery.
     - Always try to identify the feeder at the first stage. If one is not sure whether a vessel is a feeder, a temporary clip may be used on that vessel, and observation for changes in the AVM or surrounding brain can then be noted.
     - The surrounding gliotic brain presents a good cleavage plane for dissection of the nidus.
     - Avoid getting into the nidus.
     - The draining veins are taken as a last step in the resection. Again, temporary clips may be used in a similar fashion.[2,4]

6. *Describe the CT scan findings.*
   - The CT scan (**Fig. 35.3**) shows artifact from the clip placement in the left paraclinoid region; no intracranial hematoma or hypodensities are noted.
   - Ventriculostomy placement appears adequate with expected size of ventricles.
   - At the site of the previous AVM location, there is again no hemorrhage and minimal surgical artifact.

7. *What are the possible causes of this condition and how do you want to treat the patient?*
   - The most probable cause of his condition is vasospasm.
   - Other possibilities include
     - Normal pressure perfusion breakthrough (secondary to changes in autoregulation post-AVM surgery)
     - Seizure
     - Infection (meningitis, encephalitis, sepsis)
     - Electrolyte abnormalities
     - Hyperacute infarction not visible on CT scan yet

■ Answers (*continued*)

- Management should include
  - Ensure adequate oxygenation and circulation
  - Involve seizure prophylaxis
  - Check and correct electrolytes
  - Further laboratory investigations: complete blood count; electrolytes; prothrombin time/partial thromboplastin time; culture blood, urine, sputum, cerebrospinal fluid (CSF)
  - Ensure adequate antibiotic coverage
  - Monitor and control intracranial pressure (ICP)
    - Head of bed elevated 30 degrees
    - Drain CSF
    - May need to sedate or hyperventilate if ICP is elevated
  - Optimize the hematocrit
  - Nimodipine 60 mg by mouth every 4 hours
  - "Triple H maneuver" with mild hypertension, hypervolemia, and hemodilution.
  - May need to repeat the cerebral angiogram to check for vasospasm and possibly for therapeutic purposes (angioplasty or papaverine injection)
  - May also consider MRI if the clip is MRI compatible and if the patient does not improve[1,4]

- The patient is this case gradually improved with triple H therapy and physiotherapy. He had an almost complete recovery one month later, except for the left partial third nerve palsy.

■ References

1. Greenberg MS. Handbook of Neurosurgery. 6th ed. New York: Thieme Medical Publishers; 2006.
2. Winn RH. Neurological Surgery. 5th ed. Philadelphia: Saunders; 2004:1371–1387
3. Martin NA, Vinters HV. Arteriovenous malformation. In: Spetzler RF, Carter LP. Neurovascular Surgery. New York: McGraw-Hill; 1995:875–903
4. Fisher WS. Surgical treatment of arteriovenous malformations of the cerebral convexity. In: Wilkins RH, Rengachary SS, eds. Neurosurgical Operative Atlas. Vol. 3. Chicago: American Association of Neurological Surgeons; 1993

Case 36 Middle Cerebral Artery Aneurysm

Julius July and Eka Julianta Wahjoepramono

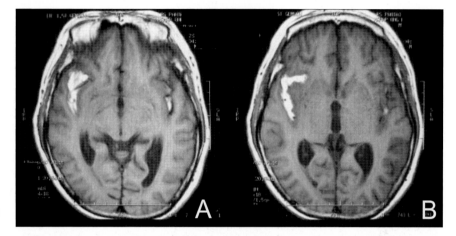

Fig. 36.1 T1-weighted magnetic resonance image without contrast performed on day 4 after patient's severe headache revealing subarachnoid blood in the sylvian fissure seen in **(A)** and **(B)**.

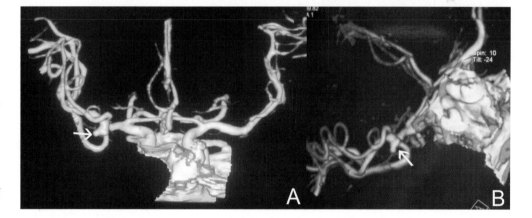

Fig. 36.2 Computed tomography angiogram with three-dimensional reconstruction confirming the presence of a right middle cerebral artery aneurysm (*arrow* in **[A]** and **[B]**). The aneurysm has a "Mickey Mouse" appearance and originates from the bifurcation of right M1 segment of the middle cerebral artery.

■ Clinical Presentation

- A 67-year-old man presented with severe headache and is admitted to another hospital for 4 days. He is then referred to the neurosurgical service in your hospital for further treatment and a magnetic resonance imaging (MRI) scan is obtained that same day (**Fig. 36.1**). There were no signs of tumor or arteriovenous malformation (AVM) on the MRI, as reviewed by the radiologist.

- Upon initial assessment, he is confused, oriented to self only. He obeys simple commands and has no obvious weakness.
- He also has a stiff neck upon examination. There was no history of smoking and the blood pressure ranged from 160–180/90–100 mm Hg.

■ Questions

1. Describe your diagnosis.

The patient obtains a computed tomography angiogram (CTA) (**Fig. 36.2**).

2. What is your definitive choice of treatment? Describe the role of endovascular treatment.
3. Describe a surgical strategy for this case.

4. What are the late complications of middle cerebral artery (MCA) aneurysm rupture?
5. What are the rates of morbidity and mortality based on treatment modality? What would these rates be if this was an unruptured aneurysm?

■ Answers

1. *Describe your diagnosis.*
   - The clinical presentation and the MRI findings favor subarachnoid hemorrhage (SAH).
   - On MRI, both sylvian fissures appear to be filled with early subacute blood, more so on the right side. Early subacute blood (day 3–7) appears on T1-weighted MRIs as very hyperintense and on T2-weighted MRIs as very hypointense, associated with the intracellular methemoglobin.[1]
   - The predominance of subarachnoid blood in the right sylvian fissure suggests that the most likely cause is a ruptured right MCA aneurysm, although aneurysms of adjacent arteries may sometimes present with similar blood distributions.

2. *What is your treatment plan? Describe the role of endovascular treatment.*
   - Aneurysms arising from the MCA almost exclusively occur at the primary bifurcation and point away from the axis of the middle cerebral artery trunk. Less commonly, MCA aneurysms may arise at the origin of the anterior temporal artery, lenticulostriate artery, secondary bifurcation, or even more distally.
   - Direct microsurgical clipping is the most common method used to treat MCA aneurysm. Even in institutions in which endovascular coiling is the preferred treatment modality, the overwhelming majority of MCA aneurysms are still treated with microsurgical clipping. MCA aneurysms are less suitable for endovascular coil packing because of both their anatomy and their frequent association with expanding hematomas. Typically, these aneurysms have wide necks with major arterial branches arising at the aneurysm base, making surgical clipping the most effective treatment. Because of their peripheral location and relatively straightforward surgical anatomy, microsurgical clipping of these aneurysms is easier than in other locations.[2]

3. *Describe a surgical strategy for this case.*
   - A right pterional craniotomy will be best suitable for this case.

   - The following are some important surgical pointers pertinent to this case:
     - Operative planning should consist of patient head positioning, extent of bony exposure, necessity of placement of a ventriculostomy to relax the brain via drainage of cerebrospinal fluid (CSF), and planning for evacuation of hematoma.
     - The patient's head is turned to the left side, around 30–45 degrees toward the floor.
     - Sharp surgical dissection of the sylvian fissure is done to identify the parent vessels, distal vessels, and the aneurysm.
     - Avoid blunt dissection around the aneurysm, as this can precipitate an intraoperative rupture. If necessary, it is better and safer to sacrifice a thin area of cortex around the aneurysm to get more working space.
     - Use of a temporary clip may be necessary, as such proximal exposure may be needed (internal carotid artery [ICA], proximal MCA). Always begin with gentle sylvian fissure dissection; the aim is to identify the parent artery for proximal control if necessary, and of course to get the aneurysm.
     - Excessive brain retraction leads to postoperative brain swelling and unsatisfactory results, regardless of how carefully the aneurysm clips are applied, and can be a significant cause of morbidity.
     - Choose the appropriate clip.[2,3]

4. *What are the late complications of MCA aneurysm rupture?*
   - Despite good technical results, patients with ruptured MCA aneurysms often have surprisingly poor outcomes. This is primarily due to the aneurysm rupture itself, which often produces both subarachnoid and intracerebral blood causing significant morbidity.
   - Late complications of MCA aneurysm rupture include
     - Seizure: The incidence varies between 7–25% with one MCA aneurysm. It can reach 27% in multiple aneurysm cases. Most MCA aneurysms that present with temporal intracerebral hematoma (ICH) develop delayed seizures.
     - Weakness with or without dysphasia: More proximal aneurysms are associated with more severe neurologic deficits.
     - Visual-field deficit: Associated with lesions in the loop of Meyer as part of the visual pathways[4,5]

5. *What are the rates of morbidity and mortality based on treatment modality? What would these rates be if this was an unruptured aneurysm?*
   - Overall surgical morbidity rates are ~30% for ruptured aneurysms.[6]
   - See **Table 36.1** for more details.[6,7]

Answers (*continued*)

Table 36.1   Morbidity and Mortality Rates Based on Treatment Modality in Cases of Ruptured and Unruptured Aneurysms

Ruptured	Surgical[6]	30%
	Endovascular[6]	23%
	Observation – 30 day mortality	45%
	Observation – serious neurologic deficit	25%
Unruptured	Surgical[7]	12%
	Endovascular[7]	9%

Source: Data from Molyneux AJ, Kerr RS, Yu LM, et al. International Subarachnoid Aneurysm Trial (ISAT) of neurosurgical clipping versus endovascular coiling in 2143 patients with ruptured intracranial aneurysms: a randomised comparison of effects on survival, dependency, seizures, rebleeding, subgroups. Lancet 2005;366(9488):809–817; Unruptured intracranial aneurysms–risk of rupture and risks of surgical intervention. International Study of Unruptured Intracranial Aneurysms Investigators. N Engl J Med 1998;339(24):1725–1733.

References

1. Osborn AG. Diagnostic Neuroradiology. St. Louis, MO: Mosby; 1994:465
2. Porterfield R, Chyatte D. Nuances of middle cerebral artery aneurysm microsurgery. Neurosurgery 2001;48(2):339–346
3. Winn RH. Neurological Surgery. 5th ed. Philadelphia: Saunders; 2004:1371–1387
4. Greenberg MS. Handbook of Neurosurgery. 6th ed. New York: Thieme Medical Publishing; 2006
5. Rinne J, Ishii K, Shen H, Kivisaari R, Hernesniemi J. Surgical management of aneurysms of the middle cerebral artery. In: Roberts DW Schmideck HH, eds. Schmidek & Sweet's Operative Neurosurgical Techniques. Indication, Methods, and Results. 5th ed. Philadelphia: Saunders Elsevier; 2006:1144–1166
6. Molyneux AJ, Kerr RS, Yu LM, et al. International Subarachnoid Aneurysm Trial (ISAT) of neurosurgical clipping versus endovascular coiling in 2143 patients with ruptured intracranial aneurysms: a randomised comparison of effects on survival, dependency, seizures, rebleeding, subgroups. Lancet 2005;366(9488):809–817
7. Unruptured intracranial aneurysms–risk of rupture and risks of surgical intervention. International Study of Unruptured Intracranial Aneurysms Investigators. N Engl J Med 1998;339(24):1725–1733

Case 37   Hypertensive Putaminal Hematoma

Remi Nader

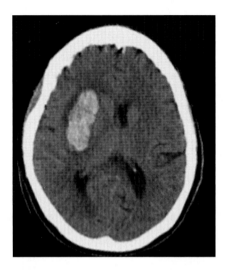

Fig. 37.1   Follow-up computed tomography scan without contrast at the level of the basal ganglia.

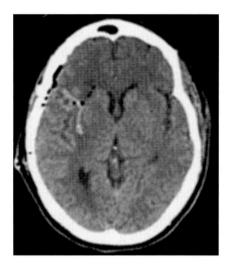

Fig. 37.2   Postoperative computed tomography scan without contrast at the same level of the basal ganglia.

■ Clinical Presentation

- A 56-year-old woman with diabetes mellitus, hypertension, and obesity presents with sudden-onset left-sided weakness.
- Initial studies show a 2-cm right-sided basal ganglia intracerebral hematoma (ICH).

- She is managed conservatively in the intensive care unit (ICU) initially; however, she starts becoming lethargic on day 5 and her weakness is more pronounced.
- A follow-up computed tomography (CT) scan is obtained (**Fig. 37.1**).

■ Questions

1. What are the criteria to operate on a basal ganglia ICH?
2. What would you recommend in this case?
3. What are the surgical and nonsurgical options?
4. What are the expected outcomes based on each option?

You decide to evacuate the ICH with a craniotomy. The procedure goes well, but postoperatively, the patient is still lethargic and hard to arouse; she remains this way for over 12 hours. A postoperative CT scan is obtained (**Fig. 37.2**).

5. Provide a differential diagnosis.
6. What is your management now?

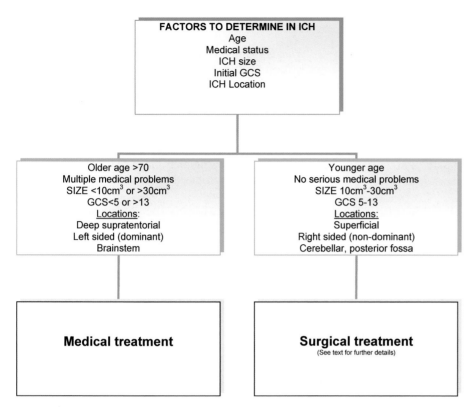

Fig. 37.3 Guidelines for the treatment of intracerebral hemorrhage. (GCS, Glasgow Coma Scale; ICH, intracerebral hemorrhage.) (Adapted from Mendelow AD, Gregson BA, Fernandes HM, et al. Early surgery versus initial conservative treatment in patients with spontaneous supratentorial intracerebral haematomas in the International Surgical Trial in Intracerebral Haemorrhage (STICH): a randomised trial. Lancet 2005;365:387–397; Broderick JP, Adams HP Jr, Barsan W, et al. Guidelines for the management of spontaneous intracerebral hemorrhage. A statement for healthcare professionals from a special writing group of the Stroke Council, American Heart Association. Stroke 1999;30:905–915.)

■ Answers

1. *What are the criteria to operate on basal ganglia ICH?*
   - The recent International Surgical Trial in Intracerebral Haemorrhage (STICH) trial[2] suggests that prophylactic removal of ICH had no clear advantage over medical management with removal only if deterioration occurs.[2]
   - Some of the reasons to favor surgery have been[1–5]:
     - Symptomatic patients with potential for acceptable recovery who seem to be worsening rapidly despite medical management
     - Moderate ICH volume (~10–30 mL)
     - Favorable location
     - Younger age
     - Edema
     - Midline shift
     - Reversible symptoms due to increase intracranial pressure (ICP)
   - Surgery has also been viewed as a more favorable option when performed relatively early.
   - These factors are, however, controversial, given more recent prospective studies.

2. *What would you recommend in this case?*
   - This patient does fit some of the current criteria:
     - She is relatively young (56 years old).
     - The location is favorable (right-sided, nondominant).
     - The size is favorable (~20–30 mL).
     - There is midline shift as well as some mass effect.
     - There has been a deterioration in her mental status.
   - Given these factors, surgery should be offered as an option to the family with clear understanding that expected outcome may only be slightly improved at best. Also observation is a reasonable option as well, given the family's wishes (**Fig. 37.3**). In this case, the family did opt for surgery.

3. *What are the surgical and nonsurgical options?*
   - Small craniotomy and resection
   - Stereotactic technique for drainage of hematoma[5]
   - Placement of catheter in the ICH ± tPA (tissue plasminogen activator) infusion
   - Ultrasound (Cavitron ultrasonic aspirator [CUSA]) aspiration

■ Answers (*continued*)

4. *What are the expected outcomes based on each option?*
   - There is no significant difference in long-term outcomes between observation and surgery in general regarding deep-seated brain ICH
   - 25% favorable outcome overall
   - 2–3% absolute difference in favorable outcome between surgery and observation (based on STICH study)[2]

5. *Provide a differential diagnosis.*
   - Swelling/edema
   - Infarction /stroke
   - Seizures
   - Metabolic deterioration (hypo/hypernatremia, hypoxia, hypercapnia)
   - Infection
   - Side effect of medications
   - Endocrinopathy

6. *What is your management now?*
   - Given the fact that the postoperative CT (**Fig. 37.2**) shows complete resolution of the hematoma with no significant mass effect, midline shift, or other evidence of increased ICP, the problem remains nonsurgical at this point.
   - Medical management in ICU
     – Laboratories: complete blood count, electrolytes, coagulation profile, drug levels, liver function tests, endocrine panel
     – Cultures: blood, urine, sputum, cerebrospinal fluid (lumbar puncture)
     – Seizure prophylaxis medications
     – Intravenous fluids
   - May consider magnetic resonance imaging if infarct is suspected

■ References

1. Donnan GA, Davis SM. Surgery for intracerebral hemorrhage: an evidence-poor zone. Stroke 2003;34(6):1569–1570
2. Mendelow AD, Gregson BA, Fernandes HM, et al. Early surgery versus initial conservative treatment in patients with spontaneous supratentorial intracerebral haematomas in the International Surgical Trial in Intracerebral Haemorrhage (STICH): a randomised trial. Lancet 2005;365:387–397
3. Auer LM, Deinsberger W, Niederkorn K, et al. Endoscopic surgery versus medical treatment for spontaneous intracerebral hematoma: a randomized study. J Neurosurg 1989;70:530–535
4. Broderick JP, Adams HP Jr, Barsan W, et al. Guidelines for the management of spontaneous intracerebral hemorrhage. A statement for healthcare professionals from a special writing group of the Stroke Council, American Heart Association. Stroke 1999;30:905–915
5. Peresedov VV. Strategy, technology, and techniques of surgical treatment of supratentorial intracerebral hematomas. Comput Aided Surg 1999;4(1):51–63

Case 38   Intraventricular Hemorrhage

Hosam Al-Jehani, Denis J. Sirhan, and Abdulrahman J. Sabbagh

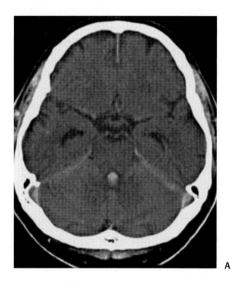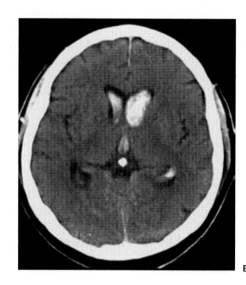

Fig. 38.1 Computed tomography scan without contrast at the level of **(A)** the 4th ventricle and **(B)** foramen of Monro revealing extensive intraventricular hemorrhage with mild ventricular dilatation.

A

B

■ Clinical Presentation

- A 34-year-old man previously healthy presents to the emergency department complaining of a headache, mild nausea, and unsteady gait.
- There are no focal neurologic deficits on physical examination.

- Coagulation profile is within normal limits.
- A computed tomography (CT) scan is done and shown in **Fig. 38.1**. It reveals an intraventricular hemorrhage with mild hydrocephalus.

■ Questions

1. How would you classify intraventricular hemorrhage (IVH)?
2. What are the pathophysiologic consequences of IVH?
3. Could the clinical picture help differentiate between primary and secondary IVH?
4. How would you grade IVH?
5. How would you grade hydrocephalus associated with IVH?
6. What are the treatment options for IVH?
7. What is the prognosis of IVH?

■ Answers

1. *How would you classify IVH?*
   - Intraventricular hemorrhage is classified into[1,2]
     - Primary IVH: in which the bleeding occurs directly into the ventricle, from a source or lesion that is in contact with or is part of the ventricular wall. This represents ~3% of all spontaneous intracerebral bleeding (intracerebral hemorrhage; ICH).
     - Secondary IVH: More common, in which the blood is introduced into the ventricular system either by dissection of an ICH or spill out of subarachnoid hemorrhage (SAH).
     - For causes of IVH see **Table 38.1**.[2]
2. *What are the pathophysiologic consequences of IVH?*
   - The cerebrospinal fluid (CSF) has limited fibrinolytic activity that renders it unable to dissolve the blood clots at critical areas of the ventricular system.
   - This will result in acute obstructive hydrocephalus that could be associated with morbidity or even mortality if the intracranial pressure (ICP) is not controlled.
   - The concept is further supported by the observation that IVH volume may be associated with a commensurate decrease in global cerebral blood flow.[1,2]
   - There is a hypothesis that the enhanced morbidity associated with IVH is attributable, at least in part, to the pressure exerted by the clot on periventricular structures. This emphasizes the possible impact of a treatment that prevents IVH or limits further IVH expansion.[1]
   - Blood degradation occurs slowly by hemolysis of erythrocytes and phagocytosis by macrophages.[3] These events lead to an increased risk of communicating hydrocephalus secondary to the blockage of the arachnoid granulations, and carry a small risk for cerebral vasospasm.[3]

Table 38.1   Causes for Intraventricular Hemorrhage (IVH)

Primary IVH	Secondary IVH
Germinal matrix H	HTN H
Vascular malformation, PV or IV	SAH (aneurysms)
AVM	ACOM aneurysms (most common IVH 25%)
Subependymal	• Forceful IPH dissect parenchyma to reach V.
Choroid plexus	PICA aneurysms 1/2 will have IVH.
Cerebral (PV)	ACOM, MCA aneurysms
• Associated with deep venous drainage	• → Frontal H → Ant horn of lateral V
Cavernous angioma	ICA aneurysm (PCOM or ACHOR)
	• Rupture into temporal horn
	Basilar apex aneurysms
	• Rupture directly to hypothalamus to 3rd V
Tumor: periventricular or intraventricular	Vascular malformation
Malignant astrocytoma *most common*	Cerebral AVMs with deep venous drainage
Papilloma	Dural AV-fistulas, cavernomas that have transcerebral venous drainage
Subependymoma	
Choroid plexus papilloma	
IV meningioma	Tumor
Neurocytoma	Pituitary apoplexy
Pituitary tumors eroding through 3rd V floor	
Granular cell tumor	
Metastasis	
Trauma	Vasculitis or amyloid angiopathy
Coagulation or platelet disorders	Coagulation or platelet disorders
Ventricular catheter insertion or removal	Trauma
Aneurysms, IV rare:	H Cerebral infarction
Lenticulostriate	
Choroidal	
Idiopathic	ETOH, illicit drug use (i.e., amphetamines)

Source: Adapted from Findlay JM. Intraventricular hemorrhage. In: Choi DW, Grotta JC, Weir B, Wolf PA, Mohr JP, eds. Stroke: Pathophysiology, Diagnosis, and Management. 4th ed. New York: Churchill Livingstone; 2004:1231–1243. Adapted with permission.

Abbreviations: ACHOR, anterior choroidal artery; ACOM, anterior communicating artery; Ant, anterior; AV, arteriovenous; AVM, arteriovenous malformation; Ch, choroid; ETOH, alcohol; H, hemorrhage or hemorrhagic; HTN, hypertensive; IPH, intraparenchymal hemorrhage; IV, intraventricular; IVH, intraventricular hemorrhage; MCA, middle cerebral artery; PICA, posterior inferior cerebellar artery; PCOM, posterior communicating artery; PV, periventricular; SAH, subarachnoid hemorrhage.

■ Answers (*continued*)

- Another interesting finding with patients who present with IVH, especially those with clinical signs of high ICP, is electrocardiographic (ECG) changes in the form of focal or generalized ST-T wave changes that could be misinterpreted as an acute myocardial infarction. This phenomenon is associated with sympathetic overdrive associated with the IVH and should be self-resolving once the ICP is under control.

3. *Could the clinical picture help differentiate between primary and secondary IVH?*
   - It is possible in certain circumstances to differentiate between the two types of IVH.
   - Clinical features of each type are summarized in **Table 38.2**.[2]

4. *How would you grade IVH?*
   - There are two grading scales.[1,4,5]
   - Graeb et al.[3] devised an IVH scale (maximum score is 12).
     - Lateral ventricles score
       1. Trace amount of blood or mild bleeding
       2. Less than half of the ventricle filled with blood
       3. More than half of the ventricle filled with blood
       4. Ventricle expanded and filled with blood
     - 3rd and 4th ventricles score
       1. Blood present without dilatation
       2. Ventricle expanded and filled with blood
     - Each ventricle is scored separately, including both lateral ventricles.
   - LeRoux et al.[6] described another IVH scale (Maximum score is 16).
     - Lateral, 3rd, and 4th ventricles score
       1. Trace of blood
       2. Less than half of the ventricle filled with blood
       3. More than half of the ventricle filled with blood
       4. Ventricle expanded and filled with blood
     - Each ventricle is scored separately, including both lateral ventricles.

5. *How would you grade hydrocephalus associated with IVH?*
   - Diringer et al.[7] described a hydrocephalus scale (Maximum score is 24.).
   - See **Table 38.3** for details of the scale.[8]

6. *What are the treatment options for IVH?*
   - The underlying cause must be treated.[8]
     - Needless to say, the primary cause of the IVH should be treated to prevent expansion or recurrence of the IVH. The blood pressure should be kept under control as appropriate for each patient, and correction of the coagulation abnormalities should be of primary importance.
     - There is no evidence that open surgical procedure will alter the natural history. On the contrary, they have been reported to portray worse prognosis. Some authors advocate the use of neuroendoscopy for the breakage and clearance of IVH followed by the insertion of unilateral or bilateral external ventricular drain (EVD) for further drainage.[9]
   - EVD[5]
     - Aids in relieving the hydrocephalus, if present, and helps the clearance of the CSF. This could be associated with the risk of catheter blockage that could necessitate replacement if irrigation and flushing of the catheter was not successful.
     - Prolonged use could be necessary in certain cases, which could increase the rate of infection. One should keep a close surveillance on CSF cell counts and cultures to detect early signs of infection and replace the drain accordingly.
     - Bilateral catheter placement might become indicated in certain 3rd ventricular clots that blocks the outflow through the foramen of Monro sequestering the lateral ventricles.

Table 38.2   Clinical Features of Primary and Secondary Intraventricular Hemorrhage (IVH)

Primary IVH	Secondary IVH
Symptoms may be surprisingly minimal (provided normal size of the ventricles and normal ICP)	Symptoms related to associated SAH or ICH Corresponds to location and size
Sudden headache	
Vomiting	
Altered LOC	
Generalized seizure	
No focal signs	

Source: From Findlay JM. Intraventricular hemorrhage. In: Choi DW, Grotta JC, Weir B, Wolf PA, Mohr JP, eds. Stroke: Pathophysiology, Diagnosis, and Management. 4th ed. New York: Churchill Livingstone; 2004:1231–1243. Reprinted with permission.

Abbreviations: ICH, intracerebral hemorrhage; ICP, intracranial pressure; IVH, intraventricular hemorrhage; LOC, level of consciousness; SAH, subarachnoid hemorrhage.

■ **Answers (***continued***)**

Table 38.3   Diringer Hydrocephalus Scale (Maximum Score Is 24)*

Score	0	1	2	3
Lateral				
Frontal horn	No dilatation	Mild	Moderate	Rounding, increasing radius, decreasing ventricular angle, and sulcal effacement of the lobe
Atrium	No dilatation	Mild	Moderate	Rounding and enlargement with sulcal effacement of the parietooccipital lobe
Temporal horn	No dilatation	Mild	Moderate	Increased width
3rd Ventricle	No dilatation	Mild	Moderate	Increased width and ballooning of the anterior recess
4th Ventricle	No dilatation	Mild	Moderate	Ballooning

Source: Adapted from Diringer MN, Edwards DF, Zazulia AR. Hydrocephalus: a previously unrecognized predictor of poor outcome from supratentorial intracerebral hemorrhage. Stroke 1998;29(7):1352–1357.

*The score depends on the amount of ventricular dilatation. The more the ventricle is dilated, the higher the score. All individual scores for each ventricle are added up, providing a final score.

- Intraventricular fibrinolytic treatment[5,10,11]
  - It has been found in animal models as well as in human studies that intraventricular thrombolysis expedites clot resolution and reestablishment of CSF flow. This is currently achieved using recombinant tissue plasminogen activator (rt-PA). This could achieve clot clearance in as fast as 3 or 4 days. It is also shown to reduce the 30-day mortality and reduces the cohort of poor outcome state (from 67% to 32%).
  - Contraindications to thrombolysis include large intraparenchymal hemorrhage (IPH) or IPH associated with deep or prominent cerebral tissue destruction. Another contraindication is a concomitant diagnosis associated with poor prognosis or evidence of brainstem dysfunction not in keeping with intracranial hypertension.
  - A practical approach to thrombolysis mandates a CT scan postinsertion of the EVD to ensure safe placement (all the holes of the catheter need to be within the ventricle). The dose of the rt-PA is 2–4 mg (1 mg/mL solution). It is injected slowly with frequent checking of the ICP. After the dose is delivered completely, the EVD should be closed for 1 hour, provided that the ICP is controlled, after which the EVD should be opened to a loop of 2 cm above the ear to allow drainage of the CSF. Some advocate alternating closure and opening of the EVD every hour for 24 hours to avoid collapse of the ventricle and delay the clearance of the thrombolytic agent.

7. *What is the prognosis for IVH?*
   - The prognosis is not necessarily poor. Poor outcome predictors include[1,2,12]
     - Secondary IVH associated with a large ICH or SAH
     - Anticoagulant treatment
     - Poor neurologic condition on presentation
     - Note that quantity of blood in the ventricles and presence of hydrocephalus do not necessarily correlate with outcome.[12]
   - Recent series reveal the following overall outcomes for IVH[2,4,12]:
     - Good outcome: ~36–54%
     - Mild to moderate disability: 39–50%
     - Severe disability: 17–35%
     - Death: 8–25%

■ References

1. Hanley DF, Naff NJ, Harris DM. Intraventricular hemorrhage: presentation and management options. Seminars in Cerebrovascular Diseases and Stroke 2005;5(3):209–216

2. Findlay JM. Intraventricular hemorrhage. In: Choi DW, Grotta JC, Weir B, Wolf PA, Mohr JP, eds. Stroke: Pathophysiology, Diagnosis, and Management. 4th ed. New York: Churchill Livingstone; 2004:1231–1243

3. Mayer SA, Lignelli A, Fink ME, et al. Perilesional blood flow and edema formation in acute intracerebral hemorrhage: a SPECT study. Stroke 1998;29(9):1791–1798

4. Graeb DA, Robertson WD, Lapointe JS, Nugent RA, Harrison PB. Computed tomographic diagnosis of intraventricular hemorrhage. Etiology and prognosis. Radiology 1982;143(1):91–96

5. LeRoux PD, Haglund MM, Newell DW, Grady MS, Winn HR. Intraventricular hemorrhage in blunt head trauma: an analysis of 43 cases. Neurosurgery 1992;31(4):678–685

6. Tuhrim S, Horowitz DR, Sacher M, Godbold JH. Volume of ventricular blood is an important determinant of outcome in supratentorial intracerebral hemorrhage. Crit Care Med 1999;27(3):617–621

7. Gerard E, Frontera JA, Wright CB. Vasospasm and cerebral infarction following isolated intraventricular hemorrhage. Neurocrit Care 2007;7(3):257–259

8. Diringer MN, Edwards DF, Zazulia AR. Hydrocephalus: a previously unrecognized predictor of poor outcome from supratentorial intracerebral hemorrhage. Stroke 1998;29(7):1352–1357

9. Longatti PL, Martinuzzi A, Fiorindi A, Maistrello L, Carteri A. Neuroendoscopic management of intraventricular hemorrhage. Stroke 2004;35(2):e35–e38

10. Findlay JM, Grace MG, Weir BK. Treatment of intraventricular hemorrhage with tissue plasminogen activator. Neurosurgery 1993;32(6):941–947

11. Findlay JM, Jacka MJ. Cohort study of intraventricular thrombolysis with recombinant tissue plasminogen activator for aneurysmal intraventricular hemorrhage. Neurosurgery 2004;55(3):532–537

12. Roos YB, Hasan D, Vermeulen M. Outcome in patients with large intraventricular haemorrhages: a volumetric study. J Neurol Neurosurg Psychiatry 1995;58(5):622–624

Case 39   Cerebellar Hemorrhage

Julius July and Eka Julianta Wahjoepramono

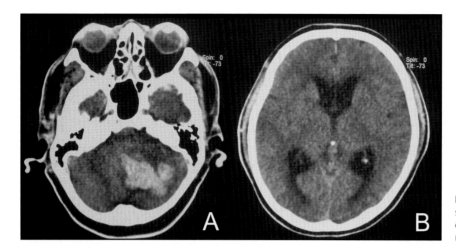

Fig. 39.1   Plain computed tomography scan showing left cerebellar hemorrhage **(A)** with effacement of 4th ventricle and **(B)** enlargement of the lateral ventricles.

■ Clinical Presentation

- A 55-year-old man with a long history of poorly controlled hypertension, diabetes mellitus, and heavy smoking presents to the emergency room with acute decreased level of conscious.
- This morning, he awakened with a headache that has progressively gotten worse.

- On physical examination, he opens his eyes spontaneously and localizes the pain. There is no obvious weakness in his extremities. Pupils are both 3 mm and responsive to light. Initial blood pressure is 200/110 mm Hg.
- A computed tomography (CT) scan is obtained and shown in **Fig. 39.1**.

■ Questions

1. What is your initial management?
2. Describe your surgical plan.

3. After you open the dura, you observe a very swollen and tight brain. What are your steps in managing intraoperative brain swelling?
4. Describe your postoperative care.

■ Answers

1. *What is your initial management?*
   - The cerebellar hemorrhage seen on CT is most likely due to hypertension.
   - A small number of patients can present with micro-aneurysm of the posterior circulation, which rupture and give a similar clinical picture.[1]
   - The frequency of cerebellar hemorrhage ranges between 5–10% of all intracranial hemorrhages (ICHs), and occurs predominantly in the older age groups, from the sixth to the eighth decades.
   - The history of diabetes in this case is also considered a general risk factor for developing a cerebellar hemorrhage.
   - Recommendation for surgical intervention on cerebellar hemorrhage include
     - Patients with Glasgow Coma Score (GCS) ≤13 or with hematoma size ≥4 cm.
     - Ventricular catheter placement is recommended for patients with hydrocephalus and no coagulopathy. Most cases with hydrocephalus also require evacuation of the hematoma.
     - The presence of the "tight posterior fossa" (TPF) concept, described by Weisberg et al.,[2] warrants surgical intervention. Weisberg defines this concept as
       - Obliteration of the basal cistern of the posterior cranial fossa
       - Enlargement of the third ventricle, lateral ventricle, and temporal horn
       - Effacement of the 4th ventricle
     - The TPF does not only depend on the size of the hematoma. A hematoma of similar size may exert widely differing amounts of compression. This is probably due to several factors including patient's age, the amount of cerebellar atrophy and the anatomy of the posterior fossa. Based on the TPF concept, the critical size for hematoma evacuation can be reduced by 5–10 mm to a size of 3 cm.[1,2]
   - Intensive therapy is not indicated in patients with absent brainstem reflexes and flaccid quadriplegia, that is, in moribund condition.[1–3]

2. *Describe your surgical plan.*
   - Initially, a ventricular catheter is inserted (one may choose the entry site at Kocher's point or a Frazier burr hole site). Two to 3 cc of cerebrospinal fluid (CSF) are drained slowly to control the intracranial pressure (ICP) then the drainage is stopped to avoid upward herniation.
   - A suboccipital craniectomy is then performed with goal of removing the ICH, decompressing the brainstem, and relieving hydrocephalus. The external drain can be opened after the dural opening.

   - A transverse incision along the folia closest to the most superficial part of the clot is performed. After removing the ICH, meticulous hemostasis should be completed. The blood clot should be sent to histopathology for examination.
   - Very often the cerebellum itself will swell after the surgery. It is better to close the dura via a duraplasty, using pericranium, fascia lata, or synthetic dura.
   - The ventricular catheter in general is kept temporarily. However, some cases necessitate conversion to a permanent ventriculoperitoneal shunt.[1,3]

3. *After you open the dura, you observe a very swollen and tight brain. What are your steps in managing intraoperative brain swelling?*
   - The following is a checklist of steps to ensure proper management of intraoperative posterior fossa swelling[4,5]:
     - Elevate the patient's head to above 30 degrees.
     - Check neck positioning for obstruction of venous return and readjust as necessary.
     - Hyperventilate to a PCO_2 of 30–35 mm Hg.
     - Infuse a dose of mannitol and/or Lasix (Aventis Pharmaceuticals, Parsippany, NJ).
     - Ensure adequate sedation and pharmacologic muscle paralysis.
     - Decompress the hematoma!
     - Drain some CSF from the ventriculostomy.
     - Open the cisterna magna and drain some more CSF.
     - One may need to resect parts of the cerebellar hemisphere.
     - Ensure that the foramen magnum is open.
     - If the swelling is still uncontrollable, then consider the following causes:
       - Intraparenchymal hematoma in a different location
       - Contralateral or supratentorial subdural or epidural hematoma
       - Cytotoxic edema from trauma
       - Venous infarction
     - In intractable cases, some of the following steps may be considered:
       - Duraplasty and quick closure
       - Keeping the bone flap out (i.e., craniectomy)
       - Obtaining an emergent CT scan of the head and considering going back to the operating room for further exploration.
       - In the past, exploratory supratentorial burr holes were suggested. However, with the advent of fast spiral CT scanners, an adequate scan can be completed within minutes eliminating the need and potential risks associated with such a procedure.

Answers (*continued*)

4. *Describe your postoperative care.*
   - Postoperatively, the patient should be monitored in the intensive care unit for at least 24 hours in anticipation of the peak of arterial blood pressure. Blood pressure should be closely monitored with an arterial line and controlled closely with intravenous (i.v.) antihypertensives (such as nitroprusside or nicardipine).
   - Patients with a critical neurologic condition remain under mechanical ventilation and receive a full dose of corticosteroid (dexamethasone 10 mg i.v. once, then 6 mg i.v. every 6 hours).
   - If required, mannitol may be administered to reduce ICP.
   - A postoperative CT scan should be completed within 24 hours (**Fig. 39.2**).
   - As the patient's neurologic condition improves, he may be transferred to the neurosurgical ward and subsequently discharged from the hospital once the blood pressure remains under control with oral antihypertensives.[1,3]

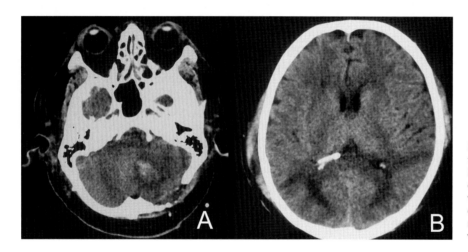

Fig. 39.2 **(A)** Postoperative computed tomography scan shows that most of the blood clot has been removed from the left cerebellum, but the posterior fossa is still very tight. **(B)** The computed tomography confirms the ventricular catheter placement, and the reduction in size of the lateral ventricles.

References

1. Raco A. Surgical management of cerebellar hemorrhage and cerebellar infarction. In: Schmideck HH, Roberts DW, eds. Schmidek & Sweet's Operative Neurosurgical Techniques. Indication, Methods, and Results. 5th ed. Philadelphia: Saunders Elsevier; 2006:859–872
2. Weisberg LA. Acute cerebellar hemorrhage and CT evidence of tight posterior fossa. Neurology 1986;36(6):858–860
3. Singh RVP, Prusmack CJ, Morcos JJ. Spontaneous intracerebral hemorrhage: non-arteriovenous malformation, nonaneurysm. In: Winn RH. Neurological Surgery. 5th ed. Philadelphia: Saunders; 2004:1371–1387
4. Greenberg MS. Handbook of Neurosurgery. 6th ed. New York: Thieme Medical Publishers; 2006
5. Horwitz NH, Rizzoli HV. Postoperative Complications of Intracranial Neurological Surgery. Baltimore: Williams & Wilkins; 1983

Case 40   **Moyamoya Disease**

Abdulrahman J. Sabbagh, Jean-Pierre Farmer, Jie Ma, Ahmad I. Lary, and José Luis Montes

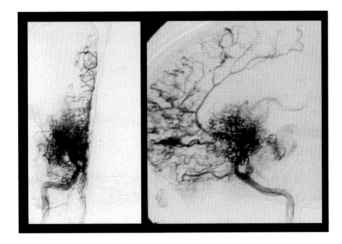

Fig. 40.1   Cerebral angiogram, internal carotid artery injection, with anteroposterior **(A)** and lateral **(B)** views.

■ Clinical Presentation

- A 2-year-old girl had been born at term through a spontaneous vaginal delivery after a noneventful pregnancy.
- She was normal up to 14 months of age, when she presented with a left-sided simple partial motor seizure that was treated with an antiepileptic.
- At 23 months of age, she developed a new aphasia and right-sided weakness.
- Magnetic resonance imaging (MRI) and magnetic resonance angiography (MRA) were performed, which prompted the ordering of an angiogram, shown in **Fig. 40.1**.

■ Questions

1. Describe the pertinent findings on the angiogram (**Fig. 40.1**).

A physician starts her on aspirin 81 mg per day; by the time she sees you, she develops a new left foot drop.

2. What would be your management strategy?
3. What is the definition of moyamoya disease (MMD)?
4. What are the clinical presentations in children for MMD?

5. What are the factors associated with MMD?
6. What are the angiographic stages of MMD?
7. What is the pathophysiology of moyamoya vessel occlusion and formation?
8. What is the natural history of MMD in the pediatric population?
9. What are examples of revascularization procedures?
10. Describe briefly the principles of an encephaloduroarteriosynangiosis (EDAS) procedure.

■ Answers

1. *Describe the pertinent findings on the angiogram* (**Fig. 40.1**).
   - Left internal carotid angiography shows
     - Occlusion of the right internal carotid artery at the anterior cerebral artery (ACA)–middle cerebral artery (MCA) bifurcation
     - Extensive hypertrophy of moyamoya vessels
2. *A physician starts her on aspirin 81 mg per day; by the time she sees you, she develops a new left foot drop. What would be your management strategy?*
   - Management of pediatric ischemic attack in a patient with MMD[1,2]:
     - Admit her to the pediatric intensive care unit.
       - Oxygenation
       - Hydration
       - Monitoring with frequent neuro checks
     - Consult pediatric neurology service to manage the new stroke.
     - Anticoagulation instead of aspirin in preparation for surgery:
       - Low-molecular-weight heparin: for example, Lovenox (Sonafi-Aventis, Bridgewater, NJ) at 0.5 mg/kg twice a day.
     - Obtain imaging studies: Computed tomography (CT) scan of the head, CT angiography or digital angiography, MRI, CT perfusion, positron emission tomography (PET) scan, etc.
     - These studies are obtained as a baseline assessment of vascular occlusion to assess extent of cerebral infarction, for documentation of new changes, and for surgical planning.
     - Preoperative planning and investigation for a revascularization procedure
3. *What is the definition of MMD?*
   - *Moyamoya* is a Japanese term that was first used by Suzuki and Takaku in 1969.[3]
   - It is a radiologic term that translates as something hazy or ill-defined, like a cloud of smoke.[2]
   - It is a form of progressive cerebral arteriopathy characterized by[2]
     - Progressive occlusion of
       - Terminal internal carotid artery (ICA)
       - ACAs or MCAs
     - Profuse lenticulostriate collateral formation (moyamoya vessels) at the base of the brain
4. *What are the clinical presentations in children for MMD?*
   - Clinical presentation in children includes[1,4]
   - Ischemic symptoms in 80%
     - Cerebral infarction
     - Transient ischemic attack

   - Epilepsy in 5%
   - Intracranial hemorrhage in 2.5%
   - Other symptoms in 12.5% (headache, movement disorders, or a mixture of symptoms)
5. *What are the factors associated with MMD?*
   - Associated factors include[4-6]
     - Asian ethnicity
     - Neurofibromatosis type I, especially if with radiation for an optic nerve glioma
     - Radiation for optic or hypothalamic pathway glioma or craniopharyngioma
     - Down syndrome
     - Renal artery stenosis
     - Hypertension
     - Thalassemia and sickle cell anemia
     - Other conditions
6. *What are the angiographic stages of MMD?*
   - MMD has six angiographic stages (**Fig. 40.2**).[3,7]
     - Stage 1: Narrowing of the carotid bifurcation
     - Stage 2: Initiation of the moyamoya vessels and dilatation of the intracerebral main arteries
     - Stage 3: Intensification of the moyamoya vessels and nonfilling of the ACAs and MCAs
     - Stage 4: Minimization of the moyamoya vessels and disappearance of the posterior cerebral artery
     - Stage 5: Reduction of the moyamoya vessels. The main arteries arising from the ICA disappear.
     - Stage 6: Complete loss of the moyamoya vessels. Only the collateral circulation from the external carotid artery is seen at this stage.
7. *What is the pathophysiology of moyamoya vessel occlusion and formation?*
   - Pathophysiology of arterial occlusion and formation in MMD are described below (**Fig. 40.3**).[8-10]
     - Angiogenic factors such as CRABP-1 (cellular retinoic acid binding protein), bFGF (fibroblast growth factor), TGF-β (transforming growth factor-β), HGF (hepatocyte growth factor), and others contribute to
       - A slow and long-term proliferation and migration of intimal smooth muscle deposition eventually causing vessel occlusion
       - Revascularization and formation of the moyamoya vessels
       - Vasodilatation of collaterals
     - Other genetic and environmental factors come into play.[8-10]
8. *What is the natural history of MMD in the pediatric population?*

■ Answers (*continued*)

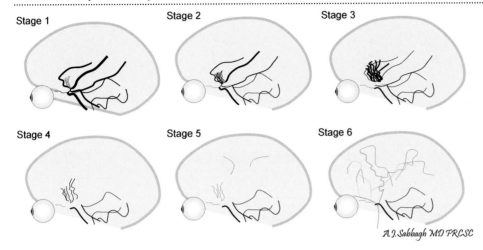

Fig. 40.2 Artist's rendering of the angiographic stages of moyamoya disease. This illustrates lateral projection angiograms at each stage, with the globe and anterior portion on the left side. See text for detailed description of each stage. Note: The thinner collection of straight black lines at the internal cerebral artery bifurcation represent the moyamoya vessels (stage 1), which become thicker at stages 2 and 3; the extracranial collaterals are illustrated in red hatched lines (stage 6).

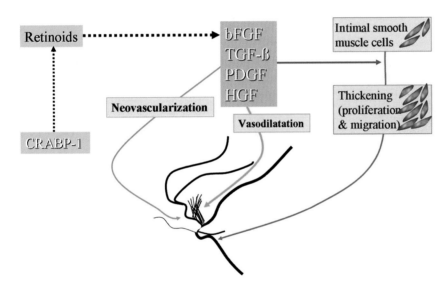

Fig. 40.3 Pathophysiology of arterial occlusion and formation in moyamoya disease. Solid arrows, cause; hatched arrows, inhibit. Thick black lines represent a lateral carotid injection arteriogram with the internal carotid artery (ICA), middle cerebral and anterior cerebral arteries illustrated. The thinner collection of straight black lines at the ICA bifurcation represent the moyamoya vessels. (bFGF, fibroblast growth factor; CRABP-1, cellular retinoic acid binding protein-1; HGF, hepatocyte growth factor; TGF-β, transforming growth factor-β.)

- The natural history of MMD in the pediatric population[11]
  - In patients who are not surgically revascularized, only around 23% subsequently improve, 20% do not change, and up to 57% get worse (these results are based on a study by Choi et al.[11] of 52 subjects with a mean follow-up of 67.2 months).
  - 65% of patients of the same age group that are revascularized improve, 23% remain unchanged, and only 12% get worse (These results are based on a study by Choi et al.[11] of 36 subjects with a mean follow-up of 28.8 months).

9. *What are examples of revascularization procedures?*
- Indirect procedures include[5,11,12]
  - EDAS: encephaloduroarteriosynangiosis
  - EMS: encephalomyosynangiosis
  - EDAMS: encephaloduroarteriomyosynangiosis
  - Modified EDAS (pial synangiosis)
  - EGS: encephalogaleosynangiosis
  - Omental transfer

- Direct procedures include[12]
  - Superficial temporal artery to middle cerebral artery (STA–MCA) bypass

10. *Describe briefly the principles of an EDAS procedure.*
- The steps of an EDAS procedure include[2] (**Fig. 40.4**)
  - After preparing the scalp, the STAs and occipital arteries (OcAs) are outlined using a Doppler ultrasound; then the skin overlying them is opened and the vessels identified.
  - The STAs and OcAs are separated from neighboring tissues along with a strip of adventitia on either side of the vessels.
  - A craniotomy or a small craniectomy is performed, and then a Z-shape durotomy is tailored.
  - The adventitia is sutured to close the durotomy edges, making the STAs and the OcAs in close proximity to pial vessels.
  - This facilitates collateral development over time, from the external to the intracranial circulation.

■ Answers (*continued*)

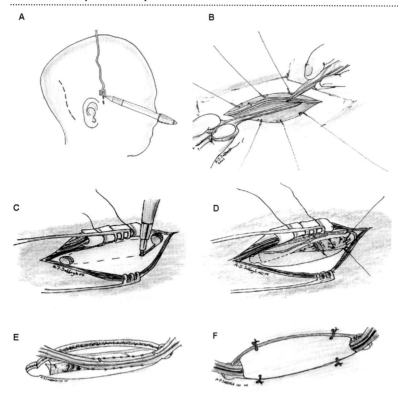

Fig. 40.4   Artist's rendering of the encephaloduroarteriosynangiosis procedure. **(A)** The superficial temporal (STAs) and occipital arteries (OcAs) are outlined. **(B)** The skin overlying them is opened and the vessels identified. **(C)** A small craniotomy is performed and then **(D)** a Z-shape durotomy is tailored. **(E)** The adventitia is sutured to close the durotomy edges, making the STAs and the OcAs in close proximity to pial vessels. **(F)** The craniotomy bone is then put back in place with careful attention not to occlude the implanted vessels.

■ References

1. Smith ER. Ischemic stroke in the pediatric population. In: Pollack IF, Adelson PD Albright AL, eds. *Principles and Practice of Pediatric Neurosurgery*. 2nd ed. New York/Stuttgart: Thieme Medical Publishers; 2008:1004–1013

2. David CA, Nottmeier E. Intracranial occlusion disease moyamoya. In: Winn HR ed. Youmans Neurological Surgery. Vol. 2. 5th ed. Philadelphia: Saunders; 2004:1715–1722

3. Suzuki J, Takaku A. Cerebrovascular "moyamoya" disease. Disease showing abnormal net-like vessels in base of brain. Arch Neurol 1969;20(3):288–299

4. Chiu D, Shedden P, Bratina P, Grotta JC. Clinical features of moyamoya disease in the United States. Stroke 1998;29(7):1347–1351

5. Scott RM, Smith JL, Robertson RL, Madsen JR, Soriano SG, Rockoff MA. Long-term outcome in children with moyamoya syndrome after cranial revascularization by pial synangiosis. J Neurosurg 2004; 100(Suppl 2)142–149

6. Wakai K, Tamakoshi A, Ikezaki K, et al. Epidemiological features of moyamoya disease in Japan: findings from a nationwide survey. Clin Neurol Neurosurg 1997;99(Suppl 2):S1–S5

7. Fukuyama Y, Umezu R. Clinical and cerebral angiographic evolutions of idiopathic progressive occlusive disease of the circle of Willis ("moyamoya" disease) in children. Brain Dev 1985;7(1):21–37

8. Yoshimoto T, Houkin K, Takahashi A, Abe H. Angiogenic factors in moyamoya disease. Stroke 1996;27(12):2160–2165

9. Nanba R, Kuroda S, Ishikawa T, Houkin K, Iwasaki Y. Increased expression of hepatocyte growth factor in cerebrospinal fluid and intracranial artery in moyamoya disease. Stroke 2004;35(12):2837–2842

10. Kim SK, Yoo JI, Cho BK, et al. Elevation of CRABP-I in the cerebrospinal fluid of patients with moyamoya disease. Stroke 2003;34(12):2835–2841

11. Choi JU, Kim DS, Kim EY, Lee KC. Natural history of moyamoya disease: comparison of activity of daily living in surgery and non surgery groups. Clin Neurol Neurosurg 1997;99(Suppl 2):S11–S18

12. Fung LW, Thompson D, Ganesan V. Revascularisation surgery for paediatric moyamoya: a review of the literature. Childs Nerv Syst 2005;21(5):358–364

Case 41   Amaurosis Fugax with Carotid Occlusion

Glenn C. Hunter and Alwin Camancho

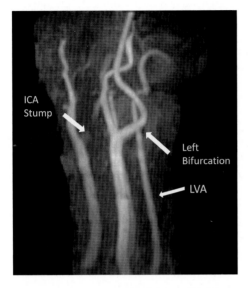

Fig. 41.1   Magnetic resonance angiography of the neck revealing right internal carotid artery (ICA) stump. (LVA, left vertebral artery.)

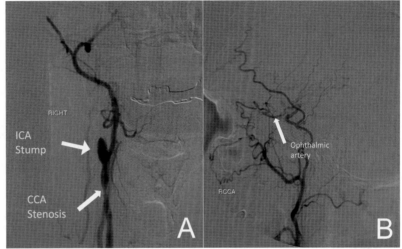

Fig. 41.2   Angiogram: **(A)** Right common carotid artery (CCA) injection showing internal carotid artery (ICA) distal stump (*arrow*) and CCA stenosis (*arrow*). **(B)** Selective external carotid artery injection showing communication between the internal and external circulation via the ophthalmic artery (*arrow*). (RCCA, right common carotid artery.)

■ Clinical Presentation

• A 70-year-old man presents to his ophthalmologist with worsening vision in the right eye.
• Three months previously he experienced an episode of amaurosis fugax.
• A funduscopic exam shows a Hollenhorst plaque and diminished flow in a branch of the retinal artery.
• He is referred for urgent neurosurgical consultation.

■ Questions

1. List the differential diagnoses.
2. What are the most common causes of monocular visual symptoms?
3. What are the most common sources of thromboembolism?
4. Physical examination reveals bilateral carotid bruits and a blood pressure of 145/95 mm Hg. What studies would you obtain?

A carotid duplex scan and magnetic resonance angiography (MRA) are ordered. The MRA shows right internal carotid artery occlusion with a patent external carotid artery (ECA) (**Fig. 41.1**). The left carotid artery appears normal.

5. Outline your plan of management.
6. During your evaluation he experiences another episode of worsening vision. What are the potential causes of this episode?

7. How may this episode alter your treatment plan?
8. In view of the results of the MRA would you order a cerebral angiogram?
9. A four-vessel angiogram is obtained (**Fig. 41.2**). Interpret the findings on the right.
10. What is the significance and importance of a residual stump?
11. You consider doing a common carotid endarterectomy and excision of the stump. What is the risk and natural history of stroke in patients who present with monocular visual symptoms versus those who present with transient ischemic attacks (TIAs)?
12. What are the risk factors for stroke in patients with monocular visual symptoms?
13. How would you treat this patient?

■ Answers

1. *List the differential diagnoses.*
   - Ocular manifestations account for 15% of transient ischemic attacks. The differential diagnoses of this patient's symptoms include[1,2]
     - Amaurosis fugax
     - Hollenhorst plaque
     - Retinal artery occlusion (central/branch)
     - Venous stasis retinopathy
     - Nonspecific visual symptoms

2. *What are the most common causes of monocular visual symptoms?*
   - Visual symptoms in patients in this age group are most often due to thromboembolism and less often due to hypoperfusion.[3,4]

3. *What are the most common sources of thromboembolism?*
   - The carotid bifurcation is the most common embolic source in these patients.[4]
   - Cardiac thromboembolism (valves/aortic arch), intravascular injection of talc, and steroidal suspensions are other potential sources.

4. Physical examination reveals bilateral carotid bruits and a blood pressure of 145/95 mm Hg. What studies would you obtain?
   - The focus of the studies should be to find an embolic source. A carotid duplex scan would be the initial screening test.[2,5]

5. *Outline your plan of management.*
   - Admission to hospital
   - Locate potential embolic sources by obtaining CT, magnetic resonance imaging (MRI), computed tomography angiography (CTA), MRA
   - Exclude cardiac sources by obtaining electrocardiogram (EKG) and echocardiogram
   - Specific laboratory tests: complete blood count (CBC), electrolytes, blood glucose, coagulation profile, type and screen
   - Antiplatelet therapy

6. *During your evaluation, he experiences another episode of worsening vision. What are the potential causes of this episode?*
   - Worsening symptoms may be due to hypoperfusion or another embolic episode.[2,3]

7. *How may this episode alter your treatment plan?*
   - In patients with carotid occlusion, control of blood pressure is an important consideration. Also, if the patient is not on antiplatelet therapy or is taking only aspirin, an additional agent should be added. Heparin should be considered if the ipsilateral occlusion is recent.[3]

8. *In view of the results of the MRA, would you order a cerebral angiogram?*
   - The presence of persistent symptoms may warrant the following studies: A four-vessel cerebral angiogram allows assessment of the ECA and ophthalmic arteries and their collateral communication and will also eliminate a "string sign."
   - An MRI/ MRA may be used instead of the angiogram in patients with renal impairment, but may miss a string sign.
   - MRA tends to overestimate the stenoses in general.
   - CTA may be a better study, and can be obtained in a shorter time. However, it has limitations in patients with renal impairment.

9. *A four-vessel angiogram is obtained (**Fig. 41.2**). Interpret the findings on the right.*
   - The four-vessel angiogram shows occlusion of the right internal carotid artery (RICA) at its origin, with a residual stump and antegrade vertebral flow.

10. *What is the significance and importance of a residual stump?*
    - The residual stump may be an embolic source and if associated with a high-grade ECA stenosis may contribute to retinal hypoperfusion.[3,6,7]

11. *You consider doing a common carotid endarterectomy and excision of the stump. What is the risk and natural history of stroke in patients who present with monocular visual symptoms versus those who present with TIAs?*
    - The 3-year risk of ipsilateral stroke is 10% for patients with transient monocular blindness versus 20% for those presenting with hemispheric symptoms.[8]

12. *What are the risk factors for stroke in patients with monocular visual symptoms?*
    - Risk factors include[8]
      - Age >70
      - Male gender
      - History of TIA
      - History of intermittent claudication
      - Ipsilateral stenosis (80–99%)
      - Number of collaterals on angiography

13. *How would you treat this patient?*
    - The patient was treated with excision of the stump and common carotid artery (CCA) endarterectomy[9] and angioplasty with only minor improvement in symptoms.
    - **Fig. 41.3** presents a treatment algorithm for patients with ophthalmic manifestations of carotid disease.

■ Answers (*continued*)

Ophthalmic Manifestations of Carotid Disease

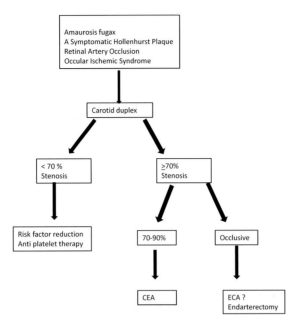

Fig. 41.3 Treatment algorithm for patients with ophthalmic manifestations of carotid disease. (Data from Wolintz RJ. Carotid endarterectomy for ophthalmic manifestations: is it ever indicated? J Neuro-Ophthalmol 2005;25(4):299-302.)

■ References

1. Ahuja RM, Chaturvedi S, Eliott D, Joshi N, Puklin J, Abrams GW. Mechanisms of retinal arterial occlusive disease in African American and Caucasian patients. Stroke 1999;30:1506–1509

2. Bull DA, Fante RG, Hunter GC, et al. Correlation of ophthalmic findings with carotid artery stenosis. J Cardiovasc Surg (Torino) 1992;33(4):401–406

3. Countee RW, Vijayanathan T, Chavis P. Recurrent retinal ischemia beyond cervical carotid occlusions: clinical-angiographic correlations and therapeutic implications. J Neurosurg 1981;55(4):532–542

4. Lawrence PF, Oderich GS. Ophthalmologic findings as predictors of carotid artery disease. Vasc Endovascular Surg 2002;36:415–424

5. McCullough HK, Reinert CG, Hynan LS, et al. Ocular findings as predictors of carotid artery occlusive disease: is carotid imaging justified? J Vasc Surg 2004;40:279–286

6. Barnett HJ, Peerless SJ, Kaufmann JC. "Stump" on internal carotid artery—a source for further cerebral embolic ischemia. Stroke 1978;9(5):448–456

7. McIntyre KE, Ely RL, Malone JM, Bernhard VM, Goldstone J. External carotid artery reconstruction: its role in the treatment of cerebral ischemia. Am J Surg 1985;150(1):58–64

8. Wolintz RJ. Carotid endarterectomy for ophthalmic manifestations: is it ever indicated? J Neuroophthalmol 2005;25(4):299–302

9. Benavente O, Eliasziw M, Streifler JY, Fox AJ, Barnett HJM, Meldrum H. Prognosis after transient monocular blindness associated with carotid-artery stenosis. N Engl J Med 2001;345(15):1084–1090

Case 42   In Tandem Extracranial and Intracranial Carotid Stenosis

Glenn C. Hunter

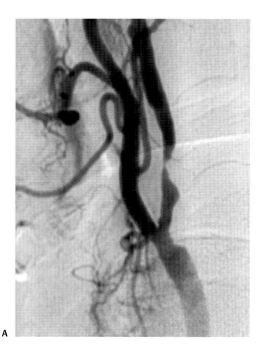 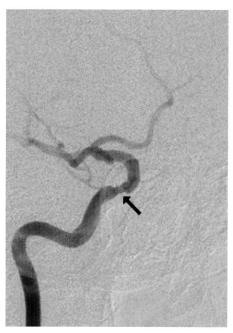

A   B

Fig. 42.1   Selective cerebral angiogram demonstrating (**A**) 70% extracranial ICA stenosis and (**B**) 50% intracranial ICA stenosis.

■ Clinical Presentation

- A 67-year-old right-handed woman presents to the emergency room (ER) with recurrent episodes of left hemispheric transient ischemic attacks (TIAs) with difficulty speaking and right-sided weakness.
- She has a history of hypertension, hyperlipidemia, type 2 diabetes mellitus, and had undergone a femoral-popliteal bypass 2 years previously.

- Pulse rate is 106/min, irregular. Blood pressure is 140/95 mm Hg. There are bilateral carotid bruits.
- Neurologic exam was intact.

■ Questions

1. What is the differential diagnosis?
2. The ER physician obtains a computed tomography (CT) scan, electrocardiogram (EKG), and orders a carotid duplex exam. Are there any further tests you would obtain at this time?
3. The EKG shows atrial fibrillation and duplex scan bilateral 50–79% internal carotid artery (ICA) stenosis. What is your initial management of this patient?
4. What are the guidelines for hospital admission of this patient?

The patient has urgent family problems and does not want to be admitted to hospital. She is already on aspirin so you add clopidogrel.

Two days later, she returns to the ER with another TIA that lasted 2 hours.

5. How does this change your management?

A four-vessel cervical and cerebral angiogram is ordered. The angiogram shows bilateral 70% ICA stenosis with a 50% siphon stenosis of the left ICA (**Fig. 42.1**). The left A-1 segment is not well visualized.

■ Questions (*continued*)

6. What are the risk factors for intracranial athero-sclerotic disease (IAD)? What are the risk factors for combined extracranial atherosclerotic disease (EAD) and IAD disease?
7. What are the causes of symptoms in patients with tandem carotid stenosis?
8. What is the distribution of an intracranial lesion?
9. What is the added risk of the presence of IAD in cases of preexisting EAD?

10. What is the recommended treatment for combined disease?
11. What is the risk of stroke, in general, in patients with carotid stenosis both symptomatic and asymptomatic? Provide your answer based on percentage of stenosis and modality of treatment (surgical vs. medical).
12. When would you perform surgery on this patient if she had had a stroke rather than a TIA?
13. What is the management of patients with inoperable disease?

■ Answers

1. *What is the differential diagnosis?*
   - The differential diagnosis should include
     - Carotid stenosis
     - Cardiac embolism
     - Carotid dissection
     - Hemiplegic migraine
     - Seizure disorder
     - Subdural hematoma
     - Tumor
     - Hypo/hyperglycemia
2. *The ER physician obtains a CT scan, EKG, and orders a carotid duplex exam. Are there any further tests you would obtain at this time?*
   - Full blood count
   - Screen electrolytes/renal function tests
   - Blood glucose, serum lipids
   - Cardiac enzymes
   - Coagulation studies
   - C-reactive protein
   - Chest x-ray
3. *The EKG shows atrial fibrillation and duplex scan bilateral 50–79% ICA stenosis. What is your initial management of this patient?*
   - Initial management of the patient should include
     - Admission to hospital for control of blood pressure, glucose, arrhythmias
     - Consider heparin if no intracranial bleeding
     - Magnetic resonance imaging (MRI)/magnetic resonance angiography (MRA)[1]
     - Cardiac echography
4. *What are the guidelines for hospital admission of this patient?*
   - Hospital admission should be considered for patients with first TIA within 24–48 hours and with:
     - Crescendo TIAs
     - Duration of symptoms >1 hour

5. *How does this change your management?*
   - Direct hospital admission
   - Repeat CT/MRI
   - Repeat duplex scan
   - Transcranial Doppler
6. *What are the risk factors for IAD? What are the risk factors for combined EAD and IAD disease?*
   - Risk factors for IAD[2]
     - Race: African American or Asian[3]
     - Gender: risk of 28.4% in females versus 16.6% in males[4]
     - Hypertension
     - Hyperlipidemia
     - Diabetes mellitus
   - Risk factors for combined EAD and IAD[2,5]
     - Diabetes mellitus
     - Coronary artery disease
7. *What are the causes of symptoms in patients with tandem carotid stenosis?*
   - Etiology of symptoms in patients with tandem disease
     - Embolism from carotid bifurcation
     - Hypoperfusion—IAD > EAD
8. *What is the distribution of an intracranial lesion?*
   - Distribution of IAD
     - ICA 49%
     - Middle cerebral artery (MCA) 20%
     - Posterior cerebral artery (PCA) 11%
     - Vertebrobasilar artery (V-B)11%
     - Anterior communicating artery (ACOM) 9%
9. *What is the added risk of the presence of IAD in cases of preexisting EAD?*
   - Deficits persist longer
   - Plaques more fibrotic[6]
   - Independent risk factor for stroke[3,7]
   - Risk of stroke is greater in IAD as compared with MCA lesions alone (36% vs. 24%).

■ Answers (*continued*)

10. *What is the recommended treatment for combined disease?*
    - Treatment of combined EAD and IAD stenosis
      - Carotid endarterectomy (CEA) in cases of 70–90% stenosis[8]
      - CEA if 50–79% EAD stenosis and 70% IAD stenosis[3,7]
      - Other options include
        - CEA and IAD angioplasty (Angioplasty and stenting are increasingly being used for intracranial disease. Long-term results and large population studies are not yet available.)
        - Carotid stenting (CAS)[9] and IAD angioplasty (32% restenosis in 6 months)
        - CEA is not beneficial if the IAD is worse than the EAD.
11. *What is the risk of stroke, in general, in patients with carotid stenosis both symptomatic and asymptomatic? Provide your answer based on percentage of stenosis and modality of treatment (surgical vs. medical).*
    - See **Table 42.1**[8,10,11] and **Table 42.2**[12-14] for a summary.

- In symptomatic cases[8]:
  - CEA is of benefit if there is 70–99% stenosis as long as surgical morbidity and mortality (M&M) is 6% or less. The stroke risk is overall decreased by ~8% per year.
  - CEA is of marginal benefit in cases of 50–69% stenosis. Consider this procedure if there are associated risk factors such as
    - Associated ulcerated lesion[7] (as in this case)
    - Contralateral ICA occlusion
    - Male gender
    - Intraluminal thrombus
    - Stroke more than transient (not TIA)
    - Younger age at presentation
- In asymptomatic cases[12]:
  - CEA is of marginal benefit in cases of 60–99% carotid stenosis.
  - Consider performing this procedure if
    - The overall operative risk (M&M) is ~3% or less
    - There are associated risk factors such as the ones described above.

Table 42.1 Comparison or Risks of Stroke between Medical and Surgical Treatment Modalities in Patients with Symptomatic Carotid Stenosis (Estimates Based on NASCET and ECST Studies)

Stenosis	Risk of Stroke at 2 Years with Medical Therapy (%)	Risk of Stroke at 2 Years with Surgical Therapy (CEA) (%)	Absolute Risk Reduction (%)	Perioperative M&M (%)
70–99% NASCET(8)	25	9	16	6
50–69% NASCET(8)	14.5	9.5	5	6
50–69% ESCT(10)	9.7	11	-1.5	10

Source: From North American Symptomatic Carotid Endarterectomy Trial Collaborators. Beneficial effect of carotid endarterectomy in symptomatic patients with high-grade carotid stenosis. N Engl J Med 1991;325(7):505–507; Randomised trial of endarterectomy for recently symptomatic carotid stenosis: final results of the MRC European Carotid Surgery Trial (ECST). Lancet 1998;351(9113):1379–1387; Mohr JP, Choi DW, Grotta JC, Weir B, Wolf PA. Stroke. Pathophysiology, Diagnosis, and Management. 4th ed. New York: Churchill Livingstone; 2004.[8,10,11]

Abbreviations: CEA, carotid endarterectomy; ECST, European Carotid Surgery Trial; M&M, morbidity and mortality; NASCET, North American Symptomatic Carotid Endarterectomy Trial.

Table 42.2 Comparison or Risks of Stroke between Medical and Surgical Treatment Modalities in Patients with Asymptomatic Carotid Stenosis (Estimates Based on ACAS and VA Studies)

Stenosis	Risk of Stroke with Medical Therapy (%)	Risk of Stroke with Surgical Therapy (%)	Absolute Risk Reduction (%)	Perioperative M&M (%)
60–99% ACAS[12] RISK at 5 years	11	5	6	1.2
50–99% VA study[13] RISK at 4 years	10	5	5	4

Source: From Executive Committee for the Asymptomatic Carotid Atherosclerosis Study. Endarterectomy for asymptomatic carotid artery stenosis. JAMA 1995;273(18):1421–1428; Hobson RW II, Weiss DG, Fields WS, et al. Efficacy of carotid endarterectomy for asymptomatic carotid stenosis. The Veterans Affairs Cooperative Study Group. N Engl J Med 1993;328(4):221–227; Findlay JM, Marchak BE, Pelz DM, Feasby TE. Carotid endarterectomy: a review. Can J Neurol Sci 2004;31(1):22–36.

Abbreviations: ACAS, Asymptomatic Carotid Atherosclerosis Study; CEA, carotid endarterectomy; M&M, morbidity and mortality; VA, Veterans Affairs.

■ Answers (*continued*)

12. *When would you perform surgery on this patient if she had had a stroke rather than a TIA?*
    - Surgery is delayed until the symptoms resolve and the deficits have plateaued.

13. *What is the management of patients with inoperable disease?*
    - Medical therapy for patients with inoperable disease
    - Control: blood pressure, blood sugar, lipids
    - Warfarin (Coumadin; Bristol-Myers Squibb, New York, NY)

■ References

1. Feldmann E, Wilterdink JL, Kosinski A, et al. The Stroke Outcomes and Neuroimaging of Intracranial Atherosclerosis (SONIA) Trial. Neurology 2007;68:2099–2106
2. Takahashi W, Ohnuki T, Ide M, Takagi S, Shinohara Y. Stroke risk of asymptomatic intra- and extracranial large-artery disease in apparently healthy adults. Cerebrovasc Dis 2006;22:263–270
3. Kappelle LJ, Eliasziw M, Fox AJ, Sharpe BL, Barnett HJM. Importance of intracranial atherosclerotic disease in patients with symptomatic stenosis of the internal carotid artery. Stroke 1999;30:282–286
4. Williams JE, Chimowitz MI, Cotsonis GE, Lynn MJ, Waddy SP. Gender differences in outcomes among patients with symptomatic intracranial arterial stenosis. Stroke 2007;38:2055–2062
5. Wong KS, Ng PW, Tang A, Liu R, Yeung V, Tomlinson B. Prevalence of asymptomatic intracranial atherosclerosis in high-risk patients. Neurology 2007;68:2035–2038
6. Lammie GA, Sandercock PAG, Dennis MS. Recently occluded intracranial and extracranial carotid arteries: relevance of the unstable atherosclerotic plaque. Stroke 1999;30:1319–1325
7. Guppy KH, Charbel FT, Loth F, Ausman JI. Hemodynamics of in-tandem stenosis of the internal carotid artery: when is carotid endarterectomy indicated? Surg Neurol 2000;54:145–154
8. North American Symptomatic Carotid Endarterectomy Trial Collaborators. Beneficial effect of carotid endarterectomy in symptomatic patients with high-grade carotid stenosis. N Engl J Med 1991;325(7):505–507
9. Gupta R, Al-Ali F, Thomas AJ, et al. Safety, feasibility, and short-term follow-up of drug-eluting stent placement in the intracranial and extracranial circulation. Stroke 2006;37:2562–2566
10. Randomised trial of endarterectomy for recently symptomatic carotid stenosis: final results of the MRC European Carotid Surgery Trial (ECST). Lancet 1998;351(9113):1379–1387
11. Mohr JP, Choi DW, Grotta JC, Weir B, Wolf PA. Stroke. Pathophysiology, Diagnosis, and Management. 4th ed. New York: Churchill Livingstone;2004
12. Executive Committee for the Asymptomatic Carotid Atherosclerosis Study. Endarterectomy for asymptomatic carotid artery stenosis. JAMA 1995;273(18):1421–1428
13. Hobson RW II, Weiss DG, Fields WS, et al. Efficacy of carotid endarterectomy for asymptomatic carotid stenosis. The Veterans Affairs Cooperative Study Group. N Engl J Med 1993;328(4):221–227
14. Findlay JM, Marchak BE, Pelz DM, Feasby TE. Carotid endarterectomy: a review. Can J Neurol Sci 2004;31(1):22–36

Case 43   Vertebral Artery Stenosis with Ischemia

Glenn C. Hunter and Rudiger Von Ritschl

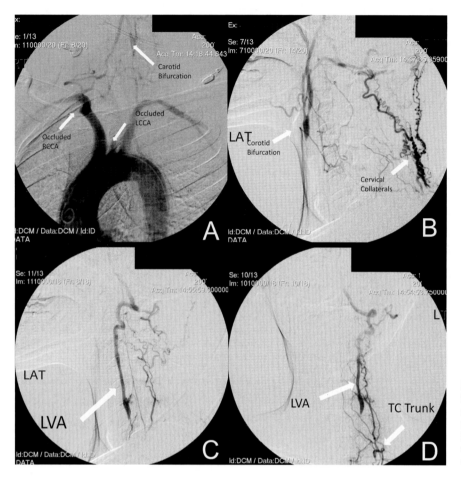

Fig. 43.1 Angiogram demonstrating the aortic arch and takeoff of the carotid, subclavian, and vertebral arteries. **(A)** More distal views demonstrating the left carotid bifurcation **(B)** and left vertebral artery (LVA) with collaterals **(C)** and **(D)**. (TC, thyrocervical trunk.)

■ Clinical Presentation

- A 56-year-old man with known hypertension and type 2 diabetes mellitus presents with a 6- to 9-month history of inability to raise his head or get out of bed. Any attempt to raise his head was accompanied by light headedness, dizziness, blurred vision, and drop attacks. His symptoms had become so severe that he was currently housebound.

- Physical examination revealed a healthy appearing man with blood pressure of 150/90 in both arms and bilateral carotid bruits.

■ Questions

1. What is the differential diagnosis?
2. What tests would you obtain?
3. A carotid duplex scan is obtained. The scan demonstrates bilateral internal carotid occlusion and no antegrade vertebral flow in the neck. Does this finding always indicate vertebral artery occlusion?
4. You have a choice between ordering magnetic resonance imaging (MRI)/magnetic resonance angiography

(MRA) or a conventional cerebral angiogram. What factors should you consider in making the decision?
5. Given the severe nature of the occlusive disease on the duplex scan, one would assume that symptoms in patients with vertebrobasilar (V-B) insufficiency are most frequently due to hypoperfusion. Is this assumption correct?

◼ Questions (*continued*)

6. A four-vessel angiogram is obtained. Describe the angiographic findings (**Fig. 43.1**).
7. How would your management differ if there was 80–99% carotid stenosis with vertebral artery occlusion?
8. What are the operative procedures for V-B insufficiency?

9. What alternative interventional therapies are available?
10. What is the medical management of the inoperable patient?
11. How would you treat this patient?

◼ Answers

1. *What is the differential diagnosis?*
   - Cardiac arrhythmias
   - Postural hypotension
   - V-B insufficiency
   - Hypoglycemia
   - Hypovolemia
   - Hyperventilation
2. *What tests would you obtain?*
   - Cardiac evaluation – electrocardiogram (EKG), cardiac echography, Holter monitoring
   - Routine blood chemistries – electrolytes, blood glucose, complete blood count (CBC), coagulation profile
   - Vascular imaging studies – Carotid duplex scan, transcranial Doppler
   - Cerebral imaging studies – MRI/MRA, computed tomography (CT), or conventional angiogram.[1]
3. *A carotid duplex scan is obtained. The scan demonstrates bilateral internal carotid occlusion and no antegrade vertebral flow in the neck. Does this finding always indicate vertebral artery occlusion?*
   - The absence of antegrade flow in one or both vertebral arteries is not diagnostic of occlusion. Anatomic variations include arch origin and hypoplasia of the vertebral arteries.[2]
4. *You have a choice between ordering an MRI/MRA or a conventional cerebral angiogram. What factors should you consider in making the decision?*
   - MRA is more effective in the diagnosis of basilar artery lesions than extracranial vertebral artery (ECVA) or intracranial vertebral artery (ICVA) disease.
   - Four-vessel cerebral angiography is the investigation of choice depending on the cause of symptoms. It is less valuable in thromboembolism of cardiac origin.
5. *Given the severe nature of the occlusive disease on the duplex scan, one would assume that symptoms in patients with V-B insufficiency are most frequently due to hypoperfusion. Is this assumption correct?*
   - No – the main causes of V-B insufficiency are listed below in order of frequency[1,3]:
     – Large vessel embolism 41%
     – Hemodynamic causes 33%
     – Cardiac embolism 24%

6. *A four-vessel angiogram is obtained. Describe the angiographic findings (**Fig. 43.1**).*
   - The angiogram shows bilateral ECVA and common carotid artery (CCA) occlusion with reconstitution of the distal ECVA.
   - There is reconstitution of the left carotid bifurcation and 60% internal carotid artery (ICA) stenosis.
7. *How would your management differ if there were 80–99% carotid stenosis with vertebral artery occlusion?*
   - The efficacy of treating concomitant asymptomatic occlusive disease is controversial.
     – If there is high grade 70–99% bilateral or unilateral symptomatic ICA stenosis then carotid endarterectomy (CEA) is done first.
     – The symptomatic hemisphere or dominant hemisphere in asymptomatic patients is treated first.
8. *What are the operative procedures for V-B insufficiency?*
   - CEA
   - Carotid subclavian bypass
   - Vertebral artery endarterectomy or bypass[4]
9. *What alternative interventional therapies are available?*
   - Carotid and vertebral artery angioplasty and stenting[3,5,6]
   - ECVA and ICVA angioplasty and stenting[3,5,6]
   - Use of thrombolytic agents[3]
10. *What is the medical management of the inoperable patient?*
    - Control risk factors for atherosclerosis
    - Optimize blood pressure control
    - Warfarin (Coumadin; Bristol-Myers Squibb, New York, NY) for obstructive lesions amenable to surgery or endovascular therapy[3]
    - Tissue plasminogen activator (TPA) and Abciximab[3]
    - Aspirin/clopidogrel (Plavix; Bristol-Myers Squibb, New York, NY) after stenting[3]
11. *How would you treat this patient?*
    - The patient was treated with a left subclavian to carotid bifurcation bypass using polytetrafluoroethylene (PTFE) graft and standard endarterectomy of the bifurcation with resolution of his symptoms.

References

1. Shin HK, Yoo K, Chang HM, Caplan LR. Bilateral intracranial vertebral artery disease in the New England Medical Center posterior circulation registry. Arch Neurol 1999;56:1353–1358
2. Horrow MM, Stassi J. Sonography of the vertebral arteries: a window to disease of the proximal great vessels. AJR Am J Roentgenol 2001;177:53–59
3. Eckert B, Koch C, Thomalla G, et al. Aggressive therapy with intravenous abciximab and intra-arterial rtPA and additional PTA/stenting improves clinical outcome in acute vertebrobasilar occlusion. Stroke 2005;36:1160–1165
4. Kieffer E, Praquin B, Chiche L, Koskas F, Bahnini A. Distal vertebral artery reconstruction: Long-term outcome. J Vasc Surg 2002;36:549–554
5. Cloud GC, Crawley F, Clifton A, McCabe DJH, Brown MM, Markus HS. Vertebral artery origin angioplasty and primary stenting: safety and restenosis rates in a prospective series. J Neurol Neurosurg Psychiatry 2003;74:586–590
6. SSYLVIA Study Investigators. Stenting of symptomatic atherosclerotic lesions in the vertebral or intracranial arteries (SSYLVIA) study results. Stroke 2004;35:1388–1392

Case 44   High-grade Carotid Stenosis and Intracranial Aneurysm

Glenn C. Hunter and Remi Nader

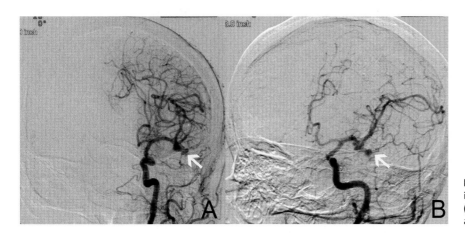

Fig. 44.1 Cerebral angiogram, left carotid injection, showing on **(A)** anteroposterior and **(B)** lateral views showing a left middle carotid artery trifurcation aneurysm of 7 mm in size.

■ Clinical Presentation

- A 74-year-old woman presents with a history of left hemispheric transient ischemic attacks (TIAs).
- She experienced one episode of right arm and leg weakness that completely resolved within 5–7 minutes ~4 weeks ago.

- Her blood pressure was 160/110 mm Hg while still on two antihypertensive medications. The blood pressure in her left arm was 30 mm Hg lower than that on the right side.
- Bilateral carotid bruits are present.

■ Questions

1. What initial studies would you order?
2. What imaging studies would assist in the diagnosis?
3. How would you manage this patient initially?

She returns 2 weeks later with complaints of having discontinued her clopidogrel (Plavix; Bristol-Myers Squibb, New York, NY) because of bruising. She has experienced two episodes of TIAs since discontinuing clopidogrel.

4. How do you manage her now?
5. A cerebral angiogram is obtained. Is this preferable to computed tomography (CT) or magnetic resonance angiography (MRA)?

The angiogram demonstrated an irregular high-grade (90%) left internal carotid artery (LICA) stenosis (not shown here) and a left 7 mm middle cerebral artery cerebral aneurysm (**Fig. 44.1**).

6. What are the prevalence and sex differences of an unruptured intracranial aneurysm (UIA)?
7. What is the incidence of a UIA on cerebral angiograms performed for carotid disease?
8. Are there any conditions associated with intracranial aneurysms?
9. How may intracranial aneurysms present?
10. What are the factors that predispose to aneurysm rupture?
11. What are the rupture rates in this case?
12. List the therapeutic options for this patient.
13. What factors need to be taken into consideration in selecting the treatment option?
14. Describe the anatomical segments of the internal carotid artery and their branches.

Answers

1. *What initial studies would you order?*
   - The patient should have a work-up for stroke.
   - Laboratory studies should include complete blood count (CBC), coagulation studies, electrolytes, and renal function tests.
   - Chest x-ray, electrocardiogram (EKG)
2. *What imaging studies would assist in the diagnosis?*
   - A carotid duplex scan
   - CT or magnetic resonance imaging (MRI) of the brain
     - The duplex scan shows 80–99% LICA stenosis with 50–79% stenosis on the right side.
     - A nonenhanced CT scan shows no evidence of hemorrhage or ischemia.
3. *How would you manage this patient initially?*
   - She is placed on aspirin and clopidogrel.
   - Arrangements should be made for an outpatient cerebral angiogram.
4. *How do you manage her now?*
   - She is experiencing more frequent TIAs; therefore, direct hospital admission is indicated.
   - Consider intravenous heparin therapy if no hemorrhage is seen on the CT scan of the brain.
5. *A cerebral angiogram is obtained. Is this preferable to CT or MRA?*
   - This patient has evidence of both subclavian and carotid stenosis. A cerebral angiogram would provide the most definitive diagnosis.
   - However, the inherent risks of this more invasive procedure (such as stroke, etc.) should be discussed with the patient prior to the study.
6. *What are the prevalence and sex differences of an UIA?*
   - The prevalence of UIA ranges from 0.8–8% (mean 5%).
   - There is a 2:1 female to male ratio.[1]
   - Incidence increases with age.[1]
7. *What is the incidence of an UIA on cerebral angiograms performed for carotid disease?*
   - Incidence: 1:40 patients with symptomatic carotid stenosis have UIAs.[2]
     - Based on the North American Symptomatic Carotid Endarterectomy Trial (NASCET) study,[3] there is a 3.1% incidence of an UIA in cerebral angiograms performed for carotid disease.
       - 96% of aneurysms are less than or equal to 10 mm in size.
       - 55% are ipsilateral to the side of the carotid stenosis.
       - These account for 6 to 16% of subarachnoid hemorrhages (SAHs)
       - 8 to 34% are multiple.
8. *Are there any conditions associated with intracranial aneurysms?*
   - UIA can have a congenital predisposition and can be associated with[1]
     - Aortic coarctation
     - Polycystic kidneys (autosomal dominant)
     - Family history of UIA/SAH
     - Fibromuscular dysplasia
     - Pseudoxanthoma elasticum
     - Moyamoya disease
     - Systemic lupus erythematosus
     - Arteriovenous malformations
9. *How may intracranial aneurysms present?*
   - Incidental
   - SAH
   - Embolism (rare)
   - Headache
   - Cranial nerve palsy[1]
10. *What are the factors that predispose to aneurysm rupture?*
    - Size
    - Location (anterior vs. posterior circulation)
    - Previous SAH (increases hemorrhage rate by 11-fold)[4]
11. *What are the rupture rates in this case?*
    - Risk of rupture in this case is less than 1%. Rupture risk depends on size and location of the aneurysm.[1,4–6]
    - See Case 31 for a detailed description of the associated risks.
12. *List the therapeutic options for this patient.*
    - Carotid endarterectomy (CEA) without UIA clipping (UIA observation)
    - Combined CEA and UIA clipping
    - CEA and aneurysm coiling
    - Carotid artery stenting (CAS) and aneurysm coiling[7]
13. *What factors need to be taken into consideration in selecting the treatment option?*
    - Determine if the symptoms are of hemodynamic or embolic origin.
    - Determine which lesion is causing the symptoms.
    - Determine the relationship between the two lesions:
      - Embolic symptoms are most often due to carotid bifurcation plaque.
      - Carotid lesions are a more common cause of symptoms (as in this case).
    - Certain factors with the treatment of one lesion may exacerbate the risks of the other:
      - CEA may increase the risk of aneurysm rupture due to an increase in BP (this is very unlikely, however).[8]
      - Hypotension necessary to clip an aneurysm may cause thrombosis of a high-grade carotid stenosis.[8]

■ Answers (*continued*)

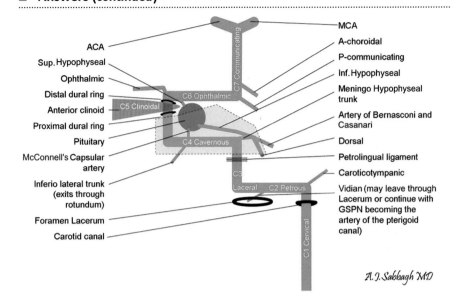

Fig. 44.2 Anatomical segments of the internal carotid artery and their branches. (ACA, anterior cerebral artery; MCA, middle cerebral artery; Sup, superior; Inf, inferior; A, anterior; P, posterior; GSPN, greater superficial petrosal nerve.)

- Based on the NASCET study,[3] the 5-year risk of rupture of UIA differs based on the treatment modality of the underlying carotid disease.
  - With CEA, it is 10%.
  - With best medical therapy, it is 22.7%.

14. *Describe the anatomical segments of the internal carotid artery and their branches.*
  - See **Fig. 44.2** for a detailed description.

■ References

1. Brisman JL, Song JK, Newell DW. Cerebral aneurysms. N Engl J Med 2006;355:928–939
2. Kappelle LJ, Eliasziw M, Fox AJ, Barnett HJ. Small, unruptured intracranial aneurysms and management of symptomatic carotid artery stenosis. North American Symptomatic Carotid Endarterectomy Trial Group. Neurology 2000;55(2):307–309
3. North American Symptomatic Carotid Endarterectomy Trial Collaborators. Beneficial effect of carotid endarterectomy in symptomatic patients with high-grade carotid stenosis. N Engl J Med 1991;325(7):505–507
4. Unruptured intracranial aneurysms–risk of rupture and risks of surgical intervention. International Study of Unruptured Intracranial Aneurysms Investigators. N Engl J Med 1998;339(24):1725–1733
5. Chen PR, Frerichs K, Spetzler R. Current treatment options for unruptured intracranial aneurysms. Neurosurg Focus 2004;17(5):E5
6. Johnston SC, Higashida RT, Barrow DL, et al. Recommendations for the endovascular treatment of intracranial aneurysms: a statement for healthcare professionals from the Committee on Cerebrovascular Imaging of the American Heart Association Council on Cardiovascular Radiology. Stroke 2002;33(10):2536–2544
7. Goldstein LB. Extracranial carotid artery stenosis. Stroke 2003;34:2767–2773
8. Ladowski JS, Webster MW, Yonas HO, Steed DL. Carotid endarterectomy in patients with asymptomatic intracranial aneurysm. Ann Surg 1984;200:70–73

Case 45   Chronic Subdural Hematoma

Remi Nader

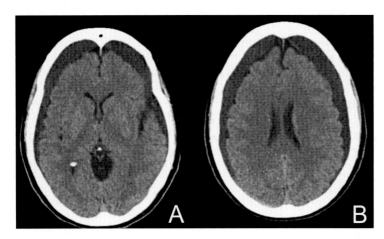

Fig. 45.1   (A,B) Computed tomography scan of the brain without contrast.

■ Clinical Presentation

- A 70-year-old woman with end-stage Alzheimer's disease, diabetes mellitus, nursing home bound, is brought to the ER for a 3-day episode of increasing confusion, agitation, and inappropriate behavior.
- The patient is confused at baseline, however, she was noted to be combative and refusing her care as well as voicing aloud her request to leave the nursing home and to go home, which is unusual behavior for her.
- She is a poor historian, but she does report having had frequent falls in the near past.
- Physical examination reveals a left-sided pronator drift and confusion. The remainder of the examination is normal.
- Computed tomography (CT) scan is obtained and shown in **Fig. 45.1**.

■ Questions

1. Interpret the CT scan.
2. What other questions or information would you like to obtain to further plan your management?
3. What further studies or investigations would you like to obtain?
4. What would you tell the family, next of kin, or caregiver?

The patient is on no anticoagulant or antiinflammatory medications. Her laboratory results including complete blood count, electrolytes, and coagulation profile are within normal limits. You had a discussion with the family about the treatment options and they opted for surgery.

5. How would you approach this case surgically? Describe all the steps of surgery including positioning, incision, bone opening, evacuation, and closure.

6. Preoperatively, as you plan the surgery, she develops hyponatremia with sodium of 118, and she becomes more lethargic. What are some causes of hyponatremia and which is the most likely in this case?
7. How would you manage this problem?

She does well from bilateral burr-hole evacuation of subdural hematomas, and is discharged home. However, she comes back 3 weeks later to your clinic. She now has some purulent discharge from the right posterior incision. She is somewhat somnolent and has a left hemiparesis slightly worse than the one she had immediately postoperatively.

8. What is your course of action now?
9. A follow-up CT scan and subsequently a magnetic resonance imaging (MRI) scan are obtained (**Fig. 45.2**). Interpret the studies and provide a differential diagnosis.
10. What is your management plan?

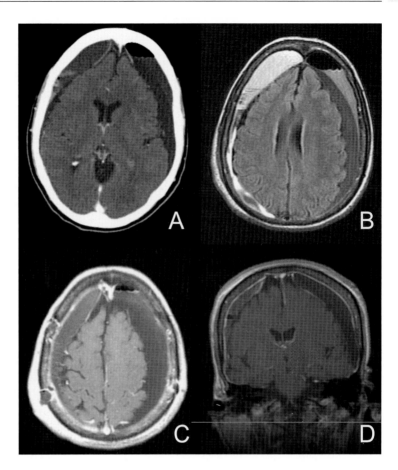

Fig. 45.2 **(A)** Computed tomography scan with contrast and **(B)** magnetic resonance imaging fluid-attenuated inversion-recovery axial image without contrast, and T1-weighted images with contrast, **(C)** axial and **(D)** coronal.

■ Answers

1. *Interpret the CT scan.*
   - CT scan of the brain reveals bilateral subdural hematomas which are mainly chronic with a very small subacute component on the right side.
   - The right subdural hematoma is close to 1.5 cm in thickness. The left subdural hematoma is ~1.3 cm in thickness. They are both mainly along the convexity in the frontal and somewhat parietal area.
   - There is some diffuse brain atrophy in both frontal lobes consistent with advanced Alzheimer's disease.
   - There also appears to be no midline shift, no obvious mass effect, and no edema. The basal cisterns are wide open.
   - There might be some effacement in the sulci along the cortical surface in the frontal lobes.

2. *What other questions or information would you like to obtain to further plan your management?*
   - Obtain current medication history, especially whether or not she is on anticoagulants.
   - Determine if there is a living will or a durable power of attorney. If so, determine the patient's wishes in a situation where lifesaving measures are needed.

3. *What further studies or investigations would you like to obtain?*

   - Laboratory tests: complete blood count, electrolytes, coagulation profile, type and screen
   - Other imaging: MRI – unlikely to change your management in this case
   - If surgical intervention is contemplated, then medical clearance may be needed (electrocardiogram [EKG], chest x-ray, cardiac echography, etc.)

4. *What would you tell the family, next of kin, or caregiver?*
   - The patient has fluid collections on the surface of her brain, and that these are likely due to old hemorrhages.
   - It is not clear whether or not these fluid collections are causing a lot of pressure on her brain.
   - She also has brain atrophy due to Alzheimer's disease.
   - She may possibly benefit from evacuation of the fluid collections.[1]
   - However, the caregiver needs to be aware that evacuation may also not help as she may be having progressive dementia due to Alzheimer's and she may also have complications from the surgery.

■ Answers (*continued*)

- Inform the caregiver of all the potential surgical complications. These include, but are not limited to pain; bleeding; infection; failure to treat presenting condition; need for further surgeries or procedures in the future; reaccumulation of the fluid collections damage to adjacent blood vessels, nerves, and tissues; additional loss of brain function including memory, stroke, changes in vision, deafness, inability to smell, coordination loss, seizures, cerebrospinal fluid leak; weakness; impaired muscle function; numbness; paralysis; death.[2-4]

5. *How would you approach this case surgically? Describe all the steps of surgery including positioning, incision, bone opening, evacuation, and closure.*
   - One operative option consists of bilateral burr hole evacuation of the subdural hematoma, with two burr holes placed on each side.[5-9]
   - Preoperative preparation includes
     - Preoperative antibiotics, cefazolin 1 g intravenously (IV) every 8 hours
     - Preoperative seizure prophylaxis with phenytoin, loading dose of 1 g IV over 1 hour, followed by a maintenance dose of 100 mg every 8 hours
     - Positioning is supine with head of bed slightly elevated
     - Anesthesia preferably conscious sedation, or general endotracheal if the patient will tolerate it (i.e., no cardiac or pulmonary risk factors)
   - Surgical steps include
     - Hair clipping and mark incisions along the convexity in-line with each other such that if the need for a bone flap arises it will suffice to connect both incisions.
     - The incisions should be ~5–6 cm away from the midline; one along the parietal boss and one just behind the hair line anteriorly — both ~3 cm in length.
     - Start by opening the right side as this is the symptomatic side.
     - Open skin, galea, and periosteum with a no. 10 blade; expose the skull and perform a burr hole with a pneumatic drill, ~2.5 cm in diameter.
     - Wax the bone edges and cauterize the dura.
     - Open the dura in cruciate fashion, then drain the blood.
     - Irrigate both burr holes profusely with normal saline until the drainage becomes clear.
     - One may place a red rubber catheter in the burr hole subdurally and further irrigate to dislodge any pockets of blood that are harder to access.
     - Closure is completed by placing a piece of Gelfoam (Pfizer, Inc., New York, NY) on top of the burr hole, close the skin and galea with 3–0 Vicryl (Ethicon, Somerville, NJ) and staples.
     - One may leave a small drain in the subgaleal space.
   - The patient is kept with the head of the bed flat postoperatively.[10]

6. *Preoperatively, as you plan the surgery, she develops hyponatremia with sodium of 118, and she becomes more lethargic. What are some causes of hyponatremia and which is the most likely in this case?*
   - Causes of hyponatremia are listed below.
   - Hypovolemic hyponatremia: sodium and free water loss with inappropriately hypotonic fluid replacement
     - Cerebral salt-wasting syndrome: traumatic brain injury, aneurysmal subarachnoid hemorrhage, subdural hematoma, and postcraniotomy — this is the most likely cause in this case
     - Gastrointestinal losses such as vomiting or diarrhea
     - Excessive sweating
     - Third spacing of fluids (peritonitis, pancreatitis, burns)
     - Acute or chronic renal insufficiency
     - Prolonged exercise in a hot environment
   - Euvolemic hyponatremia: normal sodium stores and total body excess free water
     - Psychogenic polydipsia
     - Hypotonic intravenous (i.v.) or irrigation fluids postoperatively
   - Hypervolemic hyponatremia: inappropriate increase in sodium stores
     - Hepatic cirrhosis
     - Congestive heart failure
     - Nephrotic syndrome
     - Hypothyroidism
     - Cortisol deficiency
     - Syndrome of inappropriate antidiuretic hormone (SIADH)[11]
     - Medications: acetazolamide, thiazide diuretics, angiotensin-converting enzyme inhibitors, carbamazepine, gabapentin, haloperidol, heparin, ketorolac, loop diuretics, nimodipine, opiates, proton pump inhibitors, selective serotonin reuptake inhibitors[11-13]

7. *How would you manage this problem?*
   - Ensure that the patient is stabilized first: secure airway, breathing, circulation (ABCs of trauma), place on oxygen transfer to intensive care unit (ICU), obtain i.v. access with large bore i.v., place a Foley catheter
   - Obtain laboratory studies to determine which type of hyponatremia including
     - Serum and urine sodium and osmolalities, and urine specific gravity
     - Serum electrolytes
     - Thyroid function studies
     - Adrenal function studies
   - In this case, the most likely cause is hypovolemic hyponatremia possibly from the subdural hematoma.

Answers (continued)

- If the symptoms are mild to moderate one may treat with isotonic saline.
- Monitoring of serum sodium levels needs to be done frequently to ensure that the serum sodium increases to no greater than 0.5 mEq/L/hour or 12 mEq/L/day.
- Hypertonic saline (3%) may be used as an alternative if normal saline alone is not adequate enough to correct the problem. When using this solution, care should be taken to administer it slowly (20 to 50 cc/hour drip) and frequent checks on serum sodium is required (every 2–4 hours).
- Evacuation of the subdural hematoma may resolve the hyponatremia (it did in this case).[12,13]

8. *What is your course of action now?*
   - Urgent ICU admission
   - Laboratory studies: complete blood count, electrolytes, coagulation profile, type and screen, blood, urine, sputum cultures, and culture discharge from wound
   - Obtain imaging studies: CT and MRI with and without contrast
   - May elect to wait until the cultures are sent intraoperatively before starting any broad spectrum antibiotics.
   - Antibiotics suggested:
     - Vancomycin 1 g i.v. every 12 hours, cefepime 2 g i.v. every 12 hours, and metronidazole 500 mg i.v. every 8 hours
     - Gentamycin 600 mg i.v. every 8 hours may be used instead of cefepime if the patient is allergic to penicillin.
     - Antibiotic changes are performed as culture and sensitivity results are obtained.

9. *A follow-up CT scan and subsequently an MRI are obtained (**Fig. 45.2**). Interpret the studies and provide a differential diagnosis.*

- CT scan with contrast shows some reaccumulation of fluid bilaterally. The fluid collection on the right side is partly hyperdense or enhancing, which is suggestive of acute blood or possible empyema with peripheral enhancement.
- On MRI, the subdural fluid is consistent with blood of different ages and it is seen bilaterally. On the right side there is some enhancement surrounding the subdural fluid which is possibly suggestive of infection.
- The right subdural fluid appears to be iso- to hyperintense on T1-weighted and hyperintense on T2-weighted or fluid-attenuated inversion-recovery (FLAIR) MRIs, which, if it is blood, is likely subacute to chronic (3 weeks old).
- The differential diagnosis includes
  - Reaccumulation of subdural hematoma
  - Subdural empyema
  - Subdural hygroma

10. *What is your management plan?*
   - Urgent surgical evacuation via burr hole reexploration on the right side.[14–16]
   - The exposure should be prepared in the event that a craniotomy is needed.
   - Subdural fluid needs to be sent for culture as soon as possible, after which the antibiotics are initiated.
   - Incision and sharp debridement of the posterior scalp wound is needed with irrigation and antibiotics and saline solution.
   - A drain can be left in the subgaleal space.
   - Wound closure can be done in a single layer with 2–0 Prolene (Ethicon, Somerville, NJ) vertical mattress interrupted sutures to promote better healing of infected or granulating tissues.

References

1. Ishikawa E, Yanaka K, Sugimoto K, Ayuzawa S, Nose T. Reversible dementia in patients with chronic subdural hematomas. J Neurosurg 2002;96(4):680–683
2. Pencalet P. Complications of chronic subdural hematoma in the adult. Neurochirurgie 2001;47(5):491–494
3. Zumkeller M, Höllerhage HG, Dietz H. Treatment outcome in patients with chronic subdural hematoma with reference to age and concurrent internal diseases. Wien Med Wochenschr 1997;147(3):55–62
4. Tindall GT, Payne NS II, O'Brien MS. Complications of surgery for subdural hematoma. Clin Neurosurg 1976;23:465–482
5. Gökmen M, Sucu HK, Ergin A, Gökmen A, Bezircio Lu H. Randomized comparative study of burr-hole craniotomy versus twist drill craniotomy. Surgical management of unilateral hemispheric chronic subdural hematomas. Zentralbl Neurochir 2008;69(3):129–133
6. Gurelik M, Aslan A, Gurelik B, Ozum U, Karadag O, Kars HZ. A safe and effective method for treatment of chronic subdural haematoma. Can J Neurol Sci 2007;34(1):84–87
7. Weigel R, Schmiedek P, Krauss JK. Outcome of contemporary surgery for chronic subdural haematoma: evidence based review. J Neurol Neurosurg Psychiatry 2003;74(7):937–943
8. Zakaraia AM, Adnan JS, Haspani MS, Naing NN, Abdullah JM. Outcome of 2 different types of operative techniques practiced for chronic subdural hematoma in Malaysia: an analysis. Surg Neurol 2008;69(6):608–615

■ **References** *(continued)*

9. Taussky P, Fandino J, Landolt H. Number of burr holes as independent predictor of postoperative recurrence in chronic subdural haematoma. Br J Neurosurg 2008;22(2):279–282

10. Abouzari M, Rashidi A, Rezaii J, et al. The role of postoperative patient posture in the recurrence of traumatic chronic subdural hematoma after burr-hole surgery. Neurosurgery 2007;61(4):794–797

11. Abdel Samie A, Theilmann L. Acute symptomatic hyponatremia in a 70-year-old male. case report and review on the syndrome of inadequate ADH secretion. Med Klin 2002;97:298–303

12. Greenberg MS. Handbook of Neurosurgery. 6th ed. New York: Thieme Medical Publishers; 2006

13. Craig S. Hyponatremia. emedicine 2008. Available at: http://www.emedicine.com/emerg/topic275.htm. Accessed June 10, 2009

14. Hirano A, Takamura T, Murayama N, Ohyama K, Matsumura S, Niwa J. [Subdural abscess following chronic subdural hematoma.] No Shinkei Geka 1995;23(7):643–646

15. Honda M, Tanaka K, Tanaka S, Nakayama T, Kaneko M, Ozawa T. A case of infected subdural hematoma following chronic subdural hematoma irrigation. No To Shinkei 2002;54(8):703–706

16. Sawauchi S, Saguchi T, Miyazaki Y, et al. Infected subdural hematoma. J Clin Neurosci 1998;5(2):233–237

Case 46   Mild Head Injury

Judith Marcoux and Abdulrazag Ajlan

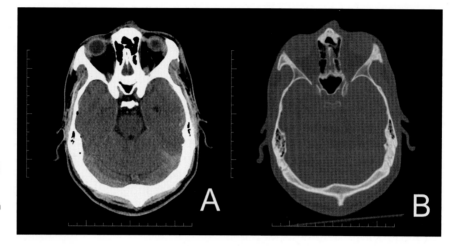

Fig. 46.1   (A) Noncontrasted head computed tomography scan showing a left temporal small contre-coup contusion in the brain window and **(B)** a right mastoid fracture with a small amount of pneumocephalus in the bone window.

■ Clinical Presentation

- A 22-year-old man is involved in a fight and is assaulted on the right side of his head.
- On clinical examination in the emergency room (ER), he opens his eyes to voice, but he is somnolent and confused.

He obeys commands and has no focal deficit. There is no sign of external trauma.
- A computed tomography (CT) scan of the head is done and depicted in **Fig. 46.1**.

■ Questions

1. How can you make the diagnosis of a mild traumatic brain injury (TBI)?
2. What are the indications for a CT scan in a mild TBI?
3. Which patient with a mild TBI will require hospital admission?
4. What is the prognosis of a mild TBI?

■ Answers

1. *How can you make the diagnosis of a mild TBI?*
   - A mild TBI is an acute brain injury resulting from a mechanical energy to the head from external physical forces.
   - To make the diagnosis of a mild TBI, you need to have at least one of the following:
     - A documented period of altered mental status (loss of consciousness or confusion)
     - Duration of the loss of consciousness less than 30 minutes
     - Duration of the posttraumatic amnesia less than 24 hours
     - Any other transitory neurologic sign or focal neurologic sign (e.g., seizure)
     - An intracranial lesion not requiring a neurosurgical intervention (if a neurosurgical intervention is required, the injury will be classified as moderate)
   - A Glasgow Coma Scale (GCS) score between 13 and 15, 30 minutes or more after the accident (sudden deterioration and signs of herniation will be classified as a moderate or severe TBI)
   - These findings should *not* be due to alcohol or drug intoxication, medication, other injuries, their treatment, other problems (e.g., psychological trauma, language barrier…), or a penetrating brain injury (classified as moderate).[1]
   - The term "concussion" should no longer be used as its definition was vague and varied considerably in the literature.[2]

2. *What are the indications for a CT scan in a mild TBI?*
   - To decide who is going to need a CT scan, you need to know which patient is at risk of developing serious complications. Two phase III studies address this question[3,4] in adults; the following criteria are a combination of the results of these studies:
     - At history:
       - Age 60 years or more
       - Dangerous mechanism of injury (see below)
       - Any vomiting
       - Headache (not specific)
       - Any seizure activity
       - Anterograde amnesia
     - On examination:
       - GCS <15
       - Drug or alcohol intoxication
       - Skull fracture (suspected open or depressed skull fracture or signs of basal skull fracture
       - Evidence of trauma above the clavicles
   - If any of these factors is positive, the patient should have a CT scan done.

   - A dangerous mechanism of injury is when the velocity or force of impact generated overcomes the human body's ability to compensate. The following mechanisms carry a high risk for intracranial injury:
     - Pedestrian struck by a motor vehicle
     - Occupant ejected from a motor vehicle
     - Fall from a height of more than 3 feet (1 m) or five stairs

3. *Which patient with a mild TBI will require hospital admission?*
   - Patients with a mild TBI requiring an admission are those with a GCS <15 or an abnormal CT scan (defined as a significant intracranial lesion).
   - Nonsignificant lesions include[4,5]
     - An isolated cerebral contusion of ≤5 mm
     - A subarachnoid hemorrhage with thickness ≤1 mm
     - A subdural hematoma with thickness ≤4 mm
     - Isolated pneumocephalus
     - Depressed skull fracture that does not extend to the inner table

4. *What is the prognosis of a mild TBI?*
   - A person presenting with a GCS score of 15 has a 0.08% risk of requiring a surgical intervention and 1% risk if the GCS is 13 or 14.
     - 0.07% of patients with a mild TBI will develop late posttraumatic epilepsy.[3]
     - The mortality rate in adults with a mild TBI is 0.01% if the GCS score is 14–15 and 1.1% if the GCS score is 13.
     - An excellent prognosis is reached.
       - In 98% of the patients with a GCS of 15
       - In 95% with a GCS of 14
       - In 76% with a GCS of 13
   - In children, the mortality rate is 0% if the GCS was 14 or 15 and 0 to 0.25% if the GCS was 13 with a postadmission deterioration.
     - The overall prognosis in children is excellent in more than 99% of the cases.[6]
     - When post-TBI symptoms are present in children, they are usually transient and are resolved by 2 weeks to 3 months.
     - Few children will have short term or long-term cognitive deficit.
   - In adults, most studies show that cognitive deficits will resolve within 3 months. Some individuals, however, will suffer from persistent symptoms.

■ Answers (*continued*)

- The main determinant for acute and late morbidity is the presence of compensation or litigation.[7]
  - Other possible factors (that are inconsistent between studies) are
    - Female gender
    - Being married
    - Being off work due to the injury
    - Not being at fault for a collision
    - Nausea or memory problems postinjury
- Other injuries
- History of preexisting physical limitations
- Prior neurologic illness or head injury
- Psychiatric problems
- Life stressors
- Being a student
- Sustaining TBI in a motor vehicle collision
- Age over 40 years

■ References

1. Carroll LJ, Cassidy JD, Holm L, Kraus J, Coronado VG. Methodological issue and research recommendations for mild traumatic brain injury: results of the WHO collaborating centre task force on mild traumatic brain injury. J Rehabil Med 2004;(Suppl 43):113–125

2. Peloso PM, Carroll LJ, Cassidy JD, et al. Critical evaluation of the existing guidelines on mild traumatic brain injury: results of the WHO collaborating centre task force on mild traumatic brain injury. J Rehabil Med 2004;(Suppl 43):106–112

3. Borg J, Holm L, Cassidy JD, et al. Diagnostic procedures in mild traumatic brain injury: results of the WHO collaborating centre task force on mild traumatic brain injury. J Rehabil Med 2004; (Suppl 43):61–75

4. Stiell IG, Wells GA, Vandemheen K, et al. The Canadian CT Head Rule for patients with minor head injury. Lancet 2001;357:1391–1396

5. Stiell IG, Clement C, Wells GA, et al. Multicenter prospective validation of the Canadian CT Head Rule. Acad Emerg Med 2003;10:539

6. Carroll LJ, Cassidy JD, Peloso PM, et al. Prognosis for mild traumatic brain injury: results of the WHO collaborating centre task force on mild traumatic brain injury. J Rehabil Med 2004;(Suppl 43):84–105

7. Cassidy JD, Carroll LJ, Côté P, Holm L, Nygren Å. Mild traumatic brain injury after traffic collisions: a population-based cohort study. J Rehabil Med 2004;(Suppl 43):11–14

Case 47   Epidural Hematoma

Abdulrazag Ajlan and Judith Marcoux

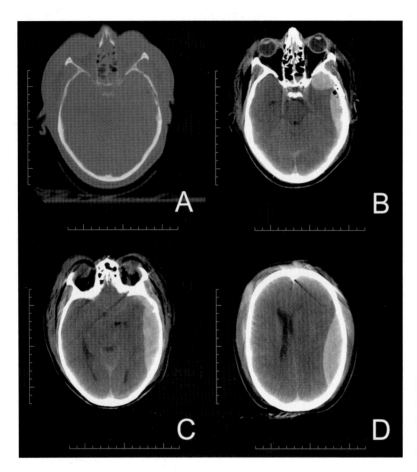

Fig. 47.1 Computed tomography scan of the head, bone window is displayed in **(A)** where a left temporal bone fracture is seen. **(B)**, **(C)** and **(D)** are brain windows showing a large epidural hematoma with significant mass effect and uncal herniation with brainstem compression and displacement **(C)** and significant midline shift **(D)**.

■ Clinical Presentation

• A 42-year-old woman fell from the third floor of a building. She presents with a Glasgow Coma Score (GCS) of 7.

• The patient is hemodynamically stable and she is quickly intubated.
• Her pupils are both reactive, but asymmetrical.

■ Questions

1. Describe what you see on the computed tomography (CT) scan (**Fig. 47.1**).
2. What is the pathophysiology of this intracranial bleed?
3. What is your initial management?
4. What are the criteria for surgical evacuation?
5. What is the prognosis?

■ Answers

1. *Describe what you see on the CT scan* (**Fig. 47.1**).
   - There is a linear nondisplaced temporal bone fracture with underlying pneumocephalus.
   - There are also hyperdense lesions in the temporal and temporoparietal areas on the same side of the fracture. The lesions are biconvex (lens shape) and are compatible with an epidural hematoma (EDH).
   - The lesions are causing a midline shift of 0.7 cm and a right-side uncal herniation.

2. *What is the pathophysiology of this intracranial bleed?*
   - Epidural hematomas are usually located in the temporoparietal areas; posterior fossa hematomas represent 5% of the EDH.
   - The source is usually a meningeal artery, which is most commonly the middle meningeal artery, but sometimes this can be a bleeding vein or an underlying sinus.
   - The bleeding in the epidural space will strip the dura from the skull causing mass effect and raising intracranial pressure.
   - Approximately 85% of cases will be associated with skull fracture.
   - 20% of patients will present in a comatose state.[1] Other presentations include localized neurologic findings and confusion. The classical presentation of transient improvement followed by sudden deterioration occurs in 47% of admissions, which is called the Lucid Interval.[2]

3. *What is your initial management?*
   - Once the airway is secured and the patient is hemodynamically stable, she needs to undergo emergency evacuation for the hematoma.
   - The patient should also be loaded with an antiepileptic drug.
   - Infusing mannitol and hyperventilation may be done as temporary measures before the evacuation.
   - This is a surgical emergency because there is a symptomatically significant mass larger than 1 cm with midline shift greater than 0.5 cm.

4. *What are the criteria for surgical evacuation?*
   - An EDH more than 30 cm³ regardless of the GCS.[2]
   - A patient with a GSC of more than 8 and a hematoma less than 30 cm³, less than 15 mm thickness, less than 0.5 cm midline shift, and without focal deficit can be managed by close observation with serial scans and placement in a monitored neurosurgical unit.[2]

5. *What is the prognosis?*
   - Outcome depends on many factors, which include GCS, CT scan findings, age, timing of surgery, and the presence of other lesions.
   - The overall mortality for patients who underwent surgical evacuation is 10%.[2] The faster the evacuation is done the better will be the outcome because the neurologic status prior to surgery is the main determinant of outcome.
   - EDH evacuation is considered one of the most "cost effective" of all surgical procedures in terms of quality of life.[3]

■ References

1. Kuday C, Uzan M, Hanci M. Statistical analysis of the factors affecting the outcome of extradural haematomas: 115 cases. Acta Neurochir (Wien) 1994;131:203–2067
2. Bullock MR, Chesnut R, Ghajar J, et al. Surgical Management of Traumatic Brain Injury Author Group. Surgical management of acute epidural hematomas. Neurosurgery 2006; 58(Suppl 3)S7–S15
3. Pickard JD. Steps towards cost-benefit analysis of regional neurosurgical care. BMJ 1990;301:629–635

Case 48   Traumatic Acute Subdural Hematoma

Abdulrazag Ajlan and Judith Marcoux

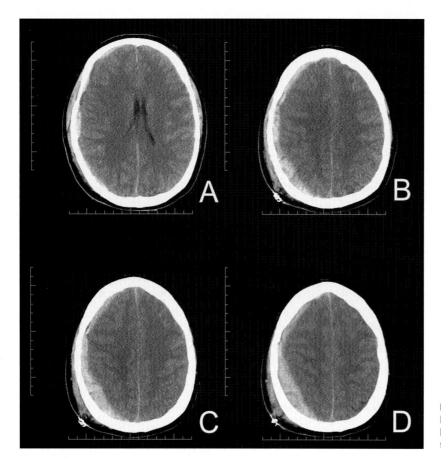

Fig. 48.1 Computed tomography scan of the head, brain windows showing a right-side subdural hematoma with associated midline shift greater than 5 mm **(A)** and brain compression **(B–D)**.

■ Clinical Presentation

- A 39-year-old man is involved in an all-terrain vehicle accident; he had no helmet on.
- His Glasgow Coma Scale (GCS) score on arrival in the emergency room was 7 (Eyes 1, Verbal 1, Motor 5).
- The patient is hemodynamically stable and is quickly intubated.

■ Questions

1. Describe what you see on the computed tomography (CT) scan (**Fig. 48.1**).
2. What is the pathophysiology of this intracranial bleed?
3. What is your management?
4. What are the criteria for surgical evacuation for acute subdural hematomas (SDHs)?
5. What is the prognosis?
6. What other types of traumatic intracranial hemorrhage can you see?
7. What are the indications for surgical evacuation in the different types of intracranial hemorrhage?
8. What are the indications for antiepileptic medication?

■ Answers

1. *Describe what you see on the CT scan (**Fig. 48.1**).*
   - There is an acute subdural hematoma over the right hemisphere which causes mass effect, compression of the brain, and a midline shift.
2. *What is the pathophysiology of this intracranial bleed?*
   - Acute subdural hematomas are usually due to torn bridging veins at the surface of the brain. Damaged cortical arteries could also produce subdural hematomas.
   - A significant degree of impact is usually required to produce a subdural hematoma.
3. *What is your management?*
   - This patient is comatose; he has a mass lesion seen on the CT scan and significant midline shift associated with it (greater than 5 mm).
   - After ensuring that there is no life-threatening injury, this patient should be taken to the operating room for quick decompression via a large frontotemporoparietal craniectomy or craniotomy.
4. *What are the criteria for surgical evacuation for acute SDHs?*
   - Indications for surgery are as follows[1]:
     – An acute SDH with a thickness greater than 10 mm or a midline shift greater than 5 mm on CT scan should be surgically evacuated, regardless of the patient's GCS score.
     – All patients with an acute SDH in a coma (GCS less than 9) should have an ICP monitor.
     – A patient with a GCS score less than 9 an acute SDH less than 1 mm, and a midline shift less than 5 mm should undergo surgical evacuation of the lesion if one of the following is present:
       ▪ Decrease in the GCS score by 2 or more points
       ▪ Asymmetric or fixed and dilated pupils
       ▪ Elevated intracranial pressure (ICP) of more than 20 mm Hg
5. *What is the prognosis?*
   - The prognosis will depend on the initial GCS score, the age, and the associated brain damage (with subsequent intracranial hypertension).
   - Early surgery may improve the outcome.

6. *What other types of traumatic intracranial hemorrhage can you see?*
   - The other types of traumatic intracranial bleeding, apart from acute subdural hemorrhage and acute epidural hemorrhage, include
     – Intraventricular hemorrhage
     – Subarachnoid hemorrhage
     – Intracerebral contusions; three subtypes:
       ▪ Coup contusion (occurs at the site of the impact)
       ▪ Contre-coup contusion (occurs at sites remote from the impact and are due to movements of the brain inside of the skull; they are most commonly found in the frontal and temporal poles and the subfrontal area)
       ▪ Gliding contusion (due to herniation or tissue tear)
     – Intracerebral hematomas (greater content of blood compared with contusions); usually caused by shearing of small vessels, but could also be caused by traumatic aneurysms.
7. *What are the indications for surgical evacuation in the different types of intracranial hemorrhage?*
   - An intraventricular hemorrhage can cause hydrocephalus requiring cerebrospinal fluid drainage. Subarachnoid hemorrhage does not require surgical evacuation; however, if it is abundant enough, it may cause vasospasm.
   - Contusions could be small and limited to the cortical layer, but they could also cause significant mass effect. Furthermore, contusions have the tendency to increase in size over the first 24–48 hours (and sometimes even longer) following a trauma. The prognosis following traumatic contusions will depend on the location and the number and the size of the contusions. Contusions may be a cause of posttraumatic seizure. Due to their location, they can also play a role in cognitive and behavioral deficit following a traumatic brain injury (TBI).

■ Answers (*continued*)

- Patients with mass effect, worsening neurologic exam, or refractory high ICP should undergo surgical evacuation. Patients with a GCS score of 6–8 with frontal or temporal contusions of greater than 20 cm^3 with a midline shift of greater than or equal to 5 mm or compression of the basal cisterns should have surgery. Any contusion with a volume greater than 50 cm^3 should be evacuated.[2] Any lesion of the posterior fossa associated with mass effect or neurologic dysfunction should be evacuated.[3]

8. *What are the indications for antiepileptic medication?*
   - Prophylaxis of late posttraumatic seizure is not recommended.
   - Prophylaxis of early posttraumatic seizure (within 7 days) is recommended, but has not been shown to change the overall outcome.[4]

■ References

1. Bullock MR, Chesnut R, Ghajar J, et al. Surgical Management of Traumatic Brain Injury Author Group, Surgical management of acute subdural hematomas. Neurosurgery 2006; 58(Suppl 3) S16–S24
2. Bullock MR, Chesnut R, Ghajar J, et al. Surgical Management of Traumatic Brain Injury Author Group, Surgical management of traumatic parenchymal lesions. Neurosurgery 2006; 58 (Suppl 3)S25–S46
3. Bullock MR, Chesnut R, Ghajar J, et al. Surgical Management of Traumatic Brain Injury Author Group, Surgical management of posterior fossa mass lesions. Neurosurgery 2006; 58(Suppl 3) S47–S55
4. Brain Trauma Foundation. American Association of Neurological Surgeons, Congress of Neurological Surgeons, Guidelines for the management of severe traumatic brain injury. Antiseizure prophylaxis. J Neurotrauma 2007;24(Suppl 1):S83–S86

Case 49   New Trends in Neurotrauma Monitoring

Judith Marcoux and Abdulrazag Ajlan

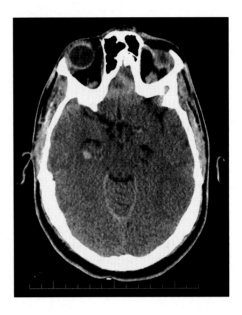

Fig. 49.1   Computed tomography scan of the head showing a very small intraparenchymal hematoma in the right hippocampal area.

■ Clinical Presentation

- A 20-year-old man is involved in a high-speed motor vehicle accident. He was the driver and was wearing his seatbelt.
- He is hemodynamically stable and his Glasgow Coma Score (GCS) before intubation is 8.
- A computed tomography (CT) scan of his head is obtained and shown in **Fig. 49.1**.
- His GCS remains 8 without sedation and he has an intraventricular drain placed to monitor his intracranial pressure (ICP). The opening pressure is 17 mm Hg.

- He is kept normothermic, normocapnic, and with a cerebral perfusion pressure (CPP) above 70 mm Hg.
- Over the course of the next 3 days, his ICP rises and he needs heavier sedation, cerebrospinal fluid (CSF) drainage, and hyperosmolar therapy.
- A repeat CT scan shows diffuse cerebral edema with effacement of the subarachnoid spaces.
- Transcranial Doppler (TCD) measurements reveal high velocities in both carotid arteries as well as the middle cerebral arteries.

■ Questions

1. What other tools can help you optimize his ICP management?

2. What is the role of continuous electroencephalography (EEG)?
3. What is the role of microdialysis?

■ Answers

1. *What other tools can help you optimize his ICP management?*
   - Jugular venous oxygen saturation ($SjvO_2$):
     - The oxygen saturation in the brain draining veins will depend on the cerebral blood flow (CBF), the metabolic rate of oxygen consumption, as well as the hemoglobin concentration. Under normal circumstances the saturation will be between 55–70%.
     - However, if the cerebral tissue does not receive enough oxygen for its metabolic demands (due to low flow or low transportation of oxygen from low hemoglobin), the $SjvO_2$ will drop, reflecting an increased extraction of oxygen from the brain.
     - On the other hand, if the metabolic rate of oxygen in the brain is decreased, or the blood flow is high, the $SjvO_2$ will increase. Therefore, a supranormal value of $SjvO_2$ could mean a state of hyperemia. But it could also reflect an impaired extraction capacity of the brain, which can be seen following a traumatic brain injury. $SjvO_2$ will detect global changes, but may miss regional abnormalities.
     - $SjvO_2$ clinical use is not simple; however, it does have some applications. Hyperventilation is very effective in lowering the ICP, but it does so by reducing the cerebral blood flow. Because brain tissue is very sensitive to ischemia following an acute traumatic brain injury, one must be careful not to overuse hyperventilation. One way to monitor the effect of hyperventilation on cerebral perfusion is by measuring the $SjvO_2$.
     - If the hyperventilation is excessive, the $SjvO_2$ will drop and the ventilator settings can be quickly adjusted (level III recommendation by the Brain Trauma Foundation).[1]
     - Low $SjvO_2$ has also been linked with poor outcome.[2]
   - Brain tissue partial pressure of oxygen (PO_2):
     - Human brain is dependent on a good oxygenation for its metabolism and a decrease in tissue oxygenation will increase the risk of ischemic cell damage, especially following a traumatic brain injury. Brain tissue oxygenation is dependent on cerebral perfusion pressure (CPP), but local hypoxia can happen despite normal CPP, intracranial pressure, and mean arterial pressure.
     - Monitoring brain tissue PO_2 can help detect an area at risk of ongoing damage. Recent evidences seem to show that aggressively treating the PO_2 will improve the outcome.[3] One must bear in mind, however, that it reflects the metabolic state of a small area of the brain only and other areas may differ significantly.
   - Cerebral blood flow (CBF)
     - Monitoring CBF when the ICP is elevated may help differentiate an ischemic state from a hyperemic state and dramatically change the therapeutic approach to the traumatic brain injury (TBI) patient.[4]
     - There are different ways to measure CBF; the most commonly used being the TCD, which is a bedside noninvasive method, but is usually noncontinuous.
     - In the current case, the increased velocities of TCD reflect hyperemia. Lowering the CPP to 60 mm Hg helped control the current patient's ICP.

2. *What is the role of continuous EEG?*
   - Posttraumatic seizures complicate a sizable percentage of TBIs. The risk will increase with the severity of the trauma.
   - In patients with moderate and severe TBI, 22.3% had electrical seizures on continuous EEG monitoring. More than half of which had no clinical manifestation of their seizures.[4]
   - In critically ill comatose patients, the duration of nonconvulsive status epilepticus and the delay to diagnosis was associated with increased mortality.[5]
   - Continuous EEG monitoring may help diagnose and treat nonconvulsive seizures, and thus prevent secondary injury to the brain. Furthermore, continuous EEG is of primary importance in the titration of barbiturate-induced coma to treat raised ICP.

3. *What is the role of microdialysis?*
   - Microdialysis gives a unique insight into the brain's metabolism by measuring tissue biochemistry.
   - It can give a warning regarding impending hypoxia/ischemia or the occurrence of secondary damage. But its measure is local and there is a great variability in the range of the values collected. Its use is still limited to research. However, a growing number of clinicians are using it. In 2004, a consensus[6] was made for its use and some of the major points are as follows:
     - The use of microdialysis should be reserved for patients with a severe TBI requiring ICP monitoring.
     - The probe should be placed in the right frontal area in patients with diffuse lesions or placed in the pericontusional area, if there is a focal lesion.
     - The best marker for secondary damage is the lactate/pyruvate ratio; glucose, glutamate, and glycerol can also be used as markers of ischemia.

■ References

1. Brain Trauma Foundation, American Association of Neurological Surgeons, Congress of Neurological Surgeons, et al. Guidelines for the management of severe traumatic brain injury. XIV. Hyperventilation. J Neurotrauma 2007;24(Suppl 1):S87–S90
2. Gopinath SP, Robertson CS, Contant CF, et al. Jugular venous desaturation and outcome after head injury. J Neurol Neurosurg Psychiatry 1994;57(6):717–723
3. Stiefel MF, Spiotta A, Gracias VH, et al. Reduced mortality rate in patients with severe traumatic brain injury treated with brain tissue oxygen monitoring. J Neurosurg 2005;103(5):805–811
4. Vespa PM, Nuwer MR, Nenov V, et al. Increased incidence and impact of nonconvulsive and convulsive seizures after traumatic brain injury as detected by continuous electroencephalographic monitoring. J Neurosurg 1999;91(5):750–760
5. Young GB, Jordan KG, Doig GS. An assessment of nonconvulsive seizures in the intensive care unit using continuous EEG monitoring: an investigation of variables associated with mortality. Neurology 1996;47(1):83–89
6. Bellander BM, Cantais E, Enblad P, et al. Consensus meeting on microdialysis in neurointensive care. Intensive Care Med 2004;30(12):2166–2169

Case 50   Intracranial Pressure Management

Abdulrazag Ajlan and Judith Marcoux

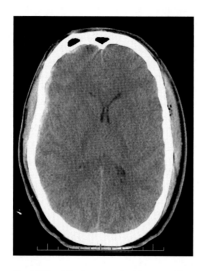

Fig. 50.1   A brain computed tomography scan showing a small right subdural hematoma with a midline shift of 4 mm. There is diffuse brain swelling and small ventricles.

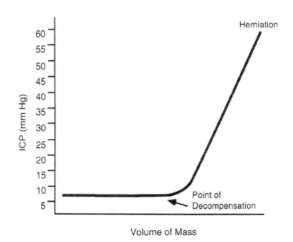

Fig. 50.2   The brain can compensate within a limited range of pressure. After the compensatory mechanisms fail, the intracranial pressure will increase dramatically.

■ Clinical Presentation

- A 26-year-old male pedestrian is hit by a car.
- Initial Glasgow Coma Score (GCS) score is 6 after resuscitation.
- A computed tomography (CT) scan is obtained and shows a small right acute subdural hematoma (SDH) with a 4 mm midline shift (**Fig. 50.1**).

- An intraventricular drain is placed to monitor the intracranial pressure (ICP).

■ Questions

1. What is the pathophysiology of raised ICP?
2. How can we monitor the ICP?
3. What are the indications for ICP monitoring?

4. How can we manage elevated ICP (describe first, second, and third tier measures)?

■ Answers

1. *What is the pathophysiology of raised ICP?*
   - The Monro-Kellie hypothesis states that the cranial compartment is incompressible, and the volume inside the cranium is a fixed volume.
   - The cranium and its constituents (blood, cerebrospinal fluid [CSF], and brain tissue) create a state of volume equilibrium, such that any increase in volume of one of the cranial constituents must be compensated by a decrease in volume of another.[1,2]
   - Small increases in brain volume does not lead to immediate high ICP because of compensatory measures such as displacement of CSF into the spinal canal, stretching of the falx cerebri and the tentorium, and decrease in venous blood volume. However, once the ICP goes beyond the compensatory phase, small increases in brain volume (or any other constituent) can lead to marked elevations in the ICP (**Fig. 50.2**).
   - Once the ICP starts to be elevated, it will affect the brain in two major ways:
     - High ICP will lead to decrease cerebral blood flow (CBF) as can be observed on the following equations:
       - CPP (cerebral perfusion pressure) = MAP (mean arterial pressure) − ICP
       - CBF = CPP / CVR (cerebral vascular resistance)
     - Any increase in the ICP will decrease the CPP. In the normal physiologic state, the CBF will be kept constant because the CVR will vary to compensate, this is called *autoregulation*. This compensation is impaired in the extreme of pressure or in abnormal states (such as brain trauma).

   - Once the ICP is high and uncompensated, the brain tissue will start shifting and herniating through dural openings. This herniation will cause brain tissue compression, disturbance in blood flow, damage to the vasculature, as well as further increase in the ICP. There are different types of herniation:
     - Uncal herniation is caused by a mass in the middle fossa that displaces the uncus between the midbrain and tentorial edge. This causes compression on the descending tract and the reticular formation in the brainstem causing a decrease in the level of consciousness and contralateral hemiparesis. The ipsilateral oculomotor nerve is also affected causing ptosis and mydriasis (**Fig. 50.3 and Fig. 50.4**).
     - Sometimes the midbrain is squeezed against the contralateral tentorial edge (Kernohan's notch) causing ipsilateral hemiparesis (**Fig. 50.3 and Fig. 50.4**). The posterior cerebral artery will be compressed causing ischemia.
     - With more severe herniation, the basilar artery will be stretched causing tearing of the brainstem perforator vessels, brainstem infarction, and bleeding (Duret's hemorrhages).
     - The Cushing triad occurs from high ICP and herniation. This triad includes hypertension, bradycardia, and respiratory irregularities.

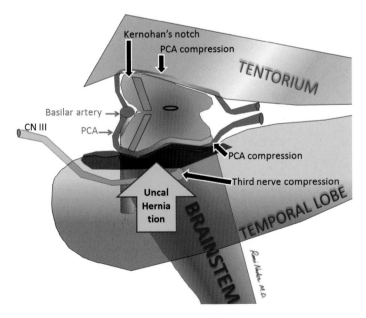

Fig. 50.3 Herniation of the uncus is causing compression of the brainstem, posterior cerebral artery (PCA), and oculomotor nerve (CN III). Compression will normally cause ipsilateral pupil dilatation and contralateral hemiparesis. If the brainstem is shifted toward the other side, structures on that other side may be compressed, giving instead a contralateral pupil dilatation and an ipsilateral hemiparesis.

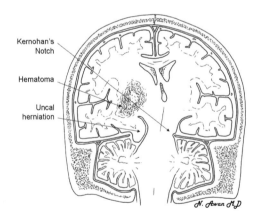

Fig. 50.4 Artist's rendering of uncal herniation.

■ Answers (continued)

2. *How can we monitor the ICP?*
   - One of the most reliable methods is the clinical picture of the patient. If the patient is awake enough to be followed clinically, this can be used as an objective parameter indicating that he is maintaining his perfusion and that his ICP is compensated. Once the clinical exam is lost for any reason (such as decrease level of consciousness or intoxication), another parameter should be used.
   - Several methods have been developed for measuring the ICP. The classical methods include
     - Intraventricular catheter placement (ventriculostomy)
     - Intraparenchymal monitoring
     - Epidural devices
     - Subdural/subarachnoid devices (bolts)
   - The ventricular catheter is the gold standard given that it is the most accurate. It is also therapeutic as well as diagnostic.

3. *What are the indications for ICP monitoring?*
   - The guidelines were revised by the Brain Trauma Foundation in 2007[3] and include
     - Patient with severe injury (GCS ≤8) after resuscitation and with an abnormal CT scan (hematoma, contusion, edema).
     - Patient with severe injury (GCS ≤8) and normal CT scan with two or more of the following:
       - Age above 40 years
       - Unilateral or bilateral motor posturing
       - Systolic blood pressure <90 mm Hg
   - ICP monitoring is not routinely indicated in mild or moderate brain trauma cases. However the treating physician can choose to monitor ICP in certain conscious patients with abnormal CT scan findings.[3]

4. *How can we manage elevated ICP (describe first, second, and third tier measures)?*
   - Brain injury from trauma results from
     - Primary injury from the first impact. This type of damage has no treatment other than prevention
     - Secondary injury, which can be due to
       - Intracranial causes such as expanding hematomas, contusions, or diffuse edema, which will cause high ICP
       - Systemic causes such as hypotension, hypoxia, and pyrexia, will cause mismatch in the metabolic demand and the blood flow.
   - Therefore, the treatment starts at the scene by preventing hypotension and hypoxia with adequate resuscitation and airway management, followed by a rapid transfer to a trauma center.
   - Once the CT scan is done and a surgical mass lesion is ruled out, an ICP monitor is inserted if indicated.
   - The goal of treatment is to keep an adequate blood flow which will match the metabolic demand of the injured brain. To reach this goal, the ICP should be kept below 20 mm Hg,[4] and the CPP between 50 and 70 mm Hg.[5] First, second, and third tier therapies have been devised for ICP treatment.
   - First tier therapies:
     - Elevation of the head to 30 degrees to enhance the venous outflow
     - Keeping the neck straight and the venous outflow patent.
     - Ventilation to normocarbia (pCO_2 = 35–40 mm Hg) to prevent cerebral vasodilatation. Hyperventilation can reduce ICP by causing cerebral vasoconstriction. On the other hand, this decrease in CBF can cause ischemia. Therefore, the use of hyperventilation as a prophylactic measure with pCO_2 <25 mm Hg is not recommended, especially in the early period after trauma. Hyperventilation is only recommended as a temporary measure in the case of high ICP until other treatments are started or with other monitoring tools for the cerebral blood flow (see Case 49, New Trends in Neurotrauma Monitoring).
     - Avoid hyperthermia because it may lead to an increase in the metabolic rate. Acetaminophen and a cooling blanket can be used to achieve this goal.
   - Second tier therapies:
     - Agitation and pain are two common causes of elevated ICP. Thus, sedation and pain control present an effective treatment modality.
     - Hyperosmolar treatment is used to decrease brain edema and subsequently the ICP. The hyperosmolar treatment will help also in cerebral perfusion.[6] Mannitol and hypertonic saline can be used as osmotic therapy agents.
     - Neuromuscular paralysis for maximal muscle relaxation and decrease muscle tone
     - CSF drainage from the intraventricular drain
   - Third tier therapies:
     - Decompressive craniectomy can be very effective in reducing the ICP. However, it is not clear if this measure improves the outcome. There are no clear guidelines about indications and timing. The only randomized clinical trial was done in a pediatric group. It shows a better outcome, but this did not reach statistical significance.[7]
     - Barbiturate coma: High-dose barbiturate therapy can result in control of ICP when all other medical and surgical treatments have failed. This effect is attributed mainly to the decrease in the cellular metabolic rate and subsequent decrease in CBF. The main side effects are hemodynamic instability and lowered immunity. It has shown no clear benefit in improving outcome and the prophylactic use in the treatment of ICP is not recommended.[8]

■ References

1. Monro A. Observations on the Structure and Function of the Nervous System. Edinburgh: Creech and Johnson, 1783
2. Kellie G. An account of the appearances observed in the dissection of two of the three individuals presumed to have perished in the storm of the 3rd, and whose bodies were discovered in the vicinity of Leith in the morning of the 4th November 1821 with some reflect. The Transactions of the Medico-Chirurgical Society of Edinburgh. 1824;1:84–169
3. Brain Trauma Foundation, American Association of Neurological Surgeons, Congress of Neurological Surgeons, et al. Guidelines for the management of severe traumatic brain injury. VI. Indications for intracranial pressure monitoring. J Neurotrauma 2007;24 (Suppl 1):S37–S44
4. Brain Trauma Foundation, American Association of Neurological Surgeons, Congress of Neurological Surgeons, et al. Guidelines for the management of severe traumatic brain injury. VIII. Intracranial pressure thresholds. J Neurotrauma 2007;24(Suppl 1):S55–S58

5. Brain Trauma Foundation, American Association of Neurological Surgeons, Congress of Neurological Surgeons, et al. Guidelines for the management of severe traumatic brain injury. IX. Cerebral perfusion thresholds. J Neurotrauma 2007;24(Suppl 1):S59–S64
6. Mendelow AD, Teasdale GM, Russell T, Flood J, Patterson J, Murray GD. Effect of mannitol on cerebral blood flow and cerebral perfusion pressure in human head injury. J Neurosurg 1985;63(1):43–48
7. Taylor A, Butt W, Rosenfeld J, et al. A randomized trial of very early decompressive craniectomy in children with traumatic brain injury and sustained intracranial hypertension. Childs Nerv Syst 2001;17(3):154–162
8. Brain Trauma Foundation, American Association of Neurological Surgeons, Congress of Neurological Surgeons, et al. Guidelines for the management of severe traumatic brain injury. XI. Anesthetics, analgesics, and sedatives. J Neurotrauma 2007;24(Suppl 1):S71–S76

Case 51   Gunshot Wound to the Head

Remi Nader

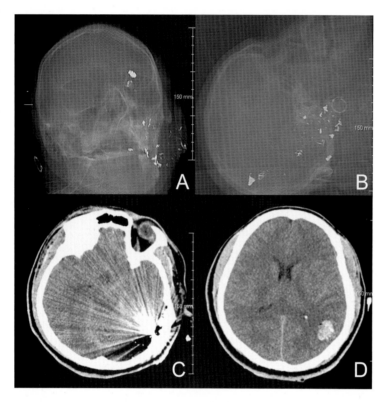

Fig. 51.1 Computed tomography scan of the head. Scout images **(A)** anteroposterior and **(B)** lateral as well as pertinent axial images **(C)** and **(D)** are shown. The bullet entry site appears to be just under the left mastoid process and the bullet fragments appear to have traveled through the mastoid air cells and are lodged up into the left parietal lobe.

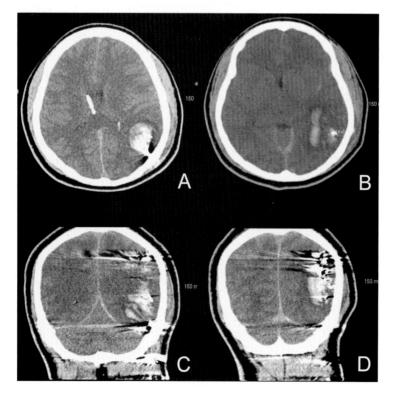

Fig. 51.2 Computed tomography scan of the head showing pertinent **(A,B)** axial and **(C,D)** coronal reconstructed images. See text for further details.

Clinical Presentation

- A 25-year-old man presents to the emergency room after sustaining a self-inflicted gunshot wound to the head ~1 hour ago. A low-caliber handgun was used.
- The patient is intubated on arrival. He is awake and agitated.
- On examination: the pupils are both 3 mm and reactive and he is moving all four extremities purposefully, localizing with both arms.
- No other pertinent findings were noted on history or examination.
- An initial computed tomography (CT) scan is obtained (**Fig. 51.1**).

Questions

1. Describe the findings on the CT scan.
2. What is your initial management?
3. Once the patient is stabilized, you elect to place a ventriculostomy. Initial intracranial pressure (ICP) is ~25 cm H_2O. What are the measures for treating ICP?

Despite appropriate medical management, he continues to deteriorate. His ICP continues to increase up to 50 cm H_2O and he develops a left dilated pupil ~4 hours after admission. An urgent CT is obtained and shown in **Fig. 51.2**.

4. Describe the CT scan findings.
5. What is your management at this time?
6. What are the indications to operate on gunshot wounds to the head?

7. What are the contraindications for surgery?

You decide to resect the hematoma and débride the bullet path. Postoperatively, the patient does well for 24 hours, while under sedation and mannitol with head of bed elevated and PCO_2 of 30. His ICP starts increasing from 20 to ~35 cm H_2O. His pupils are still equal and reactive. You cannot obtain further neurologic assessment due to the sedation. Another CT scan done postoperatively is shown in **Fig. 51.3**.

8. How would you manage the ICP problem now? What are your options?
9. What is the expected prognosis?

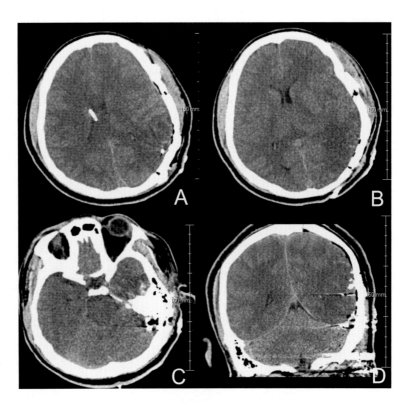

Fig. 51.3 Computed tomography scan of the head showing pertinent (**A–C**) axial and (**D**) coronal reconstructed images. The hematoma has been evacuated. There is significant diffuse brain edema, sulcal effacement, tight basal cisterns, and small ventricles. These findings may be suggestive of increased intracranial pressure.

■ Answers

1. *Describe the findings on the CT scan.*
   - Scout images show bullet fragments extending from below the left mastoid through the skull at the level of the mastoid air cells and a larger bullet fragment lodged in the left parietal lobe.
   - Axial images show tight but open quadrigeminal cisterns.
   - Rostral cuts show small (1.5 cm in diameter) intracerebral hematoma in the left parietal lobe.
   - Some diffuse subarachnoid hemorrhage is seen.
   - No significant midline shift

2. *What is your initial management?*
   - ABCs of trauma: Insure that the airway is secured, the patient is ventilated, and the blood pressure and pulse are adequate. Resuscitate if needed. Start intravenous (i.v.) line and fluids; place a Foley catheter.
   - Admit to intensive care unit (ICU).
   - Administer tetanus toxoid.
   - Start antiepileptics: load with phenytoin loading dose (1 gram over 1 hour) and give phenytoin 100 mg every 8 hours.
   - Provide broad-spectrum antibiotic coverage with both gram-negative and gram-positive coverage (such as nafcillin and ceftriaxone).
   - Administer H_2 agonists for ulcer prophylaxis.
   - Check laboratory studies: complete blood count, electrolytes, coagulation profile (prothrombin time [PT], partial thromboplastin time [PTT]), type and screen, and toxicology screen
   - Consider urgent ventriculostomy placement.[1]
   - The patient at this time does not appear to need evacuation of the hematoma or bullet fragments as there is no mass effect on the brain. However, he is likely to develop significant swelling and increased ICP in the next 24 hours and will need ICP lowering treatment.[2]

3. *Once the patient is stabilized, you elect to place a ventriculostomy. Initial ICP is ~25 cm H_2O. What are the measures for treating ICP?*
   - A detailed description of the management of ICP is outlined in Case 50, Intracranial Pressure Management. Here follows a summary of the pertinent points:
     - Elevate the head of the bed by 30 degrees.
     - Make sure there are no constrictions to the patient's jugular venous outflow (collars, etc.).
     - Avoid hypotension, hypertension, or hypoxia.
     - Hyperventilation to a PCO_2 of 30 to 35 mm Hg may be used as a short-term measure to treat surges in the ICP.[3]
     - Mannitol 0.5 to 1 g per kg i.v. infusion – this may be repeated every 4 hours, but one needs to ensure that the serum osmolality is kept lower than 320.[4]

   - Sedation with morphine and midazolam drips or alternatively with a fentanyl drip[5]
   - Pharmacological paralysis (e.g., with vecuronium)
   - If the ICP is not controlled after the above measures, serious consideration should be given to repeating the imaging studies and considering surgical evacuation of space-occupying lesions or third tier measures[2]

4. *Describe the CT scan findings.*
   - Expansion of the hematoma to a size of ~3.5 cm in diameter
   - Midline shift is now present (of at least 1 cm)

5. *What is your management at this time?*
   - The patient needs urgent surgical evacuation of the hematoma and decompression.
   - Options include:
     - Craniotomy and resection of hematoma ± debridement of the bullet tract
     - Decompressive craniectomy ± hematoma evacuation

6. *What are the indications to operate on gunshot wounds to the head?*
   - Patients with favorable neurologic exam or Glasgow Coma Score (GCS), i.e., patients with none of the contraindications described in the following questions.
   - Debridement of devitalized tissue or bone fragments
   - Evacuations of a hematoma
   - Separation of intracranial component from air sinuses[2]

7. *What are the contraindications for surgery?*
   - Bullet traveling across the midline or the geographic center of the brain
   - Bullet traveling across ventricles[6]
   - Bullets traveling across more than one contiguous lobe of the brain[2,7]

8. *How would you manage the ICP problem now? What are your options?*
   - At this time, it becomes necessary to employ second tier measures, as explained in Question 3.
   - Also consider the following surgical options:
     - Removing the bone flap by performing a craniectomy
     - Further debridement of devitalized brain in the area around the tract of the bullet

9. *What is the expected prognosis?*
   - In this case, if the patient gets through the first 72 hours with ICP better controlled, he has a chance of surviving.
   - However, he will most likely be severely disabled as the injury did involve eloquent areas of the dominant hemisphere.
   - Overall, he has a poor prognosis with survival around 30%.[8,9]

■ References

1. Brain Trauma Foundation, American Association of Neurological Surgeons, Congress of Neurological Surgeons, et al. Guidelines for the management of severe traumatic brain injury. VII. Intracranial pressure monitoring technology. J Neurotrauma 2007;24(Suppl 1):S45–S54

2. Greenberg MS. Handbook of Neurosurgery. 6th ed. New York: Thieme Medical Publishers; 2006

3. Brain Trauma Foundation, American Association of Neurological Surgeons, Congress of Neurological Surgeons, et al. Guidelines for the management of severe traumatic brain injury. XIV. Hyperventilation. J Neurotrauma 2007;24(Suppl 1):S87–S90

4. Brain Trauma Foundation, American Association of Neurological Surgeons, Congress of Neurological Surgeons, et al. Guidelines for the management of severe traumatic brain injury. II. Hyperosmolar therapy. J Neurotrauma 2007;24(Suppl 1):S14–S20

5. Brain Trauma Foundation, American Association of Neurological Surgeons, Congress of Neurological Surgeons, et al. Guidelines for the management of severe traumatic brain injury. XI. Anesthetics, analgesics, and sedatives. J Neurotrauma 2007;24(Suppl 1):S71–S76

6. Murano T, Mohr AM, Lavery RF, Lynch C, Homnick AT, Livingston DH. Civilian craniocerebral gunshot wounds: an update in predicting outcomes. Am Surg 2005;71(12):1009–1014

7. Kim TW, Lee JK, Moon KS, et al. Penetrating gunshot injuries to the brain. J Trauma 2007;62(6):1446–1451

8. Liebenberg WA, Demetriades AK, Hankins M, Hardwidge C, Hartzenberg BH. Penetrating civilian craniocerebral gunshot wounds: a protocol of delayed surgery. Neurosurgery 2005;57(2):293–299

9. Kaufman HH. Civilian gunshot wounds to the head. Neurosurgery 1993;32(6):962–964

Case 52   Other Penetrating Intracranial Trauma

Domenic P. Esposito

■ Clinical Presentation

- A 27-year-old man presents to the emergency room (ER) with a history of being struck in the head with a blunt object.
- The initial Glasgow Coma Scale (GCS) in the ER is 15.
- There are no focal neurologic deficits.
- A computed tomography (CT) scan is obtained and shown in **Fig. 52.1**.

■ Questions

1. What would be your initial work-up and management plan?
2. Other than radiologic studies, what other studies would be indicated?
3. Outline your plan of care at this point.
4. Interpret the magnetic resonance imaging (MRI) scan shown in **Fig. 52.2**.
5. Following imaging and laboratory studies, the patient develops a right hemiparesis and a speech disturbance. What is likely the cause of these findings?
6. What would be your management plan at this time?
7. What position would you use for the operative approach?
8. What special arrangements would you make preoperatively?
9. Assuming the blunt force trauma produced a very large, somewhat stellate laceration, how would you plan your skin flap?
10. What nontypical neurosurgical devices might be of value in this case?
11. Would you give your anesthesiologist any particular instructions?

You look at the anesthesiology monitor before beginning (which is usually a good idea) and see that the patient has a pulse of 120, a systolic blood pressure of 90, and the central venous pressure (CVP) line is not connected to a monitor.

12. What is your next step in the management of this patient?
13. The patient is now stable and you open the skin flap revealing the underlying depressed skull fracture, there is no excessive bleeding at this point. Would you begin removing depressed fragments, or would you plan a bone flap (if so, describe the flap)?
14. Before beginning the bone work would you consider harvesting any tissue? If so, what would be some of your choices?
15. While performing your bony removal, copious bleeding begins from a disrupted sagittal sinus. What is your next step in management?

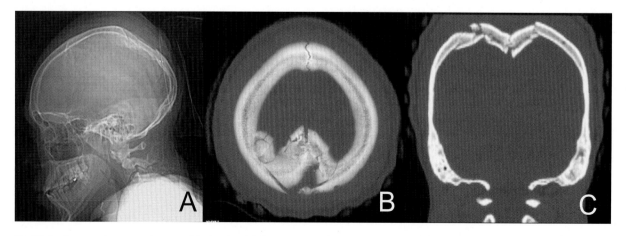

Fig. 52.1   Computed tomography scan of the head with **(A)** scout image, **(B)** axial, and **(C)** sagittal views, showing depressed skull fracture in the occipital area.

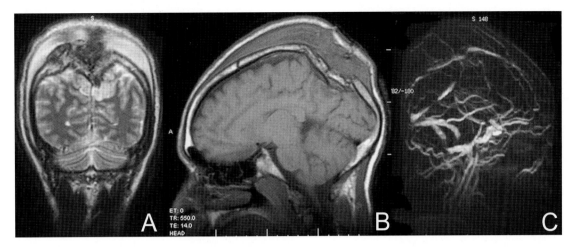

Fig. 52.2   Magnetic resonance imaging (MRI) of the brain with coronal T2-weighted **(A)** and sagittal T1-weighted **(B)** images showing the depressed skull fracture with underlying brain contusions. Magnetic resonance venography **(C)** showing disruption of the posterior portion of the superior sagittal sinus.

■ Answers

1. *What would be your initial work-up and management plan?*
   - Because the patient is currently stable, laboratory studies should be obtained including a complete blood count, electrolytes, type and screen, and coagulation profile.
   - The patient should be kept in a monitored bed while further treatment is planned.
   - Prophylactic anticonvulsants may be given.
2. *Other than radiologic studies, what other studies would be indicated?*
   - An urgent (STAT) MRI with MR venography (MRV) should be obtained; if MRV is not available a CT venogram (CTV) or angiography with late venous phases would be acceptable.
3. *Outline your plan of care at this point.*
   - Because it is highly unlikely that this lesion can be managed conservatively, preparations for surgical treatment should be initiated.
4. *Interpret the MRI scan shown in* **Fig. 52.2**.
   - The MRI reveals a large subgaleal hematoma with compromise of the superior sagittal sinus and cortical contusions.
5. *Following imaging and laboratory studies, the patient develops a right hemiparesis and a speech disturbance. What is likely the cause of these findings?*
   - The patients' neurologic deterioration is most likely due to compromise of the sagittal sinus.
6. *What would be your management plan at this time?*
   - This patient needs to be taken to the operating room for elevation of the depressed fracture and possible repair of the sagittal sinus.[1]

7. *What position would you use for the operative approach?*
   - The patient should be positioned prone with the head slightly elevated.
   - Mayfield three-point rigid fixation may be used.
8. *What special arrangements would you make preoperatively?*
   - Preoperative preparation should include
     - Type and cross-match at least 2 units of packed red blood cells
     - Precordial Doppler probe
     - Central line and arterial line
     - Preoperative antibiotics and anticonvulsants
   - This case can very easily turn into a surgical disaster. You should arrange to have competent experienced surgical hands other than your own to assist you.
9. *Assuming the blunt force trauma produced a very large somewhat stellate laceration, how would you plan your skin flap?*
   - The scalp flap was partially made by the assailant, but extension of the stellate laceration in both anteroposterior and lateral directions for good exposure is mandatory.
10. *What nontypical neurosurgical devices might be of value in this case?*
    - Some nontypical neurosurgical devices that might be of help are Fogarty catheters, cell savers, and vascular grafts.
11. *Would you give your anesthesiologist any particular instructions?*
    - The anesthesiologist needs to be aware of the possibility of extensive rapid blood loss and the blood needs to be ready in the room prior to bone removal.

■ Answers (*continued*)

12. *What is your next step in the management of this patient?*
    - After gently reminding anesthesia of the tenuous state of the patient, insist that the patient be adequately transfused, monitored, and stabilized prior to proceeding with the procedure.
    - Ensure CVP is monitored.
    - Ensure the patient is being treated for shock: fluids, blood transfusion, and pressors if necessary.

13. *The patient is now stable and you open the skin flap revealing the underlying depressed skull fracture, there is no excessive bleeding at this point. Would you begin removing depressed fragments, or would you plan a bone flap (if so, describe the flap)?*
    - Removing the depressed fragments without prior exposure and control of the proximal and distal normal sagittal sinus could easily result in the demise of this patient.
    - A circular bone flap around the depressant area with multiple burr holes on either side of the sinus as well as lateral to the fragments is mandatory.[2,3]

14. *Before beginning the bone work would you consider harvesting any tissue? If so, what would be some of your choices?*
    - Harvesting a piece of temporalis fascia to assist with possible reconstruction may be helpful.

15. *While performing your bony removal, copious bleeding begins from a disrupted sagittal sinus. What is your next step in management?*
    - Quickly remove all bone over the sinus. If proper preparations have been made, this can be hastily performed.[3,4]
    - Establish control of the sinus with digital pressure and assess the damage.
    - In this case, a large thrombus was encountered in the distal sinus (which was probably the cause of the patient's neurologic decline) and a 5 cm lateral laceration of the sinus was able to be repaired primarily. The sinus remained intact. This patient eventually made a complete recovery.[5]

■ References

1. Donovan DJ. Simple depressed skull fracture causing sagittal sinus stenosis and increased intracranial pressure: case report and review of the literature. Surg Neurol 2005;63(4):380–383
2. Donaghy RM, Wallman LJ, Flanagan MJ, Numoto M. Saggital sinus repair. Technical note. J Neurosurg 1973;38(2):244–248
3. Kapp JP, Gielchinsky I, Deardourff SL. Operative techniques for management of lesions involving the dural venous sinuses. Surg Neurol 1977;7(6):339–342
4. Pribán V, Bombic M. Compound depressed fracture of occipital bone causing laceration of left occipital lobe and injury of superior sagittal sinus–case report. Rozhl Chir 2006;85(11):541–544
5. Iskandar BJ, Kapp JP. Nonseptic venous occlusive disease. In: Rengachary SS, Wilkins RH, eds. Neurosurgery. 2nd ed. New York: McGraw-Hill; 1996:2177–2190

Case 53 Aqueductal Stenosis

Jeffrey Atkinson

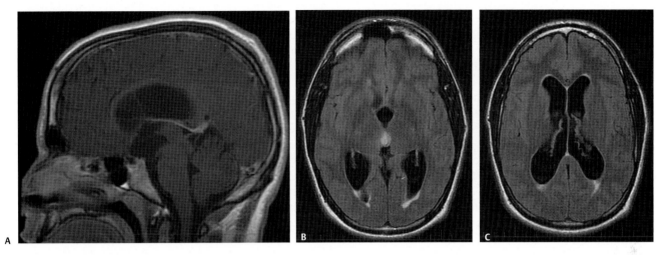

Fig. 53.1 **(A)** Midsagittal T1-weighted magnetic resonance image and **(B,C)** axial fluid-attenuated inversion-recovery image of the brain.

■ Clinical Presentation

- A 15-year-old adolescent boy presents with a long history of intermittent syncopal episodes.
- He was initially investigated at age 10 by a neurologist with normal cranial imaging, normal electroencephalogram (EEG), and normal physical examination.
- Similar episodes recurred at age 15 and although his neurologic examination remained normal, magnetic resonance imaging (MRI) was performed as part of further investigations, and was significantly different from the prior computed tomography (CT) scan.
- Representative images are presented in **Fig. 53.1**.

■ Questions

1. Describe the findings on the imaging study.
2. What advice would you give the patient in terms of management?
3. What would be the basis for intervention in this patient?
4. Describe possible surgical interventions for the management of this patient.

The patient underwent a successful endoscopic third ventriculostomy (ETV) and biopsy of the third ventricular mass. The pathology was consistent with juvenile pilocytic astrocytoma.

5. Describe the risks associated with the above procedure.
6. Are there any specific technical considerations for the procedure?
7. What is the long-term prognosis for this patient?
8. What is your management strategy for the patient given the above information?

■ Answers

1. *Describe the findings on the imaging study.*
   - The MRI demonstrates ventriculomegaly at the level of the lateral ventricles with some transependymal edema.
   - There is also an apparent mass in the posterior part of the 3rd ventricle and tegmentum of the brainstem.

2. *What advice would you give the patient in terms of management?*
   - Management strategies for this patient can be divided into observational and interventional strategies.
   - Given the relatively minor history and lack of clear relationship between the lesion and symptoms, some may argue that the patient could be followed closely.
   - However, the change in lesion and ventricles from the scan 5 years previously and the transependymal cerebrospinal fluid (CSF) on MRI, all argue for treatment of hydrocephalus.

3. *What would be the basis for intervention in this patient?*
   - The basis for intervention is the transependymal migration of CSF seen on MRI, the clear progressive dilation of the ventricles over time, both of which suggest increasing hydrocephalus, and the probable growth of the mass over the time interval between the two imaging studies.

4. *Describe possible surgical interventions for the management of this patient.*
   - This patient could receive CSF diversion by means of a ventriculoperitoneal (VP) shunt.
   - CSF diversion could also be performed by ETV.[1]
   - Consideration could be made for biopsy of the lesion at the time of ETV given the apparent location of the lesion in the posterior 3rd ventricle.[2] It is not very likely that this lesion will progress and thus consideration for resection of this lesion would not be necessary absent progressive growth or unfavorable histology on biopsy.

5. *Describe the risks associated with the above procedure.*
   - ETV presents risks of late or early failure, fornix injury, intracerebral hematoma, hypothalamic injury, basilar aneurysm or arterial injury, and uncontrolled bleeding.[3,4]

6. *Are there any specific technical considerations for the procedure?*
   - Technical considerations revolve specifically around the preferred option of ETV with lesional biopsy.
   - It would be essential that the ETV be performed first to make sure that this procedure was not aborted due to bleeding from the biopsy[2]
   - Second to perform both the ETV and the biopsy a flexible endoscope would be needed.
   - Alternately, using a rigid scope, consideration must be given to placement of a single, slightly more anterior burr hole or two burr holes to allow an appropriate trajectory to both the anterior 3rd ventricle and ventriculostomy site and the posterior 3rd ventricle for the biopsy.

7. *What is the long-term prognosis for this patient?*
   - Expectations for the long-term control of hydrocephalus in this patient are good, approximately 80%.
   - Typically tegmental, posterior 3rd ventricle lesions of this type are benign and slow growing and cause no further problems apart from the hydrocephalus.
   - If a biopsy was performed, this may further define prognosis.

8. *What is your management strategy for the patient given the above information?*
   - ETV with or without biopsy would be the best option followed by serial imaging observation of the mass lesion.[2,5]

■ References

1. de Ribaupierre S, Rilliet B, Vernet O, Regli L, Villemure JG. Third ventriculostomy vs ventriculoperitoneal shunt in pediatric obstructive hydrocephalus: results from a Swiss series and literature review. Childs Nerv Syst 2007;23(5):527–533
2. Ternier J, Wray A, Puget S, Bodaert N, Zerah M, Sainte-Rose C. Tectal plate lesions in children. J Neurosurg 2006; 104(Suppl 6)369–376
3. Drake JM, Canadian Pediatric Neurosurgery Study Group. Endoscopic third ventriculostomy in pediatric patients: the Canadian experience. Neurosurgery 2007;60(5):881–886
4. Erşahin Y, Arslan D. Complications of endoscopic third ventriculostomy. Childs Nerv Syst 2008;24(8):943–948
5. Dağlioğlu E, Cataltepe O, Akalan N. Tectal gliomas in children: the implications for natural history and management strategy. Pediatr Neurosurg 2003;38(5):223–231

Case 54 Cerebrospinal Fluid Shunt Infections

Jeffrey Atkinson

■ Clinical Presentation

- A 3-month-old child with a L5-level myelomeningocele and a ventriculoperitoneal (VP) shunt comes to the emergency department with 24 hours of progressive irritability and fever.
- The child had the spinal defect closed at 2 days of life and a VP shunt inserted for progressive macrocrania and hydrocephalus at 14 days of life.
- He has been on a program of home intermittent catheterizations since birth and no prophylactic antibiotics.

- The exam demonstrates a child with a fever of 39.5°C, bulging fontanel, somnolent, and irritable.
- The motor examination is unchanged with no plantar flexion in the feet, but otherwise normal.
- The child's incisions all look well healed.
- White blood cell (WBC) count is elevated, and the urinalysis shows positive bacteria and WBCs.

■ Questions

1. What is the differential diagnosis suggested by this child's presentation?
2. What investigations are appropriate and why?

Blood cultures are collected and urine cultures are sent. A computed tomography (CT) scan is done, which shows a stable ventricle size compared with the last scan done after the shunt was inserted. Shunt tap reveals 1500 WBCs and 10 red blood cells (RBCs) with no bacteria seen on a gram stain.

3. What is the diagnosis?

4. What are the usual organisms involved?
5. What are the treatment options for this child?
6. What antibiotic regimen would you choose?
7. What is the incidence of shunt infection after an initial procedure?
8. What is the time frame over which these infections usually develop?
9. What is the incidence of shunt infection after an initial shunt infection?
10. What maneuvers have shown benefit in reducing shunt infection?

■ Answers

1. *What is the differential diagnosis suggested by this child's presentation?*
   - This child is presenting with the clinical signs of an infectious illness, and clinical signs of shunt malfunction, though the fever itself may be causing the child's irritability independent of shunt malfunction, and a severely irritable child may present with a bulging fontanel.
   - The cause of the febrile illness may be viral or respiratory, but in this case, we would be worried about shunt infection or wound complication, as well as urosepsis.
2. *What investigations are appropriate and why?*
   - This child needs cultures of blood, urine, a complete blood count, chest x-ray as well as viral swabs of any upper respiratory tract-related secretions and a full

exam to look for skin abrasions, wound complications, or other pertinent physical findings.
   - CT scan is indicated due to the clinical signs of increased intracranial pressure (ICP).
   - A tap of the shunt reservoir to obtain cerebrospinal fluid (CSF) is clearly indicated in this child given the presentation and relatively recent shunt surgery.
3. *What is the diagnosis?*
   - The cell count of the CSF points toward shunt infection even in the absence of an initially positive gram stain.
     - The culture of CSF will probably grow eventually.
4. *What are the usual organisms involved?*
   - Shunt infections are usually from skin colonization occurring at the time of surgery – gram-positive cocci are most common.[1]

■ Answers (*continued*)

- In a child of this age, and especially one with urinary catheterizations, gram-negatives and coliforms are also possible.[2]

5. *What are the treatment options for this child?*
   - This child needs antibiotics and some type of shunt externalization procedure.
   - Very few shunt infections will respond to antibiotics alone without hardware removal.
   - Many centers will externalize the shunt by removing the distal catheter from the abdomen and then treat until the CSF is sterile before replacing the entire system.[1]
   - In the event of continued positive cultures, the entire shunt system should be converted to an external ventricular drain (EVD).[2]
   - Some centers would externalize the EVD upfront with removal of the whole shunt system.[1,2]
   - The duration of antibiotic treatment before reinternalization is debatable; it averages 10 to 14 days, but three consecutive negative CSF cultures is a common standard.[2,3]

6. *What antibiotic regimen would you choose?*
   - Initial antibiotic regimen needs to include broad spectrum CSF penetrating coverage, and good antistaphylococcal coverage until the organism is known.[1,2]
   - Typical initial regimens would include a third-generation cephalosporin with vancomycin plus or minus an aminoglycoside.

7. *What is the incidence of shunt infection after an initial procedure?*
   - Shunt infection rates per procedure after an initial shunt placement are approximately 8 to 10% in most large studies of shunt insertions in children.[1]

8. *What is the time frame over which these infections usually develop?*
   - Most shunt infections are procedure-related and present within the first 6 months of surgery.
   - Other risk factors for shunt-related infection include wound breakdown and CSF leak.[1]

9. *What is the incidence of shunt infection after an initial shunt infection?*
   - Shunt infections may occur up to 25% of the time when a shunt is replaced after an initial infection.[1]

10. *What maneuvers have shown benefit in reducing shunt infection?*
    - There are a great many studies attempting to demonstrate protocols to reduce shunt infection rates.[4]
    - Efforts to reduce shunt infection rates have included perioperative antibiotics, various procedure-related technical issues such as double gloving, short duration of surgery, surgery timing, reduced mechanical manipulation of the hardware, and more recently antibiotic-impregnated shunt catheters.[4,5,6,7]
    - Many of these techniques including antibiotic-impregnated catheters are still the subject of some debate as to their relative efficacy.[4,6,7]

■ References

1. Kestle JR, Garton HJ, Whitehead WE, et al. Management of shunt infections: a multicenter pilot study. J Neurosurg 2006; 105(Suppl 3)177–181
2. Whitehead WE, Kestle JR. The treatment of cerebrospinal fluid shunt infections. Results from a practice survey of the American Society of Pediatric Neurosurgeons. Pediatr Neurosurg 2001;35(4):205–210
3. Arthur AS, Whitehead WE, Kestle JR. Duration of antibiotic therapy for the treatment of shunt infection: a surgeon and patient survey. Pediatr Neurosurg 2002;36(5):256–259
4. Pirotte BJ, Lubansu A, Bruneau M, Loqa C, Van Cutsem N, BrotchiJ. Sterile surgical technique for shunt placement reduces the shunt infection rate in children: preliminary analysis of a prospec-tive protocol in 115 consecutive procedures. Childs Nerv Syst 2007;23(11):1251–1261
5. Drake JM, Kestle JR, Milner R, et al. Randomized trial of cerebrospinal fluid shunt valve design in pediatric hydrocephalus. Neurosurgery 1998;43(2):294–3039
6. Kan P, Kestle J. Lack of efficacy of antibiotic-impregnated shunt systems in preventing shunt infections in children. Childs Nerv Syst 2007;23(7):773–777
7. Sciubba DM, Stuart RM, McGirt MJ, et al. Effect of antibiotic-impregnated shunt catheters in decreasing the incidence of shunt infection in the treatment of hydrocephalus. J Neurosurg 2005; 103(Suppl 2)131–136

Case 55   Slit Ventricle Syndrome

Jeffrey Atkinson

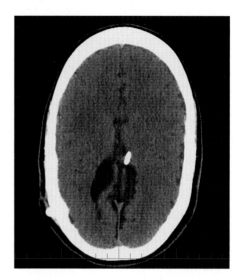

Fig. 55.1   Computed tomography scan of the brain revealing relatively small lateral ventricles and ventriculoperitoneal shunt located within the ventricle.

■ Clinical Presentation

- A 15-year-old girl with a history of myelomeningocele repaired at birth and with a ventriculoperitoneal (VP) shunted inserted shortly after birth presents with headache.
- She has a history of only one previous shunt revision.
- She is stable neurologically with a L4/L5 clinical level (both motor and sensory deficits), but presents with a new onset of disabling headaches over the past several months.
- Computed tomography (CT) scan shown in **Fig. 55.1** is no different from the routine scan done 1 year previously when she was completely asymptomatic.

■ Questions

1. What is the differential diagnosis?
2. What is the next possible step in the workup of this patient?

Shunt revision is performed, and at the time of surgery the distal and proximal catheters are changed due to "sluggish" flow. She is relieved of her headaches for a few hours, but the symptoms return shortly thereafter.

3. What are the diagnostic possibilities now?
4. What is the next step in her management?

CT scan remains unchanged; nuclear medicine shuntogram shows good flow.

5. What are other potential investigations?

Intracranial pressure (ICP) monitoring shows readings generally between 5 and 15 mm Hg depending on her position with no single reading higher than 20 mm Hg, and no reading lower than –5 mm Hg.

6. Describe the different types of syndromes associated with headaches and stable ventricle size on CT scan and outline management strategies for each.

■ Answers

1. *What is the differential diagnosis?*
   - Headache of the usual types (tension, migraine, etc.)
   - Headache related to shunt malfunction
   - Headache related to overshunting
   - It is essential to consider shunt malfunction even in the presence of unchanged or small ventricles. It may be of benefit to know the details of her last shunt revision with respect to headache history and changes seen on CT scan.

2. *What is the next possible step in the workup of this patient?*
   - Diagnostic tests should first focus on establishing whether or not there is normal shunt function.
   - There are several strategies in this regard:
     - Ophthalmology consultation might demonstrate papilledema missed on routine clinical exam.
     - In the absence of this finding, this patient is not acutely ill and might be watched expectantly with migraine medication.
     - However, with this strategy, lack of improvement in symptoms must provoke another look at the shunt.
     - Repeat CT scan after 24 to 48 hours might show some change in ventricle size.
     - Nuclear medicine shuntogram may be of some value. This test will include a shunt tap, which is a measure, though poor, of ICP at one moment in time. With good proximal reflux into the ventricle as an essential component of a normal test, some groups have reported this to be a reliable marker for shunt dysfunction.[1]
     - ICP monitoring over 24 to 48 hours may give an idea about the headache pattern and ICP management, which might prompt shunt or valve revision.
     - Finally, a semielective shunt exploration might demonstrate a poorly working component that could be replaced.[2]

3. *What are the diagnostic possibilities now?*
   - Early return of symptoms after shunt revision always prompts an appropriate workup for shunt malfunction.
   - A surgery can always convert a working shunt to a nonworking shunt. In the absence of any new signs of shunt malfunction, the same diagnostic possibilities as stated previously apply.

4. *What is the next step in her management?*
   - This patient needs an early-repeat CT scan.
   - If there is still no change in her ventricles, the management could proceed according to Question #2.

5. *What are other potential investigations?*
   - At this stage, ICP monitoring becomes the best option.

6. *Describe the different types of syndromes associated with headaches and stable ventricle size on CT scan and outline management strategies for each.*
   - Patients with VP shunts, new headaches, and no change in ventricular size on their CT scan can be broken down into four categories (variably described as part of the "slit ventricle syndrome"):
     - Shunt is malfunctioning despite CT findings – this can be determined by a shuntogram or shunt exploration, and the treatment is shunt revision.[3]
     - Shunt is overdraining – ICP monitoring may be necessary, though clinical history can be helpful and upgrading of valve to a higher resistance setting would be the appropriate treatment.[3,4]
     - Shunt is functioning maximally, but ICP is high anyway – this is rare and can only be really established with shunt exploration and ICP monitoring. In this rare instance, cranial expansion procedures would be the treatment of choice.[3]
     - Not a shunt problem – established with normal ICP tracing with ICP monitor, and treatment is neurology and/or pain service consultation, and other medical management for chronic headache relief.[2]

■ References

1. Vernet O, Farmer JP, Lambert R, Montes JL. Radionuclide shuntogram: adjunct to manage hydrocephalic patients. J Nucl Med 1996;37(3):406–4108

2. Walker ML, Fried A, Petronio J. Diagnosis and treatment of the slit ventricle syndrome. Neurosurg Clin N Am 1993;4(4):707–714

3. Olson S. The problematic slit ventricle syndrome. A review of the literature and proposed algorithm for treatment. Pediatr Neurosurg 2004;40(6):264–269

4. Kan P, Walker ML, Drake JM, Kestle JR. Predicting slitlike ventricles in children on the basis of baseline characteristics at the time of shunt insertion. J Neurosurg 2007; 106(Suppl 5)347–349

Case 56   Mega-hydrocephalus

Maqsood Ahmad and Abdulrahman J. Sabbagh

■ Clinical Presentation

- You are called to see a newborn in the neonatal intensive care unit diagnosed prenatally with severe hydrocephalus.
- The patient was delivered at 38 weeks of gestation through an elective cesarean section with normal APGAR (appearance, pulse, grimace, activity, respiration) scores.
- On exam he has a head circumference that is 4 cm above the 97th percentile, bulging fontanel, and splayed sutures. Additionally, distended scalp veins were present.
- Neonatal reflexes were present and he is spontaneously moving all limbs.
- He had no signs of spinal dysraphism or any skin manifestation of syndromic features.

■ Questions

1. Describe the CT findings (**Fig. 56.1**).
2. What are the surgical options?
3. What would be your timing of surgery?

You decide to place a ventriculoperitoneal (VP) shunt.

4. What are the shunt-type options that may be appropriate for this patient? What are the determinants that will help you to choose?
5. What are the complications specific to this patient that you will discuss with the parents?

You manage to insert a VP shunt and use a medium pressure valve.

   The patient does well and gets discharged home within a few days. You see him in clinic at 2 and 6 weeks postoperatively and he seems to be doing fine. Three months after discharge he presented to the clinic with a fluctuant subgaleal collection that is increasing in size upon coughing, crying, or simply laying in the supine position. You opt for observation for one week, but it continues to grow.

6. What do you think is happening now?
7. What are your surgical options?

You admit this child and decide to revise the shunt, downgrade the pressure setting, and repair the leak site (from the original burr hole) with fascia and tissue sealant. The patient does very well postoperatively. He is discharged home without leakage or fluid collection. Along with his follow-up with the pediatrics service for delayed milestones, he follows up with you for the VP shunt. You notice that he has started to develop progressively significant positional plagiocephaly.

8. What are the management options?

Despite multipositional stimulation the head continues to deform upward; the parietal bones grow and override the flattened occipital and frontal bones (**Fig. 56.2**). This deformity worsens with time. The fontanel remains soft. There are no associated neurologic sequelae.

   At the age of one year, the parents are offered surgery, which they opt for. Multiple cranial osteotomies and reconstruction (cranial reduction procedure) are performed to reduce the towering of the cranium and expand the anteroposterior and bilateral diameter and to correct the left-sided occipitoparietal flattening.

9. What was the purpose of a craniofacial reduction procedure in this child?
10. What are the limitations of craniofacial reduction procedures?
11. What complication risks are associated with this elective procedure?

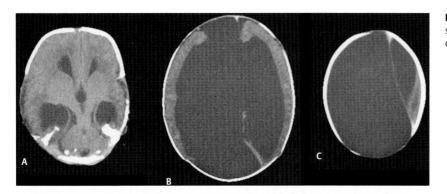

Fig. 56.1 Computed tomography scan, axial section through the 4th ventricle **(A)**, and higher cuts **(B)** and **(C)**.

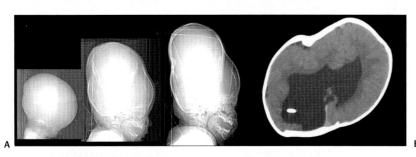

Fig. 56.2 Postshunting scout lateral images **(A)**, axial computed tomography scan through the ventricles **(B)** and three-dimensional reconstructions of CT scan **(C)**.

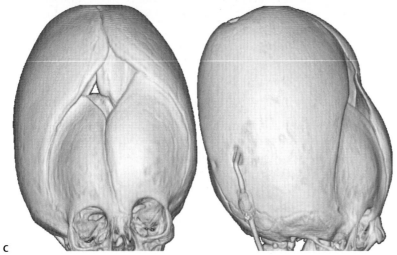

■ Answers

1. *Describe the (CT) findings* (**Fig. 56.1**).
   - This study depicts severe hydrocephalus with significantly thinned out cortical mantle.
   - The 4th ventricle is small, and this represents a case of aqueductal stenosis.
   - There is interhemispheric transcallosal schizencephaly.

2. *What are the surgical options?*
   - Surgical options include[1,2]
     – Extracranial cerebrospinal fluid (CSF) diversion procedures:
       ▪ VP shunt
       ▪ Ventriculoatrial shunt
     – Third ventriculostomy with or without choroid plexus coagulation[3]

■ Answers (*continued*)

3. *What would be your timing of surgery?*
   - As soon as the patient is medically fit for surgery – in the first few days of life

4. *What are the shunt-type options that may be appropriate for this patient? What are the determinants that will help you to choose?*
   - Shunt types include programmable vs. fixed (low or medium) pressure valves, with or without an antisiphon device.[1,2]
   - The pressure to be used will be determined during surgery from the opening pressure of the ventricle.

5. *What are the complications specific to this patient that you will discuss with the parents?*
   - Specific complications include[4–6]
     - CSF leakage around the ventricular catheter, as the cortical mantle is very thin in this case. The CSF can track through the burr hole. In addition, Laplace's law describing pressure difference over an interface in a sphere will dictate that the greater pressure in a larger skull will tend to drive further CSF out of the burr hole.
     - Overdrainage from the shunt
     - Shunt infection
     - Pressure sores, valve erosion through the skin, skin abrasions at the overriding bone edges
     - Cranial deformities due to the overriding of the floating bones that were much larger than needed preshunting.
     - Fluid and electrolyte imbalance due to the CSF shifts during surgery.
     - Occult subdural hemorrhage postoperatively: Always beware of subdural hematomas developing postshunting, especially in patients with mega-hydrocephalus. These patients will not show signs of high intracranial pressure. They may lose a large portion of their blood volume intracranially and present with hypovolemic shock.
     - General shunt complications and complications of neonatal anesthesia

6. *What do you think is happening now?*
   - CSF is leaking from the burr hole site around the ventricular catheter insertion site due to a lower resistance than that at the shunt valve.

7. *What are your surgical options?*
   - Management of a subgaleal collection postshunting:
     - Revise the shunt reservoir to a lower setting and repair the CSF leak site.
     - Repair the CSF site without revising the valve pressure. In this case, there is a risk of recurrence.

8. *What are the management options?*

- Postshunting plagiocephaly treatment options include[7,8]
  - Conservative options:
    - Multipositional stimulation
    - Frequent position changes – special care not to lie on the flat areas
    - Correction bands and helmets
- Special care not to develop abrasions from overriding skull edges
- Pressure sores at the valve and catheter sites – tailored openings in helmets at these sites
  - Surgical: Correction of deformities and remodeling

9. *What is the purpose of a craniofacial reduction procedure in this child?*
   - The purpose of surgery is to improve and ease handling, hygiene, cosmesis, and possibly mobility.[9–11]

10. *What are the limitations of craniofacial reduction procedures?*
    - Limitations include[9–11]
      - Incapability to reconstruct or change the skull base
      - Presence of a long superior sagittal sinus
      - Risk of infolding of the thinned-out cortex leading to congestion or venous infarct

11. *What complication risks are associated with this elective procedure?*
    - Complications of cranial reduction in craniofacial reconstruction procedures include[9,10]
      - Hemorrhage and complications of massive transfusion
        - Disseminated intravascular coagulation and other coagulopathies.
        - Acute respiratory distress syndrome
      - Postoperative prolonged edema that may threaten the airway and prolong the intubation period
      - Extradural collections
      - Complications of prolonged open surgical procedure
        - Anesthesia issues
        - Pressure sores
        - Infection
        - Electrolyte imbalances
      - Risk of brain injury
        - Enfolding of excess cortex causing venous infarcts
        - Manipulation of the superior sagittal sinus and risk of thrombosis or hemorrhage
        - Direct brain injury

References

1. Frim DM, Gupta N. Pediatric Neurosurgery. Georgetown, TX: Landes Bioscience; 2006

2. Winn RH. Neurological Surgery. 5th ed. Philadelphia: Saunders; 2004

3. Warf BC. Endoscopic third ventriculostomy and choroid plexus cauterization for pediatric hydrocephalus. Clin Neurosurg 2007;54:78–82

4. Lam CH, Dubuisson D. Treatment of hemispheric collapse and herniation beneath the falx in a case of shunted hydrocephalus. Surg Neurol 1990;33(3):202–205

5. Piatt JH Jr, Garton HJ. Clinical diagnosis of ventriculoperitoneal shunt failure among children with hydrocephalus. Pediatr Emerg Care 2008;24(4):201–210

6. Scott RM. Shunt complications. In: Rangachary SS, Wilkins RH, eds. Neurosurgery. New York: McGraw-Hill; 1996:3655–3664

7. Kumar R. Positional moulding in premature hydrocephalics. Neurol India 2002;50(2):148–152

8. Xia JJ, Kennedy KA, Teichgraeber JF, Wu KQ, Baumgartner JB, Gateno J. Nonsurgical treatment of deformational plagiocephaly: a systematic review. Arch Pediatr Adolesc Med 2008;162(8):719–727

9. Mathews MS, Loudon WG, Muhonen MG, Sundine MJ. Vault reduction cranioplasty for extreme hydrocephalic macrocephaly. J Neurosurg 2007;107(4, Suppl):332–337

10. Sundine MJ, Wirth GA, Brenner KA, et al. Cranial vault reduction cranioplasty in children with hydrocephalic macrocephaly. J Craniofac Surg 2006;17(4):645–655

11. Piatt JH Jr, Arguelles JH. Reduction cranioplasty for craniocerebral disproportion in infancy: indications and technique. Pediatr Neurosurg 1990;16(4–5):265–270

Case 57   Cerebellar Medulloblastoma

Ali Raja, Ian F. Pollack, and Nazer H. Qureshi

■ Clinical Presentation

- A 6-year-old boy presented with a history of clumsiness, slurred speech, and headache for the past 3 months.
- Clinical examination revealed a broad-based, ataxic gait with poor coordination.

- Computed tomography (CT) scan of the head without contrast showed a hyperdense, midline posterior fossa mass with minimal ventricular enlargement. Magnetic resonance imaging (MRI) scan of the brain is shown in **Fig. 57.1**.

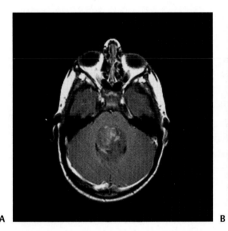
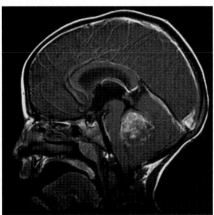
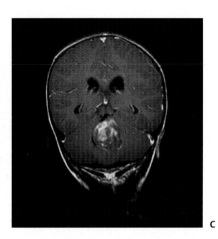

A   B   C

Fig. 57.1   T1-weighted magnetic resonance image (with gadolinium contrast) of the brain. **(A)** Axial, **(B)** sagittal, and **(C)** coronal views showing a large, contrast-enhancing 4th ventricular tumor.

■ Questions

1. What is your differential diagnosis based on clinical and imaging findings?
2. What other imaging study would you recommend?
3. Where do medulloblastomas arise and what are the different histopathologic subtypes?
4. What is the definitive management of this lesion? What is the role of surgery?
5. What surgical approaches can be used for resection of this tumor?
6. Is adjuvant treatment indicated, and if so, what would you recommend?
7. If you recommend radiation, what is the dose of radiation you would use?
8. How often is ventriculoperitoneal shunt required in patients with medulloblastomas? What can be a shunt-related complication in these patients?
9. Describe a grading system used that affects prognosis in medulloblastoma patients.

■ Answers

1. *What is your differential diagnosis based on clinical and imaging findings?*
   - Medulloblastoma, ependymoma, pilocytic astrocytoma, choroid plexus papilloma, metastasis (although metastases are rare in children, in contrast to adults)
   - Medulloblastomas, constituting ~30% of all infratentorial tumors, are the most common malignant brain neoplasms of childhood, with a gender distribution showing male preponderance (1.4 to 4.8 times higher incidence in males).[1]

2. *What other imaging study would you recommend?*
   - MRI of the entire spine with and without contrast is also indicated to evaluate for drop metastases or "sugar-coating" along the spinal cerebrospinal fluid (CSF) pathways.

3. *Where do medulloblastomas arise and what are the different histopathologic subtypes?*
   - The origin of medulloblastoma is from the roof of the 4th ventricle.
   - The World Health Organization (WHO) classification divides medulloblastomas into four histopathologic subtypes[2]:
     - Classic medulloblastoma
     - Desmoplastic medulloblastoma
     - Large cell medulloblastoma
     - Medulloblastomas with extensive nodularity

4. *What is the definitive management of this lesion? What is the role of surgery?*
   - Maximal surgical resection along with chemotherapy and craniospinal axis radiation would be the indicated treatment.
   - Gross total resection, when possible, can reduce the required radiation dose, with the caveat that the operative goal is not complete microscopic resection (which is the case for other tumors like ependymomas).

5. *What surgical approaches can be used for resection of this tumor?*
   - The surgical approach for resection of this tumor can be transvermian, transcortical, or telovelo-cerebellar, among others.[3]
   - Preoperative corticosteroids may help decrease peritumoral edema with any approach.
   - In cases with ventricular dilatation, insertion of a ventriculostomy in the operating room, via either a coronal or occipital route, immediately prior to the tumor resection, can assist in achieving brain relaxation during the resection and managing CSF diversion following the resection.

6. *Is adjuvant treatment indicated, and if so, what would you recommend?*
   - The adjunct therapy would include chemotherapy (various regimens using cisplatin, vincristine, lomustine, and cyclophosphamide are commonly used) along with radiation.

7. *If you recommend radiation, what is the dose of radiation you would use?*
   - Standard fractionated radiation regimen for medulloblastomas consists of ~3600 cGy to the entire craniospinal axis with an 1800 cGy boost to the tumor bed.[4]
   - The so-called average – or standard – risk medulloblastomas (e.g., typical histology, extensively resected, nonmetastatic [M0], posterior fossa lesions in children older than 3 years) have a significantly higher 5-year progression-free survival (60–80%) with this treatment than high-risk tumors (e.g., anaplastic histology, extensive residual disease, metastases, or nonposterior fossa tumor location, and those diagnosed in children younger than 3 years) for which it is less than 40%.[4,5]
   - The neuraxis dose may be reduced to 2340 cGy with adjuvant chemotherapy in the average-risk group.[5]
   - Accordingly, reduced-dose radiation is usually not pursued in patients with high-risk tumors, and current studies are examining ways to improve long-term survival rates.
   - Reduced doses of craniospinal radiation for the average risk group may thus diminish cognitive sequelae, although the extent to which doses can be safely reduced is currently undergoing study.
   - Enrollment of patients on multiinstitutional studies to address such issues is essential to ensure that patients receive state-of-the-art postsurgical therapy, which is constantly evolving, and to contribute to improvements in the management of these tumors.

8. *How often is ventriculoperitoneal shunt required in patients with medulloblastomas? What can be a shunt-related complication in these patients?*
   - Less than half the patients require permanent CSF shunting.[1]
   - Shunt-related intraperitoneal tumor spread is a possible complication, but is rare.[6]

9. *Describe a grading system used that affects prognosis in medulloblastoma patients.*
   - The Chang system (**Table 57.1**) may be used for evaluating tumor grade in individual patients.
   - For prognostic factors, please refer to Case 21 (Posterior Fossa Tumor).

■ Answers (*continued*)

Table 57.1 Grading of Cerebellar Medulloblastomas Using the Chang System

Tumor Stage (T)*

T1 Tumor diameter <3 cm, involving one structure in posterior fossa

T2 Tumor diameter <3 cm, involving two or more posterior fossa structures

T3a Tumor diameter >3 cm, involving two or more posterior fossa structures

T3b Tumor involving floor of the 4th ventricle

T4 Tumor spreading out of the 4th ventricle or presence of severe hydrocephalus

Metastasis (M)

M0 No tumor cells in cerebrospinal fluid (CSF)

M1 Presence of tumor cells on CSF cytology

M2 Tumor seeding in intracranial CSF pathways

M3 Tumor seeding in spinal CSF pathways

M4 Systemic spread

*T-stage is no longer used in stratification in most contemporary studies, in view of the stronger influence of postoperative (versus preoperative) tumor extent on long-term outcome.

Source: Data from Chang CH, Housepian EM, Herbert C Jr. An operative staging system and a megavoltage radiotherapeutic technic for cerebellar medulloblastomas. Radiology 1969;93(6):1351–1359.

■ References

1. Muraszko K, Brahma B, Orringer D. Medulloblastomas. In: Pollack IF, Adelson PD Albright AL, eds. Principles and Practice of Pediatric Neurosurgery. New York: Thieme Medical Publishers; 2008: 606–620

2. Louis DN, Ohgaki H, Wiestler OD, et al. The 2007 WHO classification of tumours of the central nervous system. Acta Neuropathol 2007;114(2):97–109

3. Rajesh BJ, Rao BR, Menon G, Abraham M, Easwer HV, Nair S. Telovelar approach: technical issues for large fourth ventricle tumors. Childs Nerv Syst 2007;23(5):555–558

4. Zeltzer PM, Boyett JM, Finlay JL, et al. Metastasis stage, adjuvant treatment, and residual tumor are prognostic factors for medulloblastoma in children: conclusions from the Children's Cancer Group 921 randomized phase III study. J Clin Oncol 1999;17(3):832–845

5. Packer RJ, Gajjar A, Vezina G, et al. Phase III study of craniospinal radiation therapy followed by adjuvant chemotherapy for newly diagnosed average-risk medulloblastoma. J Clin Oncol 2006;24(25):4202–4208

6. Loiacono F, Morra A, Venturini S, Balestreri L. Abdominal metastases of medulloblastoma related to a ventriculoperitoneal shunt. AJR Am J Roentgenol 2006;186(6):1548–1550

Case 58   Brainstem Glioma 1: Pons

Abdulrahman J. Sabbagh, Ayman Abdullah Albanyan, Mahmoud A. Al Yamany, Reem Bunyan, Ahmed T. Abdelmoity, and Lahbib B. Soualmi

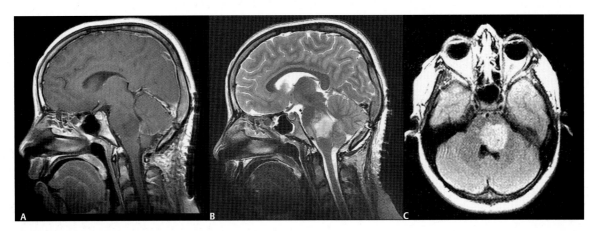

Fig. 58.1 **(A)** Brain sagittal T1-weighted magnetic resonance image (MRI) with gadolinium, **(B)** sagittal T2-weighted MRI and **(C)** axial fluid-attenuated inversion-recovery (FLAIR) image through the pons.

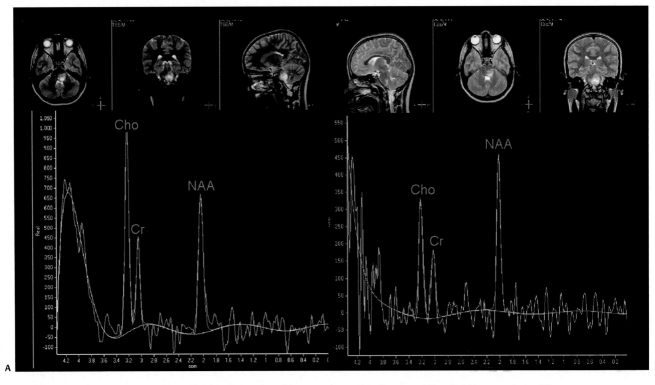

Fig. 58.2 Magnetic resonance spectroscopy showing voxel configuration taken within the tumor **(A)** and within normal pons **(B)**.

■ Clinical Presentation

- A 13-year-old right-handed girl presents to a neurologist with slowly progressive double vision and facial asymmetry.
- She complains of some balance problems toward the left side.
- Examination shows a partial left sided 6th and 7th cranial nerve (CN VI, CN VII) palsy and generalized hyperrefle-

xia. She has normal motor power but a mild right-sided pronator drift.
- A magnetic resonance imaging (MRI) scan of the brain (**Fig. 58.1**) and an MR spectroscopy (**Fig. 58.2**) are done. The initial working diagnosis is of a demyelinating process and the patient is started on corresponding treatment.

■ Questions

1. Describe the MRI.
2. Describe the MR spectroscopy images. What is your differential diagnosis?
3. How can you anatomically explain the 6th and 7th CN palsies?

Over the following months her diplopia becomes worse and on examination, her 6th and 7th CN palsy becomes complete and now she has a significant pronator drift and mild swallowing difficulties. A repeat MRI study shows that the lesion is enlarging.

4. If you chose to operate, what would be the aim of the surgery?
5. How would you approach this lesion?
6. What neurophysiologic modalities would you utilize during surgery?

7. What are the safe entry zones into the floor of the 4th ventricle?

You were able to resect close to 60% of the tumor (**Fig. 58.3** shows the postoperative MRI study). The surgery is performed in the intraoperative MRI (iMRI) suite using intraoperative neurophysiology monitoring (IOM) (IOM electrodes were tested for MRI compatibility).

Her swallowing ability returns to normal, but she has some balance issues that improve with physiotherapy. The 6th and 7th CN palsy remains. Pathologic tissue diagnosis comes back as grade II diffuse astrocytoma.

8. How would you further manage this case?
9. Classify pontine tumors.

Fig. 58.3 Comparison between **(A)** preoperative and **(B)** postoperative magnetic resonance images showing axial T2-weighted and coronal fluid-attenuated inversion-recovery images taken at the level of the pontine tumor.

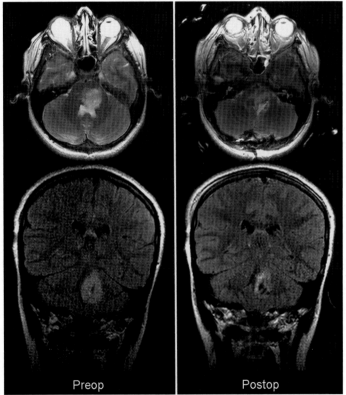

■ Answers

1. *Describe the MRI.*
   - There is a nonenhancing hypointense on T1-, hyperintense on T2-weighted images, partly defined pontine lesion that is associated with some edema and deformation of the pons.
   - Fluid-attenuated inversion-recovery (FLAIR)-weighted image (**Fig. 58.1C**) shows the pontine lesion occupying the right posterior quadrant of the pons, pointing toward the 4th ventricle.

2. *Describe the MR spectroscopy images. What is your differential diagnosis?*
   - MR spectroscopy shows increased choline/creatine (Cho/Cr) and decreased *N*-acetyl aspartate/creatine (NAA/Cr) ratio within the lesion.
   - These findings are consistent with low-grade gliomas or demyelination processes.[1,2]

3. *How can you anatomically explain the 6th and 7th CN palsies?*
   - This lesion involves the facial colliculus, which is formed by the facial motor fibers as they circle around the abducens nucleus in the dorsum of the pons.[3]
   - A lesion in the facial colliculus affects both the facial motor fibers and the abducens nucleus (**Fig. 58.4**).

4. *If you chose to operate, what would be the aim of the surgery?*
   - The aim of surgery is 2-fold:
     - Decompression of the pons
     - Obtaining tissue for diagnosis

5. *How would you approach this lesion?*
   - Suboccipital craniotomy–vermis-sparing telovelar approach
   - The infrafacial triangle may be utilized for approaching the tumor. As this lesion is occupying the facial colliculus and is pointing to the floor of the 4th ventricle, this lesion should be approached through the infrafacial triangle (that can be found by mapping or measurements) and/or the area closest to the surface of the 4th ventricle (**Fig. 58.4**).[4–6]
   - This approach would be further evaluated by use of neuronavigation and microscopy (**Fig. 58.5**).
   - In this particular case, an 8-mm area from the presumed midline and just below the striae medullares was used as the center of the infrafacial triangle and the closest part of the tumor to the 4th ventricle floor.

6. *What neurophysiologic modalities would you use during surgery?*
   - Three modalities are available to monitor this patient[7,8] (electrodes were checked and tested on a volunteer for MRI compatibility and the patient consented to monitoring):
     - Brainstem auditory evoked responses
     - Sensory evoked potentials
     - Motor evoked potentials
     - Fourth ventricular floor mapping

7. *What are the safe entry zones into the floor of the 4th ventricle?*
   - Safe entry zones into the floor of the 4th ventricle include (**Fig. 58.4**)
     - Suprafacial (supraabducental) triangle: a triangle measuring around 16 mm in longest diameter. It is located above the facial colliculus and 5 mm from the midline (to avoid the medial longitudinal fascicle [MLF]). Its upper and narrower angle is below the trochlear nucleus.[5,6]
     - Infrafacial (infraabducental) triangle: a smaller triangle measuring less than 9 mm located just below the facial colliculus. It is narrow as it is located between the MLF medially and the facial nucleus laterally.[5,6]

8. *How would you further manage this case?*
   - Management plan includes
     - For the residual tumor: conformal radiation or gamma knife treatment to the pons can be given postoperatively. This can be followed by serial MRI and close follow-ups.[9,10]
     - Note that, however, due to the relative risk and safety issues involved in using gamma knife treatments to the pons, some would not consider this option unless the lesion was exophytic from the pons.
     - For the facial palsy: teardrops and eye protection. One may resort to partial or gold-weight tarsorrhaphy in some cases to avoid corneal abrasions and ulcers. Facial-nerve reanimation procedures can also be tried.
     - For the gait disturbances: continued inpatient or outpatient rehabilitation

9. *Classify pontine tumors.*
   - Classification of pontine tumors: Pontine tumors can be classified by type of tumor or growth pattern[11]:
     - Diffused pontine tumors: usually malignant and difficult to delineate from neighboring pontine parenchyma. Usually low or isointense signal on T1-weighted MRI and may have an increased signal on T2-weighted MRI. Hyperintensity on T1-weighted MRI is usually due to hemorrhagic change. Further enhancement in these diffuse tumors may be a sign of actual malignant degeneration.
     - Focal pontine tumors: well-demarcated and hypo- or isointense signal on T1-weighted and high signal intensity on T2-weighted MRIs.
     - Exophytic pontine tumors: almost always dorsally exophytic into the 4th ventricle and may be benign or malignant.[12,13]

■ Answers (*continued*)

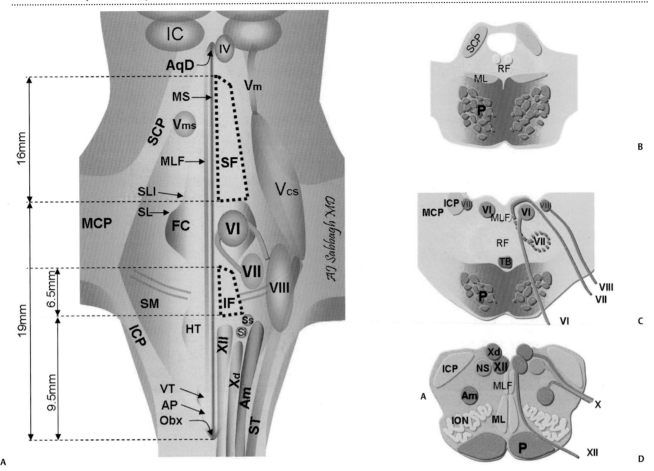

Fig. 58.4 Safe entry zones of the brainstem. Artist's rendering of the brainstem from a dorsal view **(A)** with illustrated safe entry zones and relevant nuclei and neural structures. The infrafacial and suprafacial triangles are highlighted as safe entry zones in the dorsal pons. Corresponding axial sections through the **(B)** upper, **(C)** mid, and **(D)** lower pons are illustrated. AqD, Aqueduct of Sylvius; N, nucleus; IC, inferior colliculus; MS, median sulcus; Vm, mesencephalic N. of the 5th cranial nerve (V); Vcs, chief (sensory) N. of V; Vms, motor (mastication) N. of V; MLF, medial longitudinal fascicle; FC, facial colliculus; IV, trochlear N.; CTT, central tegmental tract; SL, sulcus limitans; SLI, sulcus limitans incisure; HT, hypoglossal triangle; SM, striae medullares; SCP, MCP, SCP, superior, middle and inferior cerebellar peduncle; VT, vagal triangle; AP, area postrema; Obx, Obex; VI, Abducent N.; VII, facial N. and fiber tracks and nerve; VIII, vestibular N. and nerve; XII, hypoglossal N. and nerve; Xd, dorsal vagal N.; Am, N. ambiguus of 9th and 10th cranial nerves with parasympathetics on its medial border; Ss & Si, superior and inferior salivatory NN.; ST, spinal trigeminal tract; STT, spinothalamic tract; ML, medial lemniscus; ION, inferior olivary N.; P, Pyramid; TB, trapezoid body; Pn TPF, pontine NN and transverse pontine fibers; SF, suprafacial triangle; IF, infrafacial triangle.

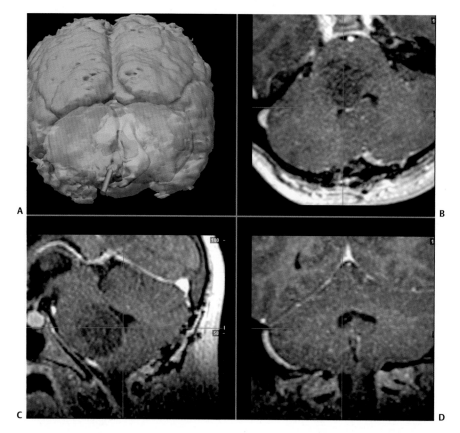

Fig. 58.5 Intraoperative neuronavigation image with three-dimensional reconstruction **(A)** highlighting tumor in green and entry trajectory with red arrow. Corresponding T1-weighted magnetic resonance images with contrast with **(B)** axial, **(C)** sagittal, and **(D)** coronal views.

■ References

1. Fan G, Sun B, Wu Z, Guo Q, Guo Y. In vivo single-voxel proton MR spectroscopy in the differentiation of high-grade gliomas and solitary metastases. Clin Radiol 2004;59(1):77–85
2. Saindane AM, Cha S, Law M, Xue X, Knopp EA, Zagzag D. Proton MR spectroscopy of tumefactive demyelinating lesions. AJNR Am J Neuroradiol 2002;23(8):1378–1386
3. Parent A. Carpenter's Human Neuroanatomy. Baltimore: Williams & Wilkins; 1996
4. Rhoton AL. Rhoton Cranial Anatomy and Surgical Approaches. Philadelphia: Lippincott Williams & Wilkins; 2008
5. Kyoshima K, Kobayashi S, Gibo H, Kuroyanagi T. A study of safe entry zones via the floor of the fourth ventricle for brain-stem lesions. Report of three cases. J Neurosurg 1993;78(6):987–993
6. Bogucki J, Czernicki Z, Gielecki J. Cytoarchitectonic basis for safe entry into the brainstem. Acta Neurochir (Wien) 2000;142(4):383–387
7. Morota N, Deletis V, Epstein FJ, et al. Brain stem mapping: neurophysiological localization of motor nuclei on the floor of the fourth ventricle. Neurosurgery 1995;37(5):922–929
8. Strauss C, Romstöck J, Nimsky C, Fahlbusch R. Intraoperative identification of motor areas of the rhomboid fossa using direct stimulation. J Neurosurg 1993;79(3):393–399
9. Farmer JP, Montes JL, Freeman CR, Meagher-Villemure K, Bond MC, O'Gorman AM. Brainstem gliomas. A 10-year institutional review. Pediatr Neurosurg 2001;34(4):206–214
10. Yen CP, Sheehan J, Steiner M, Patterson G, Steiner L. Gamma knife surgery for focal brainstem gliomas. J Neurosurg 2007;106(1): 8–17
11. Epstein FJ, Farmer JP. Brain-stem glioma growth patterns. J Neurosurg 1993;78(3):408–412
12. Hoffman HJ. Dorsally exophytic brain stem tumors and midbrain tumors. Pediatr Neurosurg 1996;24(5):256–262
13. Pollack IF, Hoffman HJ, Humphreys RP, Becker L. The long-term outcome after surgical treatment of dorsally exophytic brainstem gliomas. J Neurosurg 1993;78(6):859–863

Case 59   Brainstem Glioma 2: Medulla Oblongata

Jean-Pierre Farmer, Abdulrahman J. Sabbagh, and Ahmad Al-Jishi

■ Clinical Presentation

- A 4-year-old boy presents to the emergency room sent by his pediatrician for head tilt and nystagmus.
- He also has frequent headaches.
- Examination shows only nystagmus and head tilt toward the left side.

- There are no other cranial nerve findings, and the remainder of the neurologic exam is within normal limits.
- Computed tomography (CT) and magnetic resonance imaging (MRI) scans are done to assess his status.

■ Questions

1. Interpret the CT (**Fig. 59.1**) and the MRI (**Fig. 59.2**) scans.
2. Give a differential diagnosis.
3. What studies do you order?
4. What is the next step in the patient's management?
5. Describe approaches to intraaxial brainstem tumors, surgical principles, and adjuncts.

The patient was taken to surgery. A tumor was expanding the medulla oblongata, deforming the anatomy, and displacing the midline (**Fig. 59.3**). Using neuronavigation, the area closest to the surface was the point used for entry.

   On the frozen section, the patient's specimen confirmed a diagnosis of juvenile pilocytic astrocytoma.

6. Following completion of surgery, you obtain an MRI (**Fig. 59.4**). Given that the patient has no new neurologic sequela and given the MRI findings, what would be your recommendations for further treatment?
7. What are the treatment alternatives at this age?
8. What do you tell the family with respect to prognosis?
9. If you return, what would be the goal of the surgery?
10. What are the added risks of the second surgery?
11. What would you do assuming the histopathology remains the same following a second surgery in the presence of residual tumor?
12. Discuss favorable prognostic factors in brainstem glioma surgery.

Fig. 59.1   Computed tomography scan of the brain at the level of the **(A)** medulla and the **(B)** lateral ventricles.

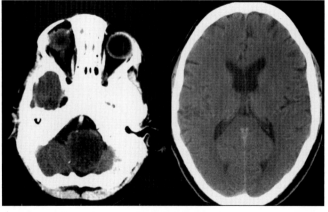

A   B

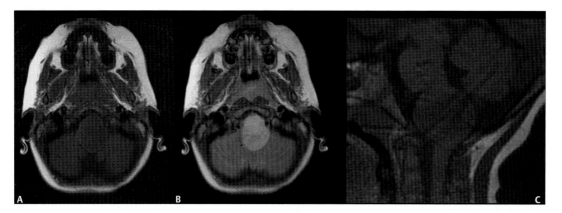

Fig. 59.2 Magnetic resonance imaging scan at the level of the medulla. **(A)** Axial cuts T1-weighted and **(B)** T2-weighted, and **(C)** midsagittal T1-weighted section.

■ Answers

1. *Interpret the CT (**Fig. 59.1**) and the MRI (**Fig. 59.2**) scans.*
   - CT scan reveals a grossly enlarged hypodense brainstem with no evidence of hydrocephalus. The hypodensity appears to be reaching the foramen magnum.
   - The MRI shows a nonenhancing lesion best seen on fluid-attenuated inversion-recovery (FLAIR) study showing a medullary epicenter with minimal if any ventral lateral medulla identified on the right side. The lesion respects the boundaries of the medulla both caudally and rostrally.
2. *Give a differential diagnosis.*
   - Differential diagnosis includes benign or malignant brainstem tumor. Benign brainstem tumor is favored by the long history without multiple cranial nerve involvement, a respect of the boundaries of the medulla, and a medullary location as opposed to a pontine location.
   - Benign masses in this location can include pilocytic astrocytoma. Less likely diagnoses include hemangioblastoma, pleomorphic xanthoastrocytoma, and a brain abscess.
   - Malignant tumors in this location include glioblastoma multiforme, metastases, and lymphoma.[1–3]
3. *What studies do you order?*
   - Important studies to obtain are swallowing studies, overnight sleep study, and vocal cord assessment by otolaryngology examination.[4]
4. *What is the next step in the patient's management?*
   - Given the probable benign nature of this lesion, despite its size based on clinical presentation and location, an initial approach should be to obtain a tissue sample (based on imaging studies, the tumor consistency appears to be different from the surrounding brainstem).

5. *Describe approaches to intraaxial brainstem tumors, surgical principles, and adjuncts.*
   - The approach should be done in prone position with some neck flexion with the use of a suitable pediatric head frame to stabilize the head for surgery.
   - Obtaining accurate neuronavigation information is essential.
   - Additionally, multimodality evoked potential monitoring should be utilized.
   - The lesion should be approached through the eroded floor of the 4th ventricle, if such an area can be identified. Otherwise, relatively safe entry zones should be used.
   - Given the extension and size of the lesion on the left side, a far lateral approach may also present a less morbid option for resection of this tumor.
   - Given the finding and the presence of a presumably acceptable distinct appearance of the tumor, a significant debulking taking care to allow for reexpansion of compressed tissue should be done with careful monitoring of vital signs and evoked potentials.
   - If the walls of the lesion appear to show pulsations that would suggest thinning of the wall, particularly on the left anterior aspect, the procedure should be terminated. A significant but subtotal resection would be sufficient in this case.[4]
6. *Following completion of surgery, you obtain an MRI (**Fig. 59.4**). Given that the patient has no new neurologic sequelae and given the MRI findings, what would be your recommendations as for further treatment?*
   - The MRI obtained postoperatively shows a central cavity of resection with a significant amount of residual tumor despite the significant reduction in the total volume of the tumor. There is reexpansion of the brainstem, particularly on the right side.

■ Answers (*continued*)

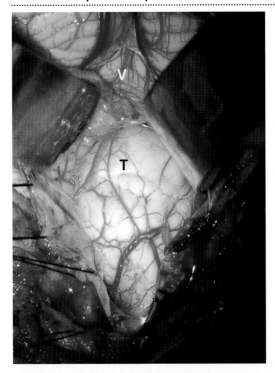

Fig. 59.3   Intraoperative image of the floor of the 4th ventricle showing entry site to the tumor (T) and cerebellar vermis (V).

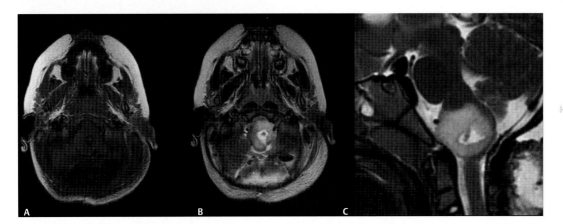

Fig. 59.4   Postoperative magnetic resonance imaging scan at the level of the medulla. **(A)** Axial cuts T1-weighted and **(B)** T2-weighted, and **(C)** midsagittal T2-weighted section.

- The patient is doing well; therefore, he may be able to sustain another surgical procedure.
- With sufficient time to allow reexpansion toward the central cavity, a second approach via the initial myelotomy tract to obtain further significant resection could be contemplated.[5]

7. *What are the treatment alternatives at this age?*
- A more expectant approach is also an option given the benign nature of the tumor (although we do not favor this option for the reasons stated above).[6]
- Alternative treatment plans also include radiotherapy and chemotherapy.
   - Both are associated with significant morbidity at this age and would not represent, at this point, a preferred option given the fact that the patient tolerated the surgery well.[5,7]

■ Answers (*continued*)

8. *What do you tell the family with respect to prognosis?*
   - Given the benign histology, the slow progression, and the fact that the brainstem is showing reexpansion, the prognosis, although guarded because of the location of the lesion, should be favorable.
   - This also favors the possibility of further intervention and close follow-up.
   - The preferred recommendation would be for return surgery through the same myelotomy approach into the brainstem.[8–10]
   - Some might recommend, prior to repeat surgery, chemotherapy in an attempt to reduce the tumor burden and then a second look at surgery. This has been advocated for choroid plexus papillomas, as well as some ependymomas.[11]

9. *If you return, what would be the goal of the surgery?*
   - The goal of a second surgery would be further debulking, taking care to avoid significant morbidity in the lower brainstem in particular.
   - Further tumor reconfiguration toward the cavity would favor a return for surgery.

10. *What are the added risks of the second surgery?*
    - Returning a second time could risk some lower cranial nerve difficulties, which can be avoided by staying in the center of the lesion.
    - Additional risks include the development of hydrocephalus following a second surgery in the posterior fossa.
    - There is an increased risk of cerebrospinal fluid fistula development in the context of a second duraplasty.
    - Additional risks include meningitis, posterior fossa hematoma, infection or abscess, poor healing, etc.

11. *What would you do assuming the histopathology remains the same following a second surgery in the presence of residual tumor?*
    - If the histology remains the same and the patient remains stable clinically after further debulking, the recommendation would be for careful observation with baseline MRI scans being done at approximately a 2-month interval. All three treatment options discussed previously remain viable for the future.[7]

12. *Discuss favorable prognostic factors in brainstem glioma surgery.*
    - Not all brainstem gliomas have the same prognosis.
    - Having the epicenter of the lesion within a nonpontine territory of the brainstem is a favorable prognostic factor.
    - A prolonged history and a focal positive neurologic examination are favorable prognostic factors.[9]
    - Uniformity of the signal within the tumor on imaging studies, either as uniform enhancement or as a FLAIR high signal, represents a favorable factor.
    - Growth pattern limited to a segment of the brainstem and, in particular, a deviation toward the floor of the 4th ventricle are favorable factors. This growth pattern may be either from a dorsal exophytic brainstem tumor or a cervicomedullary tumor, and its limitation suggests restriction of growth by existing ventral corticospinal fibers of the pons or the cervical medullary junction.[12]
    - The presence of a cyst is also a favorable factor.
    - Noninfiltrative tumors if approached with care can be significantly debulked with microsurgical technique and the use of multimodality evoked potential monitoring.

■ References

1. Osborn AG. Diagnostic Neuroradiology. St Louis: Mosby; 1994
2. Tsementzis SA. Differential Diagnosis in Neurology and Neurosurgery. A Clinician's Pocket Guide. New York: Thieme Medical Publishers; 2000
3. Shaya MR, Fowler MR, Nanda A. Pilocytic astrocytoma presenting as an intrinsic brainstem tumor: case report and review of the literature. J La State Med Soc 2004;156(1):33–36
4. Konovalov AN, Gorelyshev SK, Khuhlaeva EA. Surgical management of brain stem, thalamic and hypothalamic tumors. In: Roberts DW, Schmideck HH, eds. Schmidek and Sweet's Operative Neurosurgical Techniques: Indications, Methods and Results. Philadelphia: Saunders Elsevier; 2006
5. Bowers DC, Krause TP, Aronson LJ, et al. Second surgery for recurrent pilocytic astrocytoma in children. Pediatr Neurosurg 2001;34(5):229–234
6. Pollack IF, Hoffman HJ, Humphreys RP, Becker L. The long-term outcome after surgical treatment of dorsally exophytic brainstem gliomas. J Neurosurg 1993;78(6):859–863
7. Krieger MD, Gonzalez-Gomez I, Levy ML, McComb JG. Recurrence patterns and anaplastic change in a long-term study of pilocytic astrocytomas. Pediatr Neurosurg 1997;27(1):1–11
8. Teo C, Siu TL. Radical resection of focal brainstem gliomas: is it worth doing? Childs Nerv Syst 2008;24(11):1307–1314
9. Weiner HL, Freed D, Woo HH, Rezai AR, Kim R, Epstein FJ. Intra-axial tumors of the cervicomedullary junction: surgical results and long-term outcome. Pediatr Neurosurg 1997;27(1):12–18
10. Robertson PL, Allen JC, Abbott IR, Miller DC, Fidel J, Epstein FJ. Cervicomedullary tumors in children: a distinct subset of brainstem gliomas. Neurology 1994;44(10):1798–1803
11. Lo SS, Abdulrahman R, Desrosiers PM, et al. The role of gamma knife radiosurgery in the management of unresectable gross disease or gross residual disease after surgery in ependymoma. J Neurooncol 2006;79(1):51–56
12. Fisher PG, Breiter SN, Carson BS, et al. A clinicopathologic reappraisal of brain stem tumor classification. Identification of pilocytic astrocytoma and fibrillary astrocytoma as distinct entities. Cancer 2000;89(7):1569–1576

Case 60   **Pineal Region Tumor**

Claude-Edouard Chatillon, José-Luis Montes, and Jean-Pierre Farmer

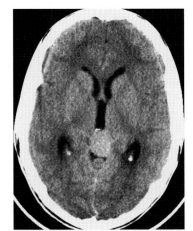

Fig. 60.1   Computed tomography scan of the head without contrast at the level of the pineal gland.

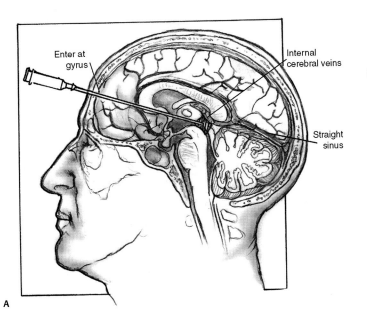

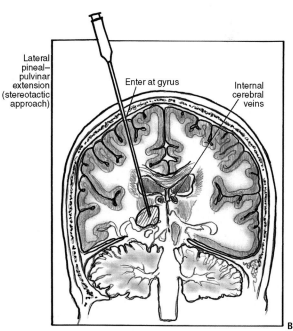

Fig. 60.2   Artist's rendering of stereotactic approaches to pineal region tumors. **(A)** Low frontal (precoronal) approach avoids the internal cerebral veins above the tumor. **(B)** The lateral pineal pulvinar approach, which is lateral to the deep veins, is depicted. (From Sekhar L, Fessler R. Atlas of Neurosurgical Techniques: Brain. New York: Thieme Medical Publishers; 2006:570–571. Reprinted with permission.)

■ Clinical Presentation

• An 18-year-old right-handed man, otherwise healthy, presents to your clinic with a one-week history of progressively increasing headaches.

• These are worse in the morning and are associated with nausea and vomiting.

• There are no other systemic symptoms.

• Physical examination is unremarkable.

• A computed tomography (CT) scan of the head is obtained and shown in **Fig. 60.1**.

■ Questions

1. Interpret the CT scan.
2. Provide a detailed differential diagnosis of pineal region tumors.
3. Describe the typical presentation patterns of pineal region tumors.
4. What studies would you order?

5. Describe the different management options – their pros and cons and approach details.
6. Describe some adjuvant treatment measures for pineal tumors.
7. What is the prognosis for pineal region tumors?

In this case, tumor markers in the serum and cerebrospinal fluid (CSF) are negative.

■ Answers

1. *Interpret the CT scan.*
   - The CT scan shows a homogeneous and slightly hyperdense mass in the pineal region with mild dilatation of the ventricles.
2. *Provide a detailed differential diagnosis of pineal region tumors.*
   - Differential diagnosis is described below.[1,2]
   - Germ cell tumors (GCTs)
     - More frequent in children (75% in teens, 95% in younger than 33 years old)
     - Male-to-female ratio is 2:1.
     - They represent about one third of cases of pineal tumors.
     - Half the cases are germinoma.
     - On imaging studies: They engulf the pineal gland and are hyperintense to gray matter.
     - World Health Organization (WHO) classification[3] consists of
       - Germinoma
       - Embryonal carcinoma
       - Yolk sac tumors (endodermal sinus tumors)
       - Choriocarcinomas
       - Teratomas
         - Mature
         - Immature
         - With malignant transformation (carcinoma or sarcoma)
       - Mixed germ cell tumors
   - Pineal cell tumors
     - They represent about one quarter of cases of pineal tumors.
     - More frequent in young adults
     - Male-to-female ratio is 1:1.
     - Genetic predisposition in Rb mutations (trilateral retinoblastoma)
     - Pineoblastoma: Most are large, greater than 3 cm with peripheral calcifications. Usually associated with obstructive hydrocephalus.
     - Pineocytoma: enhancing, well-circumscribed pineal tumor with calcifications that rarely extend into the 3rd ventricle

   - Glial tumors
     - They represent about one quarter of cases of pineal tumors.
     - They arise from midbrain tectum or thalamus, rarely from the pineal gland.
     - They include ependymoma, astrocytoma, oligodendroglioma, and glioblastoma.
   - Other miscellaneous pathologies include
     - Meningioma
     - Lymphoma
     - Metastasis
     - Sarcoidosis
     - Infectious agents (tuberculosis, Whipple disease, etc.)

3. *Describe the typical presentation patterns of pineal region tumors.*
   - Several presentation patterns have been described.[1]
   - Increased intracranial pressure
     - Morning headaches, nausea, vomiting, papilledema, obtundation, and extraocular muscle (EOM) dysfunction
   - Direct brainstem compression
     - Parinaud syndrome (superior tectum involvement)
     - Down-gaze palsy, ptosis (periaqueductal gray or third nerve involvement)
     - Rare cases of "tectal deafness" (inferior colliculus involvement)
   - Direct cerebellar compression
     - Ataxia, dysmetria (superior cerebellar peduncles or cerebellorubral fibers involvement)
   - Hydrocephalus
   - Endocrine dysfunction
     - Precocious pseudopuberty (male patients with beta human chorionic gonadotropin [β-HCG] producing tumors)
     - Hypothalamic dysfunction
   - Pineal apoplexy
     - Acute presentation of aforementioned symptoms

■ Answers (*continued*)

4. *What studies would you order?*
   - CT scan – may also be ordered with contrast.[1] Look for
     - Calcifications
     - Hydrocephalus
     - Vascularity
   - MRI scan to look for[1]
     - Signal characteristics of the tumor
     - Anatomical relationships and planes
     - Displacement of the deep venous structures
   - Serum and CSF tumor markers[1]
     - May help identify GCTs
     - Positive α fetoprotein (AFP) present in
       - Yolk sac tumors
       - Embryonal cell carcinoma
       - Immature teratoma
     - Positive β-HCG present in
       - Choriocarcinoma
       - Germinoma with syncytiotrophoblasts
       - Embryonal cell carcinoma
     - Positive placental alkaline phosphatase present in:
       - Germinoma
       - May be positive in all GCTs
     - Absence of markers does not exclude the diagnosis of GCT
     - One may have a mixed GCT (i.e., it may have multiple tumor components expressing different markers).
   - For staging purposes, all patients with malignant pineal cell tumors, GCTs, and ependymoma will need a spinal MRI and CSF cytology (which is rarely positive, even when seeding is present).

5. *Describe the different management options – their pros and cons and approach details.*
   - Management of hydrocephalus depends on the clinical status and subsequent definitive treatment plan.[1] Options include
     - Close observation while awaiting surgery
     - Ventriculostomy or external ventricular drain
     - Endoscopic third ventriculostomy (ETV)
     - Ventriculoperitoneal (VP) shunt
   - One of the goals of management includes obtaining tissue diagnosis.
     - This may not be necessary if malignant GCT markers are present.
     - Stereotactic biopsy or open biopsy/resection approached may be used.

- Stereotactic biopsy[1,4]
  - Pros and cons include
    - Relative ease of performance
    - Less complications
    - Risk of inadequate sampling in mixed GCTs
    - Report of seeding in pineoblastoma
  - Approaches include precoronal with low frontal entry point, the pathway along the antero-latero-superior portion of the tumor, inferior and lateral to internal cerebral vein, parieto-occipital and postero-latero-superior (for tumors with postero-lateral extension) (**Fig. 60.2**).
  - Serial biopsies are desirable.
  - Sample areas with different MRI signal.
- Endoscopic biopsy[1]
  - May perform ETV and biopsy during the same procedure
  - Cons include
    - Flexible endoscope or a second burr hole is required.
    - Risk of intraventricular hemorrhage
    - Obliteration of the field of view may occur.
    - Difficult to control the endoscope in inexperienced hands
- Open biopsy with possibility of resection[1,5]
  - Pros and cons include
    - More confident diagnosis
    - Reduction of tumor burden
    - Control of bleeding
    - Possibility of complete resection (teratoma, pineocytoma)
    - Increased morbidity of a major surgical procedure
  - Common approaches[5]
    - Infratentorial supracerebellar
    - Occipital transtentorial
    - Transcallosal interhemispheric
    - The best approach depends on individual tumor characteristics and the surgeon's familiarity with the approach.
  - Infratentorial supracerebellar approach[1]
    - Extraaxial pathway to the tumor via a midline approach
    - Inferior to the deep veins
    - Sitting position, which places gravity at work to the surgeon's benefit
    - Risks include blood pooling, cerebellar retraction, awkward surgical positioning, air embolism, and venous sinus injury.

■ Answers (*continued*)

- Occipital transtentorial approach
  - ¾ prone (or sitting) position, oblique trajectory
  - Excellent exposure of the quadrigeminal plate
  - Also places gravity at work to the surgeon's benefit
  - Disadvantages include working around deep veins, occipital lobe retraction, and risk of visual field deficit
- Transcallosal interhemispheric approach
  - Prone (or sitting) position, callosotomy centered around the tumor and should be limited to less than 2 cm
  - Disadvantages include working around deep veins, bridging veins may limit exposure, and risk of disconnection syndrome.
  - May be combined with the occipital transtentorial approach

6. *Describe some adjuvant treatment measures for pineal tumors.*
   - Radiation therapy (RT) is indicated for all patients with germinoma (yielding best results), malignant germ cell tumors, malignant or intermediate pineal cell tumors, anaplastic gliomas, or cases of subtotal resection of pineocytoma or ependymoma.
   - One possible regimen consists of
     - 40 Gy to the ventricular system +15 Gy to the tumor bed
     - 35 Gy to the spine empirically or if there is evidence of radiographic metastases or positive CSF cytology
     - Reduced craniospinal radiation doses in combination with chemotherapy is currently the standard treatment for germinoma in many centers.[2,6–8]
   - Chemotherapy (usually combined with radiation) is used in germinoma, nongerminomatous GCTs (NG-GCTs), germinoma with syncytiotrophoblastic cells, and recurrent or metastatic germinoma or pineal cell tumors.

- Regimens include the Einhorn regimen[9] (also used in testicular cancer), which consists of cisplatin, vinblastine, bleomycin, or etoposide replacing vinblastine–bleomycin to avoid pulmonary toxicity. Other commonly used regimens include for germinoma cisplatin, carboplatin, and etoposide. For pineoblastoma and NG-GCTs, it includes vincristine, cisplatin, cyclophosphamide, and etoposide.[9]
- Radiosurgery may be useful in the treatment of pineocytoma, but not in malignant pineal cell tumors or GCTs. It is limited to tumors smaller than 3 cm.[1,10]

7. *What is the prognosis for pineal region tumors?*
   - Prognosis is dependent on histologic diagnosis.[1]
   - In germinoma, the long-term survival rate is 90% with RT. In a study of 36 patients with germinoma by Hardenbergh et al.,[11] low-dose radiation was given to the tumor and neuraxis as well as a boost dose to the tumor bed. The 5-year disease-free survival rate was 97%. Poor prognosticators included positive CSF cytology for tumor cells and increased β-HCG levels.[2]
   - In NG-GCT, the 5-year survival rate with RT was 36%.[1] The 2-year survival with chemotherapy was 62%. There was a 10% mortality rate from toxicity of chemotherapeutic agents[1]
   - In pineocytoma, a small series of four patients was studied by Tsumanuma et al.[12] The patients underwent total or subtotal resection with a mean survival rate of 8 years.[12]
   - In pineoblastoma, Lee et al. reviewed a series of 34 patients, revealing a mean survival rate of 25 months after gross total resection and RT.[13]

■ References

1. Bruce JN. Pineal region masses: Clinical features and management. Supracerebellar approach for pineal region neoplasms. In: Schmidek HH, Roberts DW, eds. Schmidek and Sweet's Operative Neurosurgical Techniques: Indication, Methods and Results. 5th ed. Philadelphia: Saunders Elsevier; 2006: 786–797, 812–817

2. Bruce JN. Pineal tumours. In: Winn HR, ed. Youmans Neurological Surgery. 5th ed. Philadelphia: Saunders Elsevier; 2004: 1011–1026

3. Kleihues P, Cavanee WK. Pathology and Genetics of Tumors of the Nervous System. Lyon, France: World Health Organization; 2000

4. Field M, Witham TF, Flickinger JC, et al. Comprehensive assessment of hemorrhage risks and outcomes after stereotactic brain biopsy. J Neurosurg 2001;94:545–551

5. Sano K. Alternate surgical approaches to pineal region neoplasms. In: Schmidek HH, Roberts DW, eds. Schmidek and Sweet's Operative Neurosurgical Techniques: Indication, Methods and Results. 5th ed. Philadelphia: Saunders Elsevier; 2006: 798–811

6. Sawamura Y, Shirato H, Ikeda J, et al. Induction chemotherapy followed by reduced-volume radiation therapy for newly diagnosed central nervous system germinoma. J Neurosurg 1998;88(1):66–72

7. Fuller BG, Kapp DS, Cox R. Radiation therapy of pineal region tumors: 25 new cases and a review of 208 previously reported cases. Int J Radiat Oncol Biol Phys 1994;28(1):229–245

8. Osuka S, Tsuboi K, Takano S, et al. Long-term outcome of patients with intracranial germinoma. J Neurooncol 2007;83(1):71–79

9. Einhorn LH, Williams SD, Chamness A, Brames MJ, Perkins SM, Abonour R. High-dose chemotherapy and stem-cell rescue for metastatic germ-cell tumors. N Engl J Med 2007;357(4):340–348

10. Hasegawa T, Kondziolka D, Hadjipanayis CG, Flickinger JC, Lunsford LD. The role of radiosurgery for the treatment of pineal parenchymal tumors. Neurosurgery 2002;51(4):880–889

11. Hardenbergh PH, Golden J, Billet A, et al. Intracranial germinoma: the case for lower dose radiation therapy. Int J Radiat Oncol Biol Phys 1997;39(2):419–426

12. Tsumanuma I, Tanaka R, Washiyama K. Clinicopathological study of pineal parenchymal tumors: correlation between histopathological features, proliferative potential, and prognosis. Brain Tumor Pathol 1999;16(2):61–68

13. Lee JY, Wakabayashi T, Yoshida J. Management and survival of pineoblastoma: an analysis of 34 adults from the brain tumor registry of Japan. Neurol Med Chir (Tokyo) 2005;45(3):132–141

Case 61   Endoscopic Treatment of Hydrocephalus

Jeffrey Atkinson

▨ Clinical Presentation

- An 8-month-old child with normal prenatal, birth, and early infancy health history presented with increased head circumference and delayed milestones achievement.
- Her parents noticed that over several weeks she had lost the ability to crawl and the ability to sit unassisted.

- Examination revealed a head circumference at the 98th percentile compared with the 50th percentile 2 months ago and a bulging fontanel, as well as impaired upward gaze.

▨ Questions

1. What are the diagnostic possibilities in this child?
2. What are the appropriate investigations?

A magnetic resonance imaging (MRI) of her brain was performed urgently; the scan is shown in **Fig. 61.1**.

3. What are the findings on the MRI and what is the differential diagnosis?

4. What are the options for treatment of this lesion?
5. Explain what you would tell the parents in terms of risks for this procedure.
6. What is the chance of success of this procedure?
7. What would be the option if the initial procedure fails?

▨ Answers

1. *What are the diagnostic possibilities in this child?*
   - This child demonstrates typical findings for slowly progressive intracranial pressure in this age group.
   - The reasons for this could be hydrocephalus, with mass lesion as a cause.
   - Posterior fossa masses are common in this age group.
   - Arachnoid cysts occur, postinfectious or hemorrhagic hydrocephalus also occurs, and in some children subdural hematomas present in this fashion (even as a result of nonaccidental trauma).[1]
   - Benign macrocrania with benign enlargement of the subarachnoid spaces should not present with this constellation of developmental delay and neurologic exam findings.
2. *What are the appropriate investigations?*
   - This child needs urgent imaging.
   - Ultrasound, computed tomography (CT) scan, or MRI scan are all reasonable options depending on the availability, though MRI is clearly the most definitive, and might be required regardless of the result of the other studies.

3. *What are the findings on the MRI, and what is the differential diagnosis?*
   - The MRI shows a cerebrospinal fluid (CSF) density collection in the region of the suprasellar cistern and 3rd ventricle with associated obstructive hydrocephalus.
   - Typically, arachnoid cysts of the suprasellar space may extend up and compress the 3rd ventricle and obstruct the foramen of Monro causing hydrocephalus.
   - Arachnoid cysts of the 3rd ventricle may also appear with this pattern.[1]
   - Tumor cysts from craniopharyngioma or Rathke's cleft cysts may also be located in this region but should show a different density from that of CSF.
   - Tumor cysts from hypothalamic astrocytomas should demonstrate a tumor mass in addition to a cystic component.
   - Epidermoid or dermoid cysts should show a different density on fluid-attenuated inversion-recovery, but may also occur in this location.[2]

■ Answers (*continued*)

4. *What are the options for treatment of this lesion?*
   • Treatment options include[1]
     – Cyst fenestration, either open or endoscopic[3]
     – Cyst shunting procedure
5. *Explain what you would tell the parents in terms of risks for this procedure.*

   • Endoscopic fenestration might be the procedure of choice (open cyst fenestration via craniotomy usually has not worked to manage this condition).[1,3]
   • Endoscopic third ventriculostomy may also be done in the same setting. See **Fig. 61.2 and Fig. 61.3**.

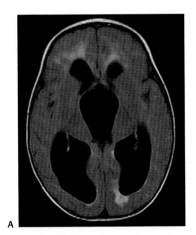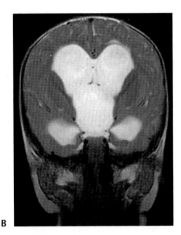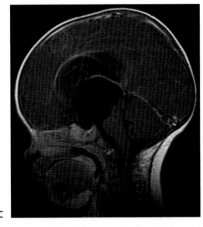

Fig. 61.1   Magnetic resonance imaging scan of the brain with **(A)** axial fluid-attenuated inversion-recovery, **(B)** coronal T2-weighted, and **(C)** sagittal T1-weighted images with contrast.

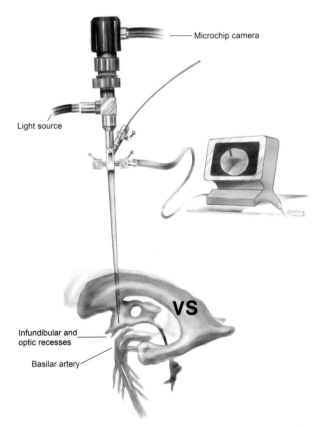

Fig. 61.2   Artist's rendering of an endoscopic third ventriculostomy procedure. The rigid endoscope has been inserted into the 3rd ventricle via the foramen of Monro. The entry point is between the infundibular recess and the mamillary bodies. The basilar artery will be visualized below the opening. (From Goodrich JT. Neurosurgical Operative Atlas. Pediatric Neurosurgery. 2nd ed. New York: Thieme Medical Publishers; 2008: 230. Reprinted with permission.)

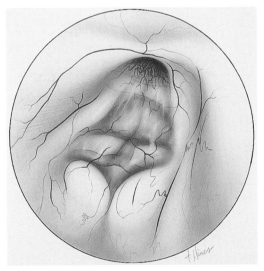

Fig. 61.3   Illustration of the floor of the 3rd ventricle as visualized through the endoscope that has penetrated through the foramen of Monro. Note the mamillary bodies caudally, the infundibular recess rostrally, and the shadow of the basilar artery termination through the floor of the ventricle. (From Sekhar L, Fessler R. Atlas of Neurosurgical Techniques: Brain. New York: Thieme Medical Publishers; 2006: 969. Reprinted with permission.)

■ Answers (*continued*)

- The risks for this include standard anesthesia risks, risks of infection, and significant bleeding; however, these are low risks as for all intracranial surgeries.
- Specific to this surgery, risks of incomplete fenestration of the cyst, and recurrence of the cyst are possible. Cortical damage; intracranial hemorrhage; risk of seizures; damage to the fornix, the hypothalamus, or the basilar artery; or other uncontrolled intraventricular bleeding are also important risks to consider.

6. *What is the chance of success of this procedure?*
   - The chance of success of this procedure is difficult to assess.

- Standard endoscopic third ventriculostomy for obstructive hydrocephalus might have a success rate as low as 40% in this age group, but successful fenestration of this cyst should have a more reliable duration of effectiveness.[3,4]

7. *What would be the option if the initial procedure fails?*
   - If the initial procedure fails, open fenestration is an option, but the surgical approach is not without significant potential morbidity.
   - Cystoperitoneal shunting of the cyst should relieve the obstructive hydrocephalus and would be the procedure of second choice.[1]

■ References

1. Pradilla G, Jallo G. Arachnoid cysts: case series and review of the literature. Neurosurg Focus 2007;22(2):E7
2. Osborn AG. Diagnostic Neuroradiology. St. Louis, MO: Mosby; 1994
3. O'Brien DF, Seghedoni A, Collins DR, Hayhurst C, Mallucci CL. Is there an indication for ETV in young infants in aetiologies other than isolated aqueduct stenosis? Childs Nerv Syst 2006;22(12):1565–1572
4. Drake JM. Canadian Pediatric Neurosurgery Study Group, Endoscopic third ventriculostomy in pediatric patients: the Canadian experience. Neurosurgery 2007;60(5):881–886

Case 62   **Neurofibromatosis Type 1**

Jean-Pierre Farmer and Abdulrahman J. Sabbagh

■ Clinical Presentation

- A 3-year-old child is referred to you because of the presence of multiple café-au-lait spots.
- His parents have a normal phenotype.
- History does not reveal any developmental delay.

- His physical examination shows macrocrania, multiple café-au-lait spots, 12 in total, greater than 0.5 cm.
- There is no scoliosis.
- He has pulsatile proptosis of the right eye without chemosis or pupillary changes.

■ Questions

1. What are the diagnostic criteria for neurofibromatosis type I (NF-1)?
2. What are other NF-1 associated conditions?
3. What are types of cutaneous neurofibromas?
4. How would you proceed with investigations?
5. Which additional consultants would you involve?
6. Which lesions, if present, would likely require more frequent surveillance and imaging in this patient?
7. What is the cause of pulsatile proptosis?
8. What is the chance of occurrence of optic pathway gliomas in NF patients?
9. What are the rates of optic glioma progression in NF patients?
10. What imaging characteristics of optic glioma might help in determining the prognosis?

11. What is the usual cause of aqueductal stenosis in NF-1 patients?
12. How frequent are academic difficulties in patients with NF?
13. Assuming the magnetic resonance imaging (MRI) of the brain and spine are normal, what would be your recommended follow-up scan frequency?
14. Is the age at diagnosis significant with respect to prognosis in patients with NF-1?
15. What is the NF-1 gene and where is it located?
16. What is neurofibromin? What are its functions?
17. Describe the Ras signaling pathway (Rat sarcoma) and its relation to neurofibromin.

■ Answers

1. *What are the diagnostic criteria for NF-1?*
   - NF-1 criteria include the following:[1]
     - Six or more café-au-lait spots (over 5 mm in prepubertal individuals, over 15 mm in postpubertal individuals)
     - Two or more neurofibromas of any type or one plexiform neurofibroma
     - Freckling in the axillary or inguinal region
     - Optic glioma
     - Two or more Lisch nodules (iris hamartomas)
     - Osseous lesions such as sphenoid dysplasia or thinning of the long bone cortex with or without pseudarthrosis
       - A first-degree relative (parent, sibling, or offspring) with NF-1 by the above criteria
2. *What are other NF-1-associated conditions?*

- NF-1 associated conditions include the following:[1,2]
  - Aqueductal stenosis
  - Macrocephaly
  - Unilateral superior orbital defect (pulsatile exophthalmos)
  - Cognitive impairment and learning disabilities
  - Kyphoscoliosis
  - Syringomyelia
  - Intracranial tumors
    - Astrocytoma, hemispheric
    - Meningioma, solitary or multicentric (adults)
  - Extracranial tumors
    - Schwann cell tumors
    - Neuroblastoma
    - Sarcoma
    - Leukemia
    - Wilms' tumor
    - Pheochromocytoma
  - Moyamoya disease

■ Answers (*continued*)

3. *What are types of cutaneous neurofibromas?*
   - Types of neurofibromata (Friedman and Riccardi classification)[3–5]:
     - Discrete cutaneous: Soft and fleshy nodules located in epidermis, dermis, and trunk mainly, but in the face and extremities as well. Usually more than a 100 lesions are seen by age 40.
     - Discrete subcutaneous: These are firm and rubbery.
     - Deep nodular (plexiform nodular): involve nerves beneath the dermis; they are fusiform; may involve the entire nerve.
     - Diffuse plexiform: congenital in origin, evident in infancy or childhood. They are locally invasive and have poorly defined margins. They may be precancerous.

4. *How would you proceed with investigations?*
   - MRI of the brain, spine, and orbits
   - Formal visual acuity, visual fields, and extraocular movement testing.
   - Genetic testing

5. *Which additional consultants would you involve?*
   - Ophthalmologist
   - Pediatrician
   - Geneticist

6. *Which lesions, if present, would likely require more frequent surveillance and imaging in this patient?*
   - Lesions requiring frequent follow-ups include[6,7]:
     - Brainstem gliomas
     - Paraspinal gliomas
     - Craniofacial neurofibromas
     - Symptomatic lesions
     - Extraoptic glioma
   - Every 2 years for asymptomatic gadolinium-enhancing lesions[7]
     - Optic pathway and parenchymal gliomas
     - Cranial nerve and visceral neurofibromas

7. *What is the cause of pulsatile proptosis?*
   - The most likely cause of pulsatile proptosis is sphenoid wing hypoplasia.

8. *What is the chance of occurrence of optic pathway gliomas in NF patients?*
   - The chance of occurrence of optic pathway gliomas in NF patients is 15 to 30%.[7,8]

9. *What are the rates of optic glioma, progression in NF patients?*
   - Optic pathway gliomas progress in 12% of NF patients that harbor them.

10. *What imaging characteristics of optic glioma might help in determining the prognosis?*

- The main characteristic that indicates a smaller chance of progression is lack of enhancement.[7]

11. *What is the usual cause of aqueductal stenosis in NF-1 patients?*
    - The usual cause of aqueductal stenosis in NF-1 patients is the occurrence of midbrain unidentified bright objects (UBOs).[9,10]

12. *How frequent are academic difficulties in patients with neurofibromatosis?*
    - Academic difficulties in patients with NF-1 are as common as 30 to 46%.[11,12]

13. *Assuming the MRI of the brain and spine are normal, what would be your recommended follow-up scan frequency?*
    - Assuming the MRI of the brain and spine are normal, young patients require annual MRIs.[13]

14. *Is the age at diagnosis significant with respect to prognosis in patients with NF-1?*
    - Age at diagnosis below 6 years carries a significantly worse prognosis in patients with NF-1.

15. *What is the NF-1 gene and where is it located?*
    - The NF-1 gene has the following characteristics[12,14]:
      - Located on chromosome 17, band q12.2
      - Base pairs 26,446,242 to 26,725,589
      - 335,000 chemical bases
      - 60 exons, alternative splicing at exons 9a, 23a, 48a
      - It is a tumor suppressor gene that encodes neurofibromin.

16. *What is neurofibromin? What are its functions?*
    - Neurofibromin[15]
      - It is a protein (2818 amino acids, molecular mass 327 kDa)[16] that is mainly expressed in
        - Astrocytes and oligodendrocytes of the central nervous system
        - Sensory neurons of the peripheral nervous system
        - Schwann cells
        - Other cells originating from the neural crest such as melanocytes
      - It functions by inactivating Ras by stimulating intrinsic Ras-GTPase to hydrolyze Ras attached guanosine triphosphate (GTP) to guanosine diphosphate (GDP).

17. *Describe the RAS signaling pathway (Rat sarcoma) and its relation to neurofibromin.*
    - RAS when activated can lead to tumor formation.
    - Neurofibromin functions to deactivate RAS.
    - See **Fig. 62.1** for further details.

Answers (*continued*)

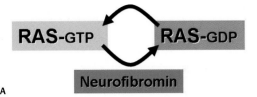

A

RAS Pathway

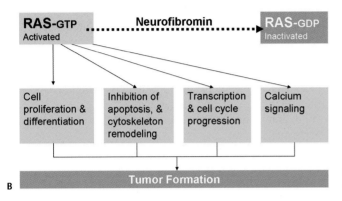

B

Fig. 62.1 Illustration of molecular genetics of Ras pathways: **(A)** Ras activation and deactivation and **(B)** Ras pathway for tumor formation

References

1. Martuza RL, Sampson JH. Neurofibromatosis and other phako-matoses. In: Rengachery SS, Wilkins RH, eds. Neurosurgery. New York: McGraw-Hill; 1996: 673–685
2. National Institutes of Health Consensus Development Conference. Neurofibromatosis: conference statement. Arch Neurol 1988;45:575–578
3. Palmer C, Szudek J, Joe H, Riccardi VM, Friedman JM. Analysis of neurofibromatosis 1 (NF1) lesions by body segment. Am J Med Genet A 2004;125A(2):157–161
4. Szudek J, Birch P, Riccardi VM, Evans DG, Friedman JM. Associations of clinical features in neurofibromatosis 1 (NF1). Genet Epidemiol 2000;19(4):429–439
5. Szudek J, Evans DG, Friedman JM. Patterns of associations of clinical features in neurofibromatosis 1 (NF1). Hum Genet 2003;112(3):289–297
6. Tucker T, Wolkenstein P, Revuz J, Zeller J, Friedman JM. Association between benign and malignant peripheral nerve sheath tumors in NF1. Neurology 2005;65(2):205–211
7. Farmer JP, Khan S, Khan A, et al. Neurofibromatosis type 1 and the pediatric neurosurgeon: a 20-year institutional review. Pediatr Neurosurg 2002;37(3):122–136
8. Lewis RA, Gerson LP, Axelson KA, Riccardi VM, Whitford RP. von Recklinghausen neurofibromatosis. II. Incidence of optic gliomata. Ophthalmology 1984;91(8):929–935
9. Lopes Ferraz Filho JR, Munis MP, Soares Souza A, Sanches RA, Goloni-Bertollo EM, Pavarino-Bertelli EC. Unidentified bright objects on brain MRI in children as a diagnostic criterion for neurofibromatosis type 1. Pediatr Radiol 2008;38(3):305–310
10. Pou Serradell A. Natural evolution of neurocutaneous syndrome in adults. Rev Neurol 1996;24(133):1085–1127
11. Bonnemaison E, Roze-Abert B, Lorette G, et al. 1 Tours-région Centre. Neurofibromatosis type 1 complications in the pediatric age: follow-up of a hundred cases. Arch Pediatr 2006;13(7):1009–1014
12. Korf BR, Rubenstein AE. Neurofibromatosis. 2nd ed. New York: Thieme Medical Publishers; 2005
13. Pinson S, Créange A, Barbarot S, et al. Neurofibromatosis 1: recommendations for management. Arch Pediatr 2002;9(1):49–60
14. Dasgupta B, Gutmann DH. Neurofibromatosis 1: closing the GAP between mice and men. Curr Opin Genet Dev 2003;13(1):20–27
15. Stephens K. Genetics of neurofibromatosis 1-associated peripheral nerve sheath tumors. Cancer Invest 2003;21(6):897–914
16. Marchuk DA, Saulino AM, Tavakko IR, et al. cDNA cloning of the type 1 neurofibromatosis gene: complete sequence of the NF1 gene product. Genomics 1991;11(4):931–940

Case 63 Epidermoid of the Sella

Abdulrahman J. Sabbagh and Jean-Pierre Farmer

■ Clinical Presentation

- An 8-year-old girl presents to the emergency room with sudden painless loss of vision in the left eye.
- She has no history of significant fever, systemic symptoms or trauma, and no symptoms of increased intracranial pressure. Her mother reports some behavioral changes.
- On examination, visual acuity:
  - Right eye: 20/25
  - Left eye: no light perception

- Pupils
  - Left: dilated nonreactive with relative afferent pupillary defect (RAPD)
- Funduscopic examination shows optic atrophy on the right side without papilledema.
- Extraocular movements are full; there is no diplopia, no pain on movement, and no nystagmus.
- Other cranial nerves are normal and the rest of the exam is normal.

■ Questions

1. Describe the available imaging studies (**Fig. 63.1**).
2. Give three differential diagnoses that would be compatible with the history and images, knowing that this lesion does not enhance on gadolinium infusion.
3. What other imaging modality would you want to see to get a more accurate diagnosis?
4. What is RAPD?
5. What are the available surgical approaches to treat this sellar-suprasellar tumor?
6. What are contraindications of the transsphenoidal approach?
7. Describe epidermoid tumors from a gross and microscopic aspect.
8. What is the difference between epidermoid and dermoid tumors?

■ Answers

1. *Describe the available imaging studies (**Fig. 63.1**).*
   - Lateral skull radiography (**Fig. 63.1A**), plain computed tomography (CT) (**Fig. 63.1B**), and magnetic resonance imaging (MRI) (**Fig. 63.1C and Fig. 63.1D**)
     - Skull x-ray shows flattened sella turcica.
     - CT: Plain axial CT shows a hypodense area in the suprasellar region.
     - MRI: This suprasellar lesion is hypointense on T1-weighted axial MRI and hyperintense on T2. It is displacing the optic chiasm posteriorly. Sagittal MRI showed that this lesion is occupying both the sellar and suprasellar regions.
2. *Give three differential diagnoses that would be compatible with the history and images, knowing that this lesion does not enhance on gadolinium infusion.*
   - Differential diagnosis includes
     - Arachnoid cyst of the sella
     - Epidermoid of the sella
     - Rathke's pouch cyst[1]

3. *What other imaging modality would you want to see to get a more accurate diagnosis?*
   - Diffusion-weighted MRI. In this case, it shows restricted diffusion signal, indicating that this is more likely to be an epidermoid cyst (**Fig. 63.2A**)
   - Contrast-enhanced MRI. In this case, it shows no uptake of gadolinium by the tumor (**Fig. 63.2B**)
   - Magnetic resonance angiography. It this case, it shows no evidence of aneurysm or arteriovenous malformation (**Fig. 63.2C**).[1]
4. *What is RAPD?*
   - Relative afferent pupillary defect (RAPD) is also known as Marcus-Gunn pupil.
   - When the pupillary reflex is tested, there is a delay in the reflex on the affected side due to damage or compression of the optic pathway causing reduction in the number of fibers subserving the light reflex on the affected side.[2]

■ Answers (*continued*)

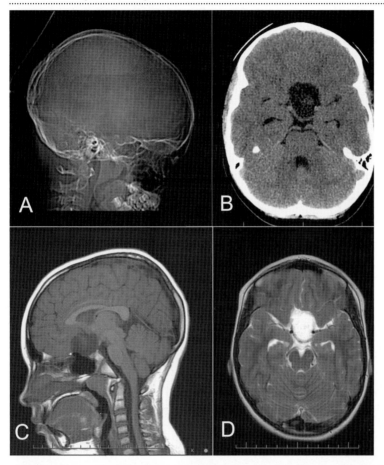

Fig. 63.1 **(A)** Imaging studies showing plain skull x-ray, **(B)** noncontrasted axial computed tomography scan through the sella, and **(C)** mid-sagittal T1-weighted magnetic resonance image and **(D)** axial T2-weighted MRI.

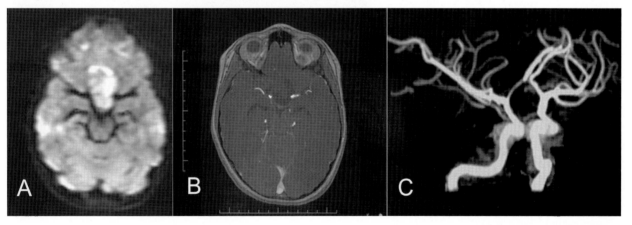

Fig. 63.2 Additional imaging studies obtained: **(A)** Diffusion-weighted magnetic resonance image (MRI) axial cut through the sella, **(B)** contrast enhanced T1-weighted MRI, and **(C)** MR angiogram.

5. *What are the available surgical approaches to treat this sellar-suprasellar tumor?*
   - Subfrontal, pterional, supraorbital (cranio-orbital),[3] or transsphenoidal approaches[4,5]

6. *What are contraindications of the transsphenoidal approach?*
   - Sphenoid sinus is not pneumatized.
   - Sella is too small to reach the suprasellar extension of the tumor.
   - Significant suprasellar extension of the tumor that cannot be reached by the transsphenoidal approach.[4]

■ Answers (*continued*)

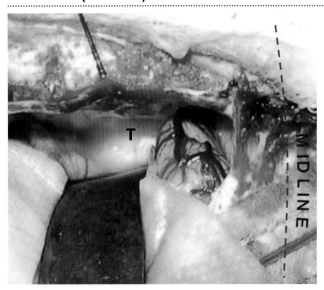

Fig. 63.3   Intraoperative picture depicting a subfrontal approach to the tumor (T) with the midline outlined by the hatched line.

7. *Describe epidermoid tumors from a gross and microscopic aspect.*
   - Gross: Epidermoid tumors envelop and take the shape of their surrounding structures, yet they are separable from them. Pearly in appearance, they can be whitish to grayish with a glistening surface (**Fig. 63.3**). When opened, they contain flaky waxy material.
   - Microscopic: The cyst lining is comprised of stratified squamous epithelium. The contents of the cyst are composed of degenerated keratinocytes. This material is of eosinophilic appearance.[6]

8. *What is the difference between epidermoid and dermoid tumors?*
   - Dermoids are usually well demarcated and contain greasy material that may contain hair and adnexal appendages such as sebaceous glands.[6]
   - Epidermoids typically do not contain such appendages.

■ References

1. Osborn AG. Diagnostic Neuroradiology. St. Louis, MO: Mosby, 1994:465
2. Kardon R, Kawasaki A, Miller NR. Origin of the relative afferent pupillary defect in optic tract lesions. Ophthalmology 2006;113(8):1345–1353
3. Al-Mefty O. Supraorbital-pteronial approach to skull base lesions. Neurosurgery 1987;21(4):474–477
4. Hardy J. Trans-sphenoidal approach to the pituitary gland. In: Wilkins RH, Rengashary SS, eds. Neurosurgery. 2nd ed. New York: McGraw-Hill;1996:1375–1384
5. Taub E, Patterson RH Jr. Transcranial approaches to the pituitary gland and sellar region. In: Wilkins RH, Rengashary SS, eds. Neurosurgery. 2nd ed. New York: McGraw-Hill; 1996:1385–1388
6. Smirniotopoulos JG, Chiechi MV. Teratomas, dermoids, and epidermoids of the head and neck. Radiographics 1995;15(6):1437–1455

Case 64   **Frontal Abscess with Sinus Involvement**

Ramez Malak and Robert Moumdjian

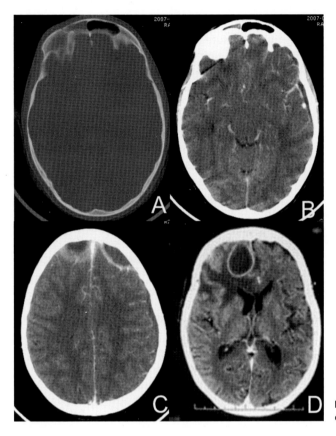

Fig. 64.1   Computed tomography scan of the brain with **(A)** bone windows and **(B–D)** brain windows contrast enhanced.

▪ Clinical Presentation

• A six-year-old girl presents with altered consciousness, left sixth nerve palsy, and fever.

• Computed tomography (CT) scan is shown in **Fig. 64.1**.

▪ Questions

1. Describe the CT scan.
2. Give a differential diagnosis.
3. Describe etiologies of cerebral abscess.
4. Provide predisposing conditions for cerebral abscess.
5. What is your initial management?

6. What are some possible complications?
7. Provide poor prognostic factors.
8. Describe treatment options and their indications.
9. Outline follow-up.

Answers

1. *Describe the CT scan.*
   - There is a ring-enhancing lesion in the left frontal subdural space and fullness of the right frontal sinus.
2. *Give a differential diagnosis.*
   - Brain abscess, neoplasm, granuloma, cerebral infarct, resolving hematoma, postoperative changes
   - The sixth nerve palsy is most likely secondary to increased intracranial pressure (ICP). The abducens nerve is often the first nerve to be compressed in cases of elevated ICP. (Alternative, but less likely causes of abducens palsy, in this case may include meningitis involving the skull base or Gradenigo syndrome.)
   - Helpful distinguishing features
     - Magnetic resonance spectroscopy: elevation of metabolites of bacterial origin including acetate, lactate, succinate, and amino acids (compared with elevated choline and decreased *N*-acetylaspartate in tumors).
     - Diffusion-weighted magnetic resonance imaging (DWI): restricted diffusion (high-signal intensity on DWI and low apparent diffusion coefficient values)[1]
3. *Describe etiologies of cerebral abscess.*
   - Between 30 and 60% of pyogenic abscesses are mixed infections, with aerobic isolates outnumbering anaerobic isolates ~2 to 1.
   - Organisms include streptococci, *Staphylococcus aureus*, and gram-negative bacilli.
   - In neutropenic patients, brain abscesses may be caused by *Candida* or *Aspergillus*.
   - In immunosuppressed patients, the causes may include *Toxoplasma gondii*, mycobacterium, *Nocardia*, *Cryptococcus*, or *Listeria*.
4. *Provide predisposing conditions for cerebral abscess.*
   - Immunosuppression, diabetes mellitus, steroid use, alcoholism, renal failure, intravenous drug abuse, meningitis (especially in children, 12% of pediatric abscess), sinusitis, mastoiditis, postoperative craniotomy, ear, nose, and throat surgery or dental surgery, cyanotic heart disease in children (tetralogy of Fallot)
   - Systemic infection
     - Skin pustules, folliculitis, pulmonary infections, osteomyelitis, dental abscess, and subacute bacterial endocarditis
   - Right-to-left shunting
   - Lung arteriovenous fistula, Osler–Weber–Rendu syndrome, patent foramen ovale
     - Removal of organisms from the systemic circulation by the lungs is bypassed.[2,3]

5. *What is your initial management?*
   - Admission
   - Septic workup: blood culture, chest radiography, urine culture, blood count
   - Sedimentation rate and C-reactive protein
   - Cardiac echography
   - Drainage of air sinus or mastoids
   - Lumbar puncture is contraindicated.
   - Antimicrobial therapy
     - If no causative pathogen is identified, initial empirical antimicrobial therapies are selected in accordance with the portal of entry and the anatomic location of the abscess (**Table 64.1**). For example, penicillin G, metronidazole, and third-generation cephalosporins are initially indicated for brain abscess associated with sinusitis.
   - Once the organism is identified, change antibiotics according to sensitivity.
   - Duration of parenteral antimicrobial therapy is 6 to 8 weeks provided that the etiologic organisms are susceptible and that adequate surgical drainage can be obtained. It is recommended that antibiotics are continued until complete disappearance of the enhancement of the capsule.
   - Corticosteroids
     - May be beneficial in patients with increased ICP from edema and potentially life-threatening complications, provided they are given after antibiotic therapy is started. However, they could delay immune responses and encapsulation and may decrease enhancement of the abscess wall on CT.
   - Anticonvulsant therapy
     - Seizures are frequent complications of brain abscess. We recommend that seizure prophylaxis or antiepileptic medication be given in every case and continued for extended periods.
6. *What are some possible complications?*
   - Vascular thrombosis
   - Brain infarctions
   - Ventriculitis (requires ventricular drainage and intraventricular and systemic antibiotics)
   - Hydrocephalus
   - Empyema of epidural or subdural spaces
   - Subdural effusions
   - Recurrence after aspiration (3–25%), after excision (0–6%)[3]
   - Death
   - Long-term sequelae: seizures, focal neurologic deficits, and cognitive dysfunction

■ **Answers (*continued*)**

Table 64.1   Mechanisms of Spread of Cerebral Abscesses

Contiguous Infection

Otogenic infection	*Streptococcus* species *Bacteroides* species *Enterobacteriaceae* *Pseudomonas* species	Penicillin G + metronidazole + third-generation cephalosporins
Paranasal sinusitis	*Streptococcus* species *Peptococcus* species *Fusobacterium* species *Bacteroides* species *Propionibacterium* species	

Hematogenous Spread

Endocarditis	*Viridans streptococci* *Staphylococcus aureus*	Oxacillin + metronidazole + third-generation cephalosporins
Intraabdominal infection	*Klebsiella pneumoniae* *Escherichia coli* Other *Enterobacteriaceae* *Streptococcus* species Anaerobes	Penicillin G + metronidazole + third generation cephalosporins

Pulmonary origin
  (Lung arteriovenous
  fistula, Osler–Weber –Rendu
  syndrome)
	Streptococcus species
	Fusobacterium species
	Corynebacterium species
	Peptococcus species	

Urinary tract infection	*Enterobacteriaceae* *Pseudomonas* species	

Postneurosurgical and Posttraumatic

Penetrating trauma	*Staphylococcus aureus* *Clostridium* species *Enterobacteriaceae* *Bacteroides* species *Fusobacterium* species *Peptostreptococcus*	Oxacillin + metronidazole + third-generation cephalosporins
Postoperative	*Staphylococcus aureus* *Enterobacteriaceae* *Staphylococcus epidermidis* *Pseudomonas* species	Vancomycin + third-generation cephalosporins

Source: Data from Lu CH, Chang WN, Lui CC. Strategies for the management of bacterial brain abscess. J Clin Neurosci 2006; 13(10):979–985.

■ Answers (*continued*)

7. *Provide poor prognostic factors.*
   - Intraventricular rupture, associated meningitis, ependymitis, empyema, unknown primary source, sterile pus or culture, large abscess, presence of hydrocephalus, metastatic abscess, neonates and infants (~10% mortality),[3] multiple deep-seated abscesses, inaccurate diagnosis, congenital cyanotic heart disease, rapid and fulminant clinical course, bad neurologic condition at presentation, *Nocardia* infection, sepsis, or meningitis.[3,4]

8. *Describe treatment options and their indications.*
   - Medical treatment
     - Nonsurgical, empirical treatment is possible and efficient in certain patients, especially when the etiologic agent is known, abscess is less than 2 cm, or at the stage of cerebritis.
   - Surgical treatment
     - Burr hole drainage, simple needle aspiration, or stereotactic aspiration
       - Advantages: simple; it can be used in the cerebritis stage; has less potential morbidity than surgical excision, especially in case of edema
       - Indications: Abscesses in the cerebritis stages, deep-seated abscesses, multiple abscesses, abscesses located in eloquent areas of the brain, abscesses extending in various sinuses and mastoids, subdural empyema
       - Risks: rupture of the abscess into the ventricle or leakage into the subarachnoid space, intracerebral hematoma
       - Contraindications: multiloculated abscesses
     - Excision
       - Advantages: lower incidence of recurrence, shorter hospitalization
       - Indications: posterior fossa abscesses, multiloculated abscesses, failure of multiple aspirations, adhesions to the dura, abscesses caused by more resistant pathogens such as fungi, abscesses containing gas, posttraumatic abscesses containing foreign bodies or contaminated retained bone fragments, abscesses resulting from fistulous communication (dermal sinus)
       - Disadvantages: higher morbidity, increased brain edema
       - Contraindications: abscesses in the cerebritis stages, deep-seated abscesses in eloquent areas, multiple abscesses

9. *Outline follow-up.*
   - The clinical improvement can precede radiologic improvement. Complete resolution of the abscess cavity will take ~12 weeks. Residual contrast enhancement should not dictate the need for additional therapy. Usually intravenous antibiotics are administered for 6 weeks, generally followed by oral intake for 3 weeks.
   - The effectiveness of the treatment of these patients should be judged according to clinical status and neuroradiographic findings. CT should show decreases in degree of ring enhancement, edema, mass effect, and size of the lesion.
   - Regular follow-up by CT should be at least every 3 months to document the therapeutic response and complete resolution of the ring-enhancing abscesses.[1,3]

■ References

1. Karampekios S, Hesselink J. Cerebral infections. Eur Radiol 2005;15(3):485–493
2. Carpenter J, Stapleton S, Holliman R. Retrospective analysis of 49 cases of brain abscess and review of the literature. Eur J Clin Microbiol Infect Dis 2007;26(1):1–11
3. Ciurea AV, Stoica F, Vasilescu G, Nuteanu L. Neurosurgical management of brain abscesses in children. Childs Nerv Syst 1999;15(6–7):309–317
4. Lu CH, Chang WN, Lui CC. Strategies for the management of bacterial brain abscess. J Clin Neurosci 2006;13(10):979–985

Case 65   Hypothalamic Hamartoma

Abdulrahman J. Sabbagh, Sandeep Mittal, Fahad Eid Alotaibi, and José Luis Montes

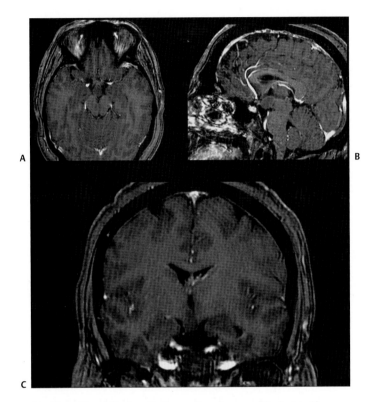

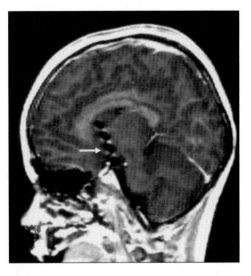

Fig. 65.2   T1-weighted sagittal magnetic resonance images of the brain showing depth electrode within the hypothalamic hamartoma.

Fig. 65.1   T1-weighted magnetic resonance images of the brain with contrast, relevant **(A)** axial, **(B)** sagittal, and **(C)** coronal slices are shown.

■ Clinical Presentation

- A 16-year-old boy is referred to you by an epileptologist. He presents with a history of progressive epilepsy that is refractory to medication.
- The seizures are described as episodes of short bouts of emotionless laughter with loss of awareness that last only a few seconds at a time and occur several times during the day now.

- He also suffers from generalized tonic-clonic seizures several times a month.
- Other pertinent findings include cognitive delay. He is able to speak. The remainder of his neurologic exam is normal (including motor, sensory, cerebellar, and gait examination).
- A magnetic resonance imaging (MRI) scan is obtained and shown in **Fig. 65.1**.

■ Questions

1. Describe the MRI (**Fig. 65.1**).
2. What is the term used for type of seizures this patient is experiencing?
3. How will you work up this patient?
4. Briefly describe the anatomy of the hypothalamus; enumerate its nuclei and their functions.
5. What seizure types are associated with hypothalamic hamartomas (HH)?

6. What symptoms other than epilepsy are associated with HH?
7. If this patient has polydactyly and hypopituitarism, what syndrome would you want to confirm?
8. How do you classify HH? What class does this patient's hamartoma belong to?
9. What treatment options can you offer to a patient with HH and intractable seizures? What are their limitations and outcomes?

■ Answers

1. *Describe the MRI (Fig. 65.1).*
   - MRI shows a small nonenhancing, isointense lesion in the hypothalamic area.
   - The mass occupies the 3rd ventricle and does not cause hydrocephalus.
   - This is most consistent with a HH.
2. *What is the term used for type of seizures this patient is experiencing?*
   - Gelastic seizures
3. *How will you work up this patient?*
   - Imaging and electrophysiologic investigations include
     - Electroencephalogram (EEG): can show slow spike and wave EEG patterns with or without multifocal epileptiform abnormalities (typically frontal or temporal)[1]
     - Computed tomography (CT) scan: may show an isodense nonenhancing lesion
     - MRI: shows an isotense to slightly hypointense lesion compared with gray matter[2]
     - Depth electrode recording: When the diagnosis is equivocal and EEG is nonspecific, specialized centers may consider this modality for diagnosis (Fig. 65.2).[3,4]
     - Positron emission tomography scan: reveals ictal hypermetabolism at the hamartoma site[5]
     - Single photon emission computerized tomography (SPECT) imaging: measures regional cerebral blood flow during seizures. Ictal SPECT scans can be done after injection of the tracer technetium-99m hexamethylpropyleneamine oxime (Tc-99m-HMPAO).
     - Magnetoencephalography (MEG): MEG maps interictal magnetic dipole sources onto MRI to produce a magnetic source image[6]
     - Magnetic resonance spectroscopy: decrease in N-acetyl aspartate/creatine and an increase in myoinositol/creatine (mI/Cr) ratios in tumor tissue when compared with values in normal gray matter of the amygdala. Choline/creatine ratios were also increased when compared with those in normal gray matter controls[7]
   - Endocrinologic workup
     - See Case 12, Pituitary Adenoma, for details
4. *Briefly describe the anatomy of the hypothalamus; enumerate its nuclei and their functions.*

- The hypothalamus is commonly subdivided into regions along its anteroposterior axis (Fig. 65.3).[8]
  - The preoptic region extends rostrally to the optic chiasm and dorsally to the anterior commissure.
  - The supraoptic region resides above the optic chiasm.
  - The tuberal region lies above and includes the tuber cinereum.
  - The mammillary region includes the mammillary bodies and the posterior hypothalamic nuclei.
5. *What seizure types are associated with HH?*
   - Seizure types include
     - Gelastic seizures (forced bouts of emotionless laughter) are considered by most authors to be characteristic of HH.
     - Multiple other seizure types exist including
       - Generalized tonic-clonic seizures
       - Partial complex seizures
       - Drop attacks
       - Atypical absences
6. *What symptoms other than epilepsy are associated with HH?*
   - Other associated symptoms can include
     - Precocious puberty
     - Psychiatric manifestations[9,10]
       - Oppositional defiant disorder (83.3%)
       - Attention deficit-hyperactivity disorder (75%)
       - Conduct disorder (33.3%)
       - Affective disorders (16.7%)
       - Progressive cognitive decline
7. *If this patient has polydactyly and hypopituitarism, what syndrome would you want to confirm?*
   - Pallister–Hall syndrome (PHS)[11]
   - The syndrome is typically characterized by the presence of a HH in association with multisystem malformations.
   - The spectrum of features also includes pituitary hypoplasia or dysfunction, central postaxial polydactyly, dysplastic nails, bifid epiglottis, and imperforate anus.
   - Additionally, cardiac anomalies, renal defects, and mild mental retardation are seen.
   - PHS is often diagnosed at birth. In familial cases it is inherited in an autosomal dominant pattern with variable expressivity.

■ Answers (*continued*)

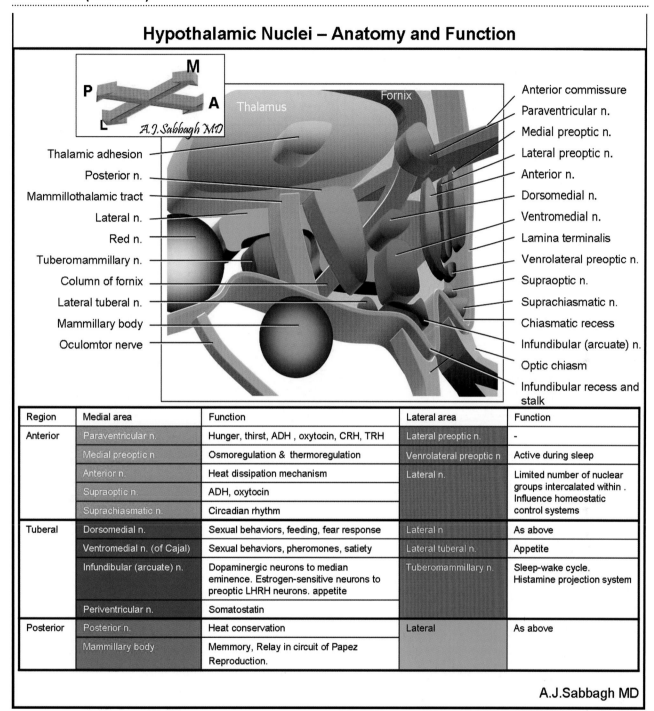

Hypothalamic Nuclei – Anatomy and Function

Labels (left side): Thalamic adhesion, Posterior n., Mammillothalamic tract, Lateral n., Red n., Tuberomammillary n., Column of fornix, Lateral tuberal n., Mammillary body, Oculomtor nerve

Labels (top/right side): Thalamus, Fornix, Anterior commissure, Paraventricular n., Medial preoptic n., Lateral preoptic n., Anterior n., Dorsomedial n., Ventromedial n., Lamina terminalis, Venrolateral preoptic n., Supraoptic n., Suprachiasmatic n., Chiasmatic recess, Infundibular (arcuate) n., Optic chiasm, Infundibular recess and stalk

Inset labels: P, L, M, A, A.J.Sabbagh MD

Region	Medial area	Function	Lateral area	Function
Anterior	Paraventricular n.	Hunger, thirst, ADH , oxytocin, CRH, TRH	Lateral preoptic n.	-
	Medial preoptic n	Osmoregulation & thermoregulation	Venrolateral preoptic n	Active during sleep
	Anterior n.	Heat dissipation mechanism	Lateral n.	Limited number of nuclear groups intercalated within . Influence homeostatic control systems
	Supraoptic n.	ADH, oxytocin		
	Suprachiasmatic n.	Circadian rhythm		
Tuberal	Dorsomedial n.	Sexual behaviors, feeding, fear response	Lateral n	As above
	Ventromedial n. (of Cajal)	Sexual behaviors, pheromones, satiety	Lateral tuberal n.	Appetite
	Infundibular (arcuate) n.	Dopaminergic neurons to median eminence. Estrogen-sensitive neurons to preoptic LHRH neurons. appetite	Tuberomammillary n.	Sleep-wake cycle. Histamine projection system
	Periventricular n.	Somatostatin		
Posterior	Posterior n.	Heat conservation	Lateral	As above
	Mammillary body	Memmory, Relay in circuit of Papez Reproduction.		

A.J.Sabbagh MD

Fig. 65.3 Hypothalamic nuclei and regions. Medial and lateral areas are illustrated in shades of red/purple or green, respectively. n, nucleus; ADH, antidiuretic hormone; CRH, corticotrophin-releasing hormone; TRH, thyrotropin-releasing hormone; LHRH, luteinizing hormone release hormone; A, anterior; P, posterior; M, medial; L, lateral. (Courtesy of the Pan Arab Journal of Neurosurgery.)

■ **Answers (continued)**

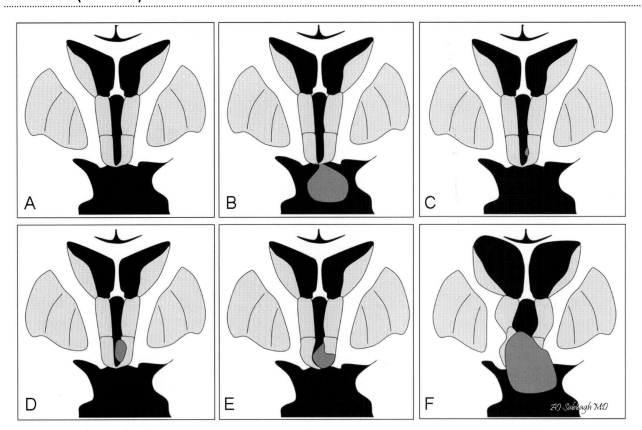

Fig. 65.4 Classification of hypothalamic hamartomas (Coronal section). **(A)** Normal; **(B)** peduncular, Delalande & Fohlen type I (horizontal insertion); **(C)** parahypothalamic, sessile Delalande & Fohlen type II (vertical insertion); **(D)** intrahypothalamic, sessile, Delalande & Fohlen type III (vertical insertion); **(E)** intrahypothalamic, Delalande & Fohlen type III (horizontal and vertical insertion); **(F)** intrahypothalamic, Delalande & Fohlen type IV (giant). (Adapted from Delalande O, Fohlen M. Disconnecting surgical treatment of hypothalamic hamartoma in children and adults with refractory epilepsy and proposal of a new classification. Neurol Med Chir (Tokyo) 2003;43(2):61-68.)

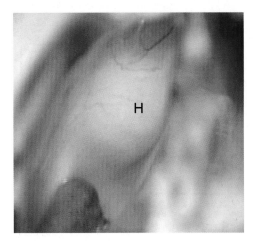

Fig. 65.5 Intraoperative endoscopic view of a hypothalamic hamartoma (H).

■ Answers (*continued*)

8. *How do you classify HH? What class does this patient's hamartoma belong to?*
   - Several classification schemes have been described.
   - The most recent and most widely used is the classification of Delalande and Fohlen (**Fig. 65.4**).[12]
   - The present patient's lesion is classified as intrahypothalamic (3E) according to Delalande and Fohlen's classification.

9. *What treatment options can you offer to a patient with HH and intractable seizures? What are their limitations and outcomes?*
   - Microsurgical resection: Seizure outcome is related to completeness of resection.[13,14]
     - Pterional and frontotemporal approach[14]
       - Advantage: shortest, most direct route to the suprasellar cistern and hamartoma
       - Disadvantage: Surgical corridor may be narrowed by the internal carotid artery, optic nerve and tracts, oculomotor nerve, and pituitary stalk.
       - Outcome: 23% of patients are seizure free, 87% have significant seizure reduction (in a study of 13 patients).
     - Transcallosal interforniceal approach[15]
       - Advantage: provides a wide exposure to the 3rd ventricle and an excellent view of the hamartoma from above; avoidance of cranial nerves and blood vessels in the suprasellar cistern and interpeduncular fossa may further reduce the risk of stroke and oculomotor nerve injury
       - Disadvantage: risk of short-term memory deficits because of potential septal, forniceal, or mammillary body injury
       - Outcome: 52% are seizure free, 24% have significant improvement (in a series of 29 patients)[15]
       - Complications: thalamic infarct in 7%, increased appetite in 33% (this is permanent in 16%), and short-term memory deficits in 50%
     - Transcallosal, subchoroidal approach: alternative to the transcallosal interforniceal route; lower risk of short-term memory deficits
     - Endoscopic transventricular approach (**Fig. 65.5** for an endoscopic view)
       - Outcome: 31% were able to sustain complete resection (14 of 44 patients), of whom 90% were seizure free.[16]
       - Complications: short-term memory difficulties (three patients) and hemiparesis (one patient).[16]
   - Disconnection procedure (open or endoscopic)[17]
     - Outcome: 58% seizure free
     - Complications (in a series of 18 patients)[17]: stroke (2 patients), diabetes insipidus (2 patients), meningitis (1 patient)
   - Stereotactic radiosurgery[18]
     - Gamma knife radiosurgery: good treatment for small- and medium-size hamartomas. The median dose recommended at the marginal isodose is 17 Gy (range is 13–26 Gy).
       - Outcome: 37% seizure free. Most had cognitive and behavioral improvement.
       - Complications: 15% transient worsening of seizures; no permanent complications mentioned.
     - Linear acceleration-based radiosurgery
     - Stereotactic brachytherapy
   - Stereotactic radiofrequency ablation
     - Outcome: 25% seizure free, 25% significant improvement (12 patients)[19]
     - Complications: 8% mortality (1 patient), 16% memory deficits
   - Vagal nerve stimulation: limited role; palliative and seizure freedom is not expected.[20]
   - Corpus callosotomy: limited role

■ References

1. Berkovic SF, Andermann F, Melanson D, Ethier RE, Feindel W, Gloor P. Hypothalamic hamartomas and ictal laughter: evolution of a characteristic epileptic syndrome and diagnostic value of magnetic resonance imaging. Ann Neurol 1988;23(5):429–439

2. Hahn FJ, Leibrock LG, Huseman CA, Makos MM. The MR appearance of hypothalamic hamartoma. Neuroradiology 1988;30(1):65–68

3. MunariC, KahaneP, FrancioneS, . Role of the hypothalamic hamartoma in the genesis of gelastic fits (a video-stereo-EEG study). Electroencephalogr Clin Neurophysiol 1995;95(3):154–160

4. Palmini A, Chandler C, Andermann F, et al. Resection of the lesion in patients with hypothalamic hamartomas and catastrophic epilepsy. Neurology 2002;58(9):1338–1347

5. Palmini A, Van Paesschen W, Dupont P, Van Laere K, Van Driel G. Status gelasticus after temporal lobectomy: ictal FDG-PET findings and the question of dual pathology involving hypothalamic hamartomas. Epilepsia 2005;46(8):1313–1316

6. Tovar-Spinoza ZS, Ochi A, Rutka JT, Go C, Otsubo H. The role of magnetoencephalography in epilepsy surgery. Neurosurg Focus 2008;25(3):E16

7. Amstutz DR, Coons SW, Kerrigan JF, Rekate HL, Heiserman JE. Hypothalamic hamartomas: correlation of MR imaging and spectroscopic findings with tumor glial content. AJNR Am J Neuroradiol 2006;27(4):794–798

8. Parent A. Carpenter's Human Neuroanatomy. Baltimore: Williams & Wilkins; 1996

9. Savard G, Bhanji NH, Dubeau F, Andermann F, Sadikot A. Psychiatric aspects of patients with hypothalamic hamartoma and epilepsy. Epileptic Disord 2003;5(4):229–234

10. Weissenberger AA, Dell ML, Liow K, et al. Aggression and psychiatric comorbidity in children with hypothalamic hamartomas and their unaffected siblings. J Am Acad Child Adolesc Psychiatry 2001;40(6):696–703

11. Hall JG, Pallister PD, Clarren SK, et al. Congenital hypothalamic hamartoblastoma, hypopituitarism, imperforate anus and post- axial polydactyly–a new syndrome? Part I: clinical, causal, and pathogenetic considerations. Am J Med Genet 1980;7(1):47–74

12. Delalande O, Fohlen M. Disconnecting surgical treatment of hypothalamic hamartoma in children and adults with refractory epilepsy and proposal of a new classification. Neurol Med Chir (Tokyo) 2003;43(2):61–68

13. Mittal S, Montes JL, Farmer JP, Sabbagh AJ. Surgical management of epilepsy related to hypothalamic hamartomas. In: Villemure JG, Baltuch G, eds. Operative Techniques in Epilepsy Surgery. New York: Thieme Medical Publishers; 2009:81–98

14. Palmini A, Paglioli-Neto E, Montes J, Farmer JP. The treatment of patients with hypothalamic hamartomas, epilepsy and behavioural abnormalities: facts and hypotheses. Epileptic Disord 2003;5(4):249–255

15. Harvey AS, Freeman JL, Berkovic SF, Rosenfeld JV. Transcallosal resection of hypothalamic hamartomas in patients with intractable epilepsy. Epileptic Disord 2003;5(4):257–265

16. Rekate HL, Feiz-Erfan I, Ng YT, Gonzalez LF, Kerrigan JF. Endoscopic surgery for hypothalamic hamartomas causing medically refractory gelastic epilepsy. Childs Nerv Syst 2006;22(8):874–880

17. Fohlen M, Lellouch A, Delalande O. Hypothalamic hamartoma with refractory epilepsy: surgical procedures and results in 18 patients. Epileptic Disord 2003;5(4):267–273

18. Régis J, Scavarda D, Tamura M, et al. Epilepsy related to hypothalamic hamartomas: surgical management with special reference to gamma knife surgery. Childs Nerv Syst 2006;22(8):881–895

19. Kuzniecky RI, Guthrie BL. Stereotactic surgical approach to hypothalamic hamartomas. Epileptic Disord 203;5(4):275–280

20. Feiz-Erfan I, Horn EM, Rekate HL, et al. Surgical strategies for approaching hypothalamic hamartomas causing gelastic seizures in the pediatric population: transventricular compared with skull base approaches. J Neurosurg 2005; 103(4, Suppl):325–332

Case 66   Vein of Galen Malformation

Samer K. Elbabaa and Sten Solander

■ Clinical Presentation

- A 1-month-old baby girl is referred to neurosurgery clinic for evaluation of enlarging head circumference since birth.
- There is no history of seizures, lethargy, or vomiting.
- Physical examination reveals a normal-looking baby girl, flat anterior fontanelle, mildly dilated scalp veins, and head circumference at the 75th percentile for age (it was at the 25th percentile at birth).

- Initial head ultrasound shows normal-sized ventricles, but with dilated vascular structures.
- Magnetic resonance imaging (MRI) of the brain is obtained and shown in **Fig. 66.1**.

■ Questions

1. Interpret the MRI findings.
2. What further diagnostic studies and workup would you like to obtain?
3. What is the most likely diagnosis?
4. Describe the incidence of this lesion.
5. What conditions do you need to evaluate when you consider your treatment options? Discuss your treatment options.
6. Interpret the provided cerebral angiogram images (**Fig. 66.2**)

7. You decide to proceed with endovascular treatment of the vascular lesion. What is the indication for treatment? What is the goal of the treatment? Does the age of presentation affect your treatment plan?
8. Interpret the provided postembolization angiogram images (**Fig. 66.3**).
9. How will you follow the patient after the treatment?
10. Provide a radiographic classification of this pathology.

■ Answers

1. *Interpret the MRI findings.*
   - MRI shows mildly dilated ventricles.
   - There is dilatation of the vein of Galen, straight sinus, and confluence of superior sagittal sinus and straight sinus.
2. *What further diagnostic studies and workup would you like to obtain?*
   - Pediatric cardiology consultation and echocardiogram to evaluate for congestive heart failure
   - Close monitoring of head circumference
   - Four-vessel angiogram and endovascular treatment in the same setting if there is clinical evidence of congestive heart failure, hydrocephalus, or change in neurologic status.
3. *What is the most likely diagnosis?*
   - Vein of Galen malformation (VOGM)
   - This is a dilatation of the median vein of the prosencephalon, which is a precursor of the vein of Galen, caused by an arteriovenous (AV) shunt from the choroidal arteries of the anterior and posterior circulation.[1]

4. *Describe the incidence of this lesion.*
   - The true incidence is unknown, but VOGM cases are rare.
   - The reported incidence is less than 1% of cerebral vascular malformations.
   - The first description of a VOGM was probably by Steinhill in the German pathology literature in 1895.[2]
5. *What conditions do you need to evaluate when you consider your treatment options? Discuss your treatment options.*
   - It is important to understand that most conditions encountered in VOGM patients are related to the degree of AV shunting.
   - Congestive heart failure (if present): Management by pediatric cardiologist is critical to evaluate the need of medical treatment (digoxin, diuretics, and ventilatory support). Emergency endovascular therapy may be necessary to reduce the AV shunt, which can improve the cardiac function.

■ Answers (*continued*)

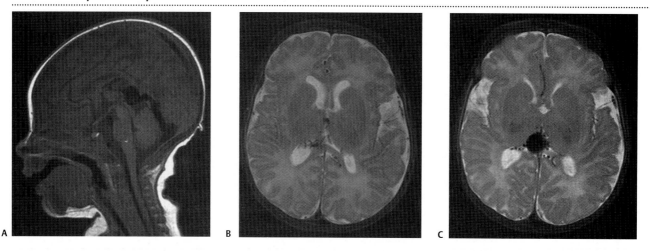

Fig. 66.1   **(A)** Initial T1-weighted sagittal and **(B,C)** T2-weighted axial magnetic resonance images (MRIs) of the brain.

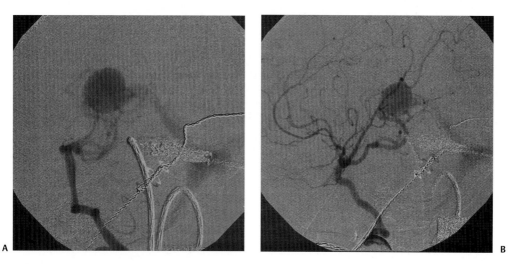

Fig. 66.2   Cerebral angiogram with lateral projection of **(A)** vertebral and **(B)** internal carotid artery.

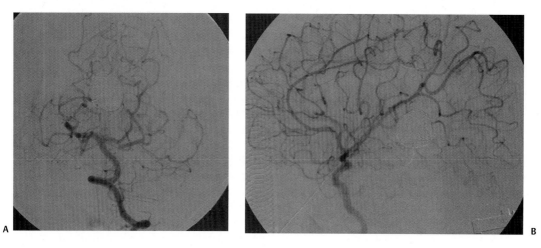

Fig. 66.3   Cerebral angiogram with **(A)** vertebral and **(B)** carotid artery injections in anteroposterior and lateral projections, respectively, after endovascular treatment.

■ Answers (*continued*)

- Ventriculomegaly: This results from the increased dural sinus pressures secondary to the AV shunting.
  - The increase in dural sinus pressure creates a resistance for cerebrospinal fluid (CSF) to enter the sinus, which may lead to hydrocephalus and intracranial hypertension.
  - Close monitoring of head circumference is important for possible signs of hydrocephalus.
  - Generally, CSF shunting without treatment of VOGM is not recommended because of the high risk of hemorrhages and seizures.
  - If the increase in head circumference seems too rapid or if the clinical follow-up period demonstrates a significant developmental delay, urgent embolization should be performed and ventricular shunting should be avoided.[3]
- Seizures (if present): There may be a need for antiepileptic therapy, likely phenobarbital in the neonatal period.
- Treatment options are discussed below.
  - Observation: Children with VOGM have a very poor prognosis if left untreated. An extensive clinical and anatomic evaluation is needed to determine the optimal timing of the treatment. A short period of observation may improve the outcome if clinically tolerated.
  - Surgical clipping: Surgical treatment was the best available therapeutic option before the era of endovascular treatment.
    - Different techniques for open microsurgical treatment of VOGM have been described.[2,4,5]
    - Yasargil et al.[4] emphasized the utility of a posterior interhemispheric approach in a sitting position.
    - The deep central fistulous communications that are characteristic for VOGM make them less amenable to excision than endovascular treatment.[6]
  - Endovascular embolization: Advances in endovascular techniques and imaging have helped us to understand the anatomy and pathophysiology of VOGM. They have also provided new treatment options with improved outcomes.

- Ciricillo et al. in 1990 retrospectively compared the outcomes of both surgical and endovascular techniques in neonatal patients and concluded that endovascular options are far safer.[7]
- Endovascular treatment has become the cornerstone for good outcomes in these challenging lesions.
- Lasjaunias et al. reported a large series of 317 patients, 233 patients were treated with endovascular embolization from 1981 to 2002. The treatment method of choice was a transfemoral arterial approach to deliver glue at the fistulous zone. In their series, mortality rate after the embolization was 10%. Of the surviving patients, moderate to severe developmental delay was seen in 26% of patients; however, 74% were neurologically normal on follow-up.[3]

6. *Interpret the provided cerebral angiogram images* (**Fig. 66.2**).
   - The images show aneurysmal dilatation of the median vein of the prosencephalon on both internal carotid and vertebral artery injections.
   - The main arterial feeders are from the posterior choroidal arteries.

7. *You decide to proceed with endovascular treatment of the vascular lesion. What is the indication for treatment? What is the goal of the treatment? Does the age of presentation affect your treatment plan?*
   - The indications for treatment include congestive heart failure, hydrocephalus, or neurologic symptoms.
   - The primary goal of the treatment is to control the AV shunt. A staged embolization is generally recommended for neonates.
     - This provides preservation of the hydrovenous equilibrium.
     - Also, it limits the high renal exposure to contrast volumes.
     - Severe encephalomalacia and multiorgan failure are associated with poor prognosis, even with a technically successful embolization.
     - In infants, normal brain development should be preserved by endovascular exclusion of the fistula, if technically feasible.[3,8]

■ Answers (*continued*)

- In 2006, Lasjaunias et al. summarized 20 years of experience in treatment of VOGM at Le Kremlin Bicetre, Paris, France, and emphasized the importance of a thorough analysis of neonatal patients with VOGM to best predict the degree of cerebral tissue impairment not evident on imaging.[3]
  - The VOGM neonatal score was developed by their group, which included cardiac, cerebral, respiratory, hepatic, and renal functions.
  - Their management decisions follow a strict protocol based on the neonatal score derived from the above information.[3]

8. *Interpret the provided postembolization angiogram images* (**Fig. 66.3**).
   - The fistula has been obliterated by a combination of transarterial catheterization of the venous pouch with coil embolization, followed by glue injection in the feeding artery.

9. *How will you follow the patients after treatment?*
   - Cardiac function by echocardiogram
   - Head circumference
   - Monitoring of ventricular size by head ultrasound or computed tomography scan
   - Follow-up cerebral angiogram at 6 months posttreatment. If contrast hyperemia is demonstrated at 6 months, even without evidence of AV shunting, additional control angiograms are recommended at 1 and 2 years later.[3]

10. *Provide a radiographic classification of this pathology.*
    - The most widely referenced angiographic classifications are those of Lasjaunias et al.[8,9,10] and Yasargil et al.[4,10]
    - Lasjaunias et al. angiographic classification includes true and secondary vein of Galen malformations.[9]

- The true VOGM occurs because of a dysembryogenic event involving the median vein of the prosencephalon.
  - As a result, a fistulous connection develops between the choroidal arteries and the veins in the wall of the dilated vein of prosencephalon.
  - The deep venous system has a separate drainage pattern without communication with the fistula.
  - Further subcategories of true VOGM include the mural type, in which the fistula is in the wall of the vein (median vein of the prosencephalon) or the choroidal type, with drainage into tributary veins of the medial vein of the prosencephalon.
- The secondary types of VOGM have adjacent arteriovenous malformation that drains selectively into the great vein of Galen.
  - These lesions are characteristically supplied by branches of the middle cerebral artery (thalamoperforating, lenticulostriate, or transsylvian branches), whereas the choroidal and mural true vein of Galen malformations are typically filled by choroidal and pericallosal vessels.[9]
- Yasargil et al. defined four types of VOGM lesions:
  - Type 1 is a simple small fistula involving branches from the pericallosal or posterior cerebral arteries.
  - Type 2 involves more feeding vessels from middle cerebral artery branches (thalamoperforating vessels).
  - Type 3 involves high-flow lesions with large numbers of fistulous connections from a wide range of feeding vessels.
  - Type 4 is a midline AVM with drainage into the vein of Galen (analogous to Lasjaunias' secondary VOGM).[10]

■ References

1. Alvarez H, Garcia Monaco R, Rodesch G, Sachet M, Krings T, Lasjaunias P. Vein of Galen aneurysmal malformations. Neuroimaging Clin N Am 2007;17(2):189–206
2. Hoffman HJ, Chuang S, Hendrick EB, Humphreys RP. Aneurysms of the vein of Galen. Experience at The Hospital for Sick Children, Toronto. J Neurosurg 1982;57(3):316–322
3. Lasjaunias PL, Chng SM, Sachet M, Alvarez H, Rodesch G, Garcia-Monaco R. The management of vein of Galen aneurysmal malformations. Neurosurgery 2006;59(5, Suppl 3):S184–S194
4. Yasargil MG, Antic J, Laciga R, Jain KK, Boone SC. Arteriovenous malformations of vein of Galen: microsurgical treatment. Surg Neurol 1976;3:195–200
5. Menezes AH, Graf CJ, Jacoby CG, Cornell SH. Management of vein of Galen aneurysms. Report of two cases. J Neurosurg 1981;55(3):457–462
6. Blount JP, Oakes WJ, Tubbs RS, Humphreys RP. History of surgery for cerebrovascular disease in children. Part II. Vein of Galen malformations. Neurosurg Focus 2006;20(6):E1
7. CiricilloSF, EdwardsMS, SchmidtKG, . Interventional neuroradiological management of vein of Galen malformations in the neonate. Neurosurgery 1990;27(1):22–27
8. LasjauniasP, Garcia-MonacoR, RodeschG, . Vein of Galen malformation. Endovascular management of 43 cases. Childs Nerv Syst 1991;7(7):360–367
9. LasjauniasP, RodeschG, PruvostP, LarocheFG, LandrieuP. Treatment of vein of Galen aneurysmal malformation. J Neurosurg 1989;70(5):746–750
10. Yasargil MG. AVM of the Brain, Clinical Considerations, General and Special Operative Techniques, Surgical Results, Nonoperative Cases, Cavernous and Venous Angiomas, Neuroanesthesia. Microneurosurgery. New York: Thieme Medical Publishers; 1988: 323–357

Case 67   Pediatric Head Trauma

Jeffrey Atkinson, José Luis Montes, and Abdulrahman J. Sabbagh

■ Clinical Presentation

- A 7-month-old child was found at home with decreased level of consciousness and no clear history of antecedent event.
- He was transported to the hospital where he had a focal seizure.

- Initial examination reveals a Glasgow Coma Score (GCS) of 5, with questionable motor asymmetry and a tense and bulging fontanel.
- He is intubated urgently and sent for a computed tomography (CT) scan. A representative image appears in **Fig. 67.1**.

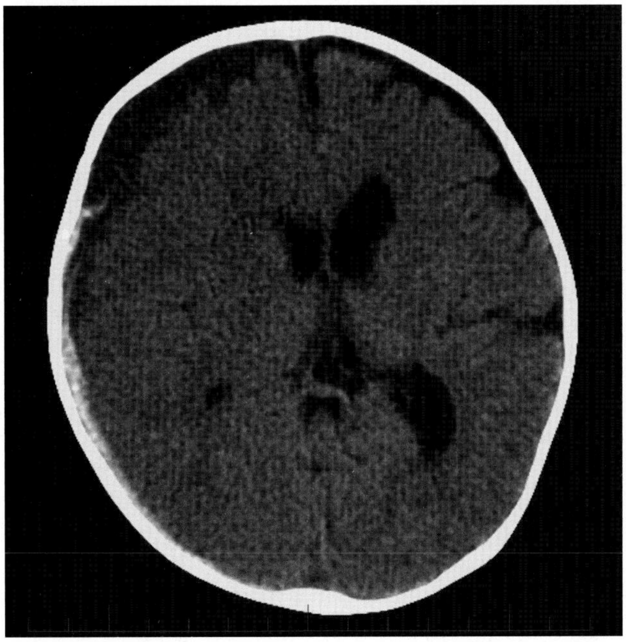

Fig. 67.1   Computed tomography scan of the brain revealing extraaxial fluid collection along the right convexity.

■ Questions

1. What are the findings on the CT scan?
2. What is the differential diagnosis?
3. What other points on history and physical examination might be important?
4. What other investigations and consultations are relevant?
5. What is the acute management of the patient?

The patient was taken urgently to the operating room for decompression and evacuation of the subdural hematoma. He recovered well from the injury.

6. What are the principles of intracranial pressure (ICP) management in a child?
7. What is the epidemiology of inflicted trauma?

8. Is there a constellation of clinical and neurologic findings that are often associated with nonaccidental trauma?
9. Are retinal hemorrhages pathognomic of nonaccidental trauma?
10. What is the differential diagnosis with the association of retinal hemorrhage and bilateral subdural hematomas?
11. What are the most common findings associated with nontraumatic head injury on CT scan?
12. What are the mechanisms of head injury involved in infants and young children?
13. What is the prognosis in a child with an abusive head injury?
14. What are the medicolegal implications of inflicted trauma?

◼ Answers

1. *What are the findings on CT scan?*
   - The CT scan of the head demonstrates subdural collections over the right hemisphere, which are both acute and chronic.
   - There is associated mass effect on the adjacent hemisphere with compression of the ipsilateral ventricle, loss of sulcations, and midline shift.

2. *What is the differential diagnosis?*
   - This subdural hematoma (SDH) is most probably traumatic.
   - The acute and chronic components may indicate hemorrhages of different ages or they may indicate an acute subdural hematoma on top of an enlarged subarachnoid space such as in the syndrome of benign extraaxial fluid collection of infancy.
   - Nontraumatic causes of SDH are very rare in infants but might include vascular malformation (of which there is no evidence on these images), coagulation disorder, or inborn error of metabolism.

3. *What other points on history and physical examination might be important?*
   - Important information obtained on history includes
     - History of trivial blunt trauma often from falling from beds or low chairs or no history of trauma at all.
     - Decreased level of consciousness from lethargy to coma.
     - Irritability, vomiting, seizures, apnea, hypoxia
   - Important findings on inspection include
     - An enlarged head
     - Unusual or patterned bruising
     - Venous engorgement
   - Important neurologic findings on examination include
     - Abnormal movements
     - Seizure activity
     - Tense fontanelle
     - Retinal hemorrhages
     - Lateralizing findings
   - Given the likely traumatic nature of this injury and the suspicion of hemorrhages of different ages, a detailed history must be taken. We need to better establish the exact nature of any traumatic injury the child might have received and establish a time line for caregivers (i.e., exactly who was caring for the child and when).[1]
   - Additionally a social history from the family would be relevant, as well as any previous history of hospital visits for suspicious injuries.[1–3]

4. *What other investigations and consultations are relevant?*
   - Consultations should be obtained from the local child abuse investigative team, which might include pediatrics and social work.[1]
   - Ophthalmology should be consulted to examine the fundi properly to look for retinal hemorrhages that might further suggest abusive injury.[4]
   - Skeletal survey or nuclear medicine bone scan should be done to look for fractures.[4]
   - Magnetic resonance imaging (MRI) of the brain might be considered to better evaluate for cortical or parenchymal injury to the brain and perhaps to better define the ages of the subdural blood.
   - A standard investigation of abnormal coagulation would also be of benefit.[1]

5. *What is the acute management of the patient?*
   - Acute management of this patient involves airway protection as already established by intubation.
   - ICP control medically can be attempted by mannitol, controlled ventilation, sedation of the child, which would imply the insertion of an ICP monitor.[5]
   - Seizure control should be obtained by an intravenous load of the antiepileptic of choice, usually phenytoin or phenobarbital.
   - In this case with the mass effect, the clinical evidence of high ICP and the clinical state of the patient, the argument for evacuation of this clot can be made. This is probably best done by craniotomy, though burr hole or transfontanel evacuation of the chronic component could be considered.
   - An ICP monitor should be inserted into the patient at the time of surgery for postoperative management.

6. *What are the principles of ICP management in a child?*
   - The principles of ICP management in a child are very much the same as those in an adult.
   - A child such as this patient with a GCS <8 and a positive CT scan should be monitored invasively.[5]
   - Even in an infant such as the one in this case, physical examination of the fontanelle is not necessarily adequate for monitoring.
   - With the clot evacuated and the monitor in place, controlled ventilation, cerebrospinal fluid (CSF) drainage if possible, sedation, and osmotic agents can be used.[6]
   - In children, there is also evidence of the benefit of continuous infusions of hypertonic saline in addition to mannitol.[7]

7. *What is the epidemiology of inflicted trauma?*
   - Population-based studies have indicated an annual incidence of 24.6 per 100,000 children younger than 1 year of age.[8]
   - The risk of suffering an inflicted head injury by 1 year of age has been established at 1 in 4065.[8]
   - In most studies, boys are slightly more at risk than girls.[9]

■ Answers (*continued*)

- Some of the risk factors include young parents, low socioeconomic status, single parents, prematurity of the infant, history of abuse to the caretaker, and a history of psychiatric or substance abuse.
- The most common perpetrators are fathers and boyfriends.
- Female babysitters account for 18% of perpetrators.

8. *Is there a constellation of clinical and neurologic findings that are often associated with nonaccidental trauma?*
    - Yes, the association consists of
        - Retinal hemorrhage and subarachnoid hemorrhage or subdural hematomas[10]
        - Bilateral chronic subdural hematomas
        - On CT scan, the association between subarachnoid hemorrhage, subdural hematoma, and interhemispheric blood is highly suspicious of this entity.

9. *Are retinal hemorrhages pathognomic of nonaccidental trauma?*
    - No, they can be associated with normal vaginal delivery.
    - Other factors associated with retinal hemorrhages include accidental trauma, coagulopathy, hypertension, subarachnoid hemorrhage, subdural hemorrhage, papilledema, arterial hypertension, and resuscitation.[11]

10. *What is the differential diagnosis with the association of retinal hemorrhage and bilateral subdural hematomas?*
    - Accidental trauma
    - Osteogenesis imperfecta
    - Blood coagulation dyscrasias
    - Metabolic disorders such as glutaric acidemia type I[11]

11. *What are the most common findings associated with nontraumatic head injury on CT scan?*
    - Acute subdural hematoma[9]
    - Interhemispheric hemorrhage, particularly posterior or layering the tentorium
    - Parenchymal hypodensities sometimes presenting as a black brain, but most common as hemispheric or patchy hypodensities

12. *What are the mechanisms of head injury involved in infants and young children?*
    - The development of acute SBH with parenchymal contusions and significant symptoms is most likely a combination of tangential acceleration, usually associated with shaking episodes and impact manipulations that are caused by hitting the head of the child against a blunt surface or throwing him against one.
    - The forces associated to impact manipulation are in the order of 20 to 30 times greater than the forces generated by shaking alone; the time lapse is significantly shorter.
    - The forces necessary to develop acute subdural hematomas, brain contusion, and diffuse axonal injury are most likely related to impact manipulation or a combination of both.
    - Low-height free-fall forces are enough to cause skull fractures or nonsymptomatic subdural hemorrhages, but not acute subdural hemorrhage accompanied by significant acute neurologic deficit as observed in most nonaccidental trauma.
    - Occasionally, low-height free falls may cause epidural hematomas that are highly symptomatic, but this represents the exception.[9,12,13]

13. *What is the prognosis in a child with abusive head injury?*
    - In general prognosis with abusive head injury is quite poor, probably due to extensive cortical and parenchymal injury of the associated brain and even cervical medullary junction.[9,14]
    - There is an overall 15 to 38% mortality rate. 30 to 50% of survivors will have cognitive or other neurological deficits, and ~30% will have no significant sequelae[9]
    - However, in this case there appears to be very little cortical damage on the CT scan. There needs to be MRI and clinical confirmation. There might be reason to be optimistic if the clinical evolution after surgery is positive.

14. *What are the medicolegal implications of inflicted trauma?*
    - The neurosurgeon is often called to establish whether there is evidence of nonaccidental trauma.
    - The neurosurgeon should be in close contact with the child protection team and ensure that all tests and studies have been done to document and support the diagnosis.
    - The neurosurgeon should be forthcoming with his or her opinion after careful consideration. Unfortunately, in medicine, answers are sometimes not clear-cut and proof of child abuse may be difficult to establish.

■ References

1. Oehmichen M, Meissner C, Saternus KS. Fall or shaken: traumatic brain injury in children caused by falls or abuse at home - a review on biomechanics and diagnosis. Neuropediatrics 2005;36(4):240–245

2. Caffey J. The whiplash shaken infant syndrome: manual shaking by the extremities with whiplash-induced intracranial and intra-ocular bleedings, linked with residual permanent brain damage and mental retardation. Pediatrics 1974;54(4):396–403

3. Kempe CH, Silverman FN, Steele BF, Droegemueller W, Silver HK. The battered-child syndrome. JAMA 1962;181:17–24

4. Duhaime AC, Gennarelli TA, Thibault LE, Bruce DA, Margulies SS, Wiser R. The shaken baby syndrome. A clinical, pathological, and biomechanical study. J Neurosurg 1987;66(3):409–415

5. Adelson PD, Bratton SL, Carney NA, et al. American Association for Surgery of Trauma, Child Neurology Society, International Society for Pediatric Neuro, Guidelines for the acute medical management of severe traumatic brain injury in infants, children, and adolescents. Chapter 5. Indications for intracranial pressure monitoring in pediatric patients with severe traumatic brain injury. Pediatr Crit Care Med 2003;4(3, Suppl):S19–S24

6. Adelson PD, Bratton SL, Carney NA, et al. American Association for Surgery of Trauma, Child Neurology Society, International Society for Pediatric Neuro, Guidelines for the acute medical management of severe traumatic brain injury in infants, children, and adolescents. Chapter 10. The role of cerebrospinal fluid drainage in the treatment of severe pediatric traumatic brain injury. Pediatr Crit Care Med 2003;4(3, Suppl):S38–S39

7. Adelson PD, Bratton SL, Carney NA, et al. American Association for Surgery of Trauma, Child Neurology Society, International Society for Pediatric Neuro, Guidelines for the acute medical management of severe traumatic brain injury in infants, children, and adolescents. Chapter 11. Use of hyperosmolar therapy in the management of severe pediatric traumatic brain injury. Pediatr Crit Care Med 2003;4(3, Suppl):S40–S44

8. Barlow KM, Minns RA. Annual incidence of shaken impact syndrome in young children. Lancet 2000;356(9241):1571–1572

9. Gerber P, Coffman K. Nonaccidental head trauma in infants. Childs Nerv Syst 2007;23(5):499–507

10. Duhaime AC, Alario AJ, Lewander WJ, et al. Head injury in very young children: mechanisms, injury types, and ophthalmologic findings in 100 hospitalized patients younger than 2 years of age. Pediatrics 1992;90(2 Pt 1):179–185

11. Aryan HE, Ghosheh FR, Jandia lR, Levy ML. Retinal hemorrhage and pediatric brain injury: etiology and review of the literature. J Clin Neurosci 2005;12(6):624–631

12. Gennarelli TA, Thibault LE. Biomechanics of head injury. In: Rengachary SS, Wilkens RH, eds. Neurosurgery. New York: McGraw-Hill; 1985:1531–1536

13. Duhaime AC, Durham S. Traumatic brain injury in infants: the phenomenon of subdural hemorrhage with hemispheric hypodensity ("big black brain"). Prog Brain Res 2007;161:293–302

14. Duhaime AC, Christian C, Moss E, Seidl T. Long-term outcome in infants with the shaking-impact syndrome. Pediatr Neurosurg 1996;24(6):292–298

Case 68   Scaphocephaly

Abdulrahman J. Sabbagh, Jeffrey Atkinson, Jean-Pierre Farmer, and José Luis Montes

◼ Clinical Presentation

- A 3-month-old child presents with an abnormal head shape since birth.
- He was born at term via a normal vaginal delivery.
- The father has a similar but more accentuated head shape.

- The physical examination is otherwise normal.
- A computed tomography (CT) scan of the head is done and shown in **Fig. 68.1**.

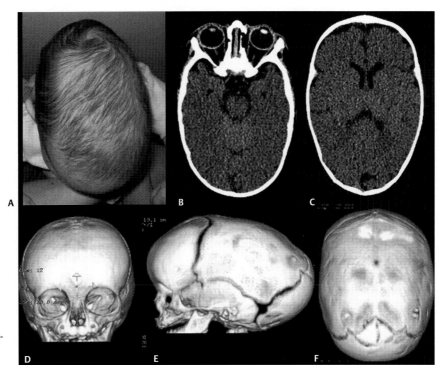

Fig. 68.1 **(A)** Head photograph, **(B,C)** axial computed tomography (CT) scan, and **(D)** three-dimensional reconstructed CT scan, **(E,F)** of a child with craniosynostosis.

◼ Questions

1. Describe the head shape and the CT scan. What is the diagnosis?
2. What is scaphocephaly?
3. How common is scaphocephaly?
4. What is the prognosis of scaphocephaly?
5. What is the risk of developing hydrocephalus in patients diagnosed with craniosynostosis? What is the risk for this patient?

6. What are some treatment options and their possible related morbidities?
7. What is the accepted hypothesis for the pathogenesis of deformities caused by craniosynostosis?
8. What is more clinically important, timing of head and brain growth or timing of normal sutural closure, and why?

■ **Answers**

1. *Describe the head shape and the CT scan. What is the diagnosis?*
   - The photograph, plain CT, and three-dimensional reconstructed CT scans show an elongated boatlike skull with a closed sagittal suture (**Fig. 68.1**).
   - Also seen is frontal and occipital bossing.
   - The diagnosis is scaphocephaly.

2. *What is scaphocephaly?*
   - Scaphocephaly can be described as a boat-shaped head, caused by synostosis of the sagittal suture, leading to a long and thin skull.[1]
   - There is bifrontal and occipital symmetric compensatory bossing.
   - There is usually a midline ridge, and there may be a saddle deformity where the synostosis began.
   - It may be evident at birth and progresses to become more pronounced with time.
   - It is the most common type of synostosis and is more common in males than females.

3. *How common is scaphocephaly?*
   - Epidemiology of scaphocephaly is described below.
     - Incidence is 2–10 per 10,000 live births.[2]
     - It comprises 55–64% of synostosis surgical cases (most common type).
     - 70–85% of patients are male.[1]
     - 6–10% of cases are familial.
     - It may follow an autosomal dominant inheritance pattern.[2]
     - There is 38% penetrance.[2]

4. *What is the prognosis of scaphocephaly?*
   - This deformity, like other forms of craniosynostosis, usually progresses with time and will have an important impact on the growing child's social and psychological status.[3]
   - These children usually would develop normally from a neurologic standpoint.
   - There is a slight risk of increased intracranial pressure (ICP).[3]

5. *What is the risk of developing hydrocephalus in patients diagnosed with craniosynostosis? What is the risk for this patient?*
   - Renier et al. in 1982 measured ICP using epidural sensor in 92 patients for 12–24 hours.[4] He found the following results as they relate to ICP.
     - In one suture synostosis, 62% were normal, 24% were borderline and 14% were high.
     - In several sutures synostosis, 19% were normal, 34% were borderline and 47% were high.
   - The incidence of hydrocephalus in sagittal craniosynostosis is remarkably rare (~0.3%), except in patients with prematurity or those who have been shunted.[5]
   - On the other hand, in syndromic craniosynostosis (Crouzon syndrome, Pfeiffer syndrome, Apert syndrome, etc.), the incidence of hydrocephalus may range from 20 to 40%.[5-7] The former two are more

likely to be associated with shunt dependent hydrocephalus than the latter.[7]

6. *What are some treatment options and their possible related morbidities?*
   - Ideally, surgical repair should be done at 2–3 months of age. When done before 3 months of age, the following options are available:
   - Midline strip craniectomy[8]
     - A 4–8 cm wide craniectomy is performed, from the coronal to just posterior to the lambdoid sutures.
     - Bilateral barrel stave osteotomies are then done (**Fig. 68.2**).
     - Blood transfusion is common.
     - There is up to a 10% chance of having a residual bone defects.
     - Good cosmetic results can be obtained (**Fig. 68.3**).
   - Pi procedure[9,10]
     - This procedure immediately provides anteroposterior shortening of the skull.
     - It may also give a better cosmetic result.
   - Endoscopic strip with molding helmet therapy
     - This method significantly lowers the rate of transfusion.[11]
   - In cases where treatment is contemplated late (after 6 months of age), the following options are available.
     - Variations of the Pi procedure[9]
     - Total cranial vault reconstruction[12]

7. *What is the accepted hypothesis for the pathogenesis of deformities caused by craniosynostosis?*
   - An older hypothesis described by Virchow (in 1851) states, "Craniosynostosis is caused by a lack of growth perpendicular to the fused suture and compensatory growth parallel to the suture in the calvarial vault."[13]
   - The currently accepted hypothesis devised by Delashaw et al. states, "The calvarial bones directly adjacent to a fused suture act as a single bone plate with decreased growth potential."[13]
   - Asymmetrical bone deposition occurs at the sutures along the perimeter of the bone plate with increased bone deposition at the outer margin.[13]
   - Nonperimeter sutures in line with the fused suture deposit bone symmetrically at their sutural edges.[13]
   - Perimeter sutures adjacent to the fused suture compensate to a greater degree than other distant sutures.[13]

8. *What is more clinically important, timing of head and brain growth or timing of normal sutural closure, and why?*
   - Timing of head and brain growth is more clinically significant than normal suture closure.[1]
     - The brain doubles in size by 6 months of age and doubles again by 2 years of age.
     - The skull is 35% of its adult size at birth, and 90% of the adult size is reached by age 7 years.

■ Answers (*continued*)

Fig. 68.2 Intraoperative photograph showing **(A,B)** incision location as well as **(C,D)** strip craniectomy with bilateral barrel stave osteotomies.

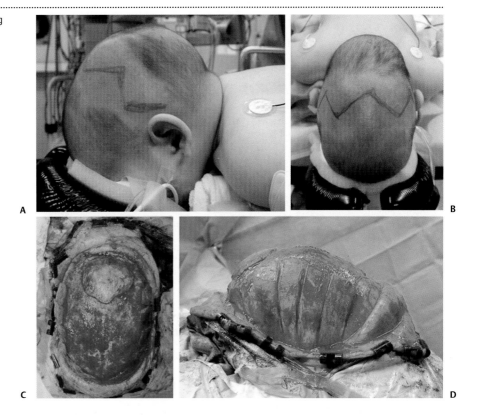

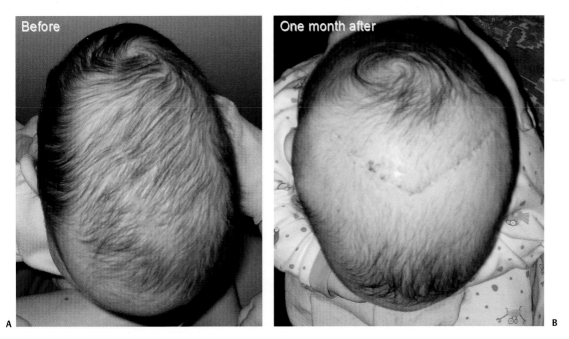

Fig. 68.3 **(A)** Preoperative and **(B)** postoperative photographs showing comparison and improvement in cosmetic result after strip craniectomy with barrel stave ostiotomies shown in **Fig. 68.2**.

■ References

1. Winston KR. Craniosynostosis. In: Rangachary SS, Wilkins RH, eds. Neurosurgery. 2nd ed. New York: McGraw-Hill; 1996:3673–3692
2. Lajeunie E, Le Merrer M, Bonaïti-Pellie C, Marchac D, Renier D. Genetic study of scaphocephaly. Am J Med Genet 1996;62(3):282–285
3. Arnaud E, Renier D, Marchac D, Brunet L, Pierre-Kahn A. Mental prognosis in scaphocephaly. Arch Pediatr 1996;3(1):16–21
4. Renier D, Sainte-Rose C, Marchac D, Hirsch JF. Intracranial pressure in craniostenosis. J Neurosurg 1982;57(3):370–377
5. Cinalli G, Sainte-Rose C, Kollar EM, et al. Hydrocephalus and craniosynostosis. J Neurosurg 1998;88(2):209–214
6. Golabi M, Edwards MS, Ousterhout DK. Craniosynostosis and hydrocephalus. Neurosurgery 1987;21(1):63–67
7. Collmann H, Sörensen N, Krauss J. Hydrocephalus in craniosynostosis: a review. Childs Nerv Syst 2005;21(10):902–912
8. Alvarez-Garijo JA, Cavadas PC, Vila MM, Alvarez-Llanas A. Sagittal synostosis: results of surgical treatment in 210 patients. Childs Nerv Syst 2001;17(1–2):64–68
9. Boulos PT, Lin KY, Jane JA Jr, Jane JA Sr. Correction of sagittal synostosis using a modified Pi method. Clin Plast Surg 2004;31(3):489–498, vii
10. Lin KY, Gampper TJ, Jane JA Sr. Correction of posterior sagittal craniosynostosis. J Craniofac Surg 1998;9(1):88–91
11. Jimenez DF, Barone CM. Early treatment of anterior calvarial craniosynostosis using endoscopic-assisted minimally invasive techniques. Childs Nerv Syst 2007;23(12):1411–1419
12. Greensmith AL, Holmes AD, Lo P, Maxiner W, Heggie AA, Meara JG. Complete correction of severe scaphocephaly: the Melbourne method of total vault remodeling. Plast Reconstr Surg 2008;121(4):1300–1310
13. Delashaw JB, Persing JA, Jane JA. Cranial deformation in craniosynostosis. A new explanation. Neurosurg Clin N Am 1991;2(3):611–620

Case 69 Spontaneous Cerebrospinal Fistula

Jeffrey Atkinson, José Luis Montes, and Abdulrahman J. Sabbagh

■ Clinical Presentation

- A 5-year-old boy presents with his third episode of bacterial meningitis.
- The child has a history of prematurity with a mild hemiparesis and mild developmental delay.
- There is no history of trauma.

- Physical examination reveals no skin defects or cutaneous markers.
- On detailed questioning, the child does recall that his nose is frequently "runny," and with prolonged forward positioning small amounts of clear fluid can be found dripping from the nose.

■ Questions

1. What are the potential causes of spontaneous cerebrospinal fluid (CSF) fistula?
2. Where are the potential sites of CSF leak?
3. What other clinical syndromes might result from CSF fistula?
4. What would be the diagnostic tests indicated in this patient?

The patient went on to have magnetic resonance imaging (MRI) and computed tomography (CT) scans following

intrathecal infusion of metrizamide that are seen in **Fig. 69.1** and **Fig. 69.2**. Ear, nose, and throat (ENT) service demonstrated a mass in the upper nasopharynx using fiberoptic endoscopy of the nasal cavity.

5. Describe the findings on the scans.
6. Describe at least two surgical approaches for repair of the above lesion.

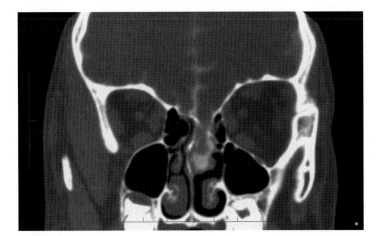

Fig. 69.1 Computed tomography coronal scan through the anterior fossa and ethmoids, with infusion of metrizamide intrathecal contrast.

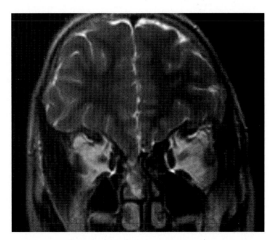

Fig. 69.2 T2-weighted coronal magnetic resonance image through the anterior cranial fossa.

Answers

1. *What are the potential causes of spontaneous CSF fistula?*
   - Spontaneous CSF fistulas may occur remotely following skull-base head trauma in any area of persistent outpouching, or dural defect through a fracture site.
   - They may occur in the spine as part of a remote trauma or pseudomeningocele or a spontaneous dural sleeve rupture.
   - Congenital arachnoid cysts, spinal Tarlov or arachnoid cysts, or congenital encephaloceles may also chronically or acutely leak CSF.
   - CSF leaks have also been reported due to congenital defects in the middle ear.[1]
2. *Where are the potential sites of CSF leak?*
   - CSF leak may occur in any area with one of the above pathologies, but obviously occult leaks into the nasal cavity or from the spine into the epidural or lumbar fascial compartments may occur and may be difficult to detect.
3. *What other clinical syndromes might result from CSF fistula?*
   - CSF fistula might result in CSF infection as in this case. Any chronic communication between the environment and meningeal space may produce acute, recurrent or chronic meningitis or other central nervous system (CNS) infections.
   - Low-pressure headache may also be attributable to a chronic CSF leak.[2]
   - Finally, superficial hemosiderosis has been reported following chronic CSF fistula into a traumatic pseudomeningocele with neovascularization and repeated hemorrhage. This could obviously present with mental deterioration, hearing, balance loss, and other cranial nerve deficits.[3,4]
4. *What would be the diagnostic tests indicated in this patient?*
   - In a patient where CSF fistula is suspected, an MRI scan of the complete neuraxis would be imperative. In some instances this may not be diagnostic.[2]
   - A CT scan can be helpful to demonstrate bone defects. Cisternal infusion of contrast media followed by a thin-cut CT, might be able to demonstrate extra CNS flow of fluid.[2]
   - In rare instances, a nuclear medicine study with lumbar cisternal infusion of radionucleotide tracer may also be used to demonstrate a small or slow communication, though with less anatomic detail.[1]
5. *Describe the findings on the scans.*
   - The coronal T2-weighted MRI scan and the coronal reconstruction of the postcisternal infusion of contrast CT scan both show a defect in the ethmoidal bone of the frontal cranial fossa with herniation of tissue and CSF through the defect into the nasal cavity.
6. *Describe at least two surgical approaches for repair of the above lesion.*
   - There are essentially two surgical approaches to this lesion.
     - A bifrontal craniotomy with repair of the defect from above using bone, muscle graft, and a vascularized pericranial flap would be possible. This might be possible entirely with an extradural approach, but an intradural inlay graft might protect better against CSF leak.[1,2]
     - Alternatively, there is significant experience in some centers with an entirely endoscopic intranasal approach to the repair of this lesion with again vascularized mucosal flap and an inlay graft if possible.[5]

References

1. Dagi TF. Management of cerebrospinal fluid leaks. In: Roberts DW, Schmidek HH, eds. Operative Neurosurgical Techniques. 5th ed. Philadelphia: Saunders/Elsevier; 2005: 130–145
2. Schievink WI. Spontaneous spinal cerebrospinal fluid leaks and intracranial hypotension. JAMA 2006;295(19):2286–2296
3. Kumar N. Superficial siderosis: associations and therapeutic implications. Arch Neurol 2007;64(4):491–496
4. Kole MK, Steven D, Kirk A, Lownie SP. Superficial siderosis of the central nervous system from a bleeding pseudomeningocele. Case illustration. J Neurosurg 2004;100(4):718
5. Marton E, Billeci D, Schiesari E, Longatti P. Transnasal endoscopic repair of cerebrospinal fluid fistulas and encephaloceles: surgical indications and complications. Minim Invasive Neurosurg 2005;48(3):175–181

Case 70   Cerebral Palsy and Selective Dorsal Rhizotomies

Jean-Pierre Farmer and Abdulrahman J. Sabbagh

■ Clinical Presentation

• A 3-year-old child is referred to you for surgical treatment of refractory spasticity.

• On examination, he is able to crawl in a reciprocal fashion predominantly and has started to use a walker.

• An earlier computed tomography (CT) scan of the head is available (**Fig. 70.1**).

Fig. 70.1   Computed tomography scan of the head showing presence of periventricular leukomalacia without hydrocephalus.

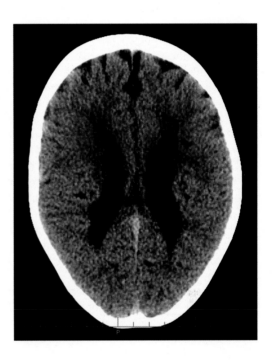

■ Questions

1. What are your surgical treatment options?
2. What key features would you like to elicit in the history to determine that this young boy is a candidate for selective dorsal rhizotomy?
3. What physical features would make you think that he is a candidate for this procedure?
4. What features, if present in the history or physical examination, would make you rule against offering rhizotomies?
5. What factors would favor offering rhizotomies in your interpretation of the imaging?
6. What other investigations would you like to obtain on this child prior to planning rhizotomies?
7. What can you tell the family with respect to the potential outcome for the child with selective dorsal rhizotomies as opposed to continuing with physiotherapy and occupational therapy alone?
8. If there is involvement in the upper extremities, how would this influence your decision in terms of offering rhizotomies versus a baclofen pump?
9. What is the relative cost of the two treatment procedures over a lifetime?
10. What are the risks and long-term sequelae following selective dorsal rhizotomies?
11. What would you recommend your anesthetist to use intraoperatively during stimulation?
12. What criteria would you use to determine your lesioning pattern?
13. What do you do to reduce the risk of sphincteric difficulties in these patients?

◾ Questions (*continued*)

14. How do you control pain and spasticity perioperatively?
15. What adjuvant treatment will the child benefit from in the 2 months following the procedure?
16. What is the expected long-term outcome with respect to lower extremity function, activities of daily living, and upper extremity fine motor control following rhizotomies?
17. Is the preoperative status of the patient a strong determinant with respect to the long-term outcome of the child?

◾ Answers

1. *What are your surgical treatment options?*
   - Selective dorsal rhizotomy[1]
   - Baclofen pump placement[2,3]
2. *What key features would you like to elicit in the history to determine that this young boy is a candidate for selective dorsal rhizotomy?*
   - A history of prematurity, low birth weight, late acquisition of motor milestones, but progress being made.[1]
   - Other key points: The absence of previous surgical interventions, the absence of movement disorders other than spasticity, the absence of a family history involving neurologic diseases, and a good collaboration with therapists are all positive features.
3. *What physical features would make you think that he is a candidate for this procedure?*
   - Candidates should show evolving locomotor skills with adequate balance in the sitting position and good protective responses in the short leg sitting position.
   - Patient should show no associated movement disorder such as chorea or choreoathetosis and should show velocity-dependent increased tone and hyperreflexia with clonus, as well as limited range of motion.[1]
   - There should be adequate underlying strength with the squat-to-stand testing.
   - Patient should show at least quadruped falling or bunny hopping.
   - If he or she shows upright locomotor function, this should be even better.
4. *What features, if present in the history or physical examination, would make you rule against offering rhizotomies?*
   - Absolute contraindications include the presence of multiple orthopedic releasing procedures for short tendons, choreoathetosis, double hemiplegia, the inability to collaborate with therapists, associated significant cognitive difficulties, and dislocated hip.[4]
   - Relative contraindications include atypical perinatal history with birth at term, but with associated confounding factors such as meningitis, trauma in the neonatal period, or other prenatal factors.[4]
   - Hydrocephalus, if well dealt with, is not an absolute contraindication.
   - Other absolute contraindications would be severe motor restrictions or the presence of severe scoliosis preoperatively.
5. *What factors would favor offering rhizotomies in your interpretation of the imaging?*
   - Imaging of the brain with a CT scan or preferably magnetic resonance imaging (MRI) should show presence of periventricular leukomalacia (**Fig. 70.1**) without hydrocephalus.
   - Presence of basal ganglia damage would be a relative contraindication.[1]
   - The spine x-rays should not show significant scoliosis.
   - The hip x-ray should show at least 50% or better femoral head coverage.
6. *What other investigations would you like to obtain on this child prior to planning rhizotomies?*
   - Other investigations would include the presence of gross motor measure scores, alignment scores, occupational therapy grading, and urodynamic testing.[5]
7. *What can you tell the family with respect to the potential outcome for the child with selective dorsal rhizotomies as opposed to continuing with physiotherapy and occupational therapy alone?*
   - The family has to be aware that randomized control trials have revealed an advantage of doing rhizotomy over simply continuing with physiotherapy and occupational therapy alone.
   - Abundant literature attests that there are persistent significant gains in gross motor function measure (GMFM), in urodynamic profile, and the upper extremity, as well as activities of daily living gains, which are durable and substantial.[1]
8. *If there is involvement in the upper extremities, how would this influence your decision in terms of offering rhizotomies versus a baclofen pump?*
   - This decision remains controversial as both intrathecal baclofen pumps and rhizotomies have been used to treat upper extremity spasticity successfully.[1-3]

■ Answers (continued)

- Because of the fact that rhizotomies have been shown to improve upper extremity function significantly, if a candidate meets the criteria for rhizotomies this may be regarded by some as the procedure of choice over baclofen pump placement.[1]
- Baclofen pump can provide effective long-term treatment of spasticity of cerebral origin, and its effects do not appear to diminish with time.[2]
- Intrathecal baclofen has been shown to reduce spasticity in the upper and lower extremities, and improve upper extremity function and activities of daily living.[3]
- However, baclofen pumps require frequent refills, change of battery packs, and repositioning of the catheters. They can occasionally produce drug toxicity, and the overall cost may be quite significant.[2,3]

9. *What is the relative cost of the two treatment procedures over a lifetime?*
   - The relative cost of the two procedures is about 4:1 (baclofen pump compared with rhizotomies).
   - Baclofen pumps remain a significantly more expensive way to treat spasticity.[1]

10. *What are the risks and long-term sequelae following selective dorsal rhizotomies?*
    - Long-term sequelae of selective dorsal rhizotomies are few if the procedure is done with stimulation and in a moderate lesioning fashion.
    - Reported problems include a higher incidence of scoliosis, which has to be compared with the natural history of the disease.[6]
    - In our experience, the rate of scoliosis is relatively high; however, the scoliosis curves are almost exclusively between 10 and 15 degrees, which present a debatably low clinical significance.[6]
    - Hyperlordosis and spinal stenosis have also been reported, although these are very rare. The clinical importance is again similar to the scoliosis cases, where cases of significance are the few ones who have undergone laminotomy or laminoplasty procedure.[6]
    - Bladder dysfunction is also a rare event.[5]

11. *What would you recommend your anesthetist to use intraoperatively during stimulation?*
    - During surgery, if done with stimulation, the anesthetist should use a combination of sufentanil or remifentanil at a low dose and propofol with nitrous oxide.
    - The neuromuscular junction transmission and the spinal cord transmission should not be altered by the anesthetic regimen during stimulation.[4]

12. *What criteria would you use to determine your lesioning pattern?*
    - The criterion most frequently used is that of spread to contralateral or upper extremity segments from stimulation of lumbosacral dorsal roots.

- Afterdischarges and amplitude of stimulus response also play a role if spread is demonstrated to contralateral or upper extremity segments.[7]

13. *What do you do to reduce the risk of sphincteric difficulties in these patients?*
    - Care has to be taken to preserve S3 and S4 roots and to limit the lesioning at S2.
    - We tend to limit lesioning to 50% of both dorsal S2 roots combined, preserving at least one third of S2 dorsal rootlets on each side.
    - With this pattern we have not identified long-term problems with bladder dysfunction and have even documented improvements in urodynamic profile.[1]

14. *How do you control pain and spasticity perioperatively?*
    - Postoperative pain is usually related to the length and depth of the incision, but also to some element of deafferentation as a result of the sectioning of the nerves.
    - An epidural catheter placed for the delivery of epidural morphine at T9–T10 that is above the surgical site is very helpful.[1]
    - Additionally, oral diazepam can be beneficial but should be given at half of the recommended dose to avoid depressant effects on respiratory drive.

15. *What adjuvant treatment will the child benefit from in the 2 months following the procedure?*
    - Most centers will recommend enhanced physiotherapy and occupational therapy with the use of a pool therapy, arts and crafts and the use of an exercise program to stretch resistant contractures, strengthen musculature, and date training.[1]

16. *What is the expected long-term outcome with respect to lower extremity function, activities of daily living, and upper extremity fine motor control following rhizotomies?*
    - Lower extremity function using objective measurement such as the GMFM score and alignment scores shows durable improvements, as do activities of daily living and upper extremity fine motor control following rhizotomies.[4,8,9]
    - These improvements have been found to last up to 5 years postoperatively and still improving at that point.[8]

17. *Is the preoperative status of the patient a strong determinant with respect to the long-term outcome of the child?*
    - Yes, the better the patient is preoperatively, the more likely the outcome will be favorable.
    - In more favorable cases, gains will bring the patient closer to the normal age-matched controls with respect to motor and upper extremity function.[1]

■ References

1. Farmer JP, Sabbagh AJ. Selective dorsal rhizotomies in the treatment of spasticity related to cerebral palsy. Childs Nerv Syst 2007;23(9):991–1002

2. Albright AL, Gilmartin R, Swift D, Krach LE, Ivanhoe CB, McLaughlin JF. Long-term intrathecal baclofen therapy for severe spasticity of cerebral origin. J Neurosurg 2003;98(2):291–295

3. Albright AL. Baclofen in the treatment of cerebral palsy. J Child Neurol 1996;11(2):77–83

4. Mittal S, Farmer JP, Al-Atassi B, et al. Functional performance following selective posterior rhizotomy: long-term results determined using a validated evaluative measure. J Neurosurg 2002;97(3):510–518

5. Houle AM, Vernet O, Jednak R, Pippi Salle JL, Farmer JP. Bladder function before and after selective dorsal rhizotomy in children with cerebral palsy. J Urol 1998;160(3 Pt 2):1088–1091

6. Golan JD, Hall JA, O'Gorman G, et al. Spinal deformities following selective dorsal rhizotomy. J Neurosurg 2007;106(6, Suppl):441–449

7. Mittal S, Farmer JP, Poulin C, Silver K. Reliability of intraoperative electrophysiological monitoring in selective posterior rhizotomy. J Neurosurg 2001;95(1):67–75

8. Mittal S, Farmer JP, Al-Atassi B, et al. Long-term functional outcome after selective posterior rhizotomy. J Neurosurg 2002;97(2):315–325

9. Mittal S, Farmer JP, Al-Atassi B, et al. Impact of selective posterior rhizotomy on fine motor skills. Long-term results using a validated evaluative measure. Pediatr Neurosurg 2002;36(3):133–141

Case 71   Neural Tube Defect

Abdulrahman J. Sabbagh, Abdulrahman Yaqub Alturki, José Luis Montes, Jean-Pierre Farmer, and Jeffrey Atkinson

■ Clinical Presentation

• A 32-year-old woman is referred to you from an obstetrician. She is 22 weeks pregnant, gravida 2 para 1 (G2P1) but otherwise healthy with a normal first daughter.
• A uterine ultrasound was done followed by a fetal magnetic resonance imaging (MRI) scan (**Fig. 71.1**).

• She has a cesarean section and a lesion is found in the midline on her infant's back.
• An MRI of the infant is done in the first few hours of its life (**Fig. 71.2**).

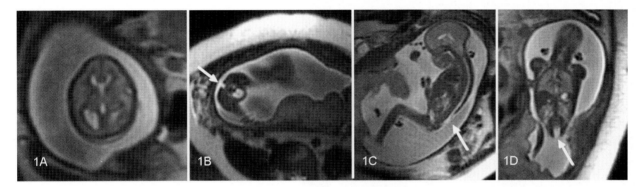

Fig. 71.1   Prenatal magnetic resonance imaging scans with **(A)** T2-weighted axial and **(B)** sagittal sections of the brain in utero. **(C)** T2-weighted sagittal and **(D)** coronal sections of the spine are also shown.

■ Questions

1. What is the diagnosis? Describe the MRI shown in **Fig. 71.1**.
2. Give five features on this MRI of the brain and spinal cord that are characteristic of this diagnosis. Why is there pneumocephalus and air in the spinal canal?
3. Describe methods of evaluation for this condition in the prenatal period.
4. What are the most common sites for neural tube defects (NTDs)?
5. How would you assess the level of the defect clinically?

6. What do you tell the parents regarding survival (with or without treatment), intelligence, ambulation, and urinary continence? What are the causes of early and late mortality?
7. Highlight a management plan.
8. When should you operate on this patient? What are the goals and principles of the surgery?
9. Describe surgical options for repair of such large defects in the skin.
10. What are the risk factors associated with NTDs?
11. How can NTDs be prevented?

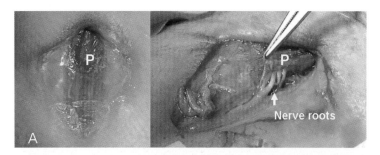

Fig. 71.2 **(A)** Preoperative and intraoperative photograph of the skin defect depicting neural placode (P) and nerve roots. **(B)** Magnetic resonance imaging scans obtained shortly after birth with sagittal T2-weighted image of the spine and T1-weighted image of the brain.

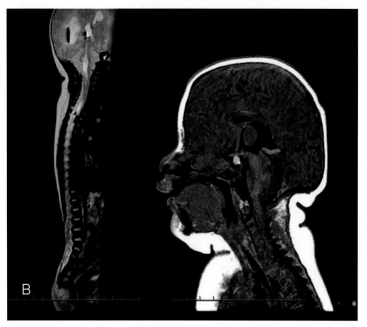

■ Answers

1. *What is the diagnosis? Describe the MRI shown in* **Fig. 71.1**.
   - The diagnosis is of Chiari II malformation with an open myelomeningocele (MMC).
   - The prenatal MRI shows a T2-weighted axial section of the brain in utero depicting asymmetrical ventriculomegaly. The axial section at the lumbar level shows an open MMC (arrow). Sagittal and coronal sections show evidence of the MMC and Chiari II.

2. *Give five features on this MRI of the brain and spinal cord that are characteristic of this diagnosis. Why is there pneumocephalus and air in the spinal canal?*
   - Characteristic findings include the following[1]:
     - Medullary kinking
     - Tectal beaking
     - Enlarged Massa intermedia
     - Elongation and/or cervicalization of the medulla
     - Low attachment of tentorium
     - Hydrocephalus
     - Syringomyelia in the area of the cervicomedullary junction
     - Dysgenesis of the corpus callosum
   - Pneumocephalus and air in the spinal canal indicate open MMC.

3. *Describe methods of evaluation for this condition in the prenatal period.*
   - Methods of evaluation include
     - Mother serum α-fetoprotein (AFP)
     - Prenatal ultrasound (high NTDs)
     - If both are positive then an amniocentesis may be performed for amniotic AFP and acetylcholinesterase levels (the diagnostic accuracy for NTD rises to more than 97%).[2]
     - Fetal MRI is an option when available, as it gives accurate information regarding associated anomalies and may help in prognostication.

4. *What are the most common sites for neural tube defects (NTDs)?*
   - Most common sites of occurrence include the lumbosacral area in 50% of cases, followed by the thoracolumbar area in 35% of cases[3]

5. *How would you assess the level of the defect clinically?*
   - The defect level is determined by assessing the lowest level of neurologic function (**Table 71.1**).

■ **Answers (*continued*)**

Table 71.1   Level of Neurologic Function and Associated Deficit

Paralysis below	Finding
T12	Complete paralysis of all muscles in the lower limbs
L1	Weak to moderate hip flexion, palpable contraction in sartorius
L2	Strong hip flexion & moderate hip adduction
L3	Normal hip adduction & almost normal knee extension
L4	Normal hip adduction, knee extension, & dorsiflexion/inversion of the foot, some hip abduction in flexion
L5	Normal adduction, flexion, & lateral rotation of the hip, normal knee extension, moderate flexion, normal foot dorsiflexion, hip extension absent; produces dorsiflexed foot & flexed thigh
S1	Normal hip flexion & abduction/adduction, moderate extension and lateral rotation; strong knee flexion & inversion/eversion of the foot, moderate plantar flexion of the foot; extension of all toes, but flexion only of terminal phalanx of the great toe; normal medial & lateral hip rotation; complete paralysis of foot intrinsic muscles (except abductor and flexor hallicis brevis); produces clawing of toes and flattening of the sole of the foot
S2	Difficult to detect abnormality clinically; with growth, this produces clawing of the toes due to weakness of intrinsic muscles of the sole of the foot (innervated by S3)

Source: Sharrard WJ. The segmental innervation of the lower limb muscles in man. Ann R Coll Surg Engl 1964;35:106–122.

6. *What do you tell the parents regarding survival (with or without treatment), intelligence, ambulation, and urinary continence? What are the causes of early and late mortality?*
   - Prognosis is described below.[5–7]
     - Survival
       - Without treatment, only 14–30% survive infancy.
       - With treatment, 85% survive.
     - Intelligence
       - 70–80% will have normal intelligence quotients.
       - Mental delays may be related to shunt malfunctions, primary microgyri, or absence of corpus callosum.
     - Ambulation
       - 50% are ambulatory.
       - Up to 80% can ambulate with bracing. However, 80% of these will decrease over time because of weight gain by the patients.
     - Urinary incontinence
       - 90–95% are incontinent but are able to stay dry with intermittent catheterizations.
     - Mortality
       - Early mortality is related to Chiari malformation complications such as aspiration and respiratory arrest
       - Late mortality may be related to shunt complications, urosepsis, as well as progressive respiratory compromise due to kyphoscoliosis.

7. *Highlight a management plan.*
   - A management plan is described below.
     - Items related to Chiari II malformation[1]
       - Measure head circumference to follow the rate of growth due to risk of hydrocephalus.
       - Obtain a head ultrasound within 24 hours of birth.
       - Check for inspiratory stridor and apneic episodes.
     - Items related to the defect[8]
       - Measure the size of the defect.
       - If the lesion is ruptured, start antibiotics.
       - Cover the lesion with a piece of sterile Telfa (Tyco Healthcare, Mansfield, MA)
       - Keep the patient in Trendelenburg position (to keep pressure off lesion).
       - Plan early surgical closure.
     - General assessment and management
       - Neonatologist assessment for other abnormalities
       - Urologic consultation and regular urinary catheterization
       - Orthopedic consultation for spine, hip, and knee deformities

8. *When should you operate on this patient? What are the goals and principles of the surgery?*
   - Timing of surgery should be within 48–72 hours.[6,9]
   - The goals of surgical repair include reconstruction of the neural tube and its coverings, avoidance of meningitis, and protection of the remaining functional tissue in the neural placode.

■ Answers (*continued*)

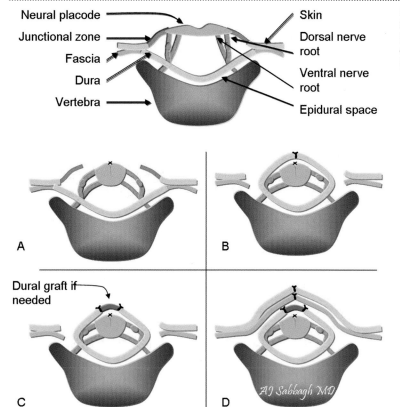

Fig. 71.3 Artist's rendering of spinal dysraphism closure. See text for detailed description. Depicted steps include **(A)** reconstruction of the neural tube, **(B)** reconstruction of the thecal sac, **(C)** dural patching of a large defect and **(D)** midline fascia and skin closure in layers.

- The principles of the surgery include
  - Reconstruction of the neural tube (**Fig. 71.3A**).
    - The placode is dissected from the surrounding tissue by incising the junctional zone.
    - All dermal remnants are resected, and the neural tube is reconstituted by closing the pia with a 7–0 monofilament suture.
  - Reconstruction of the thecal sac (**Fig. 71.3B**)
    - The dura is dissected free from its junctions with the fascia and skin.
    - The goal is a watertight closure without causing constriction of the closed neural placode.
  - Often the defect is large enough to require a dural patch (**Fig. 71.3C**)
    - Tissue sealant is preferably used at the end of dural closure.
  - Midline fascia and skin closure in layers (**Fig. 71.3D**)

9. *Describe surgical options for repair of such large defects in the skin.*
   - Several options are available and usually best done by a plastic surgeon. They include
     - Circumferential skin release dissection (used in small- to medium-sized defects)
     - Rameris procedure: medial advancement of bilateral bipedicled musculocutaneous flap based on the latissimus dorsi and maximus gluteus without any relaxing incisions or skin grafting[10]
     - Flaps used include latissimus dorsi myocutaneous flap for thoracolumbar defects and gluteus maximus myocutaneous flap for lower defects.[11]
     - The junctional zone or the cyst wall membrane can be used as a graft.
     - Alternatively, artificial dermis can be used.[12]

10. *What are the risk factors associated with NTDs?*
    - Risk factors include the following (the associated percentage risk of having a child with NTD is in brackets)[2]:

■ Answers (*continued*)

- Partner diagnosed with NTDs (2–3% risk of having a child with NTD)
- Previous pregnancy with NTDs (2–3%)
- Epileptic on carbamazepine or valproic acid (1%)
- Diabetes mellitus type I (1%)
- Close relative with NTDs (0.3–1%)
- Pregnancy with obesity and weight over 110 kg (0.2%)
- Other risk factors include exposure to radiation, pesticides, anesthetic agents, hot tubs, smoking, and occupational hazards such as nursing or part of operating room staff (exposure to anesthetic agents).

11. *How can NTDs be prevented?*
- Prevention can be achieved by supplementing expecting mothers with folic acid.
  - Expecting mothers with no known risk factors should take folic acid at the dose of 0.4 mg/day.
  - Those with a higher risk factor should take folic acid at 4 mg/day (for the duration of one month before pregnancy through the first trimester).[13]

■ References

1. Oakes WJ. Chiari malformations, hydromyelia, syringomyelia. In: Rengashary SS, Wilkins RH, eds. Neurosurgery. 2nd ed. New York: McGraw-Hill; 1996:3593–3616
2. Mclone DG. Pediatric Neurosurgery. Philadelphia: Saunders Elsevier; 2001
3. Zambelli H, Carelli E, Honorato D, et al. Assessment of neurosurgical outcome in children prenatally diagnosed with myelomeningocele and development of a protocol for fetal surgery to prevent hydrocephalus. Childs Nerv Syst 2007;23(4):421–425
4. Sharrad WJ. The segmental innervation of the lower limb muscles in man. Ann R Coll Surg Engl 1964;35:106–122
5. Soare PL, Raimondi AJ. Intellectual and perceptual-motor characteristics of treated myelomeningocele children. Am J Dis Child 1977;131(2):199–204
6. McLone DG, Dias L, Kaplan WE, Sommers MW. Concepts in the management of spina bifida. In: Humphreys RP, ed. Concepts in Pediatric Neurosurgery. Basel: Karger; 1985:97–106
7. McLone DG. Care of the neonate with a myelomeningocele. Neurosurg Clin N Am 1998;9(1):111–120

8. Humphreys RP. Spinal dysraphism. In: Rengashary SS, Wilkins RH, eds. Neurosurgery. 2nd ed. New York: McGraw-Hill;1996:3453–3463
9. Rekate HL. Comprehensive Management of Spina Bifida. Boca Raton: CRC Press; 1990
10. Bagłaj M, Ladogórska J, Rysiakiewicz K. Closure of large myelomeningocoele with Ramirez technique. Childs Nerv Syst 2006;22(12):1625–1629
11. El-khatib HA. Large thoracolumbar meningomyelocele defects: incidence and clinical experiences with different modalities of latissimus dorsi musculocutaneus flap. Br J Plast Surg 2004;57(5):411–417
12. Nakazawa H, Kikuchi Y, Honda T, Isago T, Nozaki M. Successful management of a small infant born with a large meningomyelocele using a temporary artificial dermis. Scand J Plast Reconstr Surg Hand Surg 2005;39(1):53–56
13. Committee on Genetics. Folic acid for the prevention of neural tube defects. American Academy of Pediatrics. Pediatrics 1999;104(2 Pt 1):325–327

Case 72   Tic Douloureux

Burak Sade and Joung H. Lee

■ Clinical Presentation

- An 83-year-old right-handed man presents with a 2-year history of neuralgia-like pain on the right side of his face involving the ophthalmic (V1) and maxillary (V2) divisions of the trigeminal nerve.
- He has been taking carbamazepine and topiramate, which provided minimal relief, and says he no longer wishes to use these medications.
- His neurologic evaluation is within normal limits.
- Magnetic resonance imaging (MRI) of the brain is shown in **Fig. 72.1**.

- The patient underwent a microvascular decompression (MVD) procedure. At the time of surgery, the trigeminal nerve was found to be in severe compression by a redundant vertebrobasilar complex ventrally and inferiorly and by the anterior inferior cerebellar artery superiorly. Decompression was achieved using small pieces of Teflon paddies.
- He experienced immediate and complete recovery of his pain following surgery.

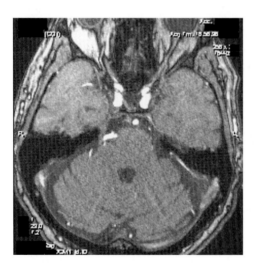

Fig. 72.1   Magnetic resonance imaging scan of the brain. Three-dimensional axial image of the Circle of Willis demonstrating a prominent vascular loop ventral to the trigeminal nerve root entry zone on the right side.

■ Questions

1. What are the different types of facial pain syndromes?
2. What are the characteristics of the pain in trigeminal neuralgia?
3. What are the main nuclei of the trigeminal nerve, and what functions do they serve?
4. What is the initial management of a patient with trigeminal neuralgia?
5. What are the surgical indications?
6. What are the other treatment options?
7. Which vessel is the most common culprit of the compression?
8. What are the efficacies of MVD and other treatment options in trigeminal neuralgia?

■ Answers

1. *What are the different types of facial pain syndromes?*
   - According to the classification proposed by Burchiel[1]:
     - Trigeminal neuralgia (type 1– predominant episodic and type 2 – predominant constant) or symptomatic trigeminal neuralgia (in multiple sclerosis)
     - Trigeminal neuropathic pain
     - Trigeminal deafferentation pain
     - Postherpetic neuralgia
     - Atypical facial pain
2. *What are the characteristics of the pain in trigeminal neuralgia?*
   - Characteristics of pain in trigeminal neuralgia[1]:
     - Sharp, shooting, electric shocklike pain
     - Momentary or lasting only a few seconds
     - Very intense
     - Common provoking factors include touching, washing the face, teeth brushing, make-up, chewing, talking, eating, a cold breeze.
     - May involve one or more branches of the trigeminal nerve
3. *What are the main nuclei of the trigeminal nerve, and what functions do they serve?*
   - The principal sensory or main nucleus: Located in the upper pons, it conveys tactile and pressure senses from the face.
   - The mesencephalic nucleus: Located near the central gray matter of the upper 4th ventricle, it conveys pressure and kinesthetic senses from the teeth, hard palate, and jaw.
   - The spinal trigeminal tract and nucleus: Extends from the upper cervical spine to the midpons, it is divided into three parts (pars caudalis, pars interpolaris, and pars oralis), which convey sensation of pain and temperature from different parts of the face (**Fig. 72.2**).
   - The motor nucleus relays fibers to the muscles of mastication and plays part in the jaw jerk reflex.
   - The ventral and dorsal trigeminothalamic tracts relay sensory information to the ventroposterior medial nucleus of the thalamus.[2]

4. *What is the initial management of a patient with trigeminal neuralgia?*
   - Initial management in trigeminal neuralgia is medical.
   - Medications that are most commonly used include carbamazepine, gabapentin, lamotrigine, and Trileptal (Novartis, East Hanover, NJ).
   - Among these, carbamazepine is the most widely used.
   - In addition, antidepressants or narcotic analgesics and steroids during severe pain episodes may provide temporary relief.
5. *What are the surgical indications?*
   - Indication for surgical treatment include failure of medical therapy, intolerance to the medications, and patients who do not like to take medications for a long time.
6. *What are the other treatment options?*
   - Other treatment options[3-5]:
     - MVD
     - Percutaneous techniques: glycerol rhizotomy (GR), balloon compression (BC), radiofrequency rhizotomy (RF)
     - Gamma knife radiosurgery (GKRS)
7. *Which vessel is the most common culprit of the compression?*
   - Superior cerebellar artery (75%)[3]
8. *What are the efficacies of MVD and other treatment options in trigeminal neuralgia?*
   - In a review by Taha and Tew,[4] the initial pain relief was 98% in MVD and RF, 93% in BC, and 91% in GR.
   - Ten years after surgery, excellent results were seen in 70% of cases who underwent MVD.[3]
   - Pain recurrence was seen in 15% of MVD, 21% in BC, 23% in RF, and 54% in GR.[4]
   - Postoperative facial numbness and corneal anesthesia incidences were 2% and none in MVD, 60% and 4% in GR, 72% and 2% in BC, 98% and 7% in RF, respectively.[4]
   - Therefore, when V1 or multiple divisions including V1 are involved, MVD is the preferred option to minimize the risk of corneal anesthesia.
   - GKRS has been reported to be effective in 50–80% of the patients, with ~25% pain recurrence.[5]
     - The risk of facial numbness and dysesthesias increase with higher radiation dose in this technique.

Fig. 72.2 Artist's rendering of the nuclei of the trigeminal nerve, their locations in the brainstem, their functions, and associated tracts. g, ganglion; n, nucleus; tr, tract.

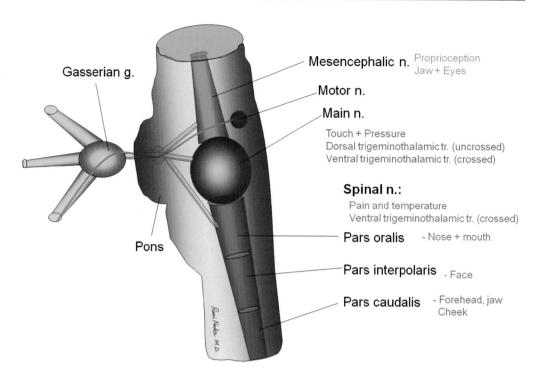

Gasserian g.

Mesencephalic n. Proprioception Jaw + Eyes

Motor n.

Main n.

Touch + Pressure
Dorsal trigeminothalamic tr. (uncrossed)
Ventral trigeminothalamic tr. (crossed)

Spinal n.:

Pain and temperature
Ventral trigeminothalamic tr. (crossed)

Pons

Pars oralis   - Nose + mouth

Pars interpolaris - Face

Pars caudalis - Forehead, jaw
Cheek

■ References

1. Burchiel KJ. A new classification for facial pain. Neurosurgery 2003;53(5):1164–1167
2. Parent A. Carpenter's Human Neuroanatomy. Baltimore: Williams & Wilkins; 1996
3. Barker FG, Jannetta PJ, Bissonette DJ, Larkins MV, Jho HD. The long-term outcome of microvascular decompression for trigeminal neuralgia. N Engl J Med 1996;334(17):1077–1083
4. Taha JM, Tew JM Jr. Comparison of surgical treatments for trigeminal neuralgia: reevaluation of radiofrequency rhizotomy. Neurosurgery 1996;38(5):865–871
5. Kanner AA, Neyman G, Suh JH, Weinhous MS, Lee SY, Barnett GH. Gamma knife radiosurgery for trigeminal neuralgia: comparing the use of 4-mm versus concentric 8-mm collimators. Stereotact Funct Neurosurg 2004;82(1):49–57

Case 73   Trigeminal Neuropathic Pain

Melanie Hood and Christopher J. Winfree

■ Clinical Presentation

- A 45-year-old woman who, 2 years previously, was in a motor vehicle accident and sustained facial injuries, including a right-sided facial laceration and an orbital fracture.
- Since the time of injury, she reports right-sided facial pain in a V1 and V2 distribution.
- The pain is constant, burning in nature, and grades 7–8/10 in severity.

- Given the persistence of pain, she was suspected of having trigeminal neuralgia. A microvascular decompression was performed at an outside institution, but this did not help.
- On physical examination, she has mildly decreased sensation in her right V1 and V2 distributions.

■ Questions

1. What is this patient's diagnosis?
2. What are her noninvasive treatment options?
3. What are her invasive treatment options?

The patient undergoes a variety of pharmacologic treatments, including nonsteroidal antiinflammatories, anticonvulsants, and antidepressants, none of which yielded acceptable pain relief. Multiple anesthetic and steroid injections along the supraorbital and infraorbital nerves likewise failed to help. Psychological evaluation reveals no psychological amplifiers of her pain syndrome, such as depression, unresolved conflicts, sleep disorders, etc. You are considering offering the patient a surgical therapy.

4. Describe the relative merits and drawbacks of each type of therapy.

■ Answers

1. *What is this patient's diagnosis?*
   - This patient has trigeminal neuropathic pain (TNP), a neuropathic pain syndrome that occurs following injury to one or more branches of the trigeminal nerve. This injury generally results in partial sensory loss within the trigeminal system.[1]
   - Although the pathophysiology of TNP is currently not well understood, deafferentation of central trigeminal pathways likely results in pathologically amplified sensory barrages that are perceived by the patient as painful.[2]
2. *What are her noninvasive treatment options?*
   - The anticonvulsant[3] and antidepressant[4] medications are the initial treatments of choice for neuropathic pain in general, although little data exist for their specific use in TNP.
   - Opiate medication, transcutaneous electrical nerve stimulation, acupuncture, and other complementary and alternative therapies may certainly be used as well, but prospective clinical data regarding their use in TNP are lacking.

3. *What are her invasive treatment options?*
   - If noninvasive measures are unhelpful, then local injections may be tried, but their efficacy in facial pain syndromes is unknown.
   - Peripheral neurectomy, in which the trigeminal branch within the painful distribution is destroyed, actually increases the trigeminal system injury, potentially exacerbating the deafferentation phenomenon and worsening the patient's pain.
   - Neurostimulation, in which electrodes are used to administer electrical impulses to the trigeminal pain pathways, may be utilized.[5]
4. *Describe the relative merits and drawbacks of each type of therapy.*
   - Although other forms of stimulation such as motor cortex stimulation could address this problem, trigeminal branch stimulation, a form of peripheral nerve stimulation, offers a less invasive and safer alternative.[6]

■ Answers (*continued*)

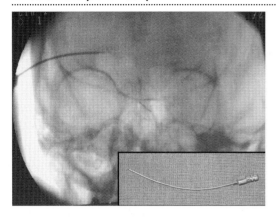

Fig. 73.1 Intraoperative anteroposterior fluoroscopic image showing the initial step used in the placement of a right-sided supraorbital electrode. First, a large gauge curved Tuohy needle is placed in the subcutaneous space just above the orbital rim. The inset shows the needle itself, which has been custom-bent by the senior author to follow the contour of the face and facilitate placement along the forehead.

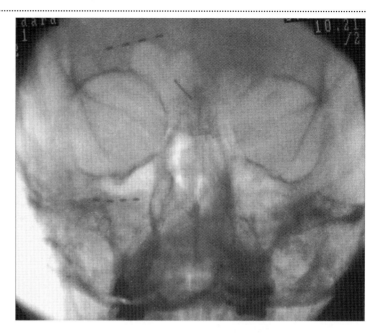

Fig. 73.2 Intraoperative anteroposterior fluoroscopic image showing final placement of right-sided supraorbital and infraorbital nerve electrodes. During a 1-week externalized trial, the patient experienced over 90% reduction in her levels of pain, and elected to undergo placement of a permanent electrode system. (From Stuart RM, Winfree CJ. Neurostimulation techniques for painful peripheral nerve disorders. Neurosurg Clin N Am 2009;20(1):111–120.)

- In this technique, percutaneous electrodes are placed in the subcutaneous space under local anesthetic; these electrodes are placed overlying either the supraorbital (V1) or infraorbital (V2) nerves depending on the particular pain distribution; stimulation paresthesias, and subsequent pain relief, occur in the respective trigeminal distribution(s) (**Fig. 73.1**).

- After a 1-week percutaneous trial, if sufficient pain relief occurs, the patient may undergo placement of a permanent electrode system (**Fig. 73.2**).

■ References

1. Burchiel KJ. Trigeminal neuropathic pain. Acta Neurochir Suppl (Wien) 1993;58:145–149
2. Eide PK, Rabben T. Trigeminal neuropathic pain: pathophysiological mechanisms examined by qualitative assessment of abnormal pain and sensory perception. Neurosurgery 1998;43:1103–1110
3. Wiffen P, Collins S, McQuay H, Carroll D, Jadad A, Moore A. Anticonvulsant drugs for acute and chronic pain. Cochrane Database Syst Rev 2005;3:CD001133
4. Saarto T, Wiffen PJ. Antidepressants for neuropathic pain. Cochrane Database Syst Rev 2005;3:CD005454
5. Osenbach R. Neurostimulation for the treatment of intractable facial pain. Pain Med 2006;7:S126–S136
6. Slavin KV, Wess C. Trigeminal branch stimulation for intractable neuropathic pain: technical note. Neuromodulation 2005;8:7–13

Case 74   Hemifacial Spasm and Microvascular Decompression

Bassem Sheikh

■ Clinical Presentation

- A 35-year-old man presents with a 10-year history of spasmodic twitching on the left side of his face.
- The twitching involves the left eyelid and causes intermittent spasmodic closure of the eye.

- The attacks of hemifacial spasm (HFS) are exacerbated by stress.
- Clinical examination did not reveal any neurologic deficit.

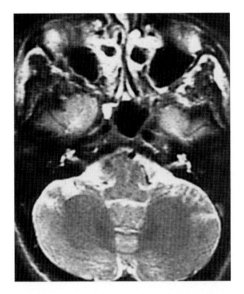

Fig. 74.1   T2-weighted magnetic resonance image at the level of the posterior fossa.

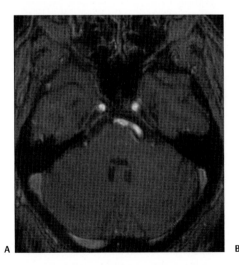
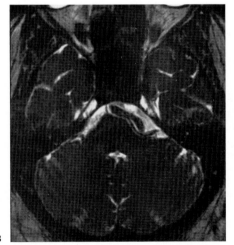
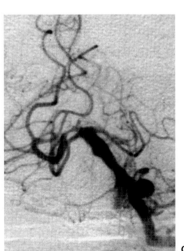

A   B   C

Fig. 74.2   (A) T1- and **(B)** T2-weighted magnetic resonance images at the level of the posterior fossa and cerebellopontine angle. **(C)** Vertebral digital subtraction angiography of the same patient.

■ Questions

1. What is the most likely diagnosis? The differential diagnosis?
2. Describe the pathophysiologic basis of HFS.
3. Interpret the magnetic resonance images (MRIs) shown in **Fig. 74.1** (which represent the current patient's findings) and **Fig. 74.2** (which represent another patient's findings, with the same diagnosis).
4. What is the underlying cause of HFS?
5. What are the surgical and nonsurgical therapeutic options?
6. Briefly describe your surgical procedure for HFS.
7. What is the expected surgical outcome?
8. What are the possible surgical complications?

■ Answers

1. *What is the most likely diagnosis? The differential diagnosis?*
   - The most likely diagnosis is HFS. Typical hemifacial spasm symptoms begin within the orbicularis oculi muscles and progress caudally. In atypical HFS, symptoms begin within the buccal muscles and progress rostrally.[1]
   - Differential diagnosis:
     – Benign essential blepharospasm
     – Craniofacial tremor
     – Facial chorea
     – Tics
     – Facial myokymia
2. *Describe the pathophysiologic basis of hemifacial spasm.*
   - HFS is a neuromuscular disorder that is characterized by paroxysmal bursts of involuntary, intermittent, or continuous clonic movements that progress to sustained tonic activity occurring in the muscles innervated by the facial nerve.
   - HFS represents a segmental myoclonus of muscles innervated by the facial nerve.
   - Irritation of the facial nerve nucleus is believed to lead to hyperexcitability of the facial nerve nucleus, whereas irritation of the proximal nerve segment may cause ephaptic transmission within the facial nerve.
   - Either mechanism explains the rhythmic involuntary myoclonic contractions observed in HFS.
   - The disorder presents usually unilaterally, although bilateral involvement may occur rarely in severe cases.
   - Typically, hemifacial spasm results secondary to vascular cross-compression of the myelinated facial nerve at or proximal to the junctional area of central and peripheral myelin (the root exit zone) of the nerve.[1]
3. *Interpret the MRIs shown in Fig. 74.1 (which represent the current patient's findings) and Fig. 74.2 (which represent another patient's findings with the same diagnosis).*
   - **Figure 74.1** reveals a T2-weighted MRI of the posterior fossa at the level of the internal auditory meatus. It reveals a flow void structure representing a blood vessel that is crossing the facial root exit level.
   - **Figure 74.2** represents another patient with hemifacial spasm. T1- and T2-weighted MRIs of the posterior fossa at the level of the cerebellopontine angle (CPA). Note the tortuous basilar artery that is compressing the left CPA at the facial exit root.
   - The same patient had a digital subtraction angiography of the vertebral artery (**Fig. 74.2C**) that confirmed the presence of dolichoectasia of the basilar artery. Note that not all HFS cases are idiopathic. The aim of investigating the patient is to rule out any underlying pathology.
4. *What is the underlying cause of HFS?*
   - The actual cause of HFS is debatable.
   - Most cases of HFS are caused by an ectatic blood vessel that irritates the facial nerve by compressing or forming a loop around the nerve at the nerve exit zone. The usual offending artery is the posterior inferior cerebellar artery complex, the anterior inferior cerebellar artery, or the vertebral artery.[2]
   - A minority of cases of HFS are caused by a venous compression.[2]
   - Rarely, the condition may be secondary to facial nerve injury, facial nerve compression by a CPA tumor, regeneration of the facial nerve following facial palsy, or it may be a result of a brainstem lesion such as a stroke or a multiple sclerosis plaque.
5. *What are the surgical and nonsurgical therapeutic options?*
   - In mild and early cases, twitching can be controlled by the use of some antiseizure medications or minor tranquillizers, such as carbamazepine (Tegretol; Novartis, East Hanover, NJ), clonazepam, and diazepam. However, results are not always satisfactory and medications need to be taken on a long-term basis.

■ Answers (*continued*)

- Botulinum toxin injection directly into the affected muscles can ablate the muscular spasm for several months, but its effect is temporary and the sensation of spasm often persists.
- The response to the latter two treatment modalities varies and their effects often attenuate over time, necessitating a surgical treatment.
- As for surgical management, the definitive procedure is a microvascular decompression. The offending blood vessel is mobilized from the nerve exit zone. This may be performed though microscopic, endoscopic, or a combined method. Use of endoscopic visualization can improve the overall outcome.[3–5]

6. *Briefly describe your surgical procedure for hemifacial spasm.*
   - Positioning and opening
     - Lateral decubitus position
     - Retromastoid craniectomy (2.0–2.5 cm in diameter)
     - Dura is incised.
     - Cerebrospinal fluid is drained slowly, allowing the structures of the posterior fossa to fall away without retraction.
     - Lateral or inferolateral cerebellar exposure of the CPA
   - Dissection and decompression
     - The acousticofacial bundle is identified.
     - The facial nerve may be stimulated for verification.
     - The offending vessel is identified, and using microdissection and gentle manipulation, the adhesions and compressions from the vessel(s) on the facial nerve are lysed, and the nerve and vessel(s) are freed from one another.
     - Small implants of shredded Teflon felt are placed to hold the vessel away from the cranial nerve root exit zone by changing the axis of the loop. Other techniques may include performing a dural sleeve to hold the artery away from the nerve or gluing the artery to the posterior fossa dura.
     - Veins are treated similarly or coagulated and divided.[3,4]

7. *What is the expected surgical outcome?*
   - Generally, patient should be informed of a possible nonresponse.
   - Excellent results (complete or nearly complete abolition of spasm) are expected in three-quarters of patients at 1 month after operation.
   - Long-term follow-up reveals more patients with total relief of their spasm.[3,4]
   - Patients having reoperation should expect lower results: 61% complete or nearly complete abolition of spasm.[4]
   - If the patient is still having spasm in the postoperative period, conservative follow-up will usually show progressive resolution of the residual spasm within the following month.

8. *What are the possible surgical complications?*
   - General complication related to posterior fossa surgery
   - Specific to facial nerve microvascular decompression:
     - Partial or complete, temporary or permanent facial palsy may result from manipulation of the facial nerve.
     - Owing to the immediate proximity of the eighth cranial nerve, microvascular decompression of the facial nerve for hemifacial spasm has a risk of producing ipsilateral hearing loss of various degrees. This may result from stretching the eighth cranial nerve between its exit from the brainstem and its entry into the internal auditory meatus as the surgeon places cerebellar retraction to expose the facial nerve root exit. This complication may be controlled if intraoperative brainstem auditory evoked potentials are monitored.[3,4]

■ References

1. Janetta P. Posterior fossa neurovascular compression syndromes other than neuralgias. In: Rengachary SS, Wilkins RH, eds. Neurosurgery. 2nd ed. New York: McGraw-Hill; 1996:3227–3233
2. Chung SS, Chang JW, Kim SH, Chang JH, Park YG, Kim DI. Microvascular decompression of the facial nerve for the treatment of hemifacial spasm: preoperative magnetic resonance imaging related to clinical outcomes. Acta Neurochir (Wien) 2000;142(8):901–906
3. Moffat DA, Durvasula VS, Stevens King A, De R, Hardy DG. Outcome following retrosigmoid microvascular decompression of the facial nerve for hemifacial spasm. J Laryngol Otol 2005;119(10):779–783
4. Barker FG II, Jannetta PJ, Bissonette DJ, Shields PT, Larkins MV, Jho HD. Microvascular decompression for hemifacial spasm. J Neurosurg 1995;82(2):201–210
5. Magnan J, Caces F, Locatelli P, Chays A. Hemifacial spasm: endoscopic vascular decompression. Otolaryngol Head Neck Surg 1997;117(4):308–314

Case 75 Postherpetic Neuralgia

Isaac Chan and Christopher J. Winfree

■ Clinical Presentation

- A 70-year-old woman on chronic prednisone therapy for polymyositis presents 5 months previously with an outbreak of herpes zoster infection along her left abdomen and groin in a T12–L1 distribution.
- She experiences severe, intractable pain radiating "like a knife" within the distribution of the zoster rash.

- Although the rash gradually resolves, the pain persists, unchanged to the present.
- The pain grades an 8/10 in severity, is ameliorated partially with cold packs, and is worsened with movement.

■ Questions

1. What is this patient's diagnosis?
2. What are her treatment options in the acute period (within 72 hours of rash onset)?
3. What are her treatment options in the chronic period (after the rash is resolved)?
4. What invasive treatment options are available if more conservative measures fail?

The patient undergoes a variety of pharmacologic treatments, including topical creams, oral anticonvulsants,

antidepressants, and opiates, none of which yielded acceptable pain relief. Multiple epidural steroid injections likewise failed to help. You are considering offering the patient either neurostimulation or a spinal infusion pump.

5. Describe the relative merits and drawbacks of each type of therapy.

■ Answers

1. *What is this patient's diagnosis?*
   - Initially, this patient had an acute herpes zoster outbreak, in which a dermatomal outbreak of pain is followed by a vesicular rash that gradually resolves over a month or so.[1]
   - Zoster pain that persists well beyond healing of the rash is called postherpetic neuralgia (PHN), and occurs following 10 to 15% of acute zoster infections.[1]
2. *What are her treatment options in the acute period (within 72 hours of rash onset)?*
   - Topical analgesics and oral anticonvulsants and antidepressants offer pain relief, but do not reduce the likelihood of developing PHN.
   - Oral antiviral agents administered within 72 hours of the onset of the acute outbreak may reduce the likelihood of developing PHN.[2]

3. *What are her treatment options in the chronic period (after the rash is resolved)?*
   - Randomized, prospective clinical trials have shown that oral antidepressants, anticonvulsants, long-acting opioids, and nonsteroidal antiinflammatory agents as well as topical anesthetic creams reduce pain in patients with PHN.[1]
   - Complementary and alternative medicine therapies such as physiotherapy and acupuncture have not been shown to be beneficial but may certainly be utilized with essentially no risk to the patient.
4. *What invasive treatment options are available if more conservative measures fail?*
   - Minimally invasive pain management techniques such as nerve blocks, sympathetic blocks, and epidural steroids have not been shown to be of benefit.[1]

■ Answers (*continued*)

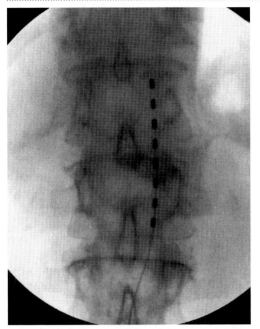

Fig. 75.1 Intraoperative fluoroscopic image showing placement of a T12–L1 intraspinal nerve root electrode in the lateral aspect of the spinal canal. In this position, the electrical stimulation focused entirely upon the left-sided T12 and L1 dermatomes, the location of the patient's pain. There were no unwanted stimulation paresthesias in the lower extremity or elsewhere. The patient experienced significant (>50%) and durable pain relief following placement of the spinal nerve root stimulator system and is quite satisfied with the result.

- Invasive surgical options such as neurectomy, cordotomy, dorsal root entry zone lesions, or other ablative therapies have been discredited and largely abandoned because of their risk of complications and lack of efficacy.[3]
- Less-invasive treatments such as intrathecal methylprednisolone infusion may be helpful.[4]
- Spinal cord stimulation, in which implanted electrodes in the spinal canal administer electrical impulses to the dorsal columns, may reduce pain and improve quality of life in PHN patients.[5]

5. *Describe the relative merits and drawbacks of each type of therapy.*
   - Spinal infusion pumps may offer dramatic pain relief for patients with chronic pain, including PHN. Implanting the devices is fairly straightforward for the practicing pain physician, and patients generally tolerate the systems fairly well. Patients generally do not perceive the effects of the infused drug(s), except for the relief of the pain.[6]
   - Nevertheless, the pumps need to be refilled every 1 to 3 months or so, and replaced every 5 to 7 years. System malfunctions may occur, prompting potentially lethal withdrawal syndromes in certain cases, and surgical revisions are sometimes required. Cere-

brospinal fluid (CSF) leaks sometimes occur, following pump implantation or revision surgery.
   - In contrast, spinal cord stimulation systems generally require less maintenance than infusion pumps, there is no risk of a withdrawal syndrome if the system malfunctions, and CSF leaks are rare.
   - Stimulation produces noticeable paresthesias that are designed to overlap with the painful areas, eliciting pain relief. Some patients find these sensations annoying, especially if the paresthesias are in unwanted areas outside of the pain distribution.[7]
   - Spinal nerve root stimulation is a neurostimulation technique similar to spinal cord stimulation, except that the electrodes are placed more laterally in the spinal canal to preferentially stimulate the dorsal rootlets (**Fig. 75.1**). This provides similar levels of pain relief within the targeted painful areas as spinal cord stimulation, while limiting unwanted stimulation paresthesias to undesired areas.[8]
   - Possible complications or drawbacks of neurostimulation implants include electrode displacement or malfunction, hematoma or pain at the site of pulse generator, requirement for battery replacement after 5 to 10 years.[7]

■ References

1. Dubinsky RM, Kabbani H, El-Chami Z, Boutwell C, Ali H. Practice parameter: treatment of postherpetic neuralgia. An evidence-based report of the Quality Standards Subcommittee of the American Academy of Neurology. Neurology 2004;63(6):959–965

2. Kost RG, Straus SE. Postherpetic neuralgia: pathogenesis, treatment, and prevention. N Engl J Med 1996;335(1):32–42

3. Watson CPN. Postherpetic neuralgia. In: Burchiel KJ, ed. Surgical Management of Pain. New York: Thieme Medical Publishers; 2002

4. Kotani N, Kushikata T, Hashimoto H, et al. Intrathecal methyl-prednisolone for intractable postherpetic neuralgia. N Engl J Med 2000;343(21):1514–1519

5. Harke H, Gretenkort P, Ladleif HU, Koester P, Rahman S. Spinal cord stimulation in postherpetic neuralgia and in acute herpes zoster pain. Anesth Analg 2002;94(3):694–700

6. Bennett G, Serafini M, Burchiel K, et al. Evidence-based review of the literature on intrathecal delivery of pain medication. J Pain Symptom Manage 2000;20(2):S12–S36

7. Kumar K, Hunter G, Demeria D. Spinal cord stimulation in treatment of chronic benign pain: challenges in treatment planning and present status, a 22-year experience. Neurosurgery 2006;58(3):481–496

8. Haque R, Winfree CJ. Spinal nerve root stimulation. Neurosurg Focus 2006;21(6):E4

Case 76 Complex Regional Pain Syndrome

Christopher P. Kellner and Christopher J. Winfree

■ Clinical Presentation

- A 47-year-old woman is walking from one commuter train car to the next, when the sliding door closes on her right arm and shoulder, trapping her for 3 to 4 minutes; during this time, she begins to experience stabbing pain throughout her right arm.
- She extricates herself, and later that day is evaluated in the Emergency Room, where no discernible injuries or neurologic deficits are discovered.

- Because her pain persists weeks after her injury, she undergoes magnetic resonance imaging of her cervical spine, which only shows some mild, nonspecific degenerative changes.
- She was treated with nonsteroidal antiinflammatory drugs and short-acting opiates, which offered partial relief of her pain.

■ Questions

1. Based on the available information, what is the differential diagnosis for this patient's pain?
2. What studies do you order?

Her electrodiagnostic studies were normal. On repeat examination a few months after injury, the patient has developed right upper extremity swelling from the shoulder to the forearm, and the entire arm is painful to touch and also to either active or passive movement.

3. What is the most likely diagnosis at this point?
4. Describe the initial, noninvasive treatment of this condition.
5. Describe the invasive treatments of this condition, for use when conservative measures fail.

The patient undergoes a comprehensive, multidisciplinary approach to treat her condition. Although she is able to tolerate physical therapy, her arm still greatly bothers her; she still has swelling and stiffness in the arm, and she cannot work. She has tried several medication trials without sufficient pain relief, and several anesthetic blocks were unhelpful. A psychological evaluation was unrevealing.

6. You now wish to employ spinal cord stimulation (SCS). Where will you place the electrodes?
7. What are the potential complications of SCS?
8. What are the outcomes for spinal cord stimulation in patients with complex regional pain syndrome (CRPS)?

■ Answers

1. *Based on the available information, what is the differential diagnosis for this patient's pain?*
   - Cervical radiculopathy
   - Brachial plexopathy
   - Peripheral nerve damage
   - CRPS
2. *What studies do you order?*
   - Electromyography with nerve conduction studies (EMG/NCS) may help distinguish a peripheral nerve injury, cervical radiculopathy, and neuralgic amyotrophy.
   - This test should be performed a minimum of 3-weeks postinjury to permit appropriate denervational changes, if any, to occur in the affected muscles.

3. *What is the most likely diagnosis at this point?*
   - CRPS is a neuropathic pain syndrome that requires
     - Persistent pain beyond that expected from an initial noxious stimulus
     - Pain that exceeds the confines of a single peripheral nerve or nerve root distribution
     - Swelling, temperature changes, abnormal coloration, or vasomotor dysfunction in the affected region
     - Absence of another condition that could reasonably explain the findings[1]
   - CRPS type I has no evidence of nerve injury, whereas in CRPS type II there is evidence of nerve injury, typically upon EMG/NCS.

■ **Answers** (*continued*)

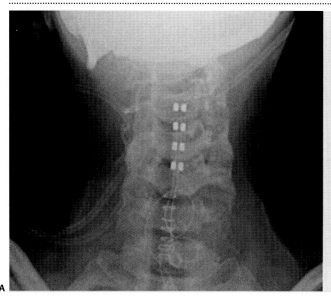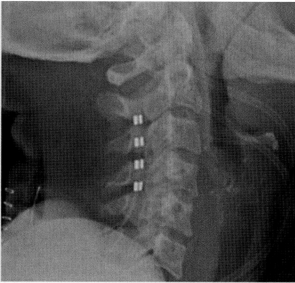

A   B

Fig. 76.1 Postoperative anteroposterior **(A)** and lateral **(B)** cervical spine x-rays following placement of a C3–4 laminectomy lead along the midline. The patient experienced significant (>50%) and durable pain relief following placement of the spinal cord stimulator system and is quite satisfied with the result.

- With negative EMG findings, this patient has CRPS type I.
4. *Describe the initial, noninvasive treatments for this condition.*
   - Effective treatment of CRPS requires a multidisciplinary, pain management-oriented approach.[2]
   - Aggressive physical therapy enables recovery of function in the affected extremity and prevents disuse changes from occurring.
   - Analgesics, typically the anticonvulsants, antidepressants, and opioids, provide pain relief to permit physical therapy (which would otherwise be too painful without them) to be undertaken.
   - Psychological evaluation, and ongoing support if needed, is performed to determine whether any psychological amplifiers of pain exist, such as stress, behavioral problems, depression, disordered coping mechanisms, etc., and treat them if necessary.
5. *Describe the invasive treatments for this condition, for use when conservative measures fail.*
   - If several weeks of the noninvasive multidisciplinary approach are insufficiently helpful, then the patient may be a candidate for anesthetic blocks to provide temporary pain relief.[3]
   - If a more aggressive approach is required, then the patient becomes a candidate for SCS.[3]
6. *You now wish to employ SCS. Where will you place the electrodes?*
   - The spinal cord stimulator array, either a percutaneous or a laminectomy paddle lead, may be placed in the dorsal epidural space from C2–C5, just off midline and eccentric to the right. C-arm radiography is used to determine the exact location (**Fig. 76.1**).
   - In this location, the stimulator will administer electricity to the dorsal columns associated with the right upper extremity. Thus, the patient should experience stimulation paresthesias in the right arm, overlapping with the painful area.
   - Ideally, this is performed in the awake patient to confirm overlap and limit unwanted stimulation paresthesias to other parts of the body such as trunk and leg.
7. *What are the potential complications of SCS?*
   - Displaced electrodes (21.5%)
   - Fractured electrode (5.9%)
   - Infection (3.4%)
   - Hardware malfunction (4.9%)
   - Subcutaneous hematoma (4.4%)
   - Discomfort over pulse generator (1.2%)
   - Cerebrospinal fluid leak (0.5%)[4,5]
8. *What are the outcomes for spinal cord stimulation in patients with CRPS?*
   - A meta-analysis of 25 case series with a median follow-up of 33 months found that 67% of CRPS patients achieved 50% or more pain relief.[6]
   - SCS is an appropriate and effective therapeutic option for patients with chronic benign pain refractory to medication.

■ References

1. Stanton-Hicks M, Janig W, Hassenbusch S, Haddox JD, Boas R, Wilson P, et al. Reflex sympathetic dystrophy: changing concepts and taxonomy. Pain 1995;63(1):127–133

2. Stanton-Hicks M, Baron R, Boas R, et al. Complex regional pain syndromes: guidelines for therapy. Clin J Pain 1998;14(2):155–166

3. Boas R. Complex regional pain syndrome. In: Burchiel KJ. Surgical Management of Pain. New York: Thieme Medical Publishers; 2002

4. Kumar K, Hunter G, Demeria D. Spinal cord stimulation in treatment of chronic benign pain: challenges in treatment planning and present status, a 22-year experience. Neurosurgery 2006;58(3):481–496

5. Lee AW, Pilitsis JG. Spinal cord stimulation: indications and outcomes. Neurosurg Focus 2006;21(6):E3

6. Taylor RS. Spinal cord stimulation in complex regional pain syndrome and refractory neuropathic back and leg pain/failed back surgery syndrome: results of a systematic review and meta-analysis. J Pain Symptom Manage 2006;31(4, Suppl):S13–S19

Case 77 Central Poststroke Pain

Deepa Danan and Christopher J. Winfree

■ Clinical Presentation

- A 45-year-old woman sustained, 3 years ago, an acute onset of right hemibody numbness, followed a few hours later by right hemibody pain and paresthesias.
- Initial brain magnetic resonance imaging scan revealed a small left thalamic infarct (**Fig. 77.1**).

- The pain has persisted to the present time and involves the right side of her face, the right arm, trunk, and leg. It is sufficiently severe enough to interfere with her ability to work and carry out activities of daily living.
- Physical examination is notable for decreased hemibody sensation in the painful distribution.

■ Questions

1. What is this patient's diagnosis?
2. What are her treatment options?

The patient undergoes a variety of pharmacologic treatments, including multiple nonsteroidal antiinflammatory drugs, anticonvulsants, antidepressants, short-acting opi-

ates, and long-acting opiates, none of which yielded sufficient pain relief. You are considering offering the patient more invasive treatment options.

3. What are some surgical options?

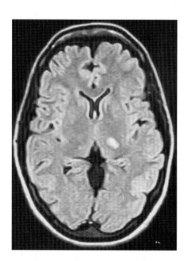

Fig. 77.1 Magnetic resonance imaging fluid-attenuated inversion-recovery without contrast of the head demonstrating the small, left-sided thalamic infarct.

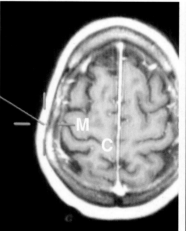 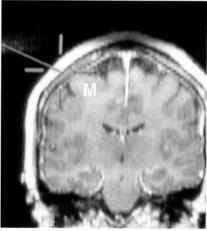

Fig. 77.2 Intraoperative frameless stereotaxis magnetic resonance image demonstrating the localization of the central sulcus (C) and motor cortex (M). Identification of these landmarks facilitates the planning of a small craniotomy directly over the area of interest. Once the craniotomy is performed, somatosensory evoked potential phase reversal is performed to confirm the exact location of the central sulcus. The location of the facial and upper extremity motor cortex is confirmed when muscle contractions are elicited by transdural electrical stimulation. Once the array of stimulator electrodes is secured to the dura overlying the motor cortex, stimulation is increased until muscle contractions are noted, confirming the motor threshold. Postoperatively, stimulation intensities are kept well below the motor threshold to reduce the risk of postoperative seizures.

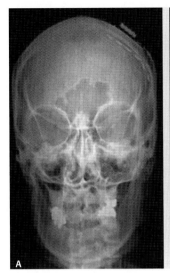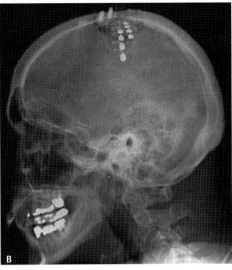

Fig. 77.3 Postoperative anteroposterior **(A)** and lateral **(B)** radiographs demonstrating the two electrode arrays placed over the motor cortex. The patient had a 90% reduction in her levels of hemibody pain postoperatively.

■ Answers

1. *What is this patient's diagnosis?*
   - *Central pain* is defined as neuropathic pain caused by a primary lesion or dysfunction within the central nervous system.
   - *Poststroke pain* is a type of central pain that occurs following a cerebrovascular accident.[1]
   - Lesions can occur nearly anywhere in the brain, but commonly involve the thalamus, brainstem, or cortex.
   - This patient has Dejerine–Roussy syndrome, a variant of central poststroke pain (CPSP) caused by infarction in the thalamus.

2. *What are her treatment options?*
   - CPSP is treated in a similar fashion as other neuropathic pain syndromes.[1]
   - Clinical trials have shown that the tricyclic antidepressants and anticonvulsants are effective first-line agents.[2]
   - Opiates, other agents, and complementary and alternative approaches may be used in refractory cases, but there is a lack of well-controlled data to support their use for CPSP.

3. *What are some surgical options?*
   - Spinal cord stimulation is a minimally invasive treatment used to treat a variety of chronic pain syndromes.[3] It utilizes a series of electrodes to administer a weak electrical current to the spinal cord. This current produces stimulation paresthesias that, through unknown mechanisms, attenuate the patient's subjective experience of pain. Although quite effective for many neuropathic pain syndromes, results have been disappointing for CPSP.[4]
   - Deep-brain stimulation is another type of neurostimulation in which pain-processing circuitry is subjected to electrical stimulation within the brain itself. Similar to spinal cord stimulation, its mechanism of action is unknown. It may be more effective than spinal cord stimulation for CPSP, but results remain dismal.[4]
   - In contrast, motor cortex stimulation fares much better as a treatment of CPSP.[4] In this procedure, a stimulation electrode is placed over the motor cortex of the brain contralateral to the side of the pain. Cortical stimulation, through cortico-cortical (and perhaps corticothalamic) pathways, inhibits the perception of pain (**Fig. 77.2 and Fig. 77.3**).[5]

■ References

1. Hansson P. Post-stroke pain case study: clinical characteristics, therapeutic options, and long-term follow-up. Eur J Neurol 2004;11(Suppl 1):22–30
2. Frese A, Husstedt IW, Ringelstein EB, Evers S. Pharmacologic treatment of central post-stroke pain. Clin J Pain 2006;22:252–260
3. Lee AW, Pilitsis JG. Spinal cord stimulation: indications and outcomes. Neurosurg Focus 2006;21(6):E3
4. Katayama Y, Yamamoto T, Kobayashi K, Kasai M, Oshima H, Fukaya C. Motor cortex stimulation for post-stroke pain: comparison of spinal cord and thalamic stimulation. Stereotact Funct Neurosurg 2001;77(1–4):183–186
5. Rasche D, Ruppolt M, Stippich C, Unterberg A, Tronnier VM. Motor cortex stimulation for long-term relief of chronic neuropathic pain: a 10 year experience. Pain 2006;121(1–2):43–52

Case 78   Stereotactic Radiosurgery Case

Carmina M. Angeles and Dennis G. Vollmer

■ Clinical Presentation

- A 72-year-old man presented to the emergency room in status epilepticus.
- He has no significant medical history.

- After loading him with fosphenytoin, a noncontrasted head computed tomography scan was obtained, which showed some abnormality prompting an magnetic resonance imaging (MRI) scan of the brain (**Fig. 78.1**).

■ Questions

1. Interpret the MRI (**Fig. 78.1**).
2. What are the differential diagnoses?
3. What is the next step in management?
4. You decide to obtain a four-vessel angiogram (**Fig. 78.2**). Interpret the images.
5. What are the management options for the lesion seen on angiography?
6. What are the management options for this patient?

This patient elected to undergo stereotactic radiosurgery (SRS) to both lesions. The treatment was planned for a dose of 22 Gy at 50% isodose line to the frontal arteriovenous malformation (AVM), and 16 Gy to the 50% isodose line for the dural based parietooccipital lesion.

7. Describe the main steps involved in the planning and completion of SRS.
8. What are the outcomes of SRS on AVMs?
9. What are the outcomes of SRS on meningiomas?
10. What are the complications of SRS?

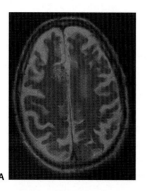 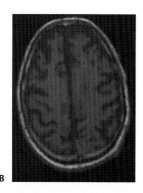 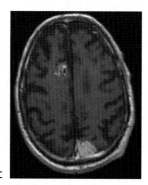

A   B   C

Fig. 78.1 Axial magnetic resonance images of the brain: **(A)** T2-weighted, **(B)** T1-weighted, and **(C)** T1-weighted with contrast.

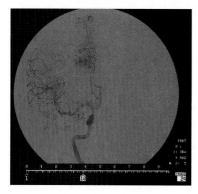

Fig. 78.2 Cerebral angiogram, left internal carotid injection, anteroposterior view.

■ **Answers**

1. *Interpret the MRI* (**Fig. 78.1**).
   - **Figure 78.1A and B** reveal noncontrasted T1- and T2-weighted images depicting two lesions. There is an ~2.6-cm nonhemorrhagic right frontal parafalcine lesion with several large flow voids.
   - There is a second nonhemorrhagic hypodense lesion on the T1-weighted image ~1.4 × 3.3 × 2.4-cm located in the left parietooccipital area.
   - In the postgadolinium T1-weighted image in **Fig. 78.1C**, the right frontal lesion is heterogeneously enhancing, whereas the left parietooccipital lesion is more homogeneous and appears to be dural-based.

2. *What are the differential diagnoses?*
   - Differential diagnoses for the right frontal lesion include
     - Arteriovenous malformation (AVM)
     - Cavernous malformation
     - Hemangiopericytoma
   - Differential diagnoses for the left parietooccipital lesion include
     - Meningioma (most likely)
     - Metastases
     - Other less likely lesions: hemangiopericytoma, lymphoma, brain abscess[1]

3. *What is the next step in management?*
   - A cerebrovascular study such as four-vessel cerebral angiography, magnetic resonance angiography, or computed tomography angiography is warranted to assess the frontal lesion. The patient did undergo in this case a cerebral angiogram.
   - In addition, an electroencephalogram (EEG) should be performed to help localize the source of the seizure. The results of the EEG, however, in this case were essentially of a normal awake person.
   - A lumbar puncture to rule out cerebrospinal fluid xanthochromia may also help delineate whether the seizure was a result of a hemorrhage from the likely AVM.

4. *You decide to obtain a four-vessel angiogram* (**Fig. 78.2**). *Interpret the image.*
   - **Figure 78.2** reveals an angiogram, right carotid artery injection, showing an AVM feeding primarily from the right pericallosal artery and appears to be draining into a right frontal cortical vein.
   - Considering the size of the lesion being less than 3 cm, location in noneloquent brain, and a superficial draining vein, this lesion is a grade I based on the Spetzler–Martin grading system (please refer to Case 28 for AVM grading).[2]

5. *What are the management options for the lesion seen on angiography?*
   - There are essentially three treatment options for an AVM: surgery, embolization, and SRS. In addition, preoperative embolization followed by surgical resection may be another option that significantly reduces the risks of surgery and can be curative compared with embolization alone.[2–4]

6. *What are the management options for this patient?*
   - Treatment options for this patient with an AVM include various combinations of open surgical resection, embolization, SRS, and observation alone, as described above.
   - Treatment options for the dural-based lesion in the parietooccipital lobe include surgical resection, biopsy, radiosurgery, or observation alone.
   - A combination of treatment modalities is possible in this case, based on the patient's preference, age, comorbidities, and other medical conditions.
   - Given the advanced age of the patient, the small size of the lesions and the convincing appearance of the lesions on MRI and angiography, some may argue that SRS alone (without having tissue biopsy specimen for pathologic diagnosis) may be a valid option in this particular case.[5]

7. *Describe the main steps involved in the planning and completion of SRS.*
   - SRS is a minimally invasive treatment technique used to deliver a focal dose of high-energy radiation to a target. This target is localized stereotactically using three-dimensional image processing. Normal surrounding tissues and structures are spared.[6]
   - A Leksell stereotactic coordinate frame is placed under local anesthetic agent and is centered on the target (tumor or AVM).[6] Other localizing frames of reference may also be used.
   - MRI or CT scan of the brain is performed and the images are then used for treatment planning with an interactive computer, which provides information on the volume of the target, dose of radiation, dose to volume ratio, isodose curves, etc.[5,6]

■ **Answers** (*continued*)

- There are two predominant types of delivery devices for SRS[6]:
  - Gamma knife (GKS)
    - A radioactive isotope such as Cobalt 60 is focused on the target by interchangeable helmets with different size collimators via 201 sources.
    - The additive effect of multiple isocenters of radiation results in a high dose of radiation delivered in a conformal manner.[5]
  - Linear accelerator (LINAC)
    - By moving a single beam of radiation in arcs around a patient's head, the amount of radiation and the size of the beam can also be collimated and tailored to the target of interest.[5]
- Steroids may be concomitantly given if there is a concern about brain edema or eloquent neural tissue damage.

8. *What are the outcomes of SRS on AVMs?*
   - 5-year AVM obliteration rate ranges from 66 to 89%.[7,8]
     - In GKS cases, it is ~72 to 89%
     - In LINAC cases, it is ~60%
9. *What are the outcomes of SRS on meningiomas?*
   - 5-year tumor control rate was 90 to 98%.[5,9–11]
   - In a series of 400 cases, tumor volume decreased in ~70%, remained the same in ~28%, and increased only in ~2.5%.[10]
   - Symptomatic complications were limited to ~5%.[9]
10. *What are the complications of SRS?*
    - Perilesional edema in 7 to 16%[10,12]
    - Damage to critical eloquent brain structures such as the optic nerves or other cranial nerves[12]
    - After SRS hemorrhage during the time before obliteration of the AVM, the rate is between 6 and 13%.[7]
    - Other potential complications include headaches, seizures, intracranial cysts,[13] and radiation necrosis.[14]

■ **References**

1. Osborn AG. Diagnostic Neuroradiology. St. Louis, MO: Mosby; 1994
2. Spetzler RF, Martin NA. A proposed grading system for arteriovenous malformations. J Neurosurg 1986;65(4):476–483
3. Veznedaroglu E, Andrews DW, Benitez RP, et al. Fractionated stereotactic radiotherapy for the treatment of large arteriovenous malformations with or without previous partial embolization. Neurosurgery 2004;55(3):519–530
4. Heros RC, Korosue K, Diebold PM. Surgical excision of cerebral arteriovenous malformations: late results. Neurosurgery 1990;26(4):570–577
5. Chin LS, Szerlip NJ, Regine WF. Stereotactic radiosurgery for meningiomas. Neurosurg Focus 2003;14(5):E6
6. Deinsberger R, Tidstrand J. Linac radiosurgery as a tool in neurosurgery. Neurosurg Rev 2005;28(2):79–88
7. Orio P, Stelzer KJ, Goodkin R, Douglas JG. Treatment of arteriovenous malformations with linear accelerator-based radiosurgery compared with Gamma Knife surgery. J Neurosurg 2006;105(Suppl):58–63
8. Fukuoka S, Takanashi M, Seo Y, Suematsu K, Nakamura J. Radiosurgery for arteriovenous malformations with gamma-knife: a multivariate analysis of factors influencing the complete obliteration rate. J Clin Neurosci 1998;5(Suppl):68–71
9. Torres RC, Frighetto L, De Salles AA, et al. Radiosurgery and stereotactic radiotherapy for intracranial meningiomas. Neurosurg Focus 2003;14(5):E5
10. Kollová A, Liscák R, Novotný J Jr, Vladyka V, Simonová G, Janousková L. Gamma Knife surgery for benign meningioma. J Neurosurg 2007;107(2):325–336
11. Elia AE, Shih HA, Loeffler JS. Stereotactic radiation treatment for benign meningiomas. Neurosurg Focus 2007;23(4):E5
12. Novotný J Jr, Kollová A, Liscák R. Prediction of intracranial edema after radiosurgery of meningiomas. J Neurosurg 2006;105(Suppl):120–126
13. Liu WM, Ye X, Zhao YL, Wang S, Zhao JZ. Clinical and pathological changes in cerebral arteriovenous malformations after stereotactic radiosurgery failure. Chin Med J 2008;121(12):1076–1079
14. Djalilian HR, Benson AG, Ziai K, Safai Y, Thakkar KH, Mafee MF. Radiation necrosis of the brain after radiosurgery for vestibular schwannoma. Am J Otolaryngol 2007;28(5):338–341

Case 79   Spasticity after Cord Injury

Remi Nader

■ Clinical Presentation

- A 64-year-old man presents 6 years after having sustained a motor vehicle accident.
- The patient is a recovered C4 partial quadriplegic who underwent a C4 corpectomy and C5–6 anterior cervical diskectomy and fusion about one year ago.
- He now presents with some upper extremity pain and bilateral shoulder pain.
- He has some persistent spasticity in both upper and lower extremities, unsteady gait, and difficulties with bladder control.

- Hyperreflexia and muscle atrophy are seen diffusely on examination.
- He has been taking baclofen, tramadol, and diazepam, but the effect of the medications seems to have worn off despite a recent increase in dosage.
- Magnetic resonance imaging (MRI) of the entire spine is done, and the only pertinent positive findings are shown in **Fig. 79.1**.

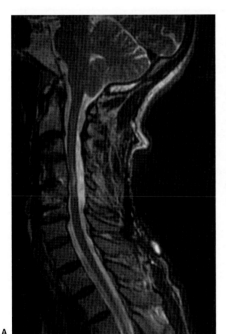

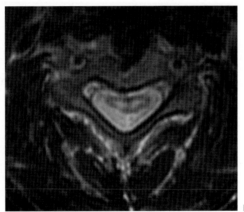

Fig. 79.1 Magnetic resonance imaging of the cervical spine: **(A)** T2-weighted images with midsagittal section and **(B)** axial section through C4–5 level.

■ Questions

1. Interpret the MRI scan.
2. How do you manage the syrinx?
3. What are some other causes of spasticity?
4. Describe a grading system for spasticity.
5. What are some other medical options to treat spasticity in this patient?
6. Name five surgical options commonly employed to treat spasticity.
7. What are the main complications of pump placements?
8. What are the main selection criteria for placement of baclofen pumps?

■ Answers

1. *Interpret the MRI scan.*
   - T2-weighted sagittal image (**Fig. 79.1A**) shows a previous C3 to C6 anterior diskectomy and fusion.
   - Cord atrophy at the level of the upper cervical cord is noted.
   - A small syrinx is seen at the level of C4–5, but it is not causing any pressure on the cord or any compression of neural elements.
   - Cerebrospinal fluid (CSF) spaces are wide open around the spinal cord.
   - There is some straightening of the normal lordosis.

2. *How do you manage the syrinx?*
   - The syrinx is managed expectantly.
   - No treatment for the syrinx is needed as it does not cause any pressure on the spinal cord or neural elements.

3. *What are some other causes of spasticity?*
   - Multiple sclerosis
   - Cerebral palsy
   - Spinal dysraphism
   - Amyotrophic lateral sclerosis
   - Traumatic brain injury
   - Stroke

4. *Describe a grading system for spasticity.*
   - Ashworth grading system[1,2]:
     0. No increase in tone
     1. Slight increase in tone with small "catch" when moving affected limb
     2. More marked increase in tone with easy passive movements
     3. Significant increase in tone with hard passive movements
     4. Rigid affected part

5. *What are some other medical options to treat spasticity in this patient?*
   - Dantrolene[3]
     - Decreases calcium influx in sarcoplasmic reticulum
   - Decreases muscle contractions
   - Progabide[3]
     - GABA A and B activator

6. *Name five surgical options commonly employed to treat spasticity.*[1–3]
   - Baclofen and morphine pumps[4]
   - Electrical stimulation via epidural electrodes
   - Selective posterior rhizotomies[5]
   - Intramuscular phenol neurolysis
   - Myelotomies
   - Stereotactic thalamotomy

7. *What are the main complications of pump placements?*
   - Mechanical[4]
     - Underinfusion
     - Catheter occlusion, kinking, dislodgment, break
   - Wound problems[4]
     - Erosion of pocket
     - Infection
     - Local pain
     - Seroma/hematoma
     - CSF collection

8. *What are the main selection criteria for placement of baclofen pumps?*
   - Selection criteria for baclofen pump are described below[4]:
     - Age 18 to 65, able to give informed consent
     - Severe chronic spasticity >6 months
     - Spasticity refractory to oral medications
     - Ashworth scale at least 3
     - No CSF block
     - Positive response to intrathecal baclofen test dose
     - No implantable device
     - Nonpregnant patient
     - No allergy to baclofen
     - No history of stroke, renal insufficiency, severe liver or gastrointestinal disease

■ References

1. Ashworth B. Preliminary trial of carisoprodol in multiple sclerosis. Practitioner 1964;192:540–542
2. Bohannon RW, Smith M. Interrater reliability of a Modified Ashworth Scale of muscle spasticity. Phys Ther 1987;67:206–207
3. Adams MM, Hicks AL. Spasticity after spinal cord injury. Spinal Cord 2005;43(10):577–586
4. Hsieh JC, Penn RD. Intrathecal baclofen in the treatment of adult spasticity. Neurosurg Focus 2006;21(2):E5
5. O'Brien DF, Park TS. A review of orthopedic surgeries after selective dorsal rhizotomy. Neurosurg Focus 2006;21(2):E2

Case 80   Neuronavigation and Intraoperative Imaging

Lahbib B. Soualmi and Abdulrahman J. Sabbagh

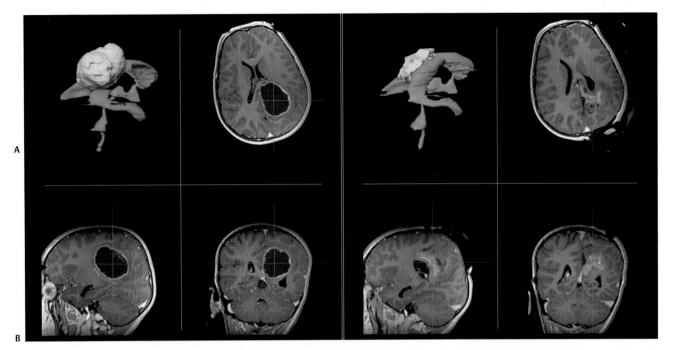

Fig. 80.1   (A) Magnetic resonance imaging (MRI) preoperative, three-dimensional (3D) reconstruction (top left) with ventricular system in purple and tumor in yellow. T1-weighted MRIs preoperative with contrast showing tumor in axial (top right), sagittal (bottom left), and coronal (bottom right) images. **(B)** MRI intraoperative, 3D reconstruction (top left) with ventricular system in purple and tumor in yellow. T1-weighted MRIs intraoperative with contrast showing tumor in axial (top right), sagittal (bottom left), and coronal (bottom right) images.

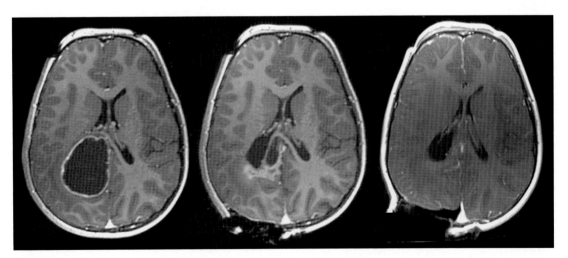

Fig. 80.2   Intraoperative axial T1-weighted magnetic resonance images with contrast showing progression of tumor resection.

■ Clinical Presentation

- A 7-year-old right-handed girl presents with slowly pro-gressive headaches and blurred vision.
- Examination is normal with the exception of early papil-ledema.

- Magnetic resonance imaging (MRI) of the brain shows a large right parietooccipital cystic lesion that is rim-enhancing (**Fig. 80.1**).
- You decide to take the patient to surgery, for diagnostic and therapeutic reasons.

■ Questions

1. How will you plan the surgery?
2. What are the characteristics of images needed for navigation in general?
3. What are the types of information that can be utilized for navigation?
4. How does neuronavigation work?
5. What are the types of registration available?

6. What are the existing types of localizers?
7. How do you classify intraoperative imaging?
8. Give examples where intraoperative imaging may be useful.
9. Compare the advantages and disadvantages of intraoperative computed tomography (iCT) and intraoperative MRI (iMRI).

■ Answers

1. *How will you plan the surgery?*
   - This patient has a cystic lesion. As the cyst leaks during surgery, the brain will shift and navigation will be very inaccurate. For this reason the surgical team may decide to use intraoperative imaging and do the following (**Fig. 80.1B**):
     - Placing the head in a rigid MRI- or CT-compatible head holder in preparation for surgery
     - Obtaining a preoperative MRI and calculating the cyst volume (**Fig. 80.1A**)
     - Performing craniotomy and frameless stereotactic aspiration of the cyst
     - Performing iMRI after cyst aspiration to compensate for the brain shift caused by cyst aspiration and craniotomy (**Fig. 80.1B**)[1,2]
     - Taking an interhemispheric approach to the lesion and complete resection (**Fig. 80.2**)
2. *What are the characteristics of images needed for navigation in general?*
   - Three-dimensional (3D) global acquisition: Contiguous slices covering the whole region of interest such as the head or spine.
     - Anatomic isotropic scan with high resolution: Fine cuts are required to be able to create an accurate volumetric data.
     - After computerized fusion, the functional data can then be superimposed on the anatomic data.

3. *What are the types of information that can be utilized for navigation?*
   - Anatomic information[3,4]
     - MRI
       - T1-weighted, ± contrast, T2-weighted, inverse recovery, fluid-attenuated inversion-recovery sequences, etc.
       - Diffusion tensor imaging, tractography
       - MR angiography, MR venography
     - CT
       - CT ± contrast,
       - CT angiography (CTA)
     - Ultrasound 3D acquisition
       - B-mode information
       - Doppler information
     - Conventional biplanar angiography
   - Functional information[5–8]
     - Positron emission tomography (PET)
     - Single photon emission computerized tomography
     - Functional MRI (fMRI)
     - Magnetoencephalography (MEG)
     - Cortical electroencephalography
     - Depth electrode recordings
     - Transcranial magnetic stimulation
   - Biochemical information
     - MR spectroscopy
     - Other chemical imaging modalities

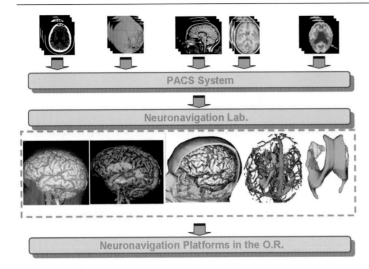

Acquisition

Transfer

Pre-surgical
Planning

Transfer

Fig. 80.3 Steps in neuronavigation (see text for further details). PACS, picture archiving and communication system; O.R., operating room.

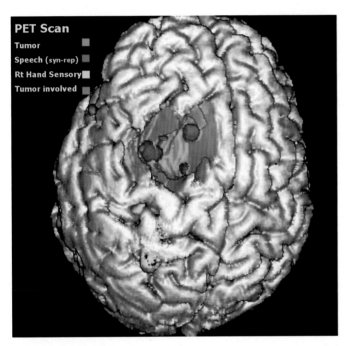

Fig. 80.4 Superimposed positron emission tomography scan with three-dimensional reconstructed magnetic resonance images delineating the eloquent brain areas.

■ Answers (*continued*)

4. *How does neuronavigation work?*
   - The following are steps required for the workings of neuronavigation.[9–12]
     - Image acquisition (**Fig. 80.3**)
     - Image data analysis: anatomical ± functional data analysis—segmentation and 3D reconstruction and volume rendering of objects of interest
     - Fusion and superimposition of different anatomical ± functional images (**Fig. 80.4**): The example given is PET data superimposed on MRI data.
     - Registration: correlating and alignment of the 3D volumetric data with the actual patient (brain or spine)
     - Tracking: The neuronavigation platform should track the patient and surgical tools through the available localizer. This is done through different available tools (**Fig. 80.5**).

5. *What are the types of registration available?*
   - Anatomic: Using anatomic landmarks (bridge of the nose, inner and outer canthi, tragus valleys, spinous processes, transverse process, etc.)[13]
   - Fiducials: Using radiopaque markers fixed before scanning the patient. These markers must be detected by the imaging modality used.[14]
   - Surface fitting: Pinpointing a mesh of points on the surface of the region of surgical interest using a probe or a laser scanning device, to be correlated with the 3D object surface (i.e., face or spine of the patient).[13,15]

■ Answers (*continued*)

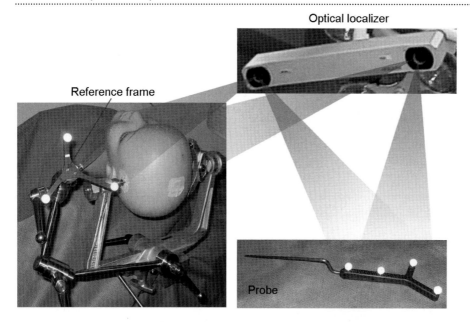

Optical localizer

Reference frame

Probe

Fig. 80.5 Navigation process involving optical localization, frame referencing, and probe.

- Automatic: Automatic recognition of geometric position of dedicated markers, which are fixed to a head-holder (in cases of iMRI) or scanner gantry (in cases of iCT) and are scanned with the patient. They are used by the navigation platform to achieve the registration.
6. *What are the existing types of localizers?*
   - Optical localizers (using an infrared camera)[14]
     - Passive tracking: Using reflective spheres that are placed on the reference frame (patient), probes, and/or any surgical instrument (**Fig. 80.5**).
     - Active tracking: The reference frame (patient) and probes are equipped with light emitting diodes.
   - Magnetic localizers: Magnetic signals that are emitted by the probe and picked up by a receiver indicating its location in space. This modality avoids the disadvantage of a clear line of sight required for optical localizers.[16]
   - Mechanical localizers: Articulated arms equipped with transducers giving the angular position.
   - Ultrasound localizers: Navigation probes transmit ultrasonic signals that are picked up by a receiver indicating its location in space.
7. *How do you classify intraoperative imaging?*
   - Real time[3,17]
     - Intraoperative ultrasound (iUS)
     - Intraoperative angiography
     - Fluoroscopy

- Preacquired[11]
  - iMRI
  - iCT
8. *Give examples where intraoperative imaging may be useful.*
   - Here are some examples of the use of intraoperative imaging.
     - iMRI, iCT, or iUS for detection or residual tumor[18]
     - iMRI, iCT, or iUS to compensate for brain shift
     - Reregister using intraoperative landmarks if the patient moves during surgery
     - iMRA, iCTA, or intraoperative angiography after clipping aneurysms or resecting arteriovenous malformations from the brain or spinal cord[17,19]
     - iUS to localize ventricles, cysts, and lesions in the brain and spinal cord
     - iUS for recalibration of navigation
     - iCT or iMRI for immediate localization of depth electrodes, strips, and grids (in epilepsy surgery), or deep brain stimulators (in functional and behavioral neurosurgery) to readjust them if needed[20]
9. *Compare the advantages and disadvantages of iCT with iMRI.*
   - See **Table 80.1**[21-24]

Table 80.1   Advantages and Disadvantages of Intraoperative Computed Tomography (iCT) and Intraoperative Magnetic Resonance Imaging (iMRI)

	iCT	iMRI
Need for nonferromagnetic tools	No	Yes (within the 5 Gauss line)
Radiation exposure to patient and medical staff	Yes	No
Soft tissue accuracy	+	+++
Bony information	+++	+
Angiography and venography	Yes	Yes
Functional imaging	No	Yes
Tractography	No	Yes
Need for different coils for different regions of the body	No	Yes
Imaging acquisition time	Seconds	Minutes
Cost	Less	More

Source: Data from Archip N, Clatz O, Whalen S, et al. Compensation of geometric distortion effects on intraoperative magnetic resonance imaging for enhanced visualization in image-guided neurosurgery. Neurosurgery 2008; 62(3, Suppl 1):209–215. Lipson AC, Gargollo PC, Black PM. Intraoperative magnetic resonance imaging: considerations for the operating room of the future. J Clin Neurosci 2001;8(4):305–310. Okudera H, Kyoshima K, Kobayashi S, Sugita K. Intraoperative CT scan findings during resection of glial tumours. Neurol Res 1994;16(4):265–267. Engle DJ, Lunsford LD. Brain tumor resection guided by intraoperative computed tomography. J Neurooncol 1987;4(4):361–370.

■ References

1. Nimsky C, Ganslandt O, von Keller B, Fahlbusch R. Preliminary experience in glioma surgery with intraoperative high-field MRI. Acta Neurochir Suppl (Wien) 2003;88:21–29

2. Nimsky C, Ganslandt O, Von Keller B, Romstöck J, Fahlbusch R. Intraoperative high-field-strength MR imaging: implementation and experience in 200 patients. Radiology 2004;233(1):67–78

3. Rasmussen IA Jr, Lindseth F, Rygh OM, et al. Functional neuronavigation combined with intra-operative 3D ultrasound: initial experiences during surgical resections close to eloquent brain areas and future directions in automatic brain shift compensation of preoperative data. Acta Neurochir (Wien) 2007;149(4):365–378

4. Berman JI, Berger MS, Chung SW, Nagarajan SS, Henry RG. Accuracy of diffusion tensor magnetic resonance imaging tractography assessed using intraoperative subcortical stimulation mapping and magnetic source imaging. J Neurosurg 2007;107(3):488–494

5. Pirotte B, Voordecker P, Neugroschl C, et al. Combination of functional magnetic resonance imaging-guided neuronavigation and intraoperative cortical brain mapping improves targeting of motor cortex stimulation in neuropathic pain. Neurosurgery 2008; 62(6, Suppl 3):941–956

6. Chakraborty A, McEvoy AW. Presurgical functional mapping with functional MRI. Curr Opin Neurol 2008;21(4):446–451

7. Sobottka SB, Bredow J, Beuthien-Baumann B, Reiss G, Schackert G, Steinmeier R. Comparison of functional brain PET images and intraoperative brain-mapping data using image-guided surgery. Comput Aided Surg 2002;7(6):317–325

8. Tovar-Spinoza ZS, Ochi A, Rutka JT, Go C, Otsubo H. The role of magnetoencephalography in epilepsy surgery. Neurosurg Focus 2008;25(3):E16

9. Fengqiang L, Jiadong Q, Yi L. Computer-assisted stereotactic neurosurgery with framework neurosurgery navigation. Clin Neurol Neurosurg 2008;110(7):696–700

10. Haberland N, Ebmeier K, Hliscs R, et al. Neuronavigation in surgery of intracranial and spinal tumors. J Cancer Res Clin Oncol 2000;126(9):529–541

11. Grunert P, Müller-Forell W, Darabi K, et al. Basic principles and clinical applications of neuronavigation and intraoperative computed tomography. Comput Aided Surg 1998;3(4):166–173

12. Matula C, Rössler K, Reddy M, Schindler E, Koos WT. Intraoperative computed tomography guided neuronavigation: concepts, efficiency, and work flow. Comput Aided Surg 1998;3(4):174–182

13. Kober H, Nimsky C, Vieth J, Fahlbusch R, Ganslandt O. Co-registration of function and anatomy in frameless stereotaxy by contour fitting. Stereotact Funct Neurosurg 2002;79(3–4):272–283

14. Lemieux L, Jagoe R. Effect of fiducial marker localization on stereotactic target coordinate calculation in CT slices and radiographs. Phys Med Biol 1994;39(11):1915–1928

15. Whalen C, Maclin EL, Fabiani M, Gratton G. Validation of a method for coregistering scalp recording locations with 3D structural MR images. Hum Brain Mapp 2008;29(11):1288–1301

16. Reinhardt H, Trippel M, Westermann B, Gratzl O. Computer aided surgery with special focus on neuronavigation. Comput Med Imaging Graph 1999;23(5):237–244

17. Ayad M, Ulm AJ, Yao T, Eskioglu E, Mericle RA. Real-time image guidance for open vascular neurosurgery using digital angiographic roadmapping. Neurosurgery 2007; 61(3, Suppl):55–61

18. Enchev YP, Popov RV, Romansky KV, Marinov MB, Bussarsky VA. Neuronavigated surgery of intracranial cavernomas–enthusiasm for high technologies or a gold standard? Folia Med (Plovdiv) 2008;50(2):11–17

19. Flasque N, Desvignes M, Constans JM, Revenu M. Acquisition, segmentation and tracking of the cerebral vascular tree on 3D magnetic resonance angiography images. Med Image Anal 2001;5(3):173–183

20. Levivier M, Wikler D, Massager N, Legros B, Van Bogaert P, Brotchi J. Intraoperative MRI and epilepsy surgery. Neurochirurgie 2008;54(3):448–452

21. Archip N, Clatz O, Whalen S, et al. Compensation of geometric distortion effects on intraoperative magnetic resonance imaging for enhanced visualization in image-guided neurosurgery. Neurosurgery 2008; 62(3, Suppl 1):209–215

22. Lipson AC, Gargollo PC, Black PM. Intraoperative magnetic resonance imaging: considerations for the operating room of the future. J Clin Neurosci 2001;8(4):305–310

23. Okudera H, Kyoshima K, Kobayashi S, Sugita K. Intraoperative CT scan findings during resection of glial tumours. Neurol Res 1994;16(4):265–267

24. Engle DJ, Lunsford LD. Brain tumor resection guided by intraoperative computed tomography. J Neurooncol 1987;4(4):361–370

Section II Spinal and Peripheral Nerve Pathology

Case 81   Lower Cervical Fracture Dislocation

Joseph A. Shehadi and Brian Seaman

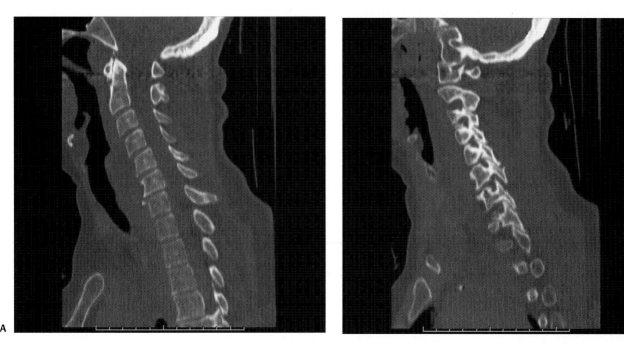

Fig. 81.1   Computed tomography scan of the cervical spine with **(A)** midsagittal view and **(B)** parasagittal view through the left-sided facet joints.

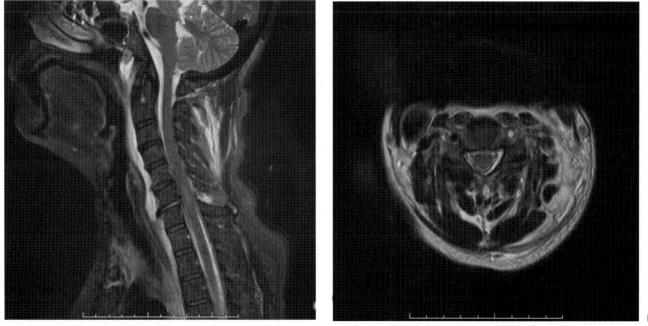

Fig. 81.2   Magnetic resonance imaging scan of the cervical spine with **(A)** sagittal T2-weighted image and **(B)** axial T2-weighted image at the level of C6.

■ Clinical Presentation

- A 60-year-old right-handed woman presents with neck pain and transient quadriplegia following a jet-ski accident.
- Her neurologic exam is significant for a grade 4/5 weakness in her left triceps, wrist flexors, wrist extensors, and intrinsic muscles of the left hand. Allodynia was present in her left hand and in the ulnar side of both forearms. Her reflexes were 2/4 throughout with the exception of her left triceps, which was absent.
- Computed tomography (CT) of the cervical spine was obtained, which is illustrated in **Fig. 81.1**.

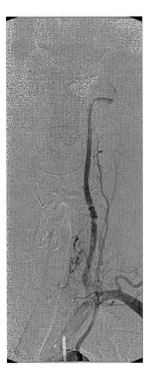

Fig. 81.3 Angiogram of the left vertebral artery demonstrating a marked luminal irregularity and filling defect which begins ~3–4 cm beyond its origin from the subclavian artery and extends cephalad ~3 cm at the level of the patient's cervical spine injury.

■ Questions

1. Interpret the CT of the cervical spine.
2. What is your initial management for this patient?
3. Are there any additional studies you would order?
4. Magnetic resonance imaging of the cervical spine is obtained (**Fig. 81.2**). Interpret the images.
5. Describe the two-column model of the subaxial cervical spine. Briefly describe the mechanistic classification of Allen et al.[3] for subaxial spine injuries.
6. What is this patient's American Spinal Injuries Association (ASIA) grade?

You decide that surgical intervention is indicated for this patient. This would allow for safe and expedient mobilization, as well as preservation of the neural elements. Prior to surgical intervention, an angiogram of the cervical vessels was completed, which demonstrated a dissected left vertebral artery (**Fig. 81.3**).

7. Discuss and justify your proposed surgical plan.
8. What recommendations would you have for the anesthesia staff prior to surgical intervention?
9. List the potential risks associated with anterior approaches to the cervical spinal column.

10. Discuss how you would proceed if you encountered an intraoperative dural tear during your anterior approach.
11. Describe the four segments of the vertebral artery. What are your treatment recommendations in regard to the patient's vertebral artery dissection?
12. During placement of one of the left lateral mass screws you encounter substantial arterial bleeding, which you presume is the vertebral artery. Describe how you would proceed if a vertebral artery were injured intraoperatively.

The patient successfully underwent a combined anterior and posterior cervical fusion. Antiplatelet therapy was initiated to treat the vertebral artery dissection. Gabapentin was initiated for the treatment of the patient's neuropathic sensory complaints.

13. Detail an outpatient follow-up plan for this patient.
14. Discuss the potential delayed surgical complications, which may occur after a cervical instrumented fusion.

■ Answers

1. *Interpret the CT of the cervical spine.*
   - CT of the cervical spine with sagittal reconstructions show widening of spinous processes and zygohypophyseal joints on the left at C6–C7, but no gross malalignment and no fracture.
   - There also appears to be a fractured osteophyte at the anterosuperior border of C7.

2. *What is your initial management for this patient?*
   - The management of airway, breathing, and circulatory stability should be maintained according to Advanced Trauma Life Support protocol.
   - Spinal precautions and cervical spine immobilization should be maintained and a rigid cervical orthosis should be implemented.
   - A thorough neurologic assessment should be completed with continued monitoring of any deficits.
   - Methylprednisolone (Solu-Medrol, Pfizer Pharmaceuticals, New York, NY) can be given intravenously if injury is less than 8 hours.

3. *Are there any additional studies you would order?*
   - Magnetic resonance imaging (MRI) is helpful in this patient to determine whether ligamentous injury is present. Injury to the anterior longitudinal ligament (ALL), posterior longitudinal ligament (PLL), posterior interspinous and supraspinous ligaments, facet capsules, and disk spaces can be appreciated. It is critical to identify injury to these structures because this affects the surgical approach.
   - Additionally, MRI is the study of choice to evaluate the neural elements if neurologic signs or symptoms are present.
   - Magnetic resonance angiography or CT angiography should be considered in these individuals to assess for cervicocephalic arterial dissections given the patient's distracting injury and complaint of occipital-based headaches and neck pain.[1,2]

4. *MRI of the cervical spine is obtained (**Fig. 81.2**). Interpret the images.*
   - Superimposed upon chronic diskogenic changes at C5–C6 and C6–C7 is an acute injury at C6–C7 with fluid in the intervertebral disk space and disruption of the interspinous ligaments.
   - There is extensive fluid beneath the ALL throughout the cervical spine.
   - A cord contusion is present at the level of C6–C7. Additionally, there is an absent left vertebral artery flow void on axial slices (**Fig. 81.2B**).
   - Significant posterolateral muscle trauma with edema is present.

5. *Describe the two-column model of the subaxial cervical spine. Briefly describe the mechanistic classification of Allen et al.[3] for subaxial spine injuries.*
   - Anterior column components include the ALL, inter-vertebral disk and annulus fibrosis, vertebral body, and PLL.
   - The posterior column components include the pedicles, posterior neural arch, and the posterior ligamentous tension band.
   - In 1982, Allen and colleagues[3] introduced a comprehensive classification system of injuries. This system includes three common mechanisms of spinal trauma: compression–flexion, distraction–flexion, and compression–extension. Distraction–extension and lateral flexion subtypes are less common. Vertical compression injury results in anterior column failure or a burst-type injury. These are further classified into stages of progressive injury.[3]

6. *What is this patient's ASIA grade?*
   - The patient's ASIA impairment scale is D–Incomplete: Motor preservation below the neurologic level (C5), and at least half of the key muscles below the neurologic level have a muscle grade of 3 or more.

7. *Discuss and justify your proposed surgical plan.*
   - Radiographically, there are multiple sites of injury including the ALL, PLL, intervertebral disk space at C6–C7, and posterior ligamentous structures.
   - The discoligamentous injury at C6–C7 in conjunction with an incomplete spinal cord injury justifies the need for a combined anterior and posterior fusion.
   - We performed an anterior cervical diskectomy with allograft bone graft and anterior cervical plating at the C6–C7 level using fluoroscopic guidance and electrophysiologic monitoring. Two days later an adjunctive posterior instrumentation was completed using polyaxial lateral mass screws and rod fixation (**Fig. 81.4**).
   - Note that posteriorly, one could have also done a C6–C7 fusion only instead of fusing C5 to C7.
   - The left-sided screws were placed first, and extra care was taken during placement secondary to the known vertebral artery injury.

8. *What recommendations would you have for the anesthesia staff prior to surgical intervention?*
   - Awake fiberoptic intubation technique should be considered, given the cervical spine instability.
   - Prevention of intraoperative hypotension and possible ischemia is critical given the patient's spinal cord injury and unilateral vertebral artery injury.

9. *List the potential risks associated with anterior approaches to the cervical spinal column.*
   - The most common complications of anterior approaches to the cervical spine include recurrent laryngeal nerve palsy with subsequent hoarseness, dysphagia, and odynophagia.[4] Complete paralysis of the vocal cords is rare and is estimated to be around 0.5%.[4]

■ Answers (*continued*)

• Other less common complications include hematoma, large vessel arterial or venous injury/thrombosis, esophageal injury, dural sac manipulation with neurologic injury, dural tear, breathing difficulties or delayed extubation secondary to soft tissue swelling, traction C5 palsy, peripheral and cranial nerve injury (hypoglossal), vertebral artery injury, Horner syndrome from sympathetic chain injury, and thoracic duct injury.[5]

10. *Discuss how you would proceed if you encountered an intraoperative dural tear during your anterior approach.*
   • One can attempt a primary repair utilizing microsurgical techniques.
   • Frequently, Gelfoam (Pfizer Pharmaceuticals, New York, NY) or collagen matrix (preferably inlay) and fibrin glue or hydrogel sealant can be placed over the defect, with care not to compress or manipulate the cord.
   • Lumbar drainage can be used as an adjunctive measure.[5]

11. *Describe the four segments of the vertebral artery. What are your treatment recommendations in regard to the patient's vertebral artery dissection?*
   • The segments of the vertebral arteries are as follows.
      – Segment I runs from the subclavian artery to the transverse foramina of cervical vertebra C5 or C6.
      – Segment II runs within the transverse foramina of C5/C6 to C2.
      – Segment III is tortuous and begins at the transverse foramen of C2 then C1, runs posterolaterally to loop around the posterior arch of C1, and passes subsequently between the atlas and the occiput.
      – Segment IV is the intracranial segment and begins as it pierces the dura at the foramen magnum and terminates at the vertebrobasilar junction.
   • Neurologic injury from posttraumatic vertebral artery dissection is often preventable with early diagnosis and therapy. Moreover, the diagnosis of a vertebral artery thrombosis may change the surgical plan, to prevent bilateral vertebral artery compromise.
   • If indicated, the use of systemic anticoagulation may be protective against cerebral thromboembolism.
   • Miller et al.[6] found that patients with vertebral artery injury treated with anticoagulation or antiplatelet therapy had a stroke rate of 2.6%, whereas untreated patients developed stroke 54% of the time.
   • If anticoagulation or antiplatelet therapy is contraindicated, then interventional embolization or surgical ligation can be considered.

12. *During placement of one of the left lateral mass screws you encounter substantial arterial bleeding, which you presume is the vertebral artery. Describe how you would proceed if a vertebral artery were injured intraoperatively.*
   • If the vertebral artery is injured from a posterior approach, then direct repair is not feasible. The screw should be kept in and intraoperative or immediate postoperative angiography is then performed.
   • Endovascular obliteration is a good option for the management of a pseudoaneurysm after vertebral artery injury as long as the vertebral artery injured is not dominant.[7]

13. *Detail an outpatient follow-up plan for this patient.*
   • The patient should initially follow up in the first 2 weeks for wound observation and preservation of spinal alignment.
   • Radiographically, fusion can be appreciated over the course of ~3 months.
   • Follow-up appointment may occur every month with plain cervical radiographs. Flexion and extension views can be performed to confirm spinal stability.
   • A hard collar should be maintained for at least 6 weeks. At the time of radiographic fusion, remove the collar and begin isometric exercises and physical therapy.

14. *Discuss the potential delayed surgical complications, which may occur after a cervical instrumented fusion.*
   • Delayed complications following cervical fusion include pseudoarthrosis, hardware failure, and postsurgical kyphosis.
   • Pseudoarthrosis is a known cause of persistent neck pain and radiculopathy following anterior cervical discectomy and fusion.[8] Pseudoarthrosis rates increase with multilevel constructs and may be as high as 50% for three-level fusions.[4] In patients who undergo anterior cervical surgery with resultant symptomatic pseudoarthrosis, a posterior fusion may be more effective than anterior revision.[9] Additionally, anterior cervical plating has reduced the incidence of pseudoarthrosis.
   • Hardware failure or screw loosening typically can be seen at the caudal end of a multilevel construct.[10] Graft displacement can be seen in 2–8% of cases.
   • These complications may be avoided by maximizing screw purchase, preparing a well-fitting graft under compression, and possibly by the use of dynamic anterior cervical plating.[4,10]
   • Postsurgical kyphosis may result in patients suffering significant two-column injuries who undergo anterior cervical surgery alone. Adjunctive-instrumented posterior fusion can reduce the incidence of this complication.
   • Adjacent segment disease can occur above or below the fusion.

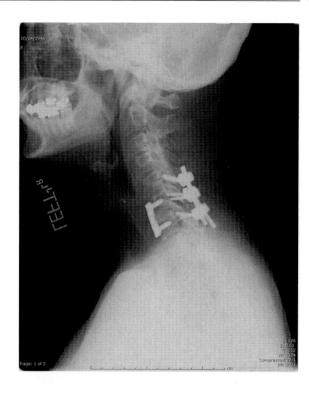

Fig. 81.4 Postoperative lateral cervical spine plain x-ray.

■ References

1. Mokri B, Piepgras DG, Houser OW. Traumatic dissections of the extracranial internal carotid artery. J Neurosurg 1988;68(2):189–197

2. De Sousa JE, Halfon MJ, Bonardo P, Reisin RC, Fernandez Pardal MM. Different pain patterns in patients with vertebral artery dissections. Neurology 2005;64(5):925–926

3. Allen BL Jr, Ferguson RL, Lehman RT, O'Brien RP. A mechanistic classification of closed, indirect fractures and dislocations of the lower cervical spine. Spine 1982;7(1):1–27

4. Winn RH, Youmans JR. Youmans Neurological Surgery. Philadelphia: Saunders; 2004

5. Nakase H, Park YS, Kimura H, Sakaki T, Morimoto T. Complications and long-term follow-up results in titanium mesh cage reconstruction after cervical corpectomy. J Spinal Disord Tech 2006;19(5):353–357

6. Miller PR, Fabian TC, Bee TK, et al. Blunt cerebrovascular injuries: diagnosis and treatment. J Trauma 2001;51(2):279–285

7. Choi JW, Lee JK, Moon KS, et al. Endovascular embolization of iatrogenic vertebral artery injury during anterior cervical spine surgery. Spine 2006;31(23):E891–E894

8. Kuhns CA, Geck MJ, Wand JC, Delamarter RB. An outcomes analysis of the treatment of cervical pseudarthrosis with posterior fusion. Spine 2005;30(21):2424–2429

9. Carreon L, Glassman SD, Dimar J, Campbell MJ. Treatment of anterior cervical pseudoarthrosis: posterior fusion versus anterior revision. Spine J 2006;6(2):154–156

10. Panjabi MM, Isomi T, Wang JL. Loosening of the screw-vertebra junction in multilevel anterior plate contructs. Spine 1999;24(22):2383–2388

Case 82 Atlantoaxial Instability

Eric P. Roger and Edward Benzel

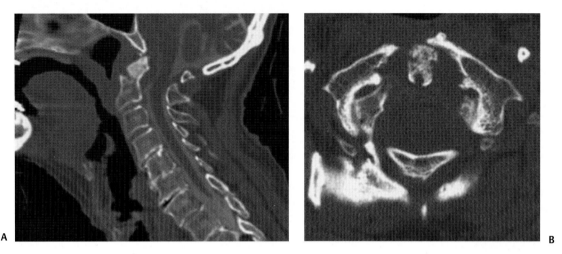

Fig. 82.1 **(A)** Sagittal computed tomography (CT) reconstruction with myelographic subarachnoid contrast injection. **(B)** Axial CT nonmyelogram cut at the level of C1 through the dens.

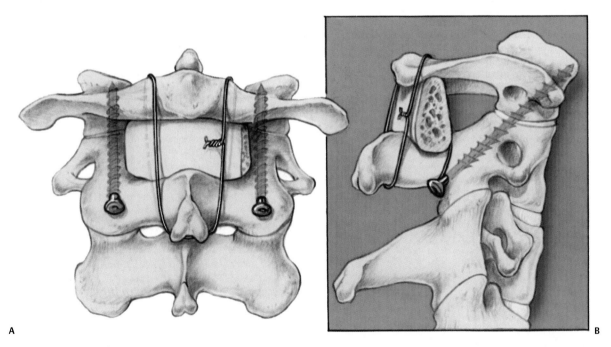

Fig. 82.2 Artist's rendering of ideal trajectory of C1–C2 transarticular screws with **(A)** anteroposterior and **(B)** lateral illustrations. Posterior wiring with interspinous iliac graft is also depicted. Note that the posterior wiring of C1 to C2 may require a structurally intact arch of C1 and may not be feasible in some cases of Jef-ferson fracture (such as possibly in this case). (From Wolfla CE, Resnick DK. Neurosurgical Operative Atlas. Spine and Peripheral Nerves. New York: Thieme/American Association of Neurological Surgeons; 2006. Reprinted with permission.)

■ Clinical Presentation

- An 83-year-old man presents with neck pain.
- He had sustained a fall 6 months prior. There was no documentation of fracture at the time. He has been experiencing neck pain since the fall.
- He denies any bladder or bowel dysfunction, gait or balance disorders.

- He is admitted for generalized weakness and shortness of breath.
- Upon further workup, he is found to be severely hyperkalemic with mental changes.
- His past medical history is remarkable for placement of a cardiac pacemaker.

■ Questions

1. What would be the sequence of radiologic investigations recommended for this patient?
2. Interpret the images in **Fig. 82.1.**
3. Is this an acute or chronic process? Why?
4. How commonly are the pathologies at C1 and C2 associated?
5. What are your therapeutic options at this point? How likely are they to be successful in achieving stability?
6. Is spinal cord decompression indicated?

7. What techniques are available for C1–C2 fixation? What factors would influence the decision making?
8. Would an odontoid screw be a good surgical option in this patient?
9. List the disadvantages of posterior C1–C2 fusion.
10. What would you do if you had pulsatile bright red blood while drilling the trajectory for the placement of the transarticular C2 screw?

■ Answers

1. *What would be the sequence of radiologic investigations recommended for this patient?*
   - The patient should be investigated with the following:
     - Chest radiograph; the patient is short of breath
     - Plain anteroposterior (AP) and lateral cervical radiographs
     - Magnetic resonance imaging (MRI) is unfortunately not possible due to the presence of a pacemaker.
     - Computed tomography (CT) myelogram is the best "second choice" instead of an MRI to assess the status of spinal cord and soft tissues (anterior soft tissue swelling and pannus). You may skip the CT myelogram if the patient is not myelopathic.
     - CT scan is best to assess bony integrity and bony anatomy. It is highly indicated preoperatively for atlantoaxial stabilization.
     - Flexion/extension radiographs should never be performed when previous imaging shows evidence of instability. These should only be used to confirm previously negative/normal imaging.[1]
2. *Interpret the images in* **Fig. 82.1**.
   - Type II odontoid fracture with minimal translation, but ~60 degrees of posterior angulation
   - Soft tissue pannus behind the odontoid, partially indenting the cerebrospinal fluid (CSF) space, but not in direct contact with the cord (at least in this static CT image in supine position)

- Axial image demonstrates anterior atlantal ring fracture consistent with a Jefferson fracture (posterior ring fracture not illustrated). This finding is suggested on **Fig. 82.1A** by the absence of the anterior ring on this midline cut.
- Various levels of degenerative changes are noted through the rest of the cervical spine, without evidence of cord compression.
3. *Is this an acute or chronic process? Why?*
   - These fractures are likely to be chronic because of the following:
     - The fracture line at the base of the dens appears sclerotic.
     - The fracture of the anterior atlantal arch is completely corticated.
     - Soft tissue pannus formation behind the odontoid is suggestive of chronic instability.
     - The patient presents with a fall 6 months prior, with neck pain since. There is no clinical evidence of an acute fall (i.e., don't forget the clues given on history!).
4. *How commonly are the pathologies at C1 and C2 associated?*
   - Axis fractures are relatively commonly associated with C1 fractures. Odontoid fractures (type II or III) are associated to C1 fractures in up to 53% of cases, and up to 26% with hangman's fractures. They are reported to have a higher morbidity and mortality rate. Treatment is primarily based on the characteristics of the C2 fracture.[2]

■ **Answers** (*continued*)

5. *What are your therapeutic options at this point? How likely are they to be successful in achieving stability?*
   - Conservative management:
     – Soft collar
     – Semirigid collar (Philadelphia, Aspen, Miami J, etc.)
     – Rigid cervicothoracic orthosis
       ▪ Minerva brace
       ▪ Halo
   - Surgical stabilization[3]
     – Occipitocervical fusion
     – Atlantoaxial fusion
     – Odontoid screw is *not* an option in chronic fractures.
   - As these fractures are chronic, they are highly unlikely to heal with any type of external immobilization. Stability can be obtained only by open fixation and bone grafting. Conservative management should be considered only for patients medically unfit for surgery or, obviously, for patients refusing surgery.
   - Halo bracing is poorly tolerated by geriatric patients. Furthermore, although solid fixation of the head and chest may be achieved, paradoxical "snaking" motion of the cervical spine may occur.
   - Open fixation with bone grafting has a high fusion rate (>90%), except in smokers or in patients on steroids.

6. *Is spinal cord decompression indicated?*
   - No. As illustrated by the CT myelogram, although there is soft tissue pannus formation with indentation onto the CSF space, there is no active cord contact or compression.
   - Furthermore, the patient does not present with any signs of myelopathy.

7. *What techniques are available for C1–C2 fixation? What factors would influence the decision making?*
   - Available techniques include the following[3,4]:
     – Spinous process wiring (requires a structurally intact arch of C1):
       ▪ Gallie fusion
       ▪ Brookes fusion
       ▪ Modified Sonntag fusion
     – C1–2 fixation:
       ▪ C1 and C2 pars screws
       ▪ C1 pars and C2 pedicle screws
       ▪ C1 pars and C2 translaminar/interlaminar screws
       ▪ C1–C2 transarticular screws
       ▪ C1–C2 Halifax clamps
     – Odontoid screw placement
     – Occiput to C2 fixation

- C1–C2 spinous process wiring (Brooks, Gallie, Sonntag) is a good adjunct to transarticular screws or to a segmented fusion but is not biomechanically a very strong construct when used as standalone.[5]
- Spinous process wiring may be performed in a variety of ways but requires the integrity of the lamina and spinous process of C2, as well as integrity of the posterior arch of C1. In this case, although no decompression is required, there is loss of integrity of the arch of C1 due to the Jefferson fracture.
- C1–C2 transarticular screw placement and C1–C2 segmental fusion (C1 lateral mass screws, C2 pars interarticularis screws/C2 pedicle screw fixation) in conjunction with spinous process wiring results in biomechanically strong constructs with higher rates of successful fusion when compared with spinous process wiring alone.[6]
- C1–C2 posterior fixation techniques do not rely on the integrity of the posterior elements. Nonetheless, they are not without risk. Specifically, the trajectory of the vertebral artery and bony anatomy of the C2 pars must be carefully studied on preoperative imaging. High-riding vertebral arteries or a thin C2 pars may preclude the placement of a transarticular screw (**Fig. 82.2** for ideal screw trajectory). If the arches of C1 or C2 are compromised (making spinous process wiring procedure not feasible), an onlay fusion laterally at the level of the articulating processes may alternatively be used in conjunction with C1–C2 transarticular screw placement.
- C2 fixation using translaminar/interlaminar screws significantly reduces the risks to the vertebral artery, although epidural cortical breach is possible.
- Preservation of C1–C2 rotation can also be achieved with a halo; however, this comes with associated morbidity in the elderly population.[7]

8. *Would an odontoid screw be a good surgical option in this patient?*
   - Odontoid screws are indicated for acute type II odontoid fractures only. The screw is intended to "pull" the free dens against the C2 body, encouraging healing by compression along the fracture line. It is not a good option in this case.

9. *List the disadvantages of posterior C1–C2 fusion.*
   - Disadvantages of C1–C2 posterior fixation include the loss of 50% of head rotation.
   - Furthermore, there is the potential for vertebral artery injury as well as significant venous plexus bleeding during lateral dissection of the C1–C2 joint.
   - The vertebral artery may be located in the path of a transarticular screw on preoperative images on at least one side in 18–23% of patients.[8]

Answers (*continued*)

- Rate of intraoperative vertebral artery injury with this approach is estimated to be 1.7–4.1%.[9]
- When C1–C2 spinous process wiring is utilized as a stand-alone technique, there is a high rate of pseudoarthrosis approaching 30% without halo fixation.[9]

10. *What would you do if you had pulsatile bright red blood while drilling the trajectory for the placement of the transarticular C2 screw?*
    - This is consistent with damage to the vertebral artery. The only way to stop the bleeding is placement of the screw. If this is the first screw (and you still need to do the other side) you should *not* place the second screw for fear of causing bilateral vertebral artery damage potentially leading to devastating neurologic sequelae including death. Unilateral fixation is then accepted. Spinous process wiring may be considered.[9]
    - If such bleeding occurs while working on the second screw, then placement of the screw is again the only way to stop the bleeding.
    - Postoperative vertebral angiogram is indicated if damage to the vertebral artery is suspected. Vertebral artery stenting may be considered.

References

1. Dickman CA, Choudhri TF, Harms J. Trauma surgery: occipitocervical junction. In: Benzel EC, ed. Spine Surgery: Techniques, Complication Avoidance, and Management. Philadelphia: Churchill Livingstone; 2004

2. Guidelines for the management of acute cervical spine and spinal cord injuries: chapter 18 - management of combination fractures of the atlas and axis in adults. Neurosurgery 2002;50(3, Suppl):S140–S147

3. Crockard HA, Soontag KH. Upper cervical and occipitocervical arthrodesis. In: Benzel EC, ed. Spine Surgery: Techniques, Complication Avoidance, and Management. Philadelphia: Churchill Livingstone; 2004

4. Wolfa CE, Resnick DK. Neurosurgical Operative Atlas. Spine and Peripheral Nerves. New York: Thieme/American Association of Neurological Surgeons; 2006

5. Sasso R, Doherty BJ, Crawford MJ, Heggeness MH. Biomechanics of odontoid fracture fixation: comparison of the one- and two-screw technique. Spine 1993;18(14):1950–1953

6. Resnick DK, Lapsiwala S, Trost G. Anatomic suitability of the C1–C2 complex for pedicle screw fixation. Spine 2002;27(14):1494–1498

7. Horn EM, Theodore N, Feiz-Erfan I, Lekovic GP, Dickman CA, Sonntag VK. Complications of halo fixation in the elderly. J Neurosurg Spine 2006;5(1):46–49

8. Paramore CG, Dickman CA, Sonntag VK. The anatomical suitability of the C1–2 complex for transarticular screw fixation. J Neurosurg 1996;85(2):221–224

9. Gluf WM, Schmidt MH, Apfelbaum RI. Atlantoaxial transarticular screw fixation: a review of surgical indications, fusion rate, complications, and lessons learned in 191 adult patients. J Neurosurg Spine 2005;2(2):155–163

Case 83 Type 2 Odontoid Fracture

Joseph A. Shehadi and Brian Seaman

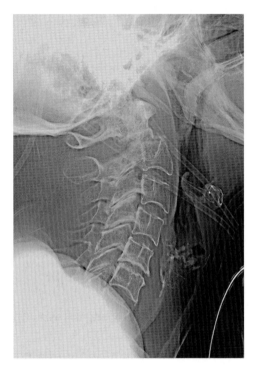

Fig. 83.1 Lateral cervical spine x-ray.

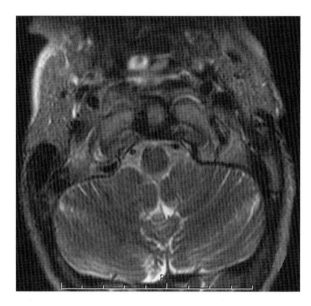

Fig. 83.2 Axial magnetic resonance imaging scan of cervical spine demonstrating transverse ligament.

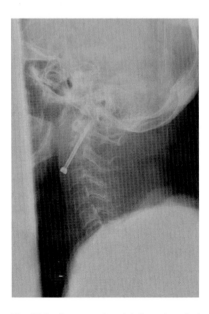

Fig. 83.3 Postoperative plain lateral cervical spine radiograph demonstrating odontoid screw in place.

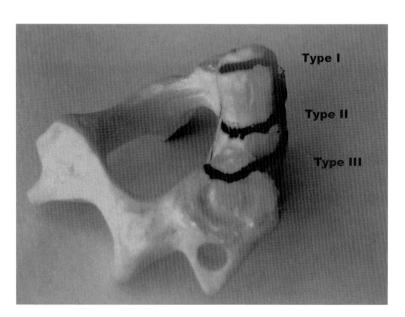

Fig. 83.4 Classification of odontoid fractures.

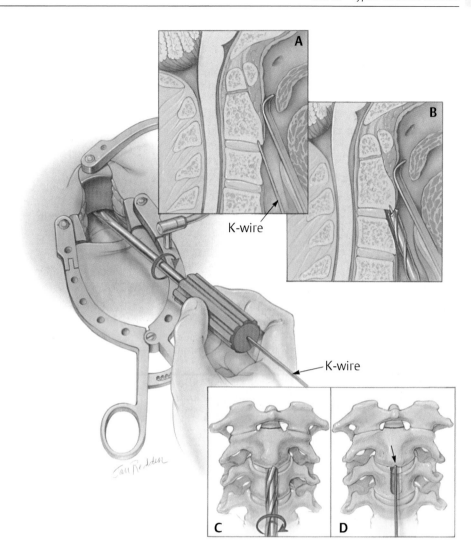

Fig. 83.5 Artist's rendering of odontoid screw placement technique. **(A)** K-wire is placed entering at the anteroinferior edge of C2 and aimed toward the odontoid tip under fluoroscopy. **(B)** This is followed by drilling a hole core over the K-wire. **(C,D)** Part of the C2–C3 anulus is removed with the coring drill. (From Wolfla CE, Resnick DK. Neurosurgical Operative Atlas. Spine and Peripheral Nerves. New York: Thieme/American Association of Neurological Surgeons; 2006:33. Reprinted with permission.)

■ Clinical Presentation

- A 76-year-old woman is involved in a motor vehicle accident. She sustained multiple rib fractures and pelvis fractures. She also complains of severe neck pain.

- Her neurologic exam is unremarkable.
- You are asked to consult on this patient regarding a cervical spine fracture seen on radiographs (**Fig. 83.1**).

■ Questions

1. Interpret the cervical spine radiograph (**Fig. 83.1**).
2. Are there any additional studies you would order and why?
3. Odontoid fracture displacement and angulation are known to be important prognostic factors of fracture healing. Classification of these fractures significantly affects management decisions. Describe the classification system of Anderson and D'Alonzo for odontoid fractures including implications for spinal stability and indications for operation.

It was decided that surgical intervention is indicated for this acute type II odontoid fracture. Magnetic resonance imaging (MRI) was performed and the transverse ligament was intact (**Fig. 83.2**). We elected against halo placement in this patient given the patient's age, associated comorbidities (multiple rib fractures), and the higher risk for nonunion with a halo.

4. Name some contraindications to anterior odontoid screw placement.
5. Explain how you would reduce the fracture segment to achieve osseous contact prior to anterior odontoid screw fixation.

6. Highlight the key procedural steps for anterior odontoid screw placement.

The patient successfully underwent placement of a single odontoid lag screw under general anesthesia (**Fig. 83.3**). The use of one screw is thought to have similar biomechanical strength as two screws side by side.[1] Successful reduction of the fracture segment was obtained during patient positioning. The patient was placed in a hard collar for 3 months. She remained neurologically intact and without neck pain. Follow-up radiographs demonstrated good bony union of the fracture segment.

7. Assume you treat a type II odontoid fracture with halo fixation. After 3 months of fixation the patient develops recurrent neck pain. Flexion–extension radiographs reveal abnormal motion of the dens fragment indicating a nonunion. How would you proceed?
8. How would you manage a patient with an odontoid screw breakage first noted on the 2-month postoperative radiograph?

■ Answers

1. *Interpret the cervical spine radiograph (**Fig. 83.1**).*
   - The sagittal radiograph of the cervical spine demonstrates a fracture of C2, at the base of the odontoid process, consistent with an acute type II odontoid fracture.
   - There is significant retrolisthesis of C1 compared with C2.
   - The atlantodens interval is within normal limits.
2. *Are there any additional studies you would order and why?*
   - MRI is indicated to assess the status of the transverse and alar ligaments as well as the tectorial membrane. The integrity of the transverse ligament in addition to the atlantoaxial distances and relationships significantly affects your management and operative approach.[2]
3. *Odontoid fracture displacement and angulation are known to be important prognostic factors of fracture healing. Classification of these fractures significantly affects management decisions. Describe the classification system of Anderson and D'Alonzo for odontoid fractures including implications for spinal stability and indications for operation.*
   - Anderson and D'Alonzo's classification is described below (**Fig. 83.4**).[3]

- Type I fractures occur through the tip of the dens above the transverse ligament. These are rare injuries and associated occipital–cervical dislocation should be excluded.[4]
- Type II fractures occur through the base of the neck and are the most common fracture subtype.
- Type IIA fractures are similar to type II, but there is comminution and large bone fragments at the fracture site.
- Type III fractures occur through the body of C2 and may involve the articulating facet and marrow space. Type III fractures may be better characterized as horizontal rostral C2 body fracture and not odontoid process fractures.[5]
   - Type I and III fractures are often treated in a conservative fashion.[3] That said, one must consider "shallow" or "high" type III odontoid fractures as potentially unstable fractures.[4,6] Furthermore, anteriorly displaced type III fractures may also be unstable.
   - Attention should be given to the extent of articulating facet injury/ distraction, which can be seen with these injuries.[7]

■ **Answers (*continued*)**

- It is generally accepted that advanced age, fracture displacement >6 mm, and angulation >10 degrees negatively influences union rates.[4,8] Other factors include chronicity of the fracture,[9] delay in diagnosis, fracture comminution,[4] or inability to maintain fracture alignment with external immobilization.[10]
- Type II odontoid fractures in patients 50 years and older should be considered for surgical stabilization and fusion.[10] This is based on a 21 times higher rate of nonunion in patients over the age of 50.[11]

4. *Name some contraindications to anterior odontoid screw placement.*
   - Contraindications for anterior odontoid screw fixation include the inability to reduce anatomically the fracture, nonunion, severe osteoporosis, transverse atlantal ligament rupture, or concomitant Jefferson-type fracture with coronal plane separation of >7 mm, or oblique fracture from anteroinferior to postero-superior.[12]
   - Furthermore, this procedure is difficult in patients with short necks, barrel chests, those unable to tolerate cervical extension (spinal stenosis), or those with tracheostomies or significant open trauma to the anterior aspect of the neck.

5. *Explain how you would reduce the fracture segment to achieve osseous contact prior to anterior odontoid screw fixation.*
   - Typically reduction of an odontoid fracture is obtained under fluoroscopy during operative positioning in the supine position with the Mayfield headholder.
   - Alternatively, Gardner-Wells tongs or manual cervical traction can be utilized to obtain reduction under fluoroscopy. Bivector traction with a flexor component is also an option.

6. *Highlight the key procedural steps for anterior odontoid screw placement.*
   - Details of the procedure are described below[13] and are illustrated in **Fig. 83.5**.[14]
   - The patient is positioned supine. The Mayfield head holder is utilized and the head is fixed in extension. Alternatively, intraoperative traction with Gardner-Wells tongs is utilized.

- High-resolution biplanar fluoroscopic imaging is utilized to ensure reduction of the anterior displaced fracture segment and to guide screw placement.
- An anteromedian neck incision is placed in the region of C5–C6.
- An avascular plane is dissected cephalad until the anteroinferior border of C2 is reached.[15]
- A Hohmann retractor may be used to aid in exposure. Then, a high-speed drill is used to make a trough in the superior portion of C3 to allow for a proper angle when drilling a pilot hole.
- A K-wire is inserted and then a long 2.5 mm cannulated drill is inserted into the trough and angled posterior to reach the dorsal portion of the odontoid tip.
- On the anteroposterior projection midline trajectory is confirmed.
- The pilot hole is drilled, and the depth of the hole is measured.
- Then the appropriate-length 3.5-mm cannulated lag screw is placed through the pilot hole to obtain bicortical purchase.[16,17] Compression of the fracture segment should be seen.

7. *Assume you treat a type II odontoid fracture with halo fixation. After 3 months of fixation, the patient develops recurrent neck pain. Flexion–extension radiographs reveal abnormal motion of the dens fragment, indicating a nonunion. How would you proceed?*
   - The development of high cervical neck pain or signs of myelopathy may signal nonunion.
   - An anterior odontoid screw is not recommended at this time secondary to fibrous scar, which is present at the fracture site.
   - In this situation, a posterior C1–C2 fusion would be indicated.[4,18,19]

8. *How would you manage a patient with an odontoid screw breakage first noted on the 2-month postoperative radiograph?*
   - Screw breakage may be a sign of nonunion. Initially, a computed tomography scan of the cervical spine and flexion–extension x-rays should be performed. If a clear lucency is appreciated near the fracture site or if there is movement of the fracture segment, then a posterior cervical C1–C2 fusion should be considered.[18,19]

References

1. Sasso R, Doherty BJ, Crawford MJ, Heggeness MH. Biomechanics of odontoid fracture fixation: comparison of the one- and two-screw technique. Spine 1993;18(14):1950–1953
2. Yuksel M, Heiserman JE, Sonntag VK, Benzel EC, Menezes AH, Shaffrey CI. Magnetic resonance imaging of the craniocervical junction at 3T: observation of the accessory atlantoaxial ligaments. Neurosurgery 2006;59(4):888–892
3. Anderson LD, D'Alonzo RT. Fractures of the odontoid process of the axis. J Bone Joint Surg Am 1974;56(8):1663–1674
4. Maak TG, Grauer JN. The contemporary treatment of odontoid injuries. Spine 2006; 31(11, Suppl):S53–S60
5. Benzel EC, Hart BL, Ball PA, Baldwin NG, Orrison WW, Espinosa M. Fractures of the C-2 vertebral body. J Neurosurg 1994;81(2):206–212
6. Carlson GD, Heller JG, Abitbol JJ. Odontoid fractures. In: Levine AM, ed. Spine Trauma. Philadelphia: WB Saunders; 1998
7. Cholavech C. Spinal injuries. In: Trieu L, Templeton J, Sherry E, eds. Trauma. Oxford: University Press; 2003
8. Papagelopoulos PJ, Currier BL, Hokari Y, et al. Biomechanical comparison of C1–C2 posterior arthrodesis techniques. Spine 2007;32(13):E363–E370
9. Jea A, Tatsui C, Farhat H, Vanni S, Levi AD. Vertically unstable type III odontoid fractures: case report. Neurosurgery 2006;58(4):E797
10. Hadley MN, Dickman CA, Browner CM, Sonntag VK. Isolated fractures of the axis in adults. Neurosurgery 2002;50(3):S125–S139
11. Lennarson PJ, Mostafavi H, Traynelis VC, Walters BC. Management of type II dens fractures: a case-control study. Spine 2000;25(10):1234–1237
12. Vaccaro AR, Albert TJ. Spine Surgery: Tricks of the Trade. New York: Thieme Medical Publishers; 2002
13. Apfelbaum RI, Lonser RR, Veres R, Casey A. Direct anterior screw fixation for recent and remote odontoid fractures. J Neurosurg 2000; 93(2, Suppl):227–236
14. Wolfa CE, Resnick DK. Neurosurgical Operative Atlas. Spine and Peripheral Nerves. New York: Thieme/American Association of Neurological Surgeons;2006: 33
15. Benzel EC, ed. Trauma Surgery: Occipitocervical Junction in Spine Surgery: Techniques, Complications, Avoidance, and Management. Philadelphia: Elsevier; 1999
16. Aebi M, Thalgott JS, Webb JK. AO ASIF Prinicples in Spine Surgery. New York: Springer/AO Publishing; 1998
17. Dickman CA, Foley KT, Sonntag VK, Smith MM. Cannulated screws for odontoid screw fixation and atlantoaxial transarticular screw fixation. Technical note. J Neurosurg 1995;83(6):1095–1100
18. Chavasiri C. Late treatment of nonunion of odontoid fracture. Tech Orthop 2006;21(2):115–120
19. Aebi M, Etter C, Coscia M. Fractures of the odontoid process: treatment with anterior screw fixation. Spine 1989;14(10):1065–1070

Case 84   Basilar Invagination

Michel Lacroix

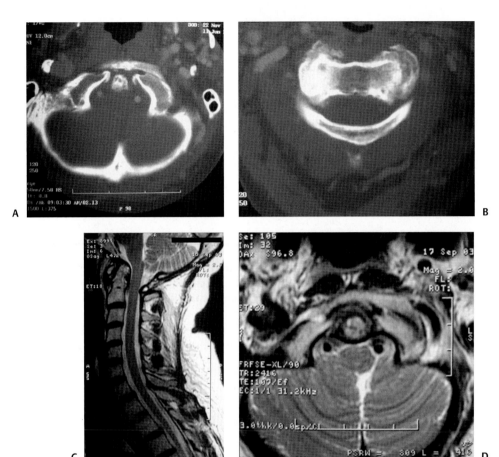

Fig. 84.1 Cervical spine imaging with **(A)** axial computed tomography at the level of the foramen magnum and **(B)** at the atlantoaxial junction. **(C)** T2-weighted sagittal magnetic resonance image (MRI) and **(D)** axial MRI at the level of the foramen magnum.

▪ Clinical Presentation

- A 55-year-old woman with rheumatoid arthritis presents with neck pain and progressive difficulty ambulating.
- She suffers from bilateral limbs paresthesias. She is showing signs of myelopathy with hyperreflexia and bilateral Babinski's signs.
- Computed tomography (CT) scan and magnetic resonance imaging (MRI) of the cervical spine are obtained (**Fig. 84.1**).

▪ Questions

1. Are there any other symptoms or signs you would like to verify?
2. Interpret the CT and the MRI scans.
3. What is your initial management?
4. What studies do you order?
5. What is your course of action?

After gradually putting her in 12 pounds of traction and mild sedation for 4 days, the CT scan shows visible reduction.

6. Describe the surgical options and select the one you would prefer.

A posterior occipitocervical fusion, in situ distraction with transarticular C1–C2 screws and iliac crest autograft fusion was performed. A postoperative radiograph is shown in **Fig. 84.2**. Solid fusion was observed and myelopathy improved.

7. After posterior fusion, what is the natural history of the basilar invagination?

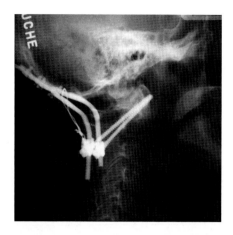

Fig. 84.2 Cervical spine lateral radiograph. An instrumented occipitocervical fusion with occipital screws and transarticular atlanto–axial screws is visible.

■ Answers

1. *Are there any other symptoms or signs you would like to verify?*
   - Hypoglossal, glossopharyngeal vagus, and trigeminal nerve deficit and neurogenic bladder are signs of severe dysfunction at the craniovertebral junction.[1,2]
   - The accentuation of the symptoms in flexion and extension may suggest an atlantooccipital segment hypermobility.
2. *Interpret the CT and the MRI.*
   - On the axial CT scan, the erosion and compression of the lateral atlantal masses as well as the penetration of the dens beyond the level of the occipital condyle in the foramen magnum are visualized. The sagittal

T2-weighted MRI image of the cervical spine clearly shows some typical findings.[3,4]
   - The downward separation of the anterior arch of the atlas from the clivus provokes a descent of the atlas arch onto the axis body.
   - The displacement of the posterior arch of the atlas rostrally and ventrally causes a decrease in the anteroposterior diameter of the spinal canal.

The inflammatory rheumatoid pannus and the resulting compression of the medulla are seen in both the axial and sagittal MRI. There is no syringomyelia or Chiari malformation. The craniometric lines[3,5] in lateral view are shown in **Fig. 84.3**.

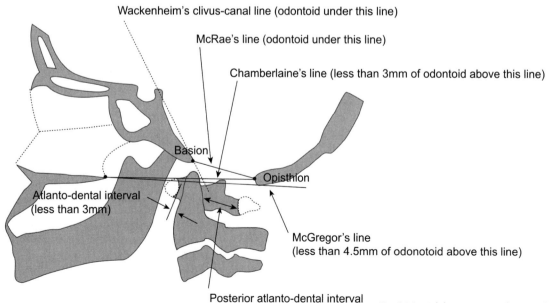

Wackenheim's clivus-canal line (odontoid under this line)

McRae's line (odontoid under this line)

Chamberlaine's line (less than 3mm of odontoid above this line)

Basion

Opisthion

Atlanto-dental interval (less than 3mm)

McGregor's line (less than 4.5mm of odonotoid above this line)

Posterior atlanto-dental interval (14mm or greater)

Fig. 84.3 Adult craniometric lines (and normal values) in lateral view.

■ **Answers (*continued*)**

3. *What is your initial management?*
   - Marks and Sharp[2] showed in 1981 that untreated myelopathic rheumatoid patients died within 6 months of presentation. Furthermore, most myelopathic rheumatoid patients (56%, $n = 18$) treated with conservative measures only (collar or traction alone) also died within 6 months.[2]
   - Treatment should be planned immediately.

4. *What studies do you order?*
   - Spinal and complete systemic workup are in order:
     - Flexion–extension cervical spine x-rays. Any increase in the atlantodental interval confirms the instability, which is consistently associated with the basilar invagination.[1,3,4]
     - Consider dynamic MRI in flexion and extension to identify instability and sites of compression.
     - Preoperative blood work including nutritional status (lymphocyte count and liver function tests).
     - Discontinue nonsteroidal antiinflammatory agents 1 week prior to surgery. Methotrexate and steroids may be used for pain management preoperatively.
     - Cardiac status, pulmonary function assessment tests, and anesthesia consult should be obtained.

5. *What is your course of action?*
   - A period of 4 to 5 days of halo traction with mild sedation and a maximum of 12 pounds of charge can reduce a basilar invagination of less than 15 mm.[4]
   - Traction is contraindicated in posterior occipitoatlantal dislocation or complex rotatory luxations.

6. *Describe the surgical options and select the one you would prefer.*

- Treatment should be designed depending on the presence of an irreducible versus reducible deformity.[4]
  - Irreducible deformity: Anterior decompression. Can be achieved through a transoral route although an endoscopic transcervical[6] or transsphenoidal (unpublished) approach have also been described. The decompression is followed by a posterior fusion.
  - Reducible deformity: Posterior occipitocervical fusion. Many posterior fusion techniques have been described for reducing the basilar invagination, restoring craniospinal alignment, and establishing fixation of the atlantoaxial joint.[7] The advance in osteosynthesis now allows for a solid instrumented fusion. Plates and screws at the occiput combined with C1 lateral masses and C2 pedicular screws, transarticular C1–C2 screws, or translaminar C2 screws and any combination thereof with autograft or mixed allograft fusion have achieved solid fusion.

7. *After posterior fusion, what is the natural history of the basilar invagination?*
   - There is evidence in the literature suggesting the regression of the soft pannus after internal fusion.[8]
   - A high rate of postoperative morbidity (42%, $n = 55$), and both early and 6 months mortality (13% and 25%, respectively) are reported for nonambulatory patients.[9]
   - Significant postoperative motor recovery was observed for a patient with a posterior atlantodental interval of more than 14 mm.[10]

■ References

1. Pellicci PM, Ranawat CS, Tsairis P. A prospective study of the progression of rheumatoid arthritis of the cervical spine. J Bone Joint Surg Am 1981;63(3):342–350
2. Marks JS, Sharp J. Rheumatoid cervical myelopathy. Q J Med 1981;50(199):307–319
3. Riew KD, Hilibrand AS, Palumbo MA, Sethi N, Bohlman HH. Diagnosing basilar invagination in the rheumatoid patient. The reliability of radiographic criteria. J Bone Joint Surg Am 2001;83-A(2):194–200
4. Winn RH. Neurological Surgery. Philadelphia: W.B Saunders; 2004
5. Greenberg MS. Handbook of Neurosurgery. New York: Thieme Medical Publishers; 2001
6. Wolinsky JP, Sciubba DM, Suk I, Gokaslan ZL. Endoscopic image-guided odontoidectomy for decompression of basilar invagination via a standard anterior cervical approach. Technical note. J Neurosurg Spine 2007;6(2):184–191
7. Kim DH, Vaccaro AR, Fessler RG. Spinal Instrumentation; Surgical Techniques. New York: Thieme Medical Publishers; 2005
8. Zygmunt S, Säveland H, Brattström H, Ljunggren B, Larsson EM, Wollheim F. Reduction of rheumatoid periodontoid pannus following posterior occipito-cervical fusion visualised by magnetic resonance imaging. Br J Neurosurg 1988;2(3):315–320
9. Casey AT, Crockard HA, Bland JM, Stevens J, Moskovich R, Ransford A. Predictors of outcome in the quadriparetic nonambulatory myelopathic patient with rheumatoid arthritis: a prospective study of 55 surgically treated Ranawat class IIIb patients. J Neurosurg 1996;85(4):574–581
10. Boden SD. Rheumatoid arthritis in the cervical spine: surgical decision making based on predictors of paralysis and recovery. Spine 1994;19(20):2275–2280

Case 85   Compression Fracture of the Thoracolumbar Spine

Eric P. Roger and Edward Benzel

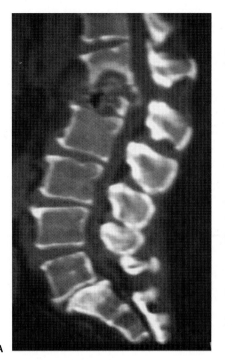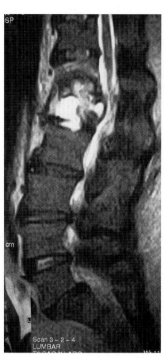

Fig. 85.1   (A) Sagittal reconstructed computed tomography of the lumbar spine and **(B)** sagittal T2-weighed magnetic resonance image of the lumbar spine are shown.

A   **B**

■ Clinical Presentation

- A 49-year-old man presents with back pain.
- He has a previous history of a fall ~3 months ago in the shower. He had no back pain prior to the fall.
- His past medical history is remarkable for arthroscopic knee surgery a few weeks prior to the fall, complicated by postoperative infection leading to sepsis. He was on intravenous (i.v.) antibiotics for 3 months.
- He denies any bladder or bowel dysfunction.
- On physical examination, he is neurologically intact and nonmyelopathic.

■ Questions

1. Please interpret the images in **Fig. 85.1**.
2. What do you think the cause of this fracture might be?
3. Assuming the fracture may be pathologic, what would be the differential diagnosis for the underlying pathology?

You are concerned about possible osteomyelitis. You obtain a computed tomography (CT) guided aspiration/biopsy of this lesion. Gram stain, final cultures, and pathology are all negative.

4. Can you rule out osteomyelitis as an underlying cause for this fracture?
5. How would osteomyelitis affect your surgical decision making?

6. What is the retropulsed bone compressing? Why does it matter?
7. What are the therapeutic options for this patient? Describe the available surgical approaches.

The patient tried a thoracolumbar spinal orthosis brace. However, when standing he experienced excruciating pain. Standing radiographs revealed progression of the kyphosis from 30 degrees to more than 60 degrees.

8. What are your surgical objectives?
9. What stabilization constructs are available to you?
10. How do you classify thoracolumbar fractures? How do you classify this fracture?
11. What is the mechanism for this fracture?

Thoracic fracture classification

Type	Group 1	Group 2	Group 3
A Compression of Anterior column	Wedge fracture	Split fracture	Burst or comminuted fracture
B anterior and posterior element injuries with distraction	ligamentous posterior flexion-distraction injury	osseous posterior flexion-distraction injury	injury involving hyperextension and shearing through the disc
C anterior and posterior element injuries with rotation	type A injury with rotation	type B injury with rotation	oblique fracture with rotational shear

ℵ-Sebbaugh MD

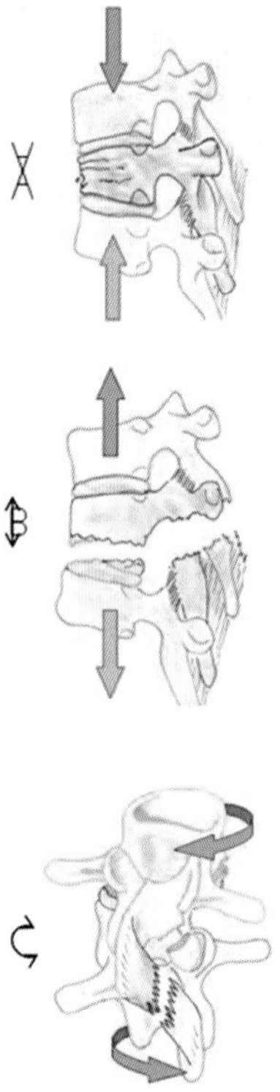

Fig. 85.2 Classification of thoracic fractures: **(A)** Type A, injury caused by compression of the anterior column; **(B)** type B, injury of the anterior column and the two posterior columns with distraction of the anterior or posterior elements; **(C)** type C, rotational injury of all three columns.

■ Answers

1. *Please interpret the images in* **Fig. 85.1**.
   - The most prominent finding is a destruction and/or a burst fracture of the L1 vertebra with involvement of the lower half of the T12 vertebral body.
   - This results in an anterior collapse, with kyphotic angulation deformity in the range of 30 degrees in these supine images.
   - There is evidence of retropulsed bony fragments into the spinal canal.
   - The T2-weighted magnetic resonance image demonstrates hyperintense signal within the T12 and L1 vertebral body, extending into the L1–L2 disk.

2. *What do you think the cause of this fracture might be?*
   - Although the patient reports that the pain initiated from a fall in the shower and therefore sounds traumatic, there might be an underlying pathology predisposing this bone to fracture.
   - The patient reported concordant sepsis from an infected knee. Underlying osteomyelitis should be suspected.

3. *Assuming the fracture may be pathologic, what would be the differential diagnosis for the underlying pathology?*
   - Differential diagnosis includes[1]
     – Infectious
       ▪ Bacterial seeding from sepsis
       ▪ Tuberculosis
     – Neoplastic
       ▪ Primary bone tumor (myeloma common)
       ▪ Metastases, lymphoma
     – Osteoporosis
     – Traumatic

4. *Can you rule out osteomyelitis as an underlying cause for this fracture?*
   - No, this cannot be entirely ruled out. This patient has been on i.v. antibiotics for 3 months. Although the biopsy or aspiration is negative, this may certainly have been an osteomyelitis initially that has now been "sterilized" by the antibiotics.
   - It has been reported that radiologic findings often "lag behind" clinical improvement and blood markers (such as C-reactive protein, erythrocyte sedimentation rate, and white blood cell count).
   - Furthermore, the lack of growth on culture does not necessarily prove that this collection is sterile. The long-term use of antibiotics may preclude culture growth, even though bacteria may still be present.[2–4]

5. *How would osteomyelitis affect your surgical decision making?*
   - Acute vertebral osteomyelitis is rarely initially treated surgically unless there is neural compromise, significant progressive deformity, or intractable pain. An aggressive course of antibiotic therapy is usually indicated (for 2 to 3 months).[2]

   - As previously mentioned, the images often "lag behind." Furthermore, successfully treated vertebral osteomyelitis will often progress to spontaneous fusion.
   - The issue with treating vertebral osteomyelitis surgically in the acute setting is one of spinal hardware contamination, although this can certainly be managed if surgery is clinically necessary.[5–7]
   - Once the osteomyelitis has been successfully "sterilized," as suspected in this patient, surgical stabilization may then be required for ongoing pain, instability, or new neurologic compromise.
   - One may consider continuing the i.v. antibiotics postoperatively for 6 weeks or more.

6. *What is the retropulsed bone compressing? Why does it matter?*
   - On **Fig. 85.1B**, it appears that the retropulsed bone is compressing the thecal sac below the level of the conus medullaris, thus affecting the cauda equina. The conus is most commonly located at L1, but may often terminate at T12.
   - The patient's lack of myelopathic findings suggests that the conus is above the retropulsed bony fragment in this case.
   - Whether the retropulsed bone is compressing the conus has a large impact on the proposed risks of the surgery, choice of approach, and ease of thecal sac decompression intraoperatively.

7. *What are the therapeutic options for this patient? Describe the available surgical approaches.*
   - Therapeutic options include
     – Conservative management: bracing[2]
     – Surgical decompression and stabilization[3–7]
       ▪ Iliac crest autograft should be harvested prior to exposing the infected level. Measurements are taken preoperatively from the CT scan.
       ▪ Anterior approach alone[8]: T12 and L1 corpectomy with intervertebral cage placement ± anterolateral plating. This would involve combined left-sided transthoracic/flank retroperitoneal approach with diaphragmatic take-down. (Note: This is a difficult approach and the assistance of an "exposure" surgeon— general or vascular—is recommended.)
       ▪ Anterior and posterior approach (combined): supplementation of the above approach with posterior pedicle fixation, one to three levels above and below
       ▪ Posterior approach alone[9,10]: transpedicular, costotransversectomy, or lateral extracavitary approach to corpectomy and cage, supplemented by pedicle screw fixation. (Note: The T12–L1 area is a junctional level; as such, it is recommended to proceed with at least two-level fixation above and below the level of involvement.)

■ Answers (*continued*)

– Kyphoplasty is *not* a valid option in this case.

8. *What are your surgical objectives?*
   - Surgical objectives[4]
     – Neural decompression from the retropulsed bony fragment
     – Restoration of alignment (i.e., correction of the kyphosis)
     – Restoration of anterior weight-bearing capacity (anterior and middle columns)
     – Fixation and fusion (arthrodesis and instrumentation)

9. *What stabilization constructs are available to you?*
   - Anterior constructs include[4,8]
     – Structural autograft or allograft such as iliac crest or tibial strut
     – Artificial cage (titanium or polyetheretherketone) filled with autograft, allograft or ceramics (β-tri-calcium-phosphate [β-TCP])
     – Expandable cages may offer an advantage in reducing the kyphosis by distracting the anterior column.
     – Anterolateral plate and screw construct
   - Posterior constructs include[4]
     – Pedicle screw fixation
     – Laminar hooks
     – Percutaneous pedicle screw fixation may be attractive if posterior decompression is not indicated (i.e., pedicle screws as a "backup").
     – Bone grafting with autograft, allograft, or β-TCP

10. *How do you classify thoracolumbar fractures? How do you classify this fracture?*
    - Fracture classification (simplified)[11,12] (**Fig. 85.2**)
      – Type A: Vertebral body compression
        ▪ A1—Impaction fractures (wedge)
        ▪ A2—Split fractures
        ▪ A3—Burst fractures
      – Type B: Anterior and posterior element injury with distraction
        ▪ B1—Posterior disruption predominantly ligamentous (ligamentous Chance injury)
        ▪ B2—Posterior disruption predominantly osseous (bony Chance injury)
        ▪ B3—Anterior disruption through disk (hyperextension shear injury)
      – Type C: Anterior and posterior element injury with rotation
        ▪ C1—Type A (compression) and rotation
        ▪ C2—Type B and rotation
        ▪ C3—Rotational shear injuries
    - This fracture would classify as an A3 (anterior column only, with burst features).

11. *What is the mechanism for this fracture?*
    - Mechanism: Axial compression with angular flexion moment arm.
    - There is no posterior element distraction associated to it.
    - There likely is underlying bone fragility from previous osteomyelitis, although this cannot be confirmed.

■ References

1. Osborn AG. Diagnostic Neuroradiology. St. Louis, MO: Mosby; 1994
2. Jaramillo-de la Torre JJ, Bohinski RJ, Kuntz CIV. Vertebral osteomyelitis. Neurosurg Clin N Am 2006;17(3):339–351
3. Aebi M, Thalgott JS, Webb JK. AO ASIF Prinicples in Spine Surgery. New York: Springer/AO Publishing; 1998
4. Benzel E. Biomechanics of Spine Stabilization. New York: Thieme/ American Association of Neurological Surgeons; 2001
5. Ruf M, Stoltze D, Merk HR, Ames M, Harms J. Treatment of vertebral osteomyelitis by radical debridement and stabilization using titanium mesh cages. Spine 2007;32(9):E275–E280
6. Dai LY, Chen WH, Jiang LS. Anterior instrumentation for the treatment of pyogenic vertebral osteomyelitis of thoracic and lumbar spine. Eur Spine J 2008;17(8):1027–1034
7. Robinson Y, Tschoeke SK, Kayser R, Boehm H, Heyde CE. Reconstruction of large defects in vertebral osteomyelitis with expandable titanium cages. Int Orthop 2008, Jul 5 Epub.
8. Rosner MK, Kuklo TR. Primary anterior treatment of thoracolumbar burst fractures. In: Resnick DK, Wolfa CE, eds. Neurosurgical Operative Atlas. Spine and Peripheral Nerves. New York: Thieme/ American Association of Neurological Surgeons; 2006
9. Ahmed A, Trost G. Costotransversectomy. In: Resnick DK, Wolfa CE, eds. Neurosurgical Operative Atlas. Spine and Peripheral Nerves. New York: Thieme/ American Association of Neurological Surgeons; 2006
10. Maiman D. Lateral extracavitary approach to the thoracolumbar spine. In: Resnick DK, Wolfa CE, eds. Neurosurgical Operative Atlas. Spine and Peripheral Nerves. New York: Thieme/American Association of Neurological Surgeons; 2006
11. Magerl F, Aebi M, Gertzbein SD, Harms J, Nazarian S. A comprehensive classification of thoracic and lumbar injuries. Eur Spine J 1994;3(4):184–201
12. McCormack T, Karaikovic E, Gaines RW. The load sharing classification of spine fractures. Spine 1994;19(15):1741–1744

Case 86   Lumbar Burst Fracture

Ahmed Jaman Alzahrani and Khalid N. Almusrea

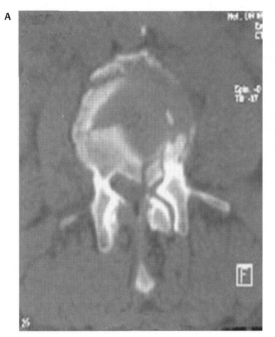
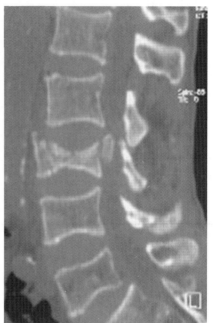

Fig. 86.1   (A) Computed tomography scan of the lumbar spine with axial section through L3 and **(B)** sagittal reconstructed image.

■ Clinical Presentation

• A 70-year-old man presents 4 days after a motor vehicle accident, transferred from a local hospital, with the complaint of severe lower back pain.
• The pain radiates to left thigh in an L3 dermatomal distribution.

• On examination he is neurologically intact.
• He has an unremarkable past medical history.
• A computed tomography (CT) scan of the lumbar spine was done at the local hospital (**Fig. 86.1**).

■ Questions

1. Describe the CT images.
2. What is your initial management?

Magnetic resonance imaging (MRI) is obtained and pertinent images are shown in **Fig. 86.2**.

3. What are the findings of the MRI of the lumbosacral spine?
4. What is your management now?

5. What are possible complications of nonoperative management in this case?
6. Describe indications for surgery in burst fractures.
7. What surgical approach will you choose and why?
8. What are the potential complications of a posterior surgical approach?
9. What are the outcomes of this approach?

A
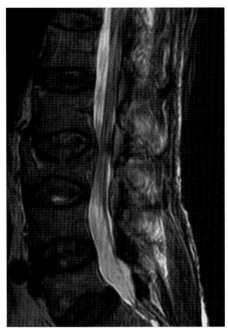

B
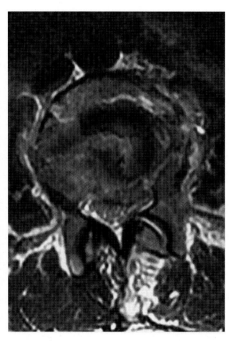

Fig. 86.2 Magnetic resonance imaging scan of the lumbar spine with **(A)** T2-weighted sagittal section and **(B)** axial section images through L3.

■ Answers

1. *Describe the CT images.*
   - There is a type A Denis burst fracture of the L3 vertebra.
   - Loss of height of ~40% and kyphosis of 15 degrees are evident.
   - There is canal compromise of ~50%.
2. *What is your initial management?*
   - Ensure the initial trauma workup has been completed (airway, breathing, circulation [ABCs], etc.).
   - Complete spinal precautions (logroll only).
   - Obtain radiographs of the rest of the spine and further CT scans if other fractures are seen.
   - Place the patient on adequate pain management.
   - Obtain basic laboratory panel including complete blood count (CBC), electrolytes, coagulation profile.
   - Obtain an MRI of lumbosacral spine to assess any neural element and ligamentous involvement.
   - You may also elect to order an external orthosis, preferably a Jewett or thoracolumbar spinal orthosis brace in this case.
3. *What are the findings of the MRI of the lumbosacral spine?*
   - The MRI confirms the severe compromise of the thecal sac.
   - There is left L3 foraminal stenosis.
4. *What is your management now?*
   - Treatment options include
     - Conservative treatment with bracing, physical therapy, and pain control.[1]
     - Surgical fixation with decompression and fusion via an anterior, posterior, or combined approach.[2,3]
   - With the presence of significant canal stenosis and root compression, surgical intervention may be a better option.
5. *What are possible complications of nonoperative management in this case?*
   - Persistent and worsening instability (mechanical, neurologic)
   - Increased kyphosis leading to neurologic deficit or intractable pain[4]
   - Further collapse of the affected vertebra with cauda equine syndrome
6. *Describe indications for surgery in burst fractures.*
   - Features of instability that lead to the requirement for surgical fixation include the following[5]:
     - Neurologic deficit
     - Canal compromise of ≥50%
     - Height loss of ≥40%
     - Kyphosis of ≥30 degrees
7. *What surgical approach will you choose and why?*
   - Posterior decompression and fixation is preferred because an anterior approach will need major exposure despite no major difference in outcome, especially in an elderly patient as in this case.[3,6] (This is our personal preference; however, the choice of the approach is debatable and remains controversial.)

■ Answers (*continued*)

8. *What are the potential complications of a posterior surgical approach?*
   - In a series of 76 patients with thoracolumbar fractures, the complication rate was ~3.6%.[7]
   - Complications include the following[7-9]:
     - Pain
     - Neurologic deficit
     - Postoperative infection
     - Progression of the kyphosis
     - Nonunion or lack of fusion
     - Rupture or loosening of the implants
     - Loss of correction and required placement of an anterior support graft
     - Vertebral arch fracture
     - Epidural hematoma
     - Inadequate decompression
     - Cerebrospinal fluid leak

9. *What are the outcomes of this approach?*
   - Results are varied and depend on the studied parameters and institution.
   - Significant differences have been shown between the immediate postoperative and late postoperative outcomes in terms of height restoration when a posterior approach is used alone.[8]

- The neurologic recovery from burst fractures is not predicted by the amount of initial canal encroachment or kyphotic deformity.[10]
- In burst fractures without a neurologic deficit, there is no superiority of conservative therapy over operative therapy.[10] One prospective trial on 80 patients without neurologic deficits showed that posterior fixation provides partial kyphosis correction and earlier pain relief, but the functional outcome at 2 years is similar to a conservatively treated group.[11]
- When there is significant neurologic involvement, operative management is advised. However, there is no obvious superiority of one approach over the other.[10]
- In a series of 28 patients treated via posterior approach, there was 82% neurologic improvement.[9]
- A retrospective review of 46 patients with encroachment of the spinal canal greater than 50% treated surgically showed that there is no significant difference in clinical outcome between those treated with a combined approach (anterior and posterior) versus those treated with a posterior approach alone. Furthermore, neurologic deficits improved by at least one Frankel grade in both cases for the most part.[12]

■ References

1. Moller A, Hasserius R, Redlund-Johnell I, Ohlin A, Karlsson MK. Nonoperatively treated burst fractures of the thoracic and lumbar spine in adults: a 23- to 41-year follow-up. Spine J 2007;7(6):701–707

2. Mahar A, Kim C, Wedemeyer M, et al. Short-segment fixation of lumbar burst fractures using pedicle fixation at the level of the fracture. Spine 2007;32(14):1503–1507

3. Hitchon PW, Torner J, Eichholz KM, Beeler SN. Comparison of anterolateral and posterior approaches in the management of thoracolumbar burst fractures. J Neurosurg Spine 2006;5(2):117–125

4. Koller H, Acosta F, Hempfing A, et al. Long-term investigation of nonsurgical treatment for thoracolumbar and lumbar burst fractures: an outcome analysis in sight of spinopelvic balance. Eur Spine J 2008;17(8):1073–1095

5. Benzel EC. Spine Surgery: Techniques, Complication Avoidance, and Management. 2nd ed. Philadelphia: Churchill Livingstone; 2004

6. Esses S. Posterior short-segment instrumentation and fusion provides better results than combined anterior plus posterior stabilization for mid-lumbar (L2 to L4) burst fractures. J Bone Joint Surg Am 2006;88(10):2311

7. Knop C, Fabian HF, Bastian L, Blauth M. Late results of thoracolumbar fractures after posterior instrumentation and transpedicular bone grafting. Spine 2001;26(1):88–99

8. Defino HL, Canto FR. Low thoracic and lumbar burst fractures: radiographic and functional outcomes. Eur Spine J 2007;16(11):1934–1943

9. Kaya RA, Aydin Y. Modified transpedicular approach for the surgical treatment of severe thoracolumbar or lumbar burst fractures. Spine J 2004;4(2):208–217

10. Dai LY, Wang XY, Jiang LS. Neurologic recovery from thoracolumbar burst fractures: is it predicted by the amount of initial canal encroachment and kyphotic deformity? Surg Neurol 2007;67(3):232–237

11. Shen WJ, Liu TJ, Shen YS. Nonoperative treatment versus posterior fixation for thoracolumbar junction burst fractures without neurologic deficit. Spine 2001;26(9):1038–1045

12. Been HD, Bouma GJ. Comparison of two types of surgery for thoraco-lumbar burst fractures: combined anterior and posterior stabilisation vs. posterior instrumentation only. Acta Neurochir (Wien) 1999;141(4):349–357

Case 87   Cervical Spondylotic Myelopathy

Remi Nader

■ Clinical Presentation

- A 53-year-old woman presents with neck pain radiating to both shoulders as well as to the left arm and right hand.
- She also complains of numbness and tingling in both upper extremities. Extending the neck slightly relieves some of the pressure; however, flexing the neck aggravates the pain.
- There is an extensive medical history of hypertension, stroke, diabetes mellitus, asthma, and congestive heart failure.

- Physical examination reveals some longstanding left-sided weakness (graded 4/5 on the Medical Research Council [MRC] motor scale) associated with her previous stroke (a few years ago).
- Sensory examination reveals decreased sensation along the left side throughout, to temperature as well as decreased sensation bilaterally in a C5–C6 distribution to temperature. Reflexes are 1–2+ symmetric with no Hoffmann and no Babinski's signs. Gait reveals a mild spasticity.
- Magnetic resonance imaging (MRI) is ordered.

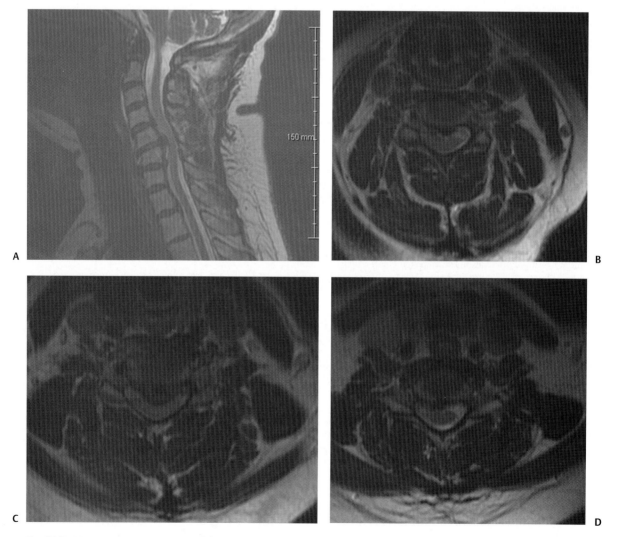

Fig. 87.1 Magnetic resonance imaging of the cervical spine with T2-weighted images: **(A)** Midsagittal cut and axial cuts through the disk spaces at **(B)** C4–C5, **(C)** C5–C6, and **(D)** C6–C7.

■ Questions

1. Interpret the MRI (**Fig. 87.1**).
2. Give a differential diagnosis. What is the most likely diagnosis?
3. What further studies would you like to obtain?
4. A computed tomography (CT) scan of the cervical spine is obtained and shown in **Fig. 87.2**. Describe the pertinent finding.
5. Briefly describe the pertinent points of your operative approach.
6. Immediately postoperatively, she awakens with bilateral upper extremity profound weakness in triceps, grips, and interossei. Lower extremity strength is unchanged. Give a differential diagnosis. What is the most likely diagnosis?
7. What is your management now?
8. You immediately obtain an MRI of the cervical spine (**Fig. 87.3**); interpret it.

9. How do you treat the patient given the MRI findings?

She improves and is discharged home after a short rehabilitation stay. She then sustains a fall 6 weeks postoperatively and presents with worsening bilateral lower extremity weakness to the point where she is unable to ambulate. You obtain the following CT scan (**Fig. 87.4**).

10. Interpret the CT scan (**Fig. 87.4**).
11. What is your management now?
12. Describe your treatment options and a surgical approach.

After a long discussion of the different treatment options with the patient, you elect to perform a multilevel corpectomy and place the patient in a halo postoperatively. She does well and her strength is improved postoperatively. You obtain a CT scan, shown in **Fig. 87.5**.

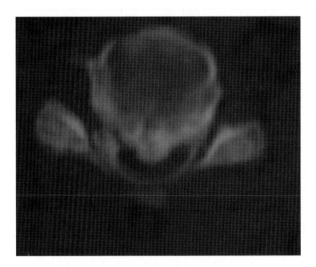

Fig. 87.2 Axial computed tomography scan at C5–C6 level.

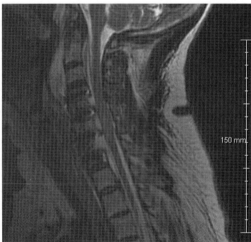

Fig. 87.3 Sagittal T2-weighted magnetic resonance image of cervical spine obtained immediately postoperatively.

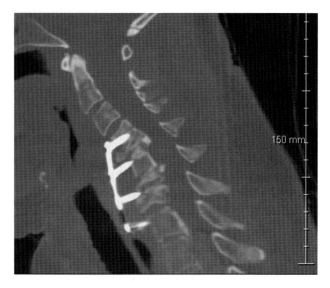

Fig. 87.4 Computed tomography scan sagittal reconstructed images through cervical spine.

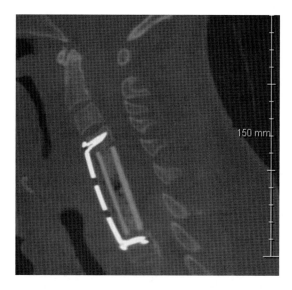

Fig. 87.5 Computed tomography scan sagittal reconstructed images through cervical spine obtained after the second procedure, showing repair of the kyphosis, alignment restoration, and decompression of the spinal cord.

■ Answers

1. *Interpret the MRI* (**Fig. 87.1**).
   - There is a large C5–C6 herniated nucleus pulposus with severe spinal cord compression at that level as well as a kyphotic deformity at the same level.
   - There is also a smaller C4–C5 and C6–C7 herniated nucleus pulposus with some cord compression at these two levels.
   - There is possibly an osteophytic spur or ossified posterior longitudinal ligament (OPLL) at C5–C6
2. *Give a differential diagnosis. What is the most likely diagnosis?*
   - Most likely diagnosis is cervical spondylotic myelopathy.
   - Differential diagnosis based on clinical presentation includes the following (mnemonic is "CITTEN DIVA")[1]:
     - Congenital: Chiari malformation, syringomyelia, narrow canal/ short pedicles, mucopolysaccharidoses, kyphosis, os odontoideum
     - Infection: syphilis (infarction), postviral (herpes, varicella, cytomegalovirus), epidural empyema, vertebral osteomyelitis, acquired immunodeficiency syndrome- [AIDS-] related myelopathy, tuberculosis (Pott disease), parasitic cyst
     - Traumatic: spinal shock, epidural hematoma, basal skull trauma, electrical injury, bony fracture
     - Tumor: spinal cord tumor (extradural, intradural extramedullary, intramedullary), metastases, carcinomatous meningitis, paraneoplastic syndrome
     - Endocrine: Cushing disease, obesity (epidural lipomatosis), acromegaly, Paget disease
     - Nutrition/toxins: vitamin B12 deficiency, local anesthetics
     - Degenerative: spondylotic myelopathy, OPLL, disk herniation
     - Inflammatory: transverse myelitis, multiple sclerosis, Devic syndrome, Guillain-Barre syndrome, amyotrophic lateral sclerosis
     - Vascular: spinal epidural, subdural, or subarachnoid hemorrhage, stroke, spinal cord infarction (syphilis, aorta-clamping intraoperatively, hypotension, aortic dissection), arteriovenous malformation, radiation necrosis (causes microvascular occlusion), contrast infusion
     - Acquired: herniated disk, OPLL
3. *What further studies would you like to obtain?*
   - Plain radiographs with flexion and extension views
   - CT scan of the cervical spine
   - Medical workup
     - Laboratory studies: complete blood count, electrolytes, coagulation profile, type and screen
     - Electrocardiogram
     - Chest radiograph
     - Cardiac echography
     - Pulmonary function tests
   - Consultation with Internal Medicine for surgical clearance

■ Answers (*continued*)

4. *A CT scan of the cervical spine is obtained and shown in* **Fig. 87.2**. *Describe the pertinent finding.*
   - There is OPLL–segmental type at the level of C5–C6
5. *Briefly describe the pertinent points of your operative approach.*
   - Anterior approach is described.
     - Anterior cervical diskectomy at C4–C5, C5–C6, C6–C7 may be performed in the standard Smith-Robinson technique.[2]
     - May need to do partial versus complete corpectomy of C5 and/or C6 for resection of OPLL[3]
     - Expect possible dural breach and anticipate its repair
     - Fusion with allograft and plate instrumentation
     - Use radiographic guidance and microscope
     - Use diamond burr on OPLL segment to avoid injuring spinal cord
     - May elect to use somatosensory and motor evoked potential monitoring intraoperatively
     - May elect to supplement with posterior C4–C7 lateral mass screws
   - Alternatively, a posterior approach may be used (however, this is not the author's preferred approach, as the pathology is located anteriorly). This may include:
     - Cervical laminoplasty from C3–4 to C7, or
     - Cervical laminectomies from C4 to C7 ± lateral mass fusion
6. *Immediately postoperatively, she awakens with bilateral upper extremity profound weakness in triceps, grips, and interossei. Lower extremity strength is unchanged. Give a differential diagnosis. What is the most likely diagnosis?*
   - Complications related to surgical technique[4,5]
     - Spinal cord edema with central cord syndrome (most likely)
     - Cord injury intraoperatively
     - Spinal epidural hematoma at surgical site
     - Graft dislodgment
     - Neck hematoma
   - Complications of anesthesia[6]
     - Spinal cord infarction due to generalized hypotension
     - Lingering effect of paralytics or anesthetics
   - Complications related to her medical conditions
7. *What is your management now?*
   - Obtain an urgent MRI of the cervical spine.
   - Start the patient on steroids (dexamethasone 10 mg intravenously (i.v.) once then 6 mg i.v. every 6 hours or use the high-dose methylprednisolone [Solu-Medrol; Pfizer Pharmaceuticals, New York, NY] spinal cord injury protocol).
   - Admit to intensive care unit for monitoring.
   - Avoid hypotension (keep mean arterial pressure >85 mm Hg).

- Call the operating room for possible return to explore the wound if a hematoma is suspected.
8. *You immediately obtain an MRI of the cervical spine* (**Fig. 87.3**); *interpret it.*
   - MRI shows diffuse cord edema and thickening as well as a cord signal at the level of C5–C6.
   - Otherwise, no obvious hematoma is seen.
   - Good alignment and good placement of grafts are visualized.
9. *How do you treat the patient given the MRI findings?*
   - Treat medically with steroids.[4]
   - There are no indications for surgical intervention.
10. *Interpret the CT scan* (**Fig. 87.4**).
    - There is collapse of the construct with extrusion of the anterior instrumentation.
    - There are compression fractures of C5, C6, and C7 vertebral bodies
    - Kyphotic deformity is seen again at C5–C6.
    - Extrusion of the graft at C4–C5 and collapse of the graft at C6–C7 is observed.
11. *What is your management now?*
    - The patient needs urgent surgical intervention (within 24 hours) for cord decompression and repair of the kyphotic deformity.
    - The extruded hardware also needs to be removed.
    - The compression fractures of the vertebral bodies need to be repaired and proper alignment needs to be restored.
    - Obtain further studies preoperatively.
      - Plain radiographs and MRI of the cervical spine
      - Preoperative medical clearance from Internal Medicine (urgent)
12. *Describe your treatment options and a surgical approach.*
    - Options include[5]
      - Anterior decompression and internal fixation with grafting followed by posterior fixation (lateral mass screws and rods/plates) down to the upper thoracic area, and placement in a cervical collar. (Given the pathology, this remains the author's preferred approach. However, this was not performed in this case due to patient-related factors and medical issues—these types of issues need to be documented in the patient's chart very clearly.)
      - Anterior decompression and internal fixation with grafting followed by placement of a halo vest (or a sterna-occipital mandibular immobilizer cervicothoracic orthosis if the patient is unable to tolerate the halo, although less ideal)
      - Posterior decompression and/or fixation alone is not a good option as the pathology is mainly anterior and the kyphotic deformity is significant.
      - Placement of a collar or other soft brace is not an option after anterior fixation alone, as there is involvement of C7 vertebral body, which places the graft at a junctional level.

■ Answers (*continued*)

- Anterior decompression and fixation would consist of[7]
  - Anterior corpectomy of C5, C6, and C7 vertebral bodies
  - Fibular strut graft placement or metallic cage placement
  - Use of bone autograft from vertebral bodies to help with arthrodesis
  - Anterior instrumentation from C4 to T1 with plate and screws
  - Intraoperative adjuncts are as described previously.

■ References

1. Tsementzis SA. Differential Diagnosis in Neurology and Neurosurgery. A Clinician's Pocket Guide. New York: Thieme Medical Publishers; 2000
2. Smith GW, Robinson RA. The treatment of certain cervical-spine disorders by anterior removal of the intervertebral disc and interbody fusion. J Bone Joint Surg Am 1958;40:607–624
3. Mizuno J, Nakagawa H. Ossified posterior longitudinal ligament: management strategies and outcomes. Spine J 2006;6(6, Suppl):282S–288S
4. Dickerman RD, Lefkowitz M, Epstein JA. A traumatic central cord syndrome occurring after adequate decompression for cervical spondylosis: biomechanics of injury: case report. Spine 2005;30(20):E611–E613
5. Benzel E. Biomechanics of Spine Stabilization. New York: Thieme/American Association of Neurological Surgeons; 2001
6. Yan K, Diggan MF. A case of central cord syndrome caused by intubation: a case report. J Spinal Cord Med 1997;20(2):230–232
7. Hukuda S, Mochizuki T, Ogata M, Shichikawa K, Shimomura Y. Operations for cervical spondylotic myelopathy. A comparison of the results of anterior and posterior procedures. J Bone Joint Surg Br 1985;67(4):609–615

Case 88   Anterior versus Posterior Approach to the Cervical Spine

Amgad S. Hanna and Remi Nader

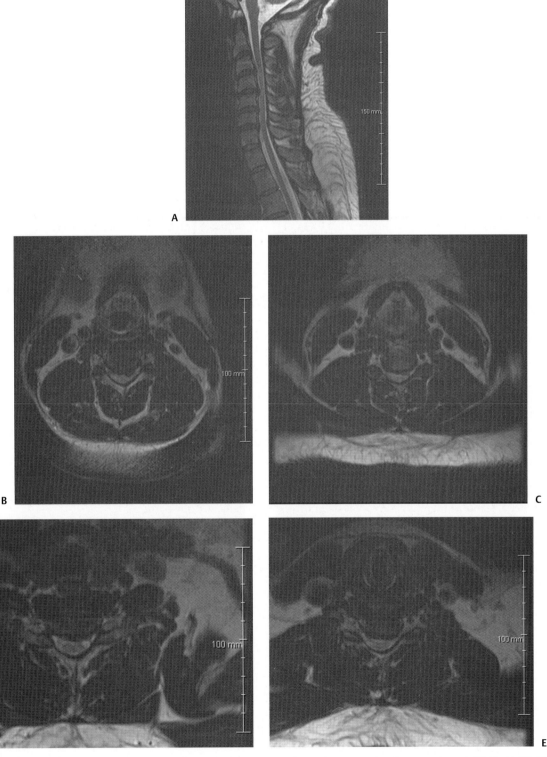

Fig. 88.1 Cervical spine T2-weighted magnetic resonance images with **(A)** midsagittal section and axial sections through **(B)** C3–C4, **(C)** C4–C5, **(D)** C5–C6, and **(E)** C6–C7, respectively.

■ Clinical Presentation

- A 37-year-old man who is human immunodeficiency virus-(HIV)-positive presents with progressive ataxia over 2 weeks, clumsiness, and dropping of objects with both hands.
- He has a longstanding history of neck pain.
- Hyperreflexia and patchy sensory loss are noted on examination.
- Magnetic resonance imaging (MRI) of the cervical spine is obtained and shown in **Fig. 88.1**.

■ Questions

1. Interpret the MRI scan.
2. What is your management?
3. What factors will favor an anterior versus a posterior surgical approach?
4. Postoperatively, the patient does not improve (no obvious intraoperative complications). What do you tell the patient?

■ Answers

1. *Interpret the MRI scan.*
   - Cervical canal stenosis is seen extending from C3 to C7 with multiple-level disk bulges, more so at C4–C5.
   - The sagittal images do not fully account for the narrowing seen in the axial cuts.
   - There is increased signal intensity of the cord on T2-weighted MRIs demonstrating damage to the spinal cord, likely from the stenosis.
   - The region of the posterior longitudinal ligament (PLL) is thickened and hypointense. This could be ossified PLL (OPLL); obtaining a computed tomography (CT) scan would confirm this finding, if present.
   - No bony changes or extradural tissues are seen to suggest the diagnosis of epidural abscess, which could well be a possibility in an HIV scenario. HIV can also lead to neuropathic changes and changes within the cord.
2. *What is your management?*
   - This patient is myelopathic in the context of significant cervical stenosis; therefore, surgery is the most appropriate treatment measure in this case.
   - In the meantime, an infectious workup for HIV should be performed (including CD4 count, viral load, etc.). Acquired immunodeficiency syndrome-(AIDS)-related myelopathy should also be in the differential diagnosis.
3. *What factors will favor an anterior versus a posterior surgical approach?*
   - Anterior approach would consist of multilevel diskectomies versus corpectomies. It would directly address the compressing pathology and correct the kyphosis. However, there is a high incidence of pseudoarthrosis if done as a stand-alone procedure.[1,2]

- Posterior approach alone would consist of laminectomies ± lateral mass fusion versus laminoplasties from C3–C6. It would not correct the kyphosis, and the cord may remain draped over the anterior pathology.[3,4]
- This stand-alone procedure needs to be supplemented by bracing with at least a hard cervical collar or halo (or SOMI brace) placement to limit motion during the healing process.
- Although it may be perfectly reasonable to perform a stand-alone anterior or posterior procedure, the ideal procedure in this patient, if medically tolerable, is a circumferential procedure. This may include C3–C4 and C4–C5 anterior diskectomies, C6 corpectomy, allograft, and plating, followed by supplementation with posterior C3–C7 lateral mass fusion (and possible posterior decompression). The C7 lateral mass is usually small (confirmation of bony landmarks with CT is important) and usually takes a pedicle screw better.[5,6]
- Anterior approach advantages and disadvantages[1,2]:
  - Pros
    - With adequate distraction, it can correct the kyphotic deformity.
    - It can address anterior pathology such as disks and bony spurs.
    - Sufficient distraction can unbuckle the ligamentum flavum and indirectly treat a posterior pathology.
  - Cons
    - There is a risk of cranial nerve (dysphagia, dysphonia) and vascular injury.

Answers (*continued*)

- It requires bony fusion and the associated morbidity of bony fusion.
- There is a high risk of subsidence in osteoporotic patients.
- There is a lesser likelihood of fusion in greater than two-level construct cases unless it is supplemented with a posterior approach procedure.
- Posterior approach advantages and disadvantages[3,4]:
  - Pros
    - It is technically easier and therefore more suitable for older and osteoporotic patients.
    - There are virtually no risks to the cranial nerves and carotids (i.e., good procedure for professional singers).
    - It can address posterior pathology such as ligamentum flavum directly.
    - There is lower risk of incidental durotomy in cases of OPLL.
  - Cons
    - There is risk of kyphotic deformities or instability in pure laminectomy cases (if too much facet is taken).

- There is an inability to directly address anterior pathology.
- C5 nerve root palsy is described more often with posterior decompressions.

4. *Postoperatively, the patient does not improve (no obvious intraoperative complications). What do you tell the patient?*
   - The main goal of surgery is to stop further deterioration.
   - Improvement rate of neurologic function is ~50% (ranging from 37 to 85%) in myelopathic patients; therefore, it is not unusual to see no change postoperatively.[6–8]
   - Also, he has myelopathic changes within the spinal cord on the MRI, and some of his symptoms may be related to HIV myelopathy and peripheral neuropathy.
   - One management approach, at this stage, would be to continue observation while initiating rehabilitative measures such as physical therapy.

References

1. Medow JE, Trost G, Sandin J. Surgical management of cervical myelopathy: indications and techniques for surgical corpectomy. Spine J 2006; 6(6, Suppl):233S–241S
2. Hillard VH, Apfelbaum RI. Surgical management of cervical myelopathy: indications and techniques for multilevel cervical discectomy. Spine J 2006; 6(6, Suppl):242S–251S
3. Komotar RJ, Mocco J, Kaiser M. Surgical management of cervical myelopathy: indications and techniques for laminectomy and fusion. Spine J 2006; 6(6, Suppl):252S–267S
4. Steinmetz MP, Resnick DK. Cervical laminoplasty. Spine J 2006; 6(6, Suppl):274S–281S
5. Kim PK, Alexander JT. Indications for circumferential surgery for cervical spondylotic myelopathy. Spine J 2006; 6(6, Suppl):299S–307S

6. Cusick JF. Pathophysiology and treatment of cervical spondylotic myelopathy. Clin Neurosurg 1991;37:661–681
7. Cheung WY, Arvinte D, Wong YW, Luk KD, Cheung KM. Neurological recovery after surgical decompression in patients with cervical spondylotic myelopathy - a prospective study. Int Orthop 2008;32(2):273–278
8. Naderi S, Ozgen S, Pamir MN, Ozek MM, Erzen C. Cervical spondylotic myelopathy: surgical results and factors affecting prognosis. Neurosurgery 1998;43(1):43–49

Case 89 Lower Back Pain — Conservative Management

Hashem Al Hashemi, Remi Nader, and Abdulrahman J. Sabbagh

■ Clinical Presentation

- A 45-year-old man presented to your clinic complaining of lower back pain for the past 3 months.
- The patient's work activities do involve heavy lifting.

- He is otherwise neurologically intact.
- Magnetic resonance imaging (MRI) of his lumbar spine was done prior to his visit; the image is shown in **Fig. 89.1**.

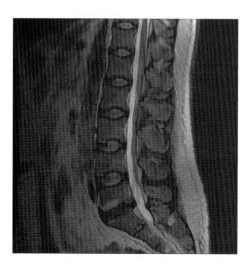

Fig. 89.1 T2-weighted sagittal magnetic resonance image of the lumbar spine demonstrating degenerative disk disease at the L5–S1 level.

Fig. 89.2 Plain radiographs taken while performing the following interventional procedures: **(A,B)** L3 medial branch neurotomy and L3 and **(C)** L4 medial branch blocks, **(D)** caudal epidural steroid injection, **(E)** L5 transforaminal epidural steroid injection, and **(F)** S1 transforaminal epidural steroid injection.

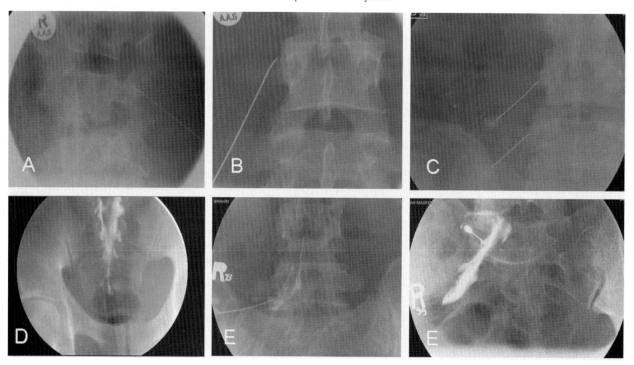

■ Questions

1. What are some common causes of lower back pain?
2. Provide a broad differential diagnosis for lower back pain.
3. What are some red flags or critical conditions that can present with lower back pain (on both history and physical examination)?
4. What imaging studies would you like to obtain?

5. What other investigations may be warranted?
6. Describe nonoperative measures of management of lower back pain.
7. What interventional procedures may be used to differentiate the types of spinal-related lower back pain?
8. Discuss interventional options for management of spinal pain.

■ Answers

1. *What are some common causes of lower back pain?*
   - Common causes include[1]
   - Poor posture
     – Poor sitting or standing posture
     – Sleeping position and/or pillow positioning
     – Bending forward too long
     – "Hiking" your shoulder to hold the phone receiver to your ear
   - Excess weight
     – Pregnancy
     – Obesity
   - Sudden or strenuous physical effort
     – Improper lifting
     – Accident, sports injury, or fall
     – Carrying a heavy purse, briefcase, or backpack
   - Stress and muscle tension
     – Lack of muscle tone
     – Deconditioning
2. Provide a broad differential diagnosis for lower back pain.
   - Differential diagnosis includes[1]
   - Congenital
     – Scoliosis, kyphosis
     – Isthmic spondylolisthesis
     – Spina bifida
     – Short pedicle syndrome
   - Infectious
     – Diskitis, osteomyelitis, tuberculosis
     – Pyelonephritis, urinary tract infections, psoas abscess
     – Endometritis
   - Traumatic
     – Lumbosacral fracture or dislocation
     – Spondylolisthesis,
     – Muscle strain or sprain
   - Tumor
     – Metastatic disease to the spine
     – Primary bone tumors of the spine
     – Abdominopelvic retroperitoneal tumors
   - Environmental
     – Repetitive heavy lifting at work
     – Poor posture, obesity
     – Prolonged riding in car or truck

   - Neurogenic
     – Herniated disk, spinal stenosis
     – Hypertrophied ligaments
     – Neuropathic pain, failed back syndrome
   - Drugs
     – Antivirals, antibiotics
     – Chemotherapeutics
     – Coumadin
   - Inflammatory
     – Ostearthritis, rheumatoid arthritis
     – Ankylosing spondylitis
     – Systemic lupus erythematosus
   - Vascular
     – Abdominal aortic aneurysm
     – Arteriovenous malformation of the spine
     – Hemangioma, hematoma
   - Gynecologic
     – Menstruating
     – Endometriosis
     – Pregnancy
     – Tumors
   - Acquired and other
3. *What are some red flags or critical conditions that can present with lower back pain (on both history and physical examination)?*
   - Clinical symptoms on history[2–4]
     – Age older than 50 years
     – Cancer: history of cancer, unexplained weight loss, pain at multiple sites
     – Pain worsening at night and not mechanical in character
     – Immunosuppression: human immunodeficiency virus (HIV), steroid use, transplant patient
     – Infection: fever, night sweats, back tenderness, limited range of motion
     – Trauma: history of significant trauma or minor trauma in osteoporotic patients
     – Intractability
     – Cauda equina syndrome: bladder or bowel dysfunction, saddle anesthesia, leg weakness or pain
     – Other neurologic symptoms

■ Answers (*continued*)

- Clinical signs on physical examination[2-4]
  - Saddle anesthesia
  - Incontinence
  - Fever (>38°C)
  - Urinary retention
  - Muscular weakness
  - Bony tenderness (vertebral)
  - Very limited range of spinal motion

4. *What imaging studies would you like to obtain?*
   - Basic imaging studies include plain x-rays of the lumbar and possibly of the thoracic spine.[5]
   - MRI of the lumbar spine[2,5]
     - Is not indicated for nonspecific low back pain.
     - Many people without symptoms show abnormalities on radiographs and MRI. The chances of finding coincidental disk prolapse increases with age.
     - MRI should be reserved for patients with red flag conditions and those with neurologic symptoms and/or signs severe enough to consider surgery.
     - In the presence of bowel and bladder incontinence, diffuse weakness suggestive of multiple roots involvement or upper motor signs, an urgent whole spine MRI is recommended.
   - Flexion and extension radiographs of the lumbar spine: recommended in cases of spondylolysis or spondylolisthesis (as there is potential spine instability)
   - Computed tomography (CT) scan of the lumbar spine recommended in trauma cases to evaluate for fracture and alignment or in certain degenerative conditions to assess pars integrity, osteophytes, etc.[5]
   - Other studies depend on the suspected pathologies.
     - Bone scan: recommended in suspected cases of malignancy (history of malignancy, history of weight loss, or night pain)
     - Abdominal x-ray and renal ultrasound (US): if kidney stones are suspected
     - Vascular studies (ankle brachial index, magnetic resonance angiography [MRA] or angiography): if the patient gives a history of vascular claudication (smokers, diabetics, history of stenting or vascular bypass).

5. *What other investigations may be warranted?*
   - Investigative measures strongly depend on the detailed history and examination obtained from the patient. Certain important tests are mentioned below. This list is, however, by no means exhaustive.
   - With history suggestive of osteoporosis (steroid use, previous osteoporotic fractures, family history of osteoporosis, or osteopenia on radiograph), a bone densimetry is recommended.

- If the clinical picture is suggestive of connective tissue disease (multiple joints or skin manifestations), a screening should be done with some laboratory tests: erythrocyte sedimentation rate (ESR), C-reactive protein (CRP), rheumatoid factor (RF), and antinuclear antibodies (ANA).
- If you suspect multiple myeloma, a skeletal survey, total proteins, and protein electrophoresis should be completed.
- If the patient is diabetic, control of blood glucose should be checked with hemoglobin A1–C.

6. *Describe nonoperative measures of management of lower back pain.*
   - Activity modification: This may involve taking 2–3 days off work, avoiding activities that provoke pain, doing a different task at work with less stress on the spine; may result in changing jobs.[6,7]
   - Pain control: This is important initially with the activity modification to allow the patient to mobilize more and do some strengthening exercises. This could be done with the help of passive therapeutic modalities while in physical therapy sessions, such as heat, cold, ultrasound, and transcutaneous electrical nerve stimulation (TENS) machines.
   - Physical therapy programs include[8,9]
     - During the first month of symptoms: low impact aerobic exercise can minimize debility due to inactivity, such as walking, bicycling, or swimming.
     - Also, conditioning exercises for trunk muscles may be done such as exercises to strengthen back extensors and abdominal muscles (the McKenzie techniques comprise a well-known set of such exercises).
     - During the first 2 weeks, these exercises may aggravate symptoms. Therefore, the recommended exercise quotas are gradually escalated, resulting in better outcomes than having patients simply stop when pain occurs.
   - Educating the patient is also important in improving and hastening recovery.
     - Explanation of the condition to the patient in understandable terms.
     - Positive reassurance that the condition will almost certainly subside.
     - Teach the patient about proper posture, sleeping positions, lifting techniques, and weight loss techniques if overweight.
   - If there is no improvement with such conservative techniques, then resorting to medications initially and later interventional procedures may be considered.

■ Answers (*continued*)

- Maintenance/ recurrence prevention programs should also be set up.
  - After some control of the pain is achieved using the activity modification and medications (±) interventions, a core strengthening program should be initiated.
  - This involves lumbar stabilization exercise: strengthening and training muscles that surround the spine can help support and protect the spine.
  - A simple way to start is with walking and performing general aerobic exercises.
  - Exercise has a good general effect on the human body that includes increasing the pain threshold and building resistance to pain.
  - The patient also has to modify unhealthy lifestyle habits and poor body mechanics that may have initiated the pain.
- Medical management includes[5,10]
  - Nonsteroidal antiinflammatory drugs (NSAIDS)
  - Acetaminophen
  - Other antiinflammatories or nonnarcotic pain medications such as tramadol and combination of the above.
  - For radicular pain that affects sleep, amitriptyline or other antidepressant-type pain medications may be used.
  - Alternatively, gabapentin or pregabalin can be employed. Both have no significant interactions with other medications, but need to be avoided in patients with significant renal dysfunction.
  - Strong narcotics may be used in the short term in cases of intractable pain. These include morphine derivatives – MS Contin, OxyContin (both Purdue Pharma, Stamford, CT), hydromorphone, etc. Fentanyl patches are contraindicated for narcotics naive patients.

7. *What interventional procedures may be used to differentiate the types of spinal-related lower back pain?*
   - For mechanical back pain, the following measures may apply.
     - Medial branch blocks may help diagnose facet-related pain in cases of whiplash injuries and degenerative disc disease.
     - Sacroiliac (SI) joint injections may help diagnose and treat SI joint pain in cases of leg length discrepancy, multiple-level fusion, or spondyloarthropathy (ankylosing spondylitis or inflammatory bowel disease).
     - Discography may be used to diagnose diskogenic pain and to narrow the level of most severe involvement if surgical fusion is contemplated.
     - Trigger point injections may aid the diagnosis and treat of muscular back pain.

8. *Discuss interventional options for management of spinal pain.*
   - Options for interventional pain management include the following (**Fig. 89.2** for illustrative intraprocedural x-rays)[11–13]:
   - Transforaminal, caudal, or interlaminal epidural injections, for radicular back pain.[14,15]
     - Transforaminal and caudal epidural carries less risk for "wet" tap with spinal fluid leakage, spinal headache, and epidural hematomas.
     - Complications during epidural injections for back pain happen due to the following mistakes[16]:
       - Performing a blind epidural injection with no radiographic guidance
       - Not using contrast
       - Using particulate steroids such as methylprednisolone (Depo-Medrol; Pfizer Pharmaceuticals, New York, NY)
       - Other faulty techniques
     - There is no definite evidence that these procedures are effective in treating acute radiculopathy or lower back pain alone.
     - Epidural injections may be an option for short-term relief of radicular pain when control on oral medications is inadequate or for patients who are not surgical candidates.
   - Radiofrequency denervation (neurotomy), for facet-related mechanical spinal pain that is proved by two positive medial branch blocks, using two different local agents of different duration.[17]
   - Spinal cord stimulators for treatment for chronic back pain[18]
   - Sacroiliac joint injection, to diagnose and treat mechanical back pain that is related to sacroiliac joint disease
   - Vertebroplasy or kyphoplasty for management of osteoporotic compression spine fractures[19]
   - In general, interventional procedures are delayed for 4–12 weeks, depending on the case. It is essential to determine if the patient responds to more conservative measures first.
   - In proven one-level diskogenic pain, after failure of conservative measures, consideration could be made to anterior lumbar interbody fusion (ALIF) versus disk arthroplasty; the latter could only be considered in the absence of facet arthropathy.

■ References

1. Greenberg MS. Handbook of Neurosurgery. 6th ed. New York: ThiemeMedical Publishers, 2006
2. Bellaïche L, Petrover D. Imaging in chronic low back pain: which one and when? Rev Prat 2008;58(3):273–278
3. Russo RB. Diagnosis of low back pain: role of imaging studies. Clin Occup Environ Med 2006;5(3):571–589
4. Lurie JD. What diagnostic tests are useful for low back pain? Best Pract Res Clin Rheumatol 2005;19(4):557–575
5. Chou R, Qaseem A, Snow V, et al. Diagnosis and treatment of low back pain: a joint clinical practice guideline from the American College of Physicians and the American Pain Society. Ann Intern Med 2007;147(7):478–491
6. Paquette S. Return to work with chronic low back pain: using an evidence-based approach along with the occupational therapy framework. Work 2008;31(1):63–71
7. Mehlum IS, Kristensen P, Kjuus H, Wergeland E. Are occupational factors important determinants of socioeconomic inequalities in musculoskeletal pain? Scand J Work Environ Health 2008;34(4):250–259
8. May S, Donelson R. Evidence-informed management of chronic low back pain with the McKenzie method. Spine J 2008;8(1):134–141
9. Busanich BM, Verscheure SD. Does McKenzie therapy improve outcomes for back pain? J Athl Train 2006;41(1):117–119
10. Rives PA, Douglass AB. Evaluation and treatment of low back pain in family practice. J Am Board Fam Pract 2004;17(Suppl):S23–S31
11. Bodduk N. Practice Guideline for Spinal Diagnostic & Treatment Procedures. Kentfield: International Spine Intervention Society; 1994
12. Boswell MV, Trescot AM, Datta S, et al. Interventional techniques: evidence-based practice guidelines in the management of chronic spinal pain. Pain Physician 2007;10(1):7–111
13. Overton EA, Kornbluth ID, Saulino MF, Holding MY, Freedman MK. Interventions in chronic pain management. 6. Interventional approaches to chronic pain management. Arch Phys Med Rehabil 2008; 89(3, Suppl 1):S61–S64
14. Benzon HT. Epidural steroid injections for low back pain and lumbosacral radiculopathy. Pain 1986;24(3):277–295
15. DePalma MJ, Bhargava A, Slipman CW. A critical appraisal of the evidence for selective nerve root injection in the treatment of lumbosacral radiculopathy. Arch Phys Med Rehabil 2005;86(7):1477–1483
16. Bogduk N, Dreyfuss P, Baker R, et al. Complications of spinal diagnostic and treatment procedures. Pain Med 2008;9(S1):S11–S34
17. Lord SM, Barnsley L, Wallis BJ, McDonald GJ, Bogduk N. Percutaneous radio-frequency neurotomy for chronic cervical zygapophyseal-joint pain. N Engl J Med 1996;335(23):1721–1726
18. Cruccu G, Aziz TZ, Garcia-Larrea L, et al. EFNS guidelines on neurostimulation therapy for neuropathic pain. Eur J Neurol 2007;14(9):952–970
19. Fourney DR, Schomer DF, Nader R, et al. Percutaneous vertebroplasty and kyphoplasty for painful vertebral body fractures in cancer patients. J Neurosurg 2003;98(1, Suppl):21–30

Case 90   Neurogenic versus Vascular Claudications

Eric P. Roger and Edward Benzel

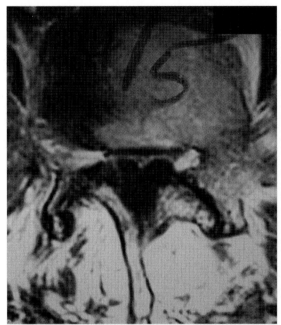 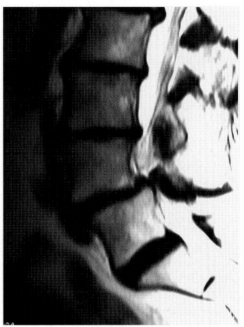

A   B

Fig. 90.1 **(A)** Axial T2-weighted magnetic resonance image (MRI) at the L4–L5 disk space. **(B)** Sagittal T2-weighted MRI of the lumbar spine at the level of the midline.

■ Clinical Presentation

• A 69-year-old man presents with difficulty ambulating.
• The patient also complains of leg "tightness" when he stands or walks, which completely resolves with sitting or leaning over a countertop.

• He has no back pain and no bladder or bowel dysfunction.
• A magnetic resonance imaging (MRI) scan is obtained and shown in **Fig. 90.1**.

■ Questions

1. Interpret the MRI.
2. What other radiologic imaging would you order?
3. What is the differential diagnosis of his leg symptoms?
4. What elements in the clinical presentation would help differentiate spinal versus vascular type of claudication?
5. What other diagnostic modality would help differentiate the two?

The patient has no evidence of arterial insufficiency on examination and has a positive "shopping cart" sign

(resolution of the leg pain when leaning on a shopping cart while walking). He is able to use a stationary bicycle without pain or symptoms. His ankle brachial indices (ABIs) are 1.10 on the right, 1.08 on the left side.

6. What therapeutic options are available to this patient?
7. What is the likelihood of destabilizing the spondylolisthesis with a simple decompressive laminectomy? What are some risk factors of this procedure?
8. Should a fusion be added to his surgical treatment? Should instrumentation also be added?

■ Answers

1. *Interpret the MRI.*
   - The images demonstrate a grade 1 spondylolisthesis of L4 over L5.
   - There is no element of pars defect, at least on these images.
   - There is resulting severe central stenosis at that level, and to a lesser extent at the level above (L3–L4).
   - Paracentral cuts would be required to fully assess the amount of foraminal stenosis present.

2. *What other radiologic imaging would you order?*
   - Plain radiographs would be essential in the evaluation of this patient. Standing anteroposterior, lateral, and oblique views should be obtained.
   - In addition, dynamic films (flexion and extension views) would be useful.
   - MRI may underestimate the degree of listhesis as the images are performed in the supine position. Standing radiographs may show an accentuation of the L4–L5 slip, therefore suggesting instability.
   - This may be confirmed by flexion/extension (flex/xt) views.
   - Oblique views may be useful to assess a pars defect, with a lysis seen across the neck of the "Scotty dog" appearance of the vertebrae.
   - Computed tomography scan of the lumbar spine can also be used to assess the pars integrity

3. *What is the differential diagnosis of his leg symptoms?*
   - Although the differential diagnosis of leg "tightening" and similar symptoms can be attributed to a vast array of etiologies, including neurodegenerative disorders, hip and/or knee pathology, metabolic causes, etc., the two most likely diagnoses are neurogenic and vascular claudications.[1]

4. *What elements of the clinical presentation would help differentiate spinal versus vascular type of claudication?*
   - Vascular claudications[1]
     - Symptoms
       - Calf pain with walking (classic)
       - Buttock, thigh, and/or foot pain may also be present
       - Brought on by walking or other activity
       - Relieved within a few minutes of rest
       - Numbness and/or weakness may be present
       - Rest pain in advanced cases
     - Signs
       - Decreased pulses and bruits
       - Skin changes of arterial insufficiency (shiny, glistening, atrophic, ulcerated, loss of hair, nail changes)
       - Pallor when elevated
       - Dusky rubor when placed in a dependent state (Buerger's sign)
   - Neurogenic claudication[1]
     - Symptoms
       - Leg pain with standing or walking

- May be described as weakness or "giving out"
- Often associated with numbness, potentially dermatomal if stenosis is foraminal
- Brought on by walking and/or standing
- Relieved relatively quickly with sitting or bending forward
     - Signs
       - Often normal on examination
       - May have diminished deep tendon reflexes
       - May have dermatomal paresthesias
       - May have positive straight leg raising (Lasègue sign)
       - Wide-based gait
   - Differentiation of neurogenic versus vascular claudications[1,2]
     - Symptoms
       - Neurogenic aggravated by standing or walking; vascular aggravated by walking but not just standing.
       - Neurogenic improves faster after sitting than does vascular.
       - Neurogenic improves by walking bent forward, as for example with the use of a shopping cart ("shopping cart sign").
       - Vascular aggravated by use of stationary bicycle; not neurogenic
     - Signs
       - Vascular claudication patients "look vasculopathic," with skin changes, nail changes, hair loss. Diminished pulses may be noted.
       - Neurogenic claudication patients often have a relatively normal examination, although neural deficits may be noted.

5. *What other diagnostic modality would help differentiate the two?*
   - ABI: ratio of Doppler-measured blood flow in upper versus lower extremities
     - Normal ratio is >1.
     - A ratio of 0.6–0.9 indicates the claudicant range.
     - A ratio ≤0.5 correlates with rest pain and ulceration.

6. *What therapeutic options are available to this patient?*
   - Conservative management[3]
     - Medications (unlikely to be beneficial): include nonsteroidal antiinflammatories, gabapentin or other antiepileptics use to treat neuropathic pain, other pain medications.
     - Therapies[4–6]
       - Physical therapy
       - Pilates therapy
       - Exercise therapy
       - Chiropractic therapy
       - Traction
     - Injections[6]
       - Epidural
       - Selective nerve root blocks

Answers (*continued*)

- Surgical management[3,7]
  - Decompression (open or minimally invasive)[8–10]
    - Laminectomies[11]
    - Laminotomies and foraminotomies[12]
    - Laminoplasty
    - Interspinous decompression via a spinous process spacer device[13]
  - Decompression and fusion[14]
- Noninstrumented
  - Facet fusion
  - Posterolateral onlay fusion
- Instrumented[15,16]
  - Posterolateral fusion (PLF)
  - Posterior lumbar interbody fusion[15]
  - Transforaminal lumbar interbody fusion (TLIF)
  - Anterior lumbar interbody fusion (indirect decompression) not generally recommended in these cases

7. *What is the likelihood of destabilizing the spondylolisthesis with a simple decompressive laminectomy? What are some risk factors of this procedure?*
   - The likelihood of destabilizing a low-grade (I or II) spondylolisthesis after laminectomy is poorly reported in the literature.
   - There are certain factors that may predispose to an increased risk of destabilization.[2]
     - Preoperative:
       - Pars defect (isthmic)
       - Evidence of instability on flexion/extension films: >4.5 mm of translation[17]
       - Presence of a tall disk space
       - Sagittally oriented facets
       - Overweight patient
     - Intraoperatively
       - Partial or generous facetectomy
       - Injury to the pars interarticularis
       - Overt evidence of instability

8. *Should a fusion be added to his surgical treatment? Should instrumentation also be added?*
   - Although the rate of spondylolisthesis progression after simple decompression is unclear, several studies have reported improved clinical outcomes after fusion (with or without instrumentation).
   - The Lumbar Fusion Guidelines[18] have therefore stated the following:
     - "Guidelines: The performance of a lumbar PLF is recommended for patients with lumbar stenosis and associated degenerative spondylolisthesis who require decompression. There is insufficient evidence to recommend a treatment guideline."[18]
   - It would appear that the addition of instrumentation to the fusion procedure increases the radiologic rate of fusion, although most studies have shown no statistical improvement in clinical outcome.
   - In this regard, the Lumbar Fusion Guidelines[18] have stated the following:
     - "Options. Pedicle screw fixation as an adjunct to lumbar PLF should be considered as a treatment option in patients with lumbar stenosis and spondylolisthesis in cases in which there is preoperative evidence of spinal instability or kyphosis at the level of the spondylolisthesis or when iatrogenic instability is anticipated."[18]
   - A prospective randomized control trial, the Spinal Laminectomy Versus Instrumented Pedicle Screw Fusion Study, is currently under way to compare decompression versus decompression and instrumented fusion in patients with stenotic grade I spondylolisthesis.[19,20]

References

1. Placide RJ, Mazenac DJ. Spinal masqueraders: nonspinal conditions mimicking spine pathology. In: Benzel EC, ed. Spine Surgery: Techniques, Complication Avoidance, and Management. 2nd ed. Philadelphia: Churchill Livingstone; 2004:144–159

2. Benzel EC, ed. Spine Surgery: Techniques, Complication Avoidance, and Management. 2nd ed. Philadelphia: Churchill Livingstone; 2004

3. Weinstein JN, Tosteson TD, Lurie JD, et al. Surgical versus nonsurgical therapy for lumbar spinal stenosis. N Engl J Med 2008;358(8):794–810

4. Goldman SM, Barice EJ, Schneider WR, Hennekens CH. Lumbar spinal stenosis: can positional therapy alleviate pain? J Fam Pract 2008;57(4):257–260

5. Markman JD, Gaud KG. Lumbar spinal stenosis in older adults: current understanding and future directions. Clin Geriatr Med 2008;24(2):369–388

6. Kalichman L, Hunter DJ. Diagnosis and conservative management of degenerative lumbar spondylolisthesis. Eur Spine J 2008;17(3):327–335

7. Katz JN, Stucki G, Lipson S, et al. Predictors of surgical outcome in degenerative lumbar spinal stenosis. Spine 1999;24:2229–2233

8. Rahman M, Summers LE, Richter B, Mimran RI, Jacob RP. Comparison of techniques for decompressive lumbar laminectomy: the minimally invasive versus the "classic" open approach. Minim Invasive Neurosurg 2008;51(2):100–105

9. Fu YS, Zeng BF, Xu JG. Long-term outcomes of two different decompressive techniques for lumbar spinal stenosis. Spine 2008;33(5):514–518

10. Costa F, Sassi M, Cardia A, et al. Degenerative lumbar spinal stenosis: analysis of results in a series of 374 patients treated with unilateral laminotomy for bilateral microdecompression. J Neurosurg Spine 2007;7(6):579–586

■ References (*continued*)

11. Andrews NB, Lawson HJ, Darko D. Decompressive laminectomy for lumbar stenosis: review of 65 consecutive cases from Tema, Ghana. West Afr J Med 2007;26(4):283–287

12. Armin SS, Holly LT, Khoo LT. Minimally invasive decompression for lumbar stenosis and disc herniation. Neurosurg Focus 2008;25(2):E11

13. Miller JD, Nader R. Treatment of combined osteoporotic compression fractures and spinal stenosis: use of vertebral augmentation and interspinous process spacer. Spine 2008;33(19):E717–E720

14. Glassman SD, Carreon LY, Djurasovic M, et al. Lumbar fusion outcomes stratified by specific diagnostic indication. Spine J 2009;9(1):13–21

15. Periasamy K, Shah K, Wheelwright EF. Posterior lumbar interbody fusion using cages, combined with instrumented posterolateral fusion: a study of 75 cases. Acta Orthop Belg 2008;74(2):240–248

16. Tsutsumimoto T, Shimogata M, Yoshimura Y, Misawa H. Union versus nonunion after posterolateral lumbar fusion: a comparison of long-term surgical outcomes in patients with degenerative lumbar spondylolisthesis. Eur Spine J 2008;17(8):1107–1112

17. White AA, Panjabi MM. Clinical Biomechanics of the Spine. 2nd ed. Philadelphia: Lippincott; 1990:30–643

18. Resnick DK, Choudhri TF, Dailey AT, et al. Guidelines for the performance of fusion procedures for degenerative disease of the lumbar spine. Part 9: fusion in patients with stenosis and spondylolisthesis. J Neurosurg Spine 2005;2(6):679–685

19. Vital Trek Clinical Trials. Spinal Laminectomy Versus Instrumented Pedicle Screw Fusion (SLIP) Study. Available at: http://www.spine-slip-study.org/2. Accessed June 21, 2009

20. Greenwich Lumbar Stenosis SLIP Study. Available at: http://www.clinicaltrials.gov/ct/show/NCT00109213. Accessed June 21, 2009

Case 91 Cauda Equina Syndrome

Cristian Gragnaniello and Remi Nader

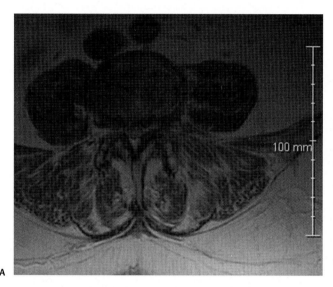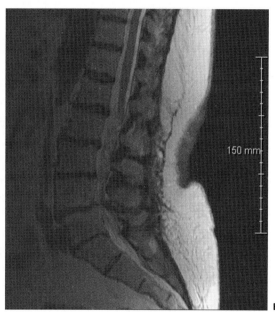

Fig. 91.1 **(A)** Axial T2-weighted magnetic resonance image (MRI) at the L5 pedicle level. **(B)** Sagittal T2-weighted MRI through the lumbar spine.

■ Clinical Presentation

- A 63-year-old woman presents with chronic lower back pain and bilateral radicular pain in an L5 distribution.
- More recently, she developed weakness in the lower extremities and episodic incontinence of urine over the past month.

- Magnetic resonance imaging (MRI) of the lumbar spine is obtained and shown in **Fig. 91.1**.

■ Questions

1. What is the clinical diagnosis? Describe the main clinical features of this diagnosis.
2. What conditions can cause these symptoms and signs?
3. Interpret the MRI findings.
4. What, if any, other imaging studies would you obtain?

5. How do you manage this condition?
6. What is the likelihood of her recovering bladder function?
7. Describe bladder micturition physiologic mechanisms.
8. If there is no relief from the pain, what is your workup and management?

■ Answers

1. *What is the clinical diagnosis? Describe the main clinical features of this diagnosis.*
   - Chronic cauda equina syndrome[1]
   - The fully developed syndrome consists of many clinical symptoms and signs that can be present in various degrees in each individual patient. This can sometimes lead to a delay in the diagnosis that can influence the outcome (**Table 91.1**).[2–4]
2. *What conditions can cause these symptoms and signs?*
   - Causes of onset of this complex syndrome must always be kept in mind when approaching the patient. They are summarized in **Table 91.2**.[5]
3. *Interpret the MRI findings.*
   - Grade 1 degenerative spondylolisthesis at L4/5 causing severe narrowing of the canal and nerve root impingement.[6]
   - The nerve root impingement correlates very well with the clinical signs of radiculopathy.[7,8]
   - A sign that the spondylolisthesis is due to degenerative changes can be found in the sagittal image that shows a malalignment of the spinous process of L4 that displaces with the vertebral body due to maintenance of the integrity of the neural arch.[6]
   - The filamentous-looking structures above L4 are just the nerve roots; they may appear that way in cases of severe stenosis.
   - Marked thickening of the ligamentum flavum is seen in the axial image.
4. *What, if any, other imaging studies would you obtain?*
   - To assess the motion of the lumbar segments that are studied, dynamic radiographs done with flexion and extension should be obtained to rule out instability.[9,10]
   - A computed tomography scan to can determine whether there is a pars defect and to assess the orientation and size of the pedicles, to study the central canal, the lateral recess, and the foramen.[11]
   - Radiographs of the thoracic and lumbar spine and MRI of the whole spine may be also obtained because even if the symptoms suggest the cauda equina syndrome, there may be a more proximal lesion (this is especially important in cases where the stenosis is mild and does not fully account for the symptoms).[12]
5. *How do you manage this condition?*
   - Decompressive bilateral laminectomies using a high-speed drill and acorn or diamond burr to avoid any possible other manipulation of the roots
   - The extent of decompression should allow access laterally to the thecal sac at the level of L4–L5.[1]
   - Timing of the surgery is essential (semiurgent, within 48 hours).[1,3,5,12–16]
   - Fusion must follow if there are instability signs on imaging. Some will elect to fuse anyway, given the significant bilateral decompression necessary here and the likely resection of the disk.[17]
6. *What is the likelihood of her recovering bladder function?*
   - Less than 50% in view of one-month history of dysfunction.
   - The recovery will be better compared with patients who suffered from a complete bladder paralysis[14]
   - Early surgical intervention within 48 hours is essential. In general, the outcome is much better compared with those operated on after 48 hours.[4,14–16,18]
7. *Describe bladder micturition physiologic mechanisms.*
   - There are two phases: bladder filling and emptying (**Fig. 91.2**).
   - Bladder-filling phase[19]
     - The bladder accumulates increasing volumes of urine.
     - The pressure within the bladder must be lower than the urethral pressure during the filling phase.
     - Bladder filling is dependent on the intrinsic viscoelastic properties of the bladder and inhibition of the parasympathetic nerves.
     - Sympathetic nerves facilitate urine storage.
     - Sympathetic input to the lower urinary tract is constantly active during bladder filling.
     - Pudendal nerve becomes excited.

Table 91.1 Most Common Symptoms and Signs of Fully Developed Cauda Equina Syndrome Reported in the Literature

Low back pain
Bilateral sciatica
Saddle anesthesia
Motor weakness of the lower extremities
Loss of reflexes (anal, bulbocavernous, medioplantar, Achilles' tendon)
Rectal and bladder sphincter's dysfunction
Sexual impotence

Source: Data from Aho AJ, Auranen A, Pesonen K. Analysis of cauda equina symptoms in patients with lumbar disc prolapse. Preoperative and follow-up clinical and cystometric studies. Acta Chir Scand 1969, 135(5):413–420. Shapiro S. Cauda equina syndrome secondary to lumbar disc herniation. Neurosurgery 1993, 32(5):743–746; Jalloh I, Minhas P. Delays in the treatment of cauda equina syndrome due to its variable clinical features in patients presenting to the emergency department. Emerg Med J 2007;24(1):33–34.

■ **Answers** *(continued)*

Table 91.2   Most Common Causes of Cauda Equina Syndrome Reported in the Literature

Type of Lesion	Etiology
Nonneoplastic compressive	Herniated lumbosacral disks
	Spinal stenosis
	Epidural abscess
	Spinal subdural hematoma
	Epidural hematoma
	Arteriovenous malformation
Neoplastic compressive	Primary spinal: Schwannomas
	Ependymomas
	Lipomas
	Teratomas
	Secondary: Lung
	Breast
	Prostate
	Kidney
	Myeloproliferative
Noncompressive	Primary Ischemic: Anterior spinal artery syndrome
	Inflammatory: Bechterew syndrome
	Spinal arachnoiditis
	Infective: Bacterial
	Viral (HSV2 seems to be selective)
	Iatrogenic: Postsurgical after intradiskal therapy
	Postchiropractic
	Postepidural anesthesia

Source: Orendácová J, Cízková D, Kafka J, Lukácová N, Marsala M, Sulla I, Marsala J, Katsube N. Cauda equina syndrome. *Prog* Neurobiol 2001;64(6):613–637.

- Bladder-emptying phase[19]
  - A voluntary signal is sent from the brain to begin urination and continues until the bladder is empty.
  - Bladder afferent signals ascend the spinal cord to the periaqueductal gray.
  - These afferents project to the pontine micturition center and to the cerebrum.[20]
  - Once the voluntary signal to begin voiding has been issued, neurons in pontine micturition center fire maximally.
  - This causes excitation of sacral preganglionic neurons leading to the wall of the bladder to contract.
  - The pontine micturition center also causes inhibition of Onuf's nucleus, leading to relaxation of the external urinary sphincter.[21]
- In cases of incontinence related to cauda equina
  - In cauda equina syndrome, afferent and efferent nerves are both lesioned, and the bladder can become flaccid and distended temporarily.
  - The detrusor muscle gradually becomes spontaneously active, with intermittent contractions that may cause dribbling.
  - The bladder then shrinks and its wall hypertrophies.
  - This mechanism is called *denervation hypersensitization.*

8. *If there is no relief from the pain, what are your workup and management?*
- In this situation, to treat refractory residual pain after all conservative therapies failed, functional neurosurgical techniques can yield good results in many cases.
- Different procedures are available and can be considered, including
  - Spinal cord stimulation
  - Ablative procedures like dorsal root entry zone (DREZ) lesioning (or DREZotomy)[22,23]

■ Answers (*continued*)

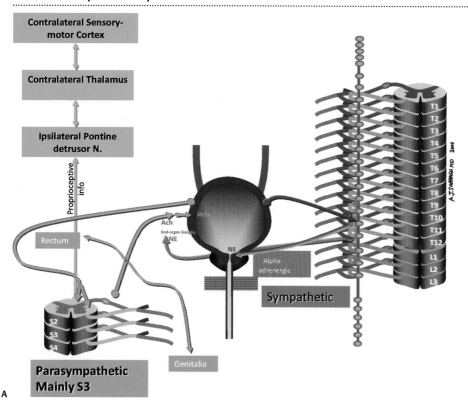

A

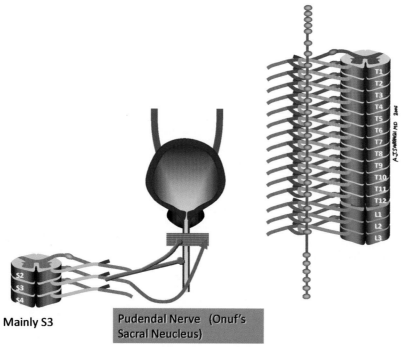

B

Fig. 91.2 Micturition physiologic mechanisms. **(A)** Bladder innervation circuits during micturition and **(B)** during relaxation phase. Ach, acetylcholine; NE, norepinephrine; N, nerve; info, information; T, thoracic; L, lumbar; S, sacral.

■ Answers

1. *What is your differential diagnosis?*
   - The differential diagnosis of spinal progressive my-elopathy is broad and includes the following[1,2] (for a more detailed diagnosis list, please refer to Case 87):
     - Syringomyelia
     - Postviral conditions
     - Vertebral osteomyelitis
     - Traumatic fracture
     - Spinal cord tumor
     - Epidural lipomatosis
     - Degenerative conditions: spondylotic myelopathy, ossified posterior longitudinal ligament, disk her-niation
     - Multiple sclerosis transverse myelitis or Guillain-Barré syndrome
     - Spinal epidural, subdural, or subarachnoid hema-toma, spinal cord infarction

2. *What studies would you like to obtain?*
   - Imaging studies
     - Plain radiographs
     - MRI
       - Study of choice
       - Noninvasive
       - >95% effective in diagnosis of myelopathy
     - Computed tomography (CT) and/or CT myelogram
       - When MRI cannot be done
       - In cases where resolution of MRI is low
       - Plain CT good for C5–C6 but poor for C6–C7 or below due to shoulder artifact
       - CT myelogram has 98% accuracy but requires overnight admission
       - In thoracic disk herniations, CT scan helps to evaluate the extent of calcifications.

3. *Give a general classification of thoracic disk herniations.*
   - Classification by level[3,4]
     - T1–T4, or upper thoracic spine
       - Thoracic outlet and superior mediastinum
     - T5–T9, or middle thoracic spine
       - Stabilizing influences of the rib cage
     - T10–T12, or thoracolumbar spine
       - Transition zone of vertebral configuration
   - Classification by laterality[4]
     - Midline
     - Paramedian
     - Lateral

4. *What are the different treatment measures?*
   - Conservative measures[4]
     - Analgesics, muscle relaxants, nonsteroidal antiin-flammatory drugs
     - Limited activity, bed rest for 1 to 2 weeks
     - Physical therapy — extension exercises and para-spinal muscle strengthening
     - Stretching and muscle relaxation with heat, ultra-sound, or transcutaneous electrical stimulation
     - Bracing (thoracolumbar spinal orthosis brace)
     - Short course of oral steroids
     - Epidural steroid injections
   - Surgical measures – indications[4,5]
     - Failure of conservative measures
     - Severe symptoms of pain or myelopathy
     - Progressive deterioration in symptoms

5. *Which one would you select in this patient and why?*
   - Surgical treatment is the most appropriate approach in this case.
   - This is due to the severity of the symptoms and signs of myelopathy.

6. *What are the different surgical approaches to a thoracic disk, their advantages and limitations?*
   - Approaches for thoracic disk herniations[4–9]
     - Posterior midline laminectomy
       - Ease and familiarity of anatomy and approach
       - Disadvantages
         - Unacceptably high failure rate in single level anterior pathology
         - Neural injury
         - Inadequate decompression
         - *Not* a generally accepted approach for most thoracic disks
   - Posterolateral approach: transpedicular or transfacet — pedicle sparing
     - Laminectomy, removal of pedicle and medial fac-etectomy
     - Good results for lateral herniated disk
     - Do not require transpleural or transmediastinal dissection
     - No violation of the rib cage or ligation of the neu-rovascular bundle
     - Potential for less operative time and bleeding
     - Familiar to most neurosurgeons
     - May be done endoscopically
     - Disadvantages
       - Limited visibility of the midline of the anterior spinal canal
       - Unable to completely remove disks that are mainly central or past the midline
       - Possible instability with removal of pedicle/facet complex

■ Answers (*continued*)

- Costotransversectomy
  - Good for lateral disk herniation
  - Resection of transverse process and 4–8 cm of rib
    - Rib that articulates with the inferior vertebra of the disk level to be treated
  - Ligation of intercostal nerve ~3 cm distal to dorsal root ganglion
  - Direct visualization of neural elements
  - Disadvantages
    - Risk of interrupting radicular artery, which supplies blood to spinal cord
    - Risk of intercostal neuralgia or anesthesia dolorosa
    - Manipulation of intercostals muscles
- Lateral extracavitary approach
  - Enables total resection of centrally located disks
  - Good for central soft and calcified disks
  - Ease of multilevel exposure
  - No need for chest tube drainage if pleura preserved
  - Disadvantages
    - Extensive procedures and bony resection
    - High operating times, blood loss
    - Significant perioperative pain and physiologic stress to the patient
- Anterolateral transthoracic approach
  - Good for central disk or when myelopathy is present → best operative results
  - Good exposure obtained from T4–5 to T11–T12
  - Right-sided thoracotomy preferred for midthoracic because heart does impede access
  - Left-sided preferred for lower thoracic (easier to mobilize aorta than vena cava)
  - Low risk of mechanical cord injury
  - Little compromise of stability
  - Disadvantages
    - Requires thoracic surgeon
    - Extensive, time-demanding procedure
    - Risk of vascular cord injury
    - Pulmonary complications and cerebrospinal fluid (CSF) pleural fistula
    - Postthoracotomy pain syndrome
    - Closed chest drainage is required postoperatively.
    - Mediastinal structures are at increased risk.
    - Hard to access disks above T4–T5
- Video-assisted thoracoscopic approach
  - Minimally invasive
  - Avoids pulmonary complications and morbidities
  - Less blood loss
  - Can access centrally located disk herniations
  - Prevents denervation of paraspinal musculature
  - Less bone resection
  - Disadvantages
    - Requires thoracic surgeon
    - High level of technical skill and steep learning curve
    - Limited ability to strut graft or fuse anteriorly
    - Difficult to repair CSF leak

7. *Which approach would you select in this case?*
   - Any of the approaches described above are appropriate except for laminectomy.
   - In this case, a posterolateral approach via costotransversectomy was selected. Postoperative MRI is shown in **Fig. 92.2 and Fig. 92.3** for illustration of the approach.
   - The reasoning behind this selection: the patient is young and the disk is more likely noncalcified and the disk is lateral to paramedian.
8. *What are the general outcomes of each approach?*
   - Overall outcomes[9–12]
     - Posterior midline laminectomy: 32% worse outcome, 57% improved or stayed the same
     - Posterolateral approach: 7% worse outcome, 82% improved or stayed the same
     - Endoscopic transpedicular: 90% improvement ($n = 25$)[9]
     - Costotransversectomy: 0% worse, 12% same, 88% improved
     - Anterolateral transthoracic approach: 0% worse, 94% pain improved, 97% myelopathy improvement
9. *What are the indications for fusion after diskectomy?*
   - Indications for fusion[4]
     - Multilevel disk resection
     - Kyphosis
     - Wide vertebral body segment resection affecting stability
     - Junctional level (T12–L1)

■ **Answers (*continued*)**

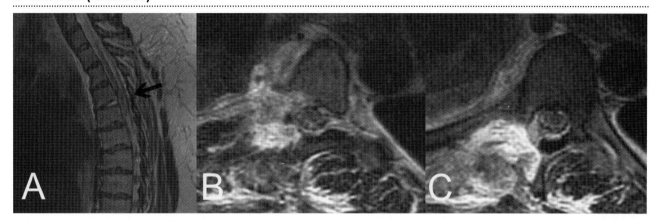

Fig. 92.2   (A) Sagittal and **(B** and **C)** axial T2-weighted magnetic resonance images of the thoracic spine showing herniated disk resection (*arrow*) at the T4–T5 level via a costotransversectomy approach.

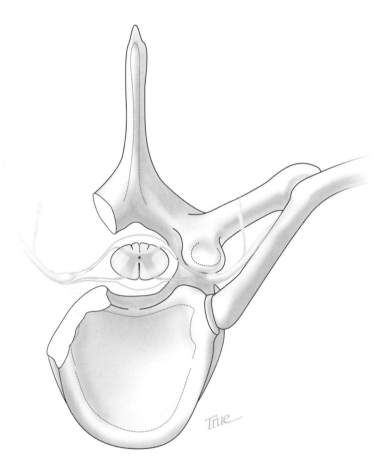

Fig. 92.3   Artist's rendering of the costotransversectomy approach, showing the maximal extent of bony removal. This includes part of the vertebral body, the lamina, transverse process, and pars interarticularis. (From Wolfla CE, Resnick DK. Neurosurgical Operative Atlas. Spine and Peripheral Nerves. New-York: Thieme Medical Publishers/ American Association of Neurological Surgeons; 2007:151. Reprinted with permission.)

■ References

1. Greenberg MS. Handbook of Neurosurgery. 6th ed. New York: Thieme Medical Publishers; 2006
2. Tsementzis SA. Differential Diagnosis in Neurology and Neurosurgery. A Clinician's Pocket Guide. New York: Thieme Medical Publishers; 2000
3. Dietze DD, Fessler RG. Thoracic disc herniations. Neurosurg Clin N Am 1993;4:75–90
4. Vanichkachorn JS, Vaccaro AR. Thoracic disk disease: diagnosis and treatment. J Am Acad Orthop Surg 2000;8(3):159–169
5. Stillerman CB, Chen TC, Couldwell WT, Zhang W, Weiss MH. Experience in the surgical management of 82 symptomatic herniated thoracic discs and review of the literature. J Neurosurg 1998;88(4):623–633
6. Krauss WE, Edwards DA, Cohen-Gadol AA. Transthoracic discectomy without interbody fusion. Surg Neurol 2005;63(5):403–408
7. Dinh DH, Tompkins J, Clark SB. Transcostovertebral approach for thoracic disc herniations. J Neurosurg 2001;94(1, Suppl):38–44
8. Stillerman CB, Chen TC, Day JD, Couldwell WT, Weiss MH. The transfacet pedicle-sparing approach for thoracic disc removal: cadaveric morphometric analysis and preliminary clinical experience. J Neurosurg 1995;83(6):971–976
9. Jho HD. Endoscopic transpedicular thoracic discectomy. J Neurosurg 1999; 91(2, Suppl):151–156
10. Arce CA, Dohrmann GJ. Thoracic disc herniation. Improved diagnosis with computed tomographic scanning and a review of the literature. Surg Neurol 1985;23(4):356–361
11. Greenberg MS. Handbook of Neurosurgery. 6th ed. New York: Thieme Medical Publishers; 2006:923–924
12. Winn RH. Neurological Surgery. 5th ed. Philadelphia: Saunders; 2004:1371–1387

Case 93   **Intradural Spinal Tumor**

Adam Sauh Gee Wu and Stephen J. Hentschel

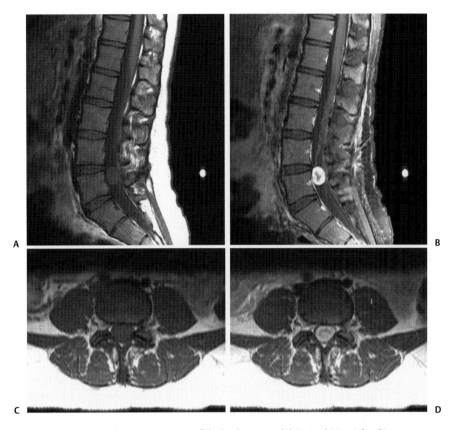

Fig. 93.1   Magnetic resonance images of the lumbar spine. **(A)** Sagittal T1-weighted image, **(B)** sagittal T1-weighted image with gadolinium, **(C)** axial T1-weighted image, **(D)** axial T1-weighted image with gadolinium through the lesion at L5.

■ Clinical Presentation

- A 25-year-old woman presented with a 1-year history of persistent bilateral leg pain radiating from the low back to the posterior thigh and lateral ankle.
- The pain is more severe on the left side than it is on the right.

- Physical examination reveals decreased pinprick sensation over the left lateral leg and ankle. Otherwise, she is neurologically intact.
- A noncontrast computed tomography (CT) scan of the lumbar spine was obtained and was within normal limits.

■ Questions

1. Is further imaging necessary? What are you looking for?
2. A magnetic resonance imaging scan is obtained (**Fig. 93.1**). Describe the findings and exact location of the abnormality.
3. What is your differential diagnosis?
4. What are the indications for and goals of surgery in this case? Is there any role for nonsurgical management?
5. Describe the surgical procedure you would perform. What intraoperative findings would you expect with respect to the relationships to neural structures and the site of origin of the mass?

6. What operative adjuncts might you consider?
7. What are the potential complications of surgery in this case, and what can you do during surgery to reduce the risk of complications?
8. Hematoxylin and eosin stains of the specimen at low and high power are shown (**Fig. 93.2**). Describe the histopathology. What is the diagnosis?
9. Describe the cytogenetics associated with this tumor.
10. What is the expected outcome of surgery in this case, and what is the potential for recurrence?

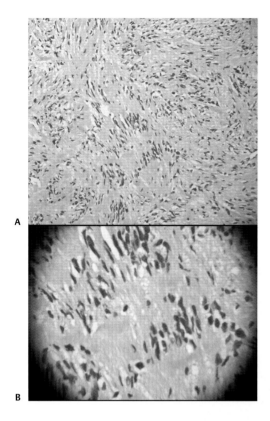

A

B

Fig. 93.2 Hematoxylin and eosin stains of pathology specimen: representative **(A)** low and **(B)** high power views are shown.

■ Answers

1. *Is further imaging necessary? What are you looking for?*
   - Although the CT scan is normal, an MRI scan is needed to rule out intradural pathology.
2. *An MRI scan is obtained (**Fig. 93.1**). Describe the findings and exact location of the abnormality.*
   - There is an intradural mass at the L5 level.
   - It is isodense on T1-weighted images, with intense gadolinium enhancement but no obvious dural tail.
3. *What is your differential diagnosis?*
   - The most common intradural neoplasms of the spinal cord and cauda equina with the MRI characteristics seen in this case are meningiomas, schwannomas, neurofibromas, and myxopapillary ependymomas.
   - Metastases, hemangiopericytomas, and lipomas are less likely.[1–3]
4. *What are the indications for and goals of surgery in this case? Is there any role for nonsurgical management?*
   - The indications for surgery are cytoreduction to relieve mass effect, and to obtain tissue for pathologic analysis.[1,4]
   - The goal of surgery is complete resection of the tumor with preservation of neurologic function,[1] but subtotal resection is preferred over aggressive tumor removal, which risks neurologic injury, as most tumors are benign.

- Nonsurgical management may be considered if the patient has high surgical risk or limited life expectancy.
5. *Describe the surgical procedure you would perform. What intraoperative findings would you expect with respect to the relationships to neural structures and the site of origin of the mass?*
   - The mass can be accessed with a standard L5 laminectomy.
   - Bone may be removed from the pedicles and facets to facilitate exposure in some cases, but that is unlikely to be necessary here.
   - The dura should be opened with preservation of the underlying arachnoid to prevent rapid cerebrospinal fluid (CSF) release, which may obscure the operative field, increase the amount of epidural bleeding, and increase the risk of neurologic injury.
   - The dural edges are tacked back and the arachnoid is opened sharply and clipped to the dura with vascular clips.
   - The expected intraoperative findings will vary with the tumor type.

■ Answers (*continued*)

- Meningiomas commonly arise lateral or posterior to the neural elements, which are usually pushed aside.[2]
  - Invasion of neural structures is very rare.
  - If there is no risk of neurologic injury from doing so, the tumor should be removed en bloc to prevent spillage of neoplastic cells.
  - The dural attachment is variably extensive and should be coagulated thoroughly or excised if possible.
- Schwannomas tend to arise from dorsal nerve roots and come from a single fascicle that can be seen entering and exiting the tumor mass.
  - Surrounding fascicles associated with the tumor's pseudocapsule can often be dissected free.
  - If not, the tumor may be debulked, leaving the pseudocapsule and adherent fascicles behind.
- In contrast, neurofibromas often arise from ventral nerve roots and may involve and invade multiple adjacent fascicles.[1,2]
  - The involved nerve root is usually nonfunctional and frequently must be sacrificed to achieve a gross total resection.
- Myxopapillary ependymomas generally arise from the conus area[5] and are surrounded by lumbosacral nerve roots, requiring piecemeal removal.

6. *What operative adjuncts might you consider?*
  - Intraoperative ultrasound can be used to determine the limits of the tumor prior to dural opening.
  - An operating microscope should always be used.
  - Direct electrical stimulation of nerve roots with bipolar stimulation and electromyography may be used to identify important functional roots.
  - Electrophysiological monitoring with somatosensory evoked potentials (sensitivity 87%, specificity 90%) and motor evoked potentials (MEPs) (sensitivity 100%, specificity 75%) can be used to detect potentially reversible neurologic injuries.[1]
  - A cavitating ultrasonic aspirator can be used to help debulk the interior of the tumor.

7. *What are the potential complications of surgery in this case, and what can you do during surgery to reduce the risk of complications?*

- The risk of neurologic morbidity is 15% and that of mortality is 3%.
- The risk of neurologic worsening is minimized by avoiding manipulation of the nerve roots, spinal cord, and other neural elements and by utilizing aggressive bony removal when necessary.
- The CSF spaces should be cleared of blood by thorough irrigation prior to dural closure to reduce the risk of postoperative headache, arachnoiditis, and aseptic meningitis.
- A watertight dural closure using dural patch grafts when necessary will decrease the risk of CSF leak and pseudomeningocele formation.
- The risk of spinal instability in cases requiring extensive bone removal can be reduced by concurrent instrumentation and fusion.[1]

8. *Hematoxylin and eosin stains of the specimen at low and high power are shown* (**Fig. 93.2**). *Describe the histopathology. What is the diagnosis?*
  - Multiple spindle-shaped cells with tapering nuclei are seen arranged in compactly associated parallel streams. This is typical of the Antoni A pattern.
  - More loosely textured Antoni B areas are also visible, primarily in the upper left corner of the image.
  - Verocay bodies are apparent in the higher magnification image.
  - These features are all consistent with the diagnosis of schwannoma.[5]

9. *Describe the cytogenetics associated with this tumor.*
  - Alterations of chromosome 22q, including loss of the entire chromosome, LOH of 22q, or loss of function mutations of the *NF2* gene found at 22q, are the only consistent genetic alterations found in schwannomas.[6]

10. *What is the expected outcome of surgery in this case, and what is the potential for recurrence?*
  - Significant relief of pain and improvement of neurologic symptoms are seen in 80 to 90% of cases.[1,7]
  - Schwannomas have a 6 to 12% recurrence rate with a mean time to recurrence of 5 years.
  - Subtotal resections have a recurrence rate of less than 15%.[1,2]

■ References

1. Hentschel SJ, McCutcheon IE. Intradural extramedullary spinal tumors. In: Fehlings MG, Gokaslan ZL, Dickman CA, eds. Spinal Cord and Spinal Column Tumors: Principles and Practice. New York: Thieme Medical Publishers; 2006: 335–348

2. Traul DE, Shaffrey ME, Schiff D. Part 1: Spinal-cord neoplasms — intradural neoplasms. Lancet Oncol 2007;8:35–45

3. Wager M, Lapierre F, Blanc JL, Listrat A, Bataille B. Cauda equina tumors: a French multicenter retrospective review of 231 adult cases and review of literature. Neurosurg Rev 2000;23:119–129

4. Chanda A, Guha A. Cauda equina, paraspinal, and peripheral nerve tumors. In: Fehlings MG, Gokaslan ZL, Dickman CA, eds. Spinal Cord and Spinal Column Tumors: Principles and Practice. New York: Thieme Medical Publishers; 2006: 349–368

5. Coons SW. Pathology of tumors of the spinal cord, spine, and paraspinous soft tissue. In: Fehlings MG, Gokaslan ZL, Dickman CA, eds. Spinal Cord and Spinal Column Tumors: Principles and Practice. New York: Thieme Medical Publishers; 2006: 41–110

6. Shapiro J. Cellular and molecular biology of central nervous system spinal and peripheral nerve neoplasms. In: Fehlings MG, Gokaslan ZL, Dickman CA, eds. Spinal Cord and Spinal Column Tumors: Principles and Practice. New York: Thieme Medical Publishers; 2006: 111–133

7. Jinnai T, Koyama T. Clinical characteristics of spinal nerve sheath tumors: analysis of 149 cases. Neurosurgery 2005;56:510–515

Case 94   Intramedullary Spinal Tumor

Amgad S. Hanna and William E. Krauss

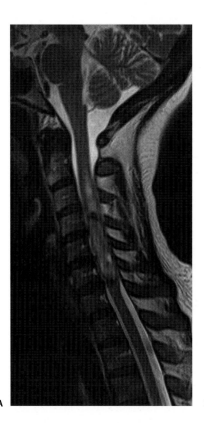

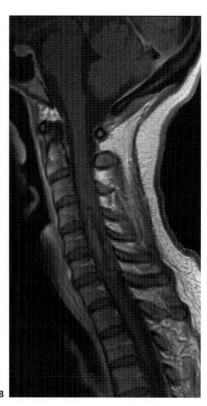

Fig. 94.1   (A) Sagittal magnetic resonance imaging of the C-spine with T2-weighted image and **(B)** T1-weighted image with gadolinium revealing an intramedullary tumor. On T2-weighted images, the tumor is isointense to the spinal cord, with hypointensity (hemosiderin deposits) above and below the tumor and a hyperintense overlying syrinx. There is heterogeneous enhancement after gadolinium.

A   B

■ Clinical Presentation

- A 47-year-old woman presents with a 4-year history of intermittent tingling of the left hand that has progressively gotten worse and is now also involving the left lower extremity.
- There was no loss of bowel or bladder function and no headaches.

- The medical history is remarkable for mitral valve prolapse and two breast biopsies for benign lesions.
- Neurologic examination was completely normal.

■ Questions

1. What is the differential diagnosis?
2. What studies do you need to order?
3. The study you ordered is in **Fig. 94.1**. Describe the findings and the current differential diagnosis.
4. What treatment would you recommend to the patient? What are the risks?
5. What equipment do you need? Describe the surgical procedure. **Figure 94.2** is an intraoperative view; how would you proceed?

6. The pathology is shown in **Fig. 94.3**. What is your diagnosis?
7. **Figure 94.4** is the postoperative magnetic resonance image (MRI); what is her prognosis? What treatment do you recommend at this point?
8. Eight months later, she complains of sagging of her head and weakness and spasticity of the left leg. The radiograph is shown in **Fig. 94.5**. What would you do?

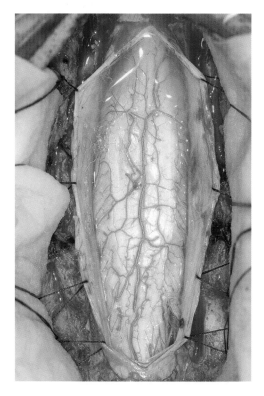

Fig. 94.2   Magnified operative view using the microscope. Note the swollen cord and grayish discoloration.

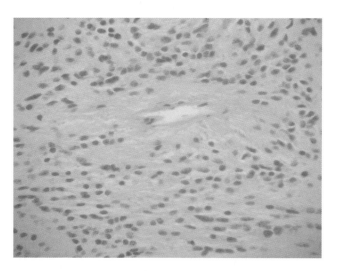

Fig. 94.3   Histological section revealing perivascular pseudorosettes, characteristic of ependymoma.

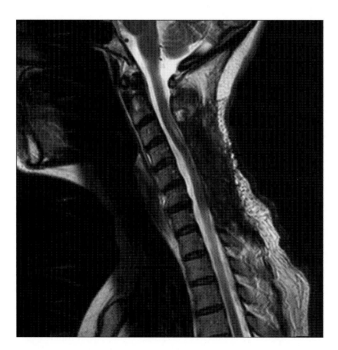

Fig. 94.4   Postoperative T2-weighted magnetic resonance imaging reveals no tumor mass.

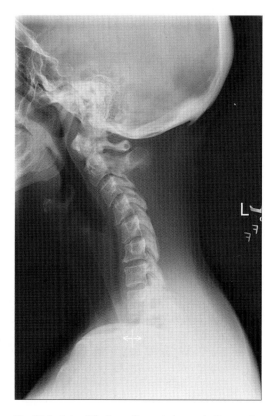

Fig. 94.5   Lateral C-spine radiograph demonstrating postlaminectomy kyphosis.

■ Answers

1. *What is the differential diagnosis?*
   - Anatomic
     - The sensory symptoms involving the left upper and lower extremities localize the lesion to the cervical spine, brainstem, or right parietal lobe.
     - The absence of headache and facial symptoms makes it less likely to be the parietal lobe.
     - The absence of cranial nerve involvement makes it less likely to be the brainstem.
     - This is probably a cervical spine lesion.
   - Etiological[1]
     - Degenerative: disk herniation, synovial cyst, cervical stenosis usually associated with pain and/or myelopathy
     - Neoplastic: extradural (metastasis, primary bone tumor), intradural extramedullary (meningioma, schwannoma, neurofibroma, ganglioneuroma), or intramedullary (ependymoma, astrocytoma, hemangioblastoma). The chronic progressive symptoms fit with a benign neoplastic etiology.
     - Vascular: cavernoma. Arteriovenous malformations (AVMs) usually present acutely or subacutely. Spinal cord infarcts present acutely, usually with motor symptoms.
     - Demyelinating: multiple sclerosis (MS). The remittent course fits with an MS plaque, although the age of onset in MS is usually younger. Transverse myelopathy presents acutely or subacutely with more dramatic deficits.
     - Others: trauma, radiation myelopathy, epidural abscess, and acquired immunodeficiency syndrome (AIDS) are less likely from the history. Toxic/metabolic — alcoholism, vitamin B12 deficiency. Syringomyelia usually presents with bilateral loss of pain and temperature sensation in the upper extremities and spastic paraparesis. Enterogenous cysts, dural ectasia, and arachnoid cysts are rare.

2. *What studies do you need to order?*
   - Cervical spine MRI with gadolinium.
   - Laboratory work: vitamin B12 level; methyl malonic acid and homocysteine levels; serum and urine protein electrophoresis; complete blood count; electrolytes

3. *The study you ordered is in* **Fig. 94.1**. *Describe the findings and the current differential diagnosis.*
   - Sagittal MRI of the cervical (C-) spine reveals an intramedullary tumor.
   - On T2-weighted images, the tumor is isointense to the spinal cord, with hypointensity (hemosiderin deposits) above and below the tumor, and a hyperintense overlying syrinx.
   - There is heterogeneous enhancement after gadolinium.
   - The commonest intramedullary tumor in this age group is ependymoma followed by astrocytoma.

Others include hemangioblastoma, schwannoma, and metastasis.
   - The hypointensities on T2-weighted images above and below the tumor are characteristic (though not pathognomonic) of ependymoma.[1]

4. *What treatment would you recommend to the patient? What are the risks?*
   - We recommend surgical resection of the tumor (given the extent and appearance of the lesion on MRI and the progressive nature of the symptoms).
   - Risks include neurologic deficits like paraplegia or quadriplegia, loss of bowel or bladder function, respiratory failure, tracheostomy, and ventilator dependency, cerebrospinal fluid leak, neck pain, cervical instability, tumor recurrence, hematoma, infection, and spinal cord ischemia.[2]

5. *What equipment do you need? Describe the surgical procedure.* **Figure 94.2** *is an intraoperative view; how would you proceed?*
   - Equipment needed intraoperatively includes the following:
     - Mayfield (or other kind) head holder
     - Jackson radiolucent table or chest rolls
     - Neurophysiologic monitoring with motor evoked potentials and somatosensory evoked potentials
     - Intraoperative ultrasonography (US) for tumor localization
     - Operative microscope and microinstruments
     - Ultrasonic surgical aspirator[3]
   - Details of the surgery are as follows:
     - After cervical laminectomy, the dura is opened and tacked (**Fig. 94.2**).
     - A midline myelotomy is performed starting in the area of grayish discoloration.
     - If the tumor is hard to find, intraoperative US could help.
     - A specimen for frozen section should be immediately sent.
     - Tumor debulking is then started using suction or ultrasonic aspiration.
     - If pathology reveals ependymoma, and a good margin is visualized between the tumor and the spinal cord, every effort should be made for gross total resection.
     - In the case of astrocytoma, the margins are usually difficult to define; the goal is to remove as much as can safely be removed.
     - After careful hemostasis, the dura is closed with or without patching.
     - One may argue to fuse the laminectomized levels.

6. *The pathology is shown in* **Fig. 94.3**. *What's your diagnosis?*
   - **Figure 94.3** reveals perivascular pseudorosettes, which are characteristic of ependymoma.[4]

■ Answers (*continued*)

7. **Figure 94.4** *is the postoperative MRI; what is her prognosis? What treatment do you recommend at this point?*
   - Postoperative T2-weighted MRI reveals no residual tumor.
   - If this is confirmed by gadolinium-enhanced MRI, the prognosis is very good because complete resection can be curative.
   - Clinical as well as radiologic observation should be recommended at this point.
   - Radiation therapy should be recommended only in cases of incomplete resection.[5–8]

8. *Eight months later, she complains of sagging of her head and weakness and spasticity of the left leg. The radiograph is shown in* **Fig. 94.5**. *What would you do?*

   - Lateral C-spine x-ray reveals a postlaminectomy kyphosis.
   - For this reason, one may argue for fusing prophylactically after a laminectomy.[9]
   - At this point, the patient may be put in traction to correct the cervical alignment.
   - Traction is followed by a posterior fusion (in this case with lateral mass screws and rod fixation) (**Fig. 94.6**).
   - If reduction is not possible, a combined anterior and posterior approach may be required. This can involve a multilevel anterior cervical diskectomy and fusion, followed by posterior release of the facet joints.[10]

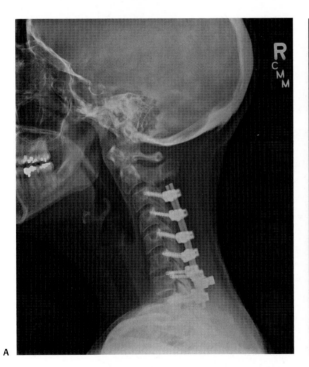
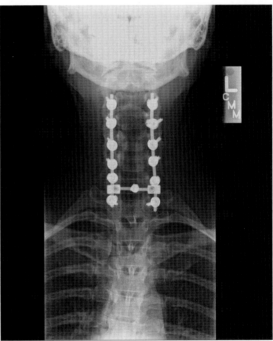

Fig. 94.6 **(A)** Lateral **(B)** and anteroposterior C-spine x-rays after reduction and stabilization using screws and rods.

■ References

1. Osborn AG. Diagnostic Neuroradiology. St. Louis, MO: Mosby, 1994: 465
2. McCormick PC, Stein B. Intramedullary tumors in adults. Neurosurg Clin N Am 1990;1(3):609–630
3. Simeone FA, Eshaghi GE. Intradural tumors. In: Garfin S, Eismont FJ, Bell GR, Balderston RA, Herkowitz H, eds. Rothman-Simeone The Spine. 5th ed. Philadelphia: Saunders-Elsevier; 2006
4. Ellison D, Love S, Chimell L, Harding B, Lowe JS, Vinters HV. Neuropathology – A reference text to CNS pathology. St. Louis, MO: Mosby; 2004
5. Cooper PR. Outcome after operative treatment of intramedullary spinal cord tumors in adults: intermediate and long-term results in 51 patients. Neurosurgery 1989;25(6):855–859
6. Epstein FJ, Farmer JP, Freed D. Adult intramedullary spinal cord ependymomas: the result of surgery in 38 patients. J Neurosurg 1993;79(2):204–209
7. Brotchi J, Dewitte O, Levivier M, et al. A survey of 65 tumors within the spinal cord: surgical results and the importance of preoperative magnetic resonance imaging. Neurosurgery 1991;29(5):651–656
8. Isaacson SR. Radiation therapy and the management of intramedullary spinal cord tumors. J Neurooncol 2000;47:231–238
9. Butler JC, Whitecloud TS III. Postlaminectomy kyphosis. Causes and surgical management. Orthop Clin North Am 1992;23(3):505–511
10. Deutsch H, Haid RW, Rodts GE, Mummaneni PV. Postlaminectomy cervical deformity. Neurosurg Focus 2003;15(3):E5

Case 95   Spinal Metastases

Brian Seaman and Joseph A. Shehadi

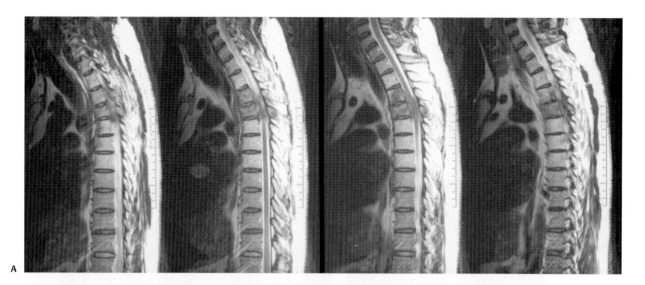

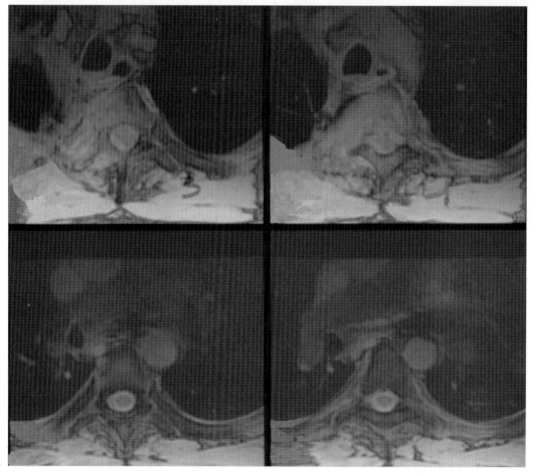

Fig. 95.1 **(A)** Thoracic spine sagittal T2-weighted and **(B)** axial T2-weighted magnetic resonance images through T3–T6: Upper two images — T3 and T4, lower two images — T5 and T6.

Clinical Presentation

- A 34-year-old man has a known history of non-small cell adenocarcinoma of the lung (NSCLC). His cancer treatment consisted of a right upper lobectomy, radiation, and chemotherapy 18 months prior to admission.
- The patient presents with progressively worsening midthoracic pain, right leg weakness, and bilateral lower extremities sensory disturbances.

- His neurologic examination was significant for ⅗ strength in the right lower extremity (based on the Medical Research Council scoring system) and a sensory level at T4 to pinprick.
- Long track signs were present in the lower extremities with hyperreflexia, bilateral upgoing toes, and clonus.
- Postvoid residual was elevated at 600 mL and rectal tone was normal.

Questions

1. Interpret the magnetic resonance imaging (MRI) of the thoracic spine (**Fig. 95.1**).
2. What is your initial management for this patient? What additional studies would you order?
3. List the most common tumors to metastasize to the spinal column in the adult population.

Computed tomography (CT) of the chest, abdomen, and pelvis failed to reveal visceral metastasis. Bone scan and MRI of the spinal axis revealed the lesions at T3 and T4 to be isolated. Karnofsky performance status was 80 prior to his recent neurologic decline.

4. List the treatment options for this patient.
5. Select a surgical treatment strategy for this lesion.
6. What spinal tumors tend to be radiosensitive? What is the typical fractionation schedule for individuals with spinal metastasis?
7. What is the efficacy of radiation therapy for preservation and restoration of neurologic function in patients with spinal cord metastasis and epidural compression?
8. What are the benefits of surgical decompression in addition to radiation compared with radiation therapy alone?
9. Is there a role for percutaneous vertebroplasty and kyphoplasty in metastatic disease?

The patient acutely underwent surgical intervention. The goals of surgery were to prevent neurologic decline, alleviate pain, stabilize the affected motion segments, and possibly restore lost neurologic function. Also, surgical intervention was a good option given that the vertebral and epidural metastases were from radioresistant NSCLC. The patient underwent single-stage transpedicular vertebrectomies at T3 and T4 with circumferential decompression and fixation. Anterior vertebral body reconstruction was completed with polymethylmethacrylate (PMMA). Posterior segmental instrumented fusion was completed via pedicle screws and rods from T1–T6 (**Fig. 95.2**). Local radiotherapy and systemic chemotherapy were initiated after the wound healed. The patient was ambulatory after treatment with significant pain relief. His survival was 6 months.

10. List the clinical factors that affect survival in patients with thoracic spine metastases and cord compression. Can these criteria reliably be used to guide surgical decision making?
11. Prior to the consideration of surgical intervention, what clinical data can be used to help determine prognosis in patients with spinal metastases specifically from lung cancer?
12. What factors should be considered when choosing the appropriate graft material for anterior spinal reconstruction?
13. What complications must you consider in individuals who are considered for surgical intervention who have previously been treated with radiation therapy?

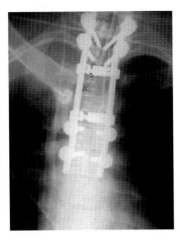

Fig. 95.2 Postoperative anteroposterior thoracic x-ray.

■ Answers

1. *Interpret the MRI of the thoracic spine (**Fig. 95.1**).*
   - T2-weighted sagittal images (**Fig. 95.1A**) demonstrate hypointense lesions at T3 and T4 level involving the vertebral bodies, pedicles, and posterior elements. There is evidence of signal changes within the spinal cord.
   - There is circumferential epidural involvement with spinal cord compression.
   - The osseous and epidural infiltration are further demonstrated on axial T2-weighted images (**Fig. 95.1B**).

2. *What is your initial management for this patient? What additional studies would you order?*
   - Corticosteroids are indicated for the prevention of neurologic deterioration and analgesia.[1]
   - Additionally, there may be an oncolytic effect for certain histology types (such as breast cancer and lymphoma).[2]
   - The patient should be admitted to the hospital and placed on high-dose intravenous steroids such as dexamethasone (50 mg once followed by 10 mg every 6 hours) with gastrointestinal prophylaxis.
   - Additionally, a Foley catheter may be placed given the elevated postvoid residuals.
   - A CT scan of the chest, abdomen, and pelvis and a radiograph of the chest should be performed to restage the cancer.
   - A total body bone scan, using technetium-99m (Tc-99m) labeled phosphate compounds, can be used to determine whether a lesion is solitary or multifocal. Uptake depends on local blood flow and osteoblastic activity; therefore, malignancies such as multiple myeloma are not usually detected via this method.

3. *List the most common tumors to metastasize to the spinal column in the adult population.*
   - More than 90% of spinal tumors are metastatic.
   - Breast, lung, and prostate cancer make up 60–70% of neoplasms that metastasize to the spinal column and cause symptomatic spinal cord compression.[3,4]
   - Less frequently, lymphoma, renal cell carcinoma, colon carcinoma, melanoma, and sarcomas metastasize to the spinal column.[2,5]

4. *List the treatment options for this patient.*
   - The prognosis and survival rates are poor in lung cancer patients with metastasis to the spine.[3,4,6]
   - Conservative nonoperative treatment consists of radiation and/or chemotherapy.
   - However, others believe advanced NSCLC in patients with symptomatic spinal cord compression is worth treating aggressively, especially young patients.[7]
   - Surgical treatment can be justified on the basis of palliation, preservation or improvement of neurological function, and/or spinal stabilization to improve mobility.[8]
   - Surgical therapy can be followed by radiation therapy, chemotherapeutic drugs, and targeted therapeutic agents.

5. *Select a surgical treatment strategy for this lesion.*
   - For a circumferential metastatic lesion in the thoracic spine, there are a few surgical options.
   - Surgical approaches include an anterior transthoracic vertebrectomy or a posterior transpedicular vertebrectomy with instrumented stabilization.[8]
   - Chen et al.[7] reviewed surgical results of metastatic spinal cord compression secondary to NSCLC.
     - Patients underwent palliative surgery using a posterolateral transpedicular approach or combined anterior and posterior procedures.
     - 68% regained the ability to walk; overall 74% of patients were able to walk after surgery.
     - Median survival was 8.8 months.

■ **Answers (*continued*)**

- Dagnew et al.[9] achieved a high success rate with respect to functional outcome and pain relief in individuals with spinal metastasis who underwent a single-stage transpedicular vertebrectomy with circumferential decompression and fixation.

6. *What spinal tumors tend to be radiosensitive? What is the typical fractionation schedule for individuals with spinal metastasis?*
   - Radiosensitive tumors include breast, prostate, small cell lung cancer, lymphoma, and multiple myeloma.
   - Renal cell carcinoma, melanoma, and NSCLC are relatively radioresistant.[1]
   - Typically, total radiation dose ranges from 2500–3600 cGy. It is usually given in 10–15 fractions to avoid significant side effects.[10]

7. *What is the efficacy of radiation therapy for preservation and restoration of neurologic function in patients with spinal cord metastasis and epidural compression?*
   - Kovner et al.[11] demonstrated that motor strength before radiation therapy was predictive of ambulatory function.
   - 90% of patients who were ambulatory before treatment remained so; 33% of the nonambulatory patients regained their ability to walk.
   - Among the nonambulatory patients, 50% of those who were paretic became ambulatory, whereas only 14% of those who were plegic became ambulatory.

8. *What are the benefits of surgical decompression in addition to radiation compared with radiation therapy alone?*
   - A randomized trial[12] assigned 101 patients with cord compressions to either radiotherapy alone (*n* = 51) or decompression surgery followed by radiotherapy (*n* = 50).
   - Results demonstrated that surgery plus radiotherapy is superior to radiotherapy alone in the treatment of spinal cord compression caused by metastasis.
   - Patients who underwent surgery were able to walk more than 3.5 times longer than those who received radiotherapy alone: a median of 126 days versus 35 days, respectively (*p* = 0.006).
   - Of the 16 patients in each group who entered the trial unable to walk, 56% of those in the surgery arm regained mobility, compared with 19% of patients who received radiation alone (*p* = 0.03).
   - Overall survival was not affected.[10]

9. *Is there a role for percutaneous vertebroplasty and kyphoplasty in metastatic disease?*
   - Percutaneous vertebroplasty and kyphoplasty represent a successful option for the palliative treatment of intractable spinal pain associated with malignant spinal tumors and metastases.[13]

10. *List the clinical factors that affect survival in patients with thoracic spine metastases and cord compression.*

Can these criteria reliably be used to guide surgical decision making?
- In general, vertebral column metastatic disease survival rates are highest in patients with radiosensitive tumors, single spinal metastasis, and individuals with preserved ambulation.[1]
- The presence of two or more poor prognostic indicators (leg strength 0/5–3/5, lung or colon cancer, multiple vertebral body involvement) usually predicts shorter survival rates.[1,3]
- Currently, there are two major grading systems that can be used to guide surgical decision making for spinal metastasis: these were derived by Tokuhashi et al. in 1990 and Tomita et al. in 2001.[14,15]
- Tomita et al.[15] designed a scoring system based on three prognostic factors: grade of malignancy (rate of growth), visceral metastasis (treatable versus untreatable), and bone metastasis (solitary or multiple).
- The lower scores suggested a wide or marginal excision for long-term local control. The highest scores indicated nonoperative supportive care. Intermediate scores justified intralesional excision or palliative surgery.
- Survival and extent of local control correlated well with the treatment strategy.
- Of note, a recent large series of spinal metastasis from breast cancer did not show prognostic value for the presence of visceral metastasis or multiplicity of spinal lesions.[16]

11. *Prior to the consideration of surgical intervention, what clinical data can be used to help determine prognosis in patients with spinal metastases specifically from lung cancer?*
    - Ogihara et al.[6] conducted a retrospective study of 114 patients to identify prognostic factors of patients with spinal metastases from lung cancer.
    - Multivariate analysis showed that the significant prognostic factors for survival after spinal metastases from NSCLC were performance status, calcium levels, and albumin.
    - Among SCLC patients, calcium levels, albumin, and a history of chemotherapy were significant (*p* = 0.05) in univariate analysis.[6]

12. *What factors should be considered when choosing the appropriate graft material for anterior spinal reconstruction?*
    - PMMA bone cement is a load-sharing entity, which is resistant to compressive forces and offers an immediate stabilizing construct when used in the anterior spine.
    - In patients with a short life span undergoing palliative surgery or postoperative radiation, PMMA is recommended.[10]
    - On the other hand, in patients with a prolonged life expectancy, allograft or autograft bone is preferred and is used when possible.[10,17]

■ **Answers** (*continued*)

13. *What complications must you consider in those individuals who are considered for surgical intervention who have previously been treated with radiation therapy?*
    • Spinal radiation before surgical decompression for metastatic spinal cord compression is associated with a significantly higher wound complication rate.[18]
    • Risk of wound infection may be up to 3-fold higher than in those individuals undergoing surgery de novo.[10]

■ **References**

1. Gabriel K, Schiff D. Metastatic spinal cord compression by solid tumors. Semin Neurol 2004;24(4):375–383

2. Posner J. Neurologic Complications of Cancer. Philadelphia: FA Davis; 1995

3. Sioutos PJ, Arbit E, Meshulam CF, Galicich JH. Spinal metastases from solid tumors. Analysis of factors affecting survival. Cancer 1995;76(8):1453–1459

4. Weigel B, Maghsudi M, Neumann C, Kretschmer R, Müller FJ, Nerlich M. Surgical management of symptomatic spinal metastases. Postoperative outcome and quality of life. Spine 1999;24(21):2240–2246

5. Shedid D, Benzel EC. Clinical presentation of spinal tumors. Neurosurg Q 2004;14:224–228

6. Ogihara S, Seichi A, Hozumi T, et al. Prognostic factors for patients with spinal metastases from lung cancer. Spine 2006;31(14):1585–1590

7. Chen YJ, Chang GC, Chen HT, et al. Surgical results of metastatic spinal cord compression secondary to non-small cell lung cancer. Spine 2007;32(15):E413–E418

8. Shehadi JA, Sciubba DM, Suk I, et al. Surgical treatment strategies and outcome in patients with breast cancer metastatic to the spine: a review of 87 patients. Eur Spine J 2007;16(8):1179–1192

9. Dagnew E, Mendel E, Rhines L, Lang F, Gokasian Z, McCutcheon I. Single-stage transpedicular vertebrectomy with circumferential decompression and fixation for the management of spinal metastasis: a 10-year experience. Neurosurgery 2005;57(2):399

10. Mut M, Schiff D, Shaffrey ME. Metastasis to nervous system: spinal epidural and intramedullary metastases. J Neurooncol 2005;75(1):43–56

11. Kovner F, Spigel S, Rider I, et al. Radiation therapy of metastatic spinal cord compression. Multidisciplinary team diagnosis and treatment. J Neurooncol 1999;42(1):85–92

12. Regine W, Tibbs P, Young A, et al. Metastatic spinal cord compression: a randomized trial of direct decompressive surgical resection plus radiotherapy vs. radiotherapy alone. Abstract presented at: the 45th Annual ASTRO Meeting, October 19–23, 2003; Salt Lake City, UT

13. Fourney DR, Schomer DF, Nader R, et al. Percutaneous vertebroplasty and kyphoplasty for painful vertebral body fractures in cancer patients. J Neurosurg 2003; 98(1, Suppl):21–30

14. Tokuhashi Y, Matsuzaki H, Toriyama S, Kawano H, Ohsaka S. Scoring system for the preoperative evaluation of metastatic spine tumor prognosis. Spine 1990;15(11):1110–1113

15. Tomita K, Kawahara N, Kobayashi T, Yoshida A, Murakami H, Akamaru T. Surgical strategy for spinal metastases. Spine 2001;26(3):298–306

16. Sciubba DM, Gokaslan ZL, Suk I, et al. Positive and negative prognostic variables for patients undergoing spine surgery for metastatic breast disease. Eur Spine J 2007;16(10):1659–1667

17. Walker MP, Yaszemski MJ, Kim CW, Talac R, Currier BL. Metastatic disease of the spine: evaluation and treatment. Clin Orthop Relat Res 2003; (415, Suppl):S165–S175

18. Ghogawala Z, Mansfield FL, Borges LF. Spinal radiation before surgical decompression adversely affects outcomes of surgery for symptomatic metastatic spinal cord compression. Spine 2001;26(7):818–824

Case 96   Spinal Arteriovenous Malformation

Bassem Sheikh

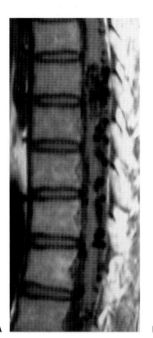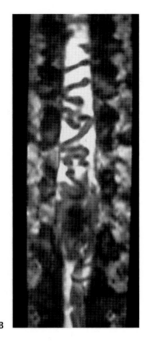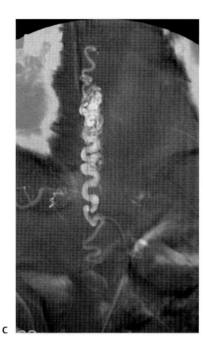

Fig. 96.1   (A) T1-weighted and **(B)** myelographic magnetic resonance imaging, and **(C)** selective spinal digital subtraction angiography.

A   B   C

■ Clinical Presentation

- A 32-year-old man presents with a 2-year history of progressive paraparesis.
- He has weakness involving both lower limbs that is progressively increasing.
- The patient also complains of back pain and bilateral leg numbness.

- Disturbance of bladder function started 3 weeks prior to presentation.
- He also shows loss of superficial sensation below the umbilicus. The vibration and position sensations are disturbed in both lower extremities.

■ Questions

1. Provide a clinical explanation to the patient's presentation.
2. What is your differential diagnosis?
3. Describe a classification of spinal arteriovenous malformations (AVMs).
4. What is your diagnostic workup for spinal AVMs?

5. Imaging studies are obtained and shown in **Fig. 96.1**. Describe the radiologic findings in these images.
6. What are the therapeutic modalities that may be suggested for this patient?
7. The patient asked you whether he would regain normal neurologic function after treatment. What is your answer to the patient?

■ Answers

1. *Provide a clinical explanation for the patient's presentation.*
   - This patient is suffering from a progressive myelopathy.
   - The myelopathy is most likely originating in the thoracic spine area given the clinical presentation.
2. *What is your differential diagnosis?*
   - The differential diagnosis of spinal progressive myelopathy is broad and includes the following[1,2]:
     – Congenital conditions: Chiari malformation, syringomyelia, narrow canal/short pedicles, mucopolysaccharidoses, kyphosis, os odontoideum
     – Infections: syphilis (infarction), postviral (herpes, varicella, cytomegalovirus), epidural empyema, vertebral osteomyelitis, acquired immunodeficiency syndrome (AIDS)-related myelopathy, tuberculosis (Pott disease), parasitic cyst
     – Traumatic conditions: spinal shock, epidural hematoma, electrical injury, bone fracture
     – Tumors: spinal cord tumor (extradural, intradural extramedullary, intramedullary), metastases, carcinomatous meningitis, paraneoplastic syndrome
     – Endocrine conditions: Cushing disease, obesity (epidural lipomatosis), acromegaly, Paget disease
     – Nutritional conditions or toxins: vitamin B12 deficiency, local anesthetics
     – Degenerative conditions: spondylotic myelopathy, ossified posterior longitudinal ligamen, disk herniation
     – Inflammatory or demyelinating conditions: transverse myelitis, multiple sclerosis, Devic syndrome, Guillain-Barre, amyotrophic lateral sclerosis
     – Vascular diseases: spinal epidural, subdural or subarachnoid hematoma, spinal cord infarction (syphilis, aorta clamping intraoperatively, hypotension, aortic dissection), AVM, radiation exposure, reaction to contrast infusion
3. *Describe a classification of spinal AVMs.*
   - There have been several classification systems for spinal vascular malformation in the literature, however, they are broadly categorized into the following three sections[3–6]:

- Dural arteriovenous fistula (DAVF): This is the most common type of malformation (**Fig. 96.2**).
  – It typically presents in older men.
  – It is usually found in the lumbar and thoracic spine.
  – This lesion consists of a small arteriovenous fistula within or just beneath the dura at the point where a feeding radicular artery enters the dura at the nerve root sleeve (at the level of the intervertebral foramen).
  – The venous outflow from the fistula, carrying arterialized blood, drains into the intradural venous plexus via the radiculomedullary vein along the dorsal surface of the spinal cord.
  – These low-flow fistulae produce venous hypertension (Foix-Alajouanine syndrome), which results in decreased spinal cord perfusion, resulting in intermittent and progressive neurologic deficits.
- Perimedullary fistulas: located intradurally but in the extramedullary space
  – They usually present at the thoracolumbar region.
  – They are characterized by a single shunt without a nidus.
  – They occur between the spinal artery (anterior or posterolateral artery) and the spinal vein.
  – They may ascend rostrally forming craniocervical shunts, reaching even into the posterior cranial fossa.
  – They are located either on the ventral or dorsal surface of the spinal cord.
- Intramedullary AVMs: These lesions are rare (**Fig. 96.2**).
  – They are supplied by the radiculomedullary artery or the spinal artery.
  – They are found partially or entirely within the substance of the spinal cord.
  – They are further subclassified according to their size and the location within the spinal cord.
    - Large complex metameric AVMs
    - Juvenile type
    - Combined intradural and extradural (intraspinal)

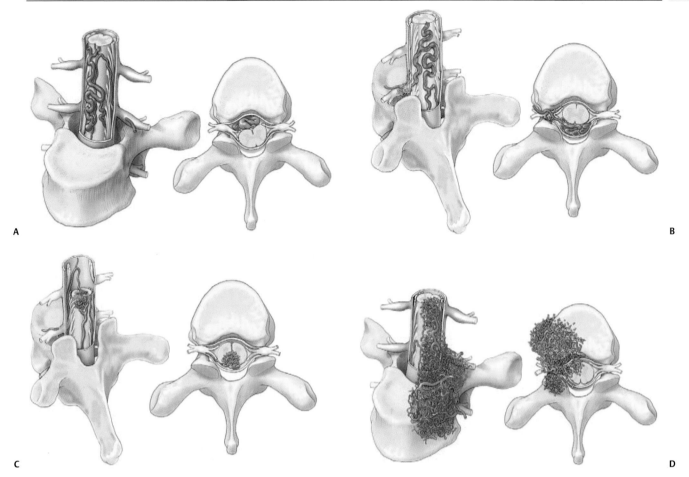

Fig. 96.2   Classification of spinal arteriovenous malformations (AVMs). **(A)** Anterior and **(B)** dorsal examples of dural arteriovenous fistulas. **(C)** Small compact intranidal spinal AVM and **(D)** large complex metameric spinal AVM. (From Gonzalez LF, Spetzler RF. Surgical technique for resection of vascular malformations within the spinal cord. In: Resnick DK, Wolfla CE, eds. Neurosurgical Operative Atlas. Spine and Peripheral Nerves. New York: Thieme Medical Publishers/American Association of Neurological Surgeons; 2006:136–144. Reprinted with permission.)

■ Answers (*continued*)

4. *What is your diagnostic workup for spinal AVMs?*
   - Diagnostic evaluation includes the following:
     - Magnetic resonance imaging (MRI): Visualization of dilated spinal veins is possible, but is difficult in cases of DAVF because the only slightly dilated vessels and the fistula itself cannot be visualized. Increased intramedullary signal in T2-weighted images can reflect the edema due to chronic venous hypertension. Serpiginous areas of low signal owing to signal void in the draining vein may be demonstrated.
     - Magnetic resonance angiography
     - Myelography: has been replaced by the more informative MRI combined with MR myelographic effect. Computed tomography (CT) myelography can help define the feeding pedicle location.
     - Selective spinal angiography: This study remains the gold standard evaluation for spinal AVMs and is the only way of diagnosing and localizing the nidus in dural fistulae. It requires detailed catheterization of thoracic and lumbar arteries. If angiographic results are routinely negative, but there is a strong clinical suggestion of a fistula, it may be necessary to extend the investigation to the vertebral, the external carotid, or the sacral arteries.

5. *Imaging studies are obtained and shown in* **Fig. 96.1**. *Describe the radiologic findings in these images.*
   - These images demonstrate the presence of an intradural, intramedullary AVM that is filling from a spinal artery and draining rostrally and caudally into draining veins.
   - Part of the nidus is present within the spinal cord substance.

6. *What are the therapeutic modalities that may be suggested for this patient?*
   - Successful treatment in each individual spinal vascular malformation requires correct understanding of the lesion's anatomic location and its angioarchitecture.
   - The therapeutic modality that should be suggested depends on the type of spinal vascular malformation.
   - The limitations of both surgery and endovascular embolization should be considered.

■ **Answers** (*continued*)

- The following summarizes each treatment modality based on type of spinal AVM.[3,7,8]
  - DAVF
    - Surgical technique: surgical exposure to excise the fistula is a simple and successful treatment of spinal DAVFs.
    - Endovascular technique: As an alternative to surgical therapy, injection of *N*-butyl cyanoacrylate can be done after superselective catheterization of the radicular artery. This method has been reported to be successful and definitive in ~75% of cases. If the occlusion of the fistula is attained endovascularly with definitive embolization material, an operation is not necessary. Otherwise, removal of the partially embolized fistula has to be performed.
  - Perimedullary fistulas
    - Surgical elimination: This is an option for posteriorly located accessible small fistula.
    - Endovascular embolization: may be used in the case of ventrally situated fistulae that are inaccessible surgically and giant fistulae with multiple dilated feeders and draining veins
  - Intramedullary AVMs
    - Endovascular embolization: This is the modality of choice in the management of intramedullary AVMs. Most techniques use particulate embolization materials that result in reduction in the flow through the malformation, thus lowering the steal and ischemic effects on the spinal cord and the venous hypertension. However, particulate embolization is noncurative and revascularization of the malformation should be expected.
    - Surgical technique: Microsurgical therapy alone is sometimes technically difficult owing to the intramedullary and ventral location of the AVM. **Figure 96.3** illustrates an intraoperative view of such an AVM.

7. *The patient asked you whether he would regain normal neurologic function after treatment. What is your answer to the patient?*
   - Postoperative improvement of patients with neurologic deficits depends on preoperative duration of signs and symptoms and on the degree of disability.[7,8]
   - Improvements may usually involve both sensory and motor deficits.
   - The genitosphincteric disturbances have a much more severe prognosis and persist more often.
   - Because of progressive ischemic lesions of the spinal cord caused by chronic venous congestion, the shunt should be eliminated as early as possible.[9]

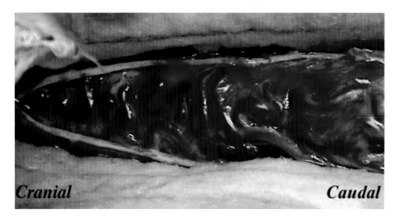

Cranial   **Caudal**

Fig. 96.3 Intraoperative view of spinal arteriovenous malformation.

■ References

1. Greenberg MS. Handbook of Neurosurgery. 6th ed. New York: Thieme Medical Publishers; 2006
2. Tsementzis SA. Differential Diagnosis in Neurology and Neurosurgery. A Clinician's Pocket Guide. New York: Thieme Medical Publishers; 2000
3. Berenstein A, Lasjaunias P. Endovascular Treatment of Spine and Spinal Cord Lesions. Surgical Neuroangiography. Berlin: Springer; 1992
4. Rodesch G, Hurth M, Alvarez H, Tadié M, Lasjaunias P. Classification of spinal cord arteriovenous shunts: proposal for a reappraisal–the Bicêtre experience with 155 consecutive patients treated between 1981 and 1999. Neurosurgery 2002;51(2):374–379
5. Spetzler RF, Detwiler PW, Riina HA, Porter RW. Modified classification of spinal cord vascular lesions. J Neurosurg 2002;96(2, Suppl):145–156
6. Gonzalez LF, Spetzler RF. Surgical technique for resection of vascular malformations within the spinal cord. In: Resnick DK, Wolfa CE, eds. Neurosurgical Operative Atlas. Spine and Peripheral Nerves. New York: Thieme Medical Publishers/American Association of Neurological Surgeons; 2006: 136–144
7. Mourier KL, Gelbert F, Rey A, et al. Spinal dural arteriovenous malformations with perimedullary drainage. Indications and results of surgery in 30 cases. Acta Neurochir (Wien) 1989;100(3–4):136–141
8. Connolly ES Jr, Zubay GP, McCormick PC, Stein BM. The posterior approach to a series of glomus (type II) intramedullary spinal cord arteriovenous malformations. Neurosurgery 1998;42(4): 774–785
9. Kataoka H, Miyamoto S, Nagata I, Ueba T, Hashimoto N. Venous congestion is a major cause of neurological deterioration in spinal arteriovenous malformations. Neurosurgery 2001;48(6):1224–1229

Case 97   Spinal Arteriovenous Fistula

Pascal M. Jabbour and Erol Veznedaroglu

■ Clinical Presentation

- A 77-year-old woman with a history of high blood pressure and diabetes presents to the emergency room for progressive weakness in her lower extremities.
- The weakness has been ongoing for the last 8 months, associated with episodes of bladder incontinence the last 3 weeks.
- She denies any lower back pain or radicular pain. There is no history of trauma.
- Neurologic examination reveals weakness in her proximal lower extremities' muscle groups graded at 3/5 with spasticity. Distally, her strength is graded 4/5 on the Medical Research Council scoring system. Sensation is intact. She has increased deep tendon reflexes and a right Babinsky. Her rectal tone is normal. She has normal strength in the upper extremities.
- Magnetic resonance imaging (MRI) of the thoracic spine is shown in **Fig. 97.1**.

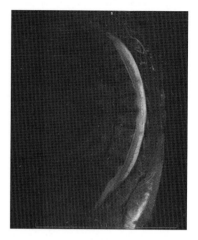

Fig. 97.1 T2-weighted magnetic resonance image (MRI), mid-sagittal section.

■ Questions

1. Where do you localize the lesion according to her examination?
2. Describe the MRI and angiogram findings.
3. What is the next imaging test to perform?
4. What are some clinical differences in spinal dural arteriovenous fistulas (DAVFs) and spinal intradural arteriovenous malformations (AVMs)?
5. What are the different treatment options for this patient?
6. What are some complications of management of spinal DAVFs?
7. What are the outcomes of treatment of spinal DAVFs?

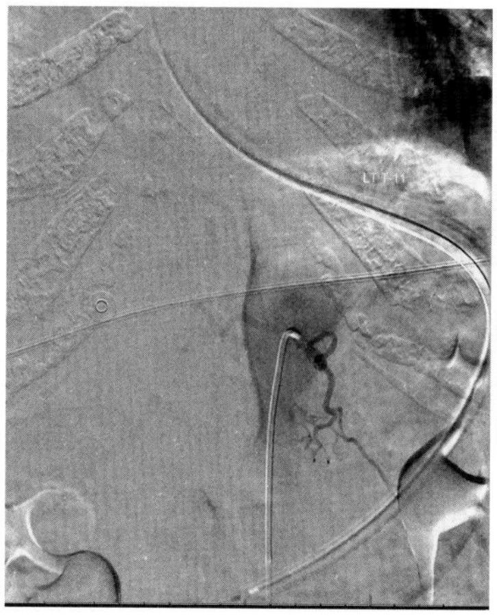

Fig. 97.2 Thoracic spine angiogram, anteroposterior view with selective injection of thoracic artery.

■ Answers

1. *Where do you localize the lesion according to her examination?*
   - She has upper motor neuron signs with increased reflexes, Babinski, and spasticity. Her upper extremities are normal; therefore, the lesion is probably located at the level of her thoracic spine.
2. *Describe the MRI and angiogram findings.*
   - The MRI shows edema in the spinal cord, with prominent flow voids representing engorged vessels surrounding the spinal cord.
   - The angiogram demonstrates a DAVF, which is also a type I spinal AVM.
3. *What is the next imaging test to perform?*
   - A spinal computed tomography (CT) angiogram or a spinal formal angiogram should be performed. Spinal angiogram is shown in **Fig. 97.2**.
4. *What are some clinical differences in spinal DAVFs and spinal intradural arteriovenous malformations?*
   - Spinal DAVFs occur predominantly in male patients, whereas intradural AVMs are more equally distributed in both genders.
   - The age of occurrence in spinal DAVFs is older than in intradural AVMs (46 years versus 24 years).
   - Onset of symptoms is more gradual in spinal DAVFs.

■ Answers (*continued*)

- The first symptom is more likely to be paresis in spinal DAVFs whereas in intradural AVMs it is more commonly related to subarachnoid hemorrhage.
- Exacerbation of symptoms by activity is more common in spinal DAVFs.
- The upper extremities are more commonly affected in intradural AVMs.[1]

5. *What are the different treatment options for this patient?*
   - The goals of treatment consist of interrupting the vein draining the AVF as it penetrates the inner dural layer.[2]
   - Her options include
     - Open surgery with clipping of the fistula, which usually resides in the sleeve of a nerve root. Laminectomies one level above and one below are usually performed. The dura can be opened in the midline and retraced laterally. The site of the fistula is identified and correlated with imaging studies. The arterialized vein is then coagulated and a limited resection is performed.[2,3]
     - Endovascular embolization of the fistula[4,5]

6. *What are some complications of management of spinal DAVFs?*

- Acute neurologic deficit postsurgery or postembolization
  - This necessitates immediate imaging studies via MRI, administration of steroids, followed by possible reexploration.
- Hematoma
- Postoperative infection
- Residual malformation or fistula on postoperative angiography (may require reoperation)
  - It is recommended to perform an angiogram ~1 week after surgical treatment.[2]

7. *What are the outcomes of treatment of spinal DAVFs?*
   - In general, safe and successful treatment is achievable.
   - In most cases, there is improvement of neurologic function or treatment – it usually arrests the progression of the symptoms. These good results can be seen in ~80–90% of patients.[1,3]
   - Most patients can ambulate after treatment.
   - Bladder symptoms are often improved.
   - Outcome correlates very much with initial neurologic condition upon presentation: patients with less neurologic deficit on presentation will fare better.[1,3]

■ References

1. Oldfield EH. Spinal vascular malformations. In: Wilkins RH, Rengashary SS, eds. Neurosurgery. 2nd ed. New York: McGraw-Hill; 1996:2541–2558
2. Oldfield EH. Spinal vascular malformations. In: McDonald RL, ed. Vascular Neurosurgery. New York: Thieme Medical Publishers; 2009:190–199
3. Post KD, Bederson J, Perin N, Stein BM. Surgical management of spinal cord tumors and arteriovenous malformations. In: Roberts DW, Schmidek HH, eds. Schimidek & Sweet Operative Neuro-surgical Techniques. 5th ed. Philadelphia: Saunders Elsevier; 2006:1337–1355
4. Veznedaroglu E, Nelson P, Jabbour P. Endovascular treatment of spinal cord arteriovenous malformations. Neurosurgery 2006; 59(5, Suppl 3):S202–S209
5. Harrop J, Jabbour P, Malone J, Przybylski G. Vascular malformations of the spinal cord. 2006. Available at: http://www.emedicine.com/Med/topic2896.htm. Accessed April 22, 2009

Case 98   Lumbar Epidural Hematoma

Remi Nader

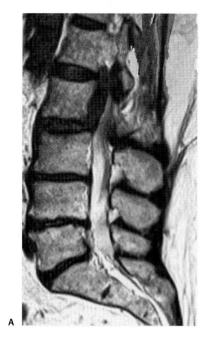

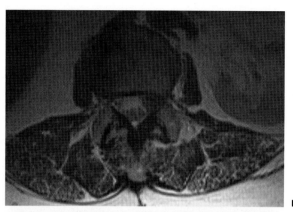

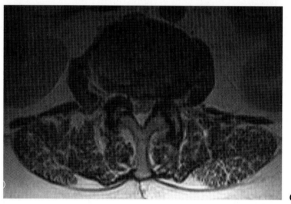

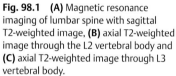

Fig. 98.1   (A) Magnetic resonance imaging of lumbar spine with sagittal T2-weighted image, **(B)** axial T2-weighted image through the L2 vertebral body and **(C)** axial T2-weighted image through L3 vertebral body.

■ Clinical Presentation

• An 86-year-old woman presents with a longstanding history of lower back pain, exacerbated over the past 12 days.

• This is associated with a 12-day history of left leg pain in a radicular pattern, mainly affecting the left thigh area and radiating down to the foot.

• On examination, she has diffuse weakness in the left leg (about 4/5 motor strength throughout all muscle groups as determined by the Medical Research Council scoring system) and some sensory loss in the L2–L3 distribution. She is unable to ambulate because of the pain.

• She does have a medical history of hypertension, diabetes, and stroke. She is currently medicated with aspirin, oral hypoglycemics, and antihypertensives.

■ Questions

1. What is your differential diagnosis?
2. Magnetic resonance imaging (MRI) is obtained and shown in **Fig. 98.1**. Interpret the MRI and provide the most likely diagnosis.
3. How do you want to manage the patient now?
4. What initial procedures would you recommend?
5. What is the next step (management and investigations)?

She undergoes an epidural steroid injection (ESI) after a failed course of physical therapy and antiinflammatory medications. However, the back pain is worsened after the injection and it now is intractable. She is admitted to the hospital for pain management.

6. You obtain another MRI while she is hospitalized (**Fig. 98.2**). Interpret it.
7. Provide a differential diagnosis based on the specific MRI findings.
8. What is your management now?
9. Describe the surgical intervention including the important perioperative points to consider.

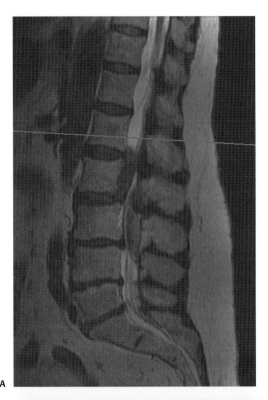

A

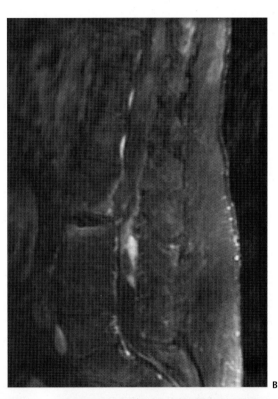

B

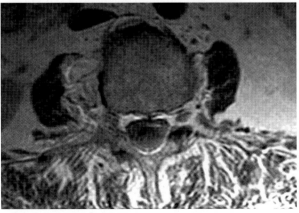

C

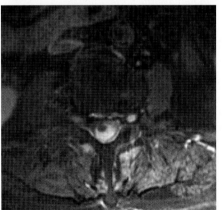

D

Fig. 98.2   (A) Magnetic resonance imaging of lumbar spine with sagittal T2-weighted image, **(B)** sagittal T1-weighted image with gadolinium contrast infusion (T1W+C), **(C)** axial T2-weighted image through lower L3 vertebral body, and **(D)** axial T1W+C image through lower L3 vertebral body.

■ Answers

1. *What is your differential diagnosis?*
   - Differential diagnosis includes the following[1,2]:
     - Congenital: scoliosis with compression of nerve root, short pedicle syndrome
     - Infectious: diskitis, osteomyelitis, urinary tract infection, pyelonephritis
     - Traumatic: compression or burst fracture (possible with history of minor trauma in elderly patient)
     - Tumor: multiple myeloma, bony metastases to the spine, intradural mass
     - Endocrine: diabetic neuropathy, other disorders of calcium, paraneoplastic syndrome
     - Neural compression: herniated disk, lateral recess stenosis, foraminal stenosis, mechanical instability, spondylolisthesis
     - Neuropathic pain
     - Degenerative: compression fracture, spondylosis with osteophytes
     - Inflammatory: arachnoiditis, perineural fibrosis, ankylosing spondylitis, scar formation
     - Vascular: abdominal aortic aneurysm
     - Myofascial: injury of musculoligamentous soft tissue structures innervated by the posterior primary ramus of the exiting spinal nerve
     - Psychosocioeconomic
2. *MRI is obtained and shown in* **Fig. 98.1**. *Interpret the MRI and provide the most likely diagnosis.*
   - MRI shows an extradural intracanalicular mass at the level of the L2 vertebral body on the left side, extending from L2–L3 disk space to L1–L2 disk space.
   - The mass is consistent with a large extruded disk fragment likely originated from the L2–L3 disk space and causing severe compression of the left lateral recess and nerve roots.
   - Other possible but less likely diagnoses include tumor (metastases, schwannoma, meningioma, neurofibroma), abscess, vascular anomaly.
3. *How do you want to manage the patient now?*
   - Given the patient's age and medical condition, conservative therapy would be the first choice in this case, consisting of[3–5]
     - Physical therapy
     - Nonsteroidal antiinflammatory medications
     - Muscle relaxants
     - Other pain medications
     - Bracing such as a lumbosacral orthosis
4. *What initial procedures would you recommend?*
   - If physical therapy fails, one may recommend an epidural steroid and analgesic mixture injection at the level of the involved nerve root.[6]
   - This procedure may require medical clearance and discontinuation of aspirin.

5. *What is the next step (management and investigations)?*
   - First, one needs to obtain further investigative studies such as MRI of the lumbar spine and laboratory studies to rule out infection or coagulopathy.
     - Complete blood count; electrolytes; coagulation profile; liver function tests; culture of urine, blood, and sputum; erythrocyte sedimentation rate; C-reactive protein level
   - Depending on the cause, proceed with indicated treatment: evacuation of hematoma or abscess, administration of antibiotics
6. *You obtain another MRI while she is hospitalized (**Fig. 98.2**). Interpret it.*
   - There is now an extradural posterior mass at the level of L3–L4, which causes severe compression centrally of the nerve roots and is consistent with either an acute to subacute hematoma or epidural abscess.
   - The fact that the mass is enhancing on contrast makes it more consistent with an abscess. The previously seen extruded disk fragment is still present.
7. *Give a differential diagnosis based on the specific MRI findings.*
   - Epidural hematoma
   - Epidural abscess
   - Both diagnoses are likely linked to the fact that she had an ESI in the face of possibly being immunocompromised from diabetes or old age and coagulopathy from aspirin.[7,8]
8. *What is your management now?*
   - She will require evacuation of the extradural mass (and the extruded disk fragment may also be removed in the same sitting).
   - She will also likely need to be started on intravenous antibiotics, broad spectrum, until final culture results are available (e.g., vancomycin, cefepime, and metronidazole).
   - Medical clearance needs to be obtained prior to surgery given her age and complicated medical history
9. *Describe the surgical intervention including the important perioperative points to consider:*
   - Surgery may consist of a laminectomy from L2–L4 with decompression of the epidural collection.
   - This will be followed by possible medial facetectomy and resection of the extruded disk fragment at L2–L3.
   - The epidural collection needs to be sent for culture and Gram stain.
   - Antibiotics may be withheld until a culture specimen is obtained intraoperatively.
   - Surgery needs to be done on an urgent basis, within 24 hours (i.e., do not wait one week for effects of aspirin to reverse), but make sure to transfuse platelets preoperatively.

■ References

1. Greenberg MS. Handbook of Neurosurgery. 6th ed. New York: Thieme Medical Publishers; 2006
2. Tsementzis SA. Differential Diagnosis in Neurology and Neurosurgery. A Clinician's Pocket Guide. New York: Thieme Medical Publishers; 2000
3. Chou R, Huffman LH. American Pain Society, American College of Physicians, Nonpharmacologic therapies for acute and chronic low back pain: a review of the evidence for an American Pain Society/American College of Physicians Clinical Practice Guideline. Ann Intern Med 2007;147(7):492–504
4. Markman JD, Gaud KG. Lumbar spinal stenosis in older adults: current understanding and future directions. Clin Geriatr Med 2008;24(2):369–388
5. Atlas SJ, Keller RB, Wu YA, Deyo RA, Singer DE. Long-term outcomes of surgical and nonsurgical management of lumbar spinal stenosis: 8 to 10 year results from the Maine Lumbar Spine Study. Spine 2005;30(8):936–943
6. Abdi S, Datta S, Trescot AM, et al. Epidural steroids in the management of chronic spinal pain: a systematic review. Pain Physician 2007;10(1):185–212
7. Snarr J. Risk, benefits and complications of epidural steroid injections: a case report. AANA J 2007;75(3):183–188
8. Hooten WM, Mizerak A, Carns PE, Huntoon MA. Discitis after lumbar epidural corticosteroid injection: a case report and analysis of the case report literature. Pain Med 2006;7(1):46–511

Case 99 Spinal Epidural Abscess

Cristian Gragnaniello and Remi Nader

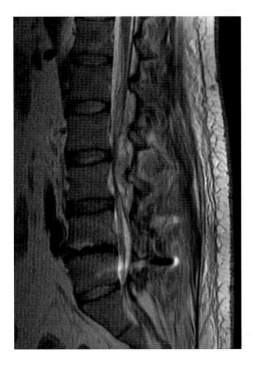

Fig. 99.1 Sagittal T2-weighted magnetic resonance image through the lumbar spine.

■ Clinical Presentation

- A 39-year-old man presents to your office 2 weeks after he has undergone a hemilaminectomy at L3–L4 for degenerative spinal stenosis.
- He has a previous history of L4–5 and L5–S1 posterolateral fusion with pedicle screw fixation.
- He presents now with a 2-day history of severe back pain radiating to the buttocks bilaterally.

- There is mild erythema around the recent surgical wound.
- There are no deficits or pain in his lower extremities.
- Magnetic resonance imaging (MRI) of the lumbar spine is obtained (**Fig. 99.1**).

■ Questions

1. Interpret the MRI and give a differential diagnosis.
2. What are the characteristics of epidural abscess on MRI?
3. What are the risk factors for this condition?
4. What are the most common microorganisms involved in epidural abscesses in the immunocompetent patient?
5. What is the incidence of this condition in the postsurgical patient?
6. How do you manage this condition?

You decide to operate. You decompress the thecal sac and perform a sharp debridement of the wound. During surgery, you send cultures and are told that there are numerous Gram-positive cocci. Once down to the thecal sac, you notice that, for the most part, there is thick granulation tissue over the sac. As you tease this tissue off the dura, you get a dural tear.

7. How do you handle a dural tear in this specific setting?
8. Why do you not remove the instrumentation of the previous fusion?

After you decompress the thecal sac, you notice a piece of floating bone, you remove it, and you notice that it comprises the inferior facet joint of L3 that is detached and free floating (you did not detach it during your current decompression).

9. Why is the piece of facet detached?
10. What condition do you now worry about, given the detached facet, and how do you manage it?

■ Answers

1. *Interpret the MRI and give a differential diagnosis.*
   - There is a posterior epidural collection from L2–L4, hyperintense on T2-weighted images. This could be a cerebrospinal fluid (CSF) collection, abscess, or infected hematoma.[1–4]
   - The disk space looks normal, and so do the vertebral bodies. This finding is important to assess the radiographic presence of concomitant osteomyelitis.
   - There is loss of lumbar lordosis.
   - Given the clinical presentation, the most likely diagnosis is epidural abscess.
2. *What are the characteristics of epidural abscess on MRI?*
   - On T1-weighted images, it has the same intensity as spinal cord or neural elements.
   - On T2-weighted images, it shows increased signal.
   - On fat-saturated sequences, edema and soft tissue inflammation are clearly visible and bright.
   - Contrast-enhanced images often show a peripheral rim of enhancement due to granulation tissue and hypervascularity.[1]
3. *What are the risk factors for this condition?*
   - Presence of hardware and instrumentation
   - Repeated surgery
   - Use of steroids
   - Diabetes or other underlying medical problems such as renal failure, previous trauma, and urinary tract infections
   - Intravenous drug abuse[3–5]
4. *What are the most common microorganisms involved in epidural abscesses in the immunocompetent patient?*
   - Gram-positive bacteria such as *Staphylococcus* (S.) *aureus* (reported in 60% of cases) or *S. epidermidis*[4,5]
   - Gram-negative bacteria such as *Escherichia coli* and *Pseudomonas aeruginosa*[4,5]

5. *What is the incidence of this condition in the postsurgical patient?*
   - The generally accepted incidence is less than 10%.
   - The incidence is reportedly increased with higher complexity procedures. It is in the range of 0.6–3.7% after microdiscectomy and of 3.7–20% after instrumented lumbar cases.[2]
6. *How do you manage this condition?*
   - Look for any discharge so it can be cultured before starting antibiotics.
   - Explore the wound to see if you find a purulent collection or CSF.
   - Drain the abscess, sampling tissue, and purulent material for culture.
   - Perform a sharp debridement and lavage.[3]
   - Place on broad-spectrum intravenous antibiotics until final culture results are available. Vancomycin for the gram-positive covering including methicillin-resistant Gram-positive cocci and cefepime for Gram-negative bacteria are among the most common medications used.[4]
   - The closure of the wound is very important and can be done in different ways, but the key concept is the obliteration of the dead space caused by the removal of the infected tissue restoring the blood supply and postoperative drainage by outflow drain or suction/irrigation device.[6,7]
7. *How do you handle a dural tear in this specific setting?*
   - A tear in this specific condition can lead to a spreading of the infection in the subdural space because of the disruption of the normal dural barrier.[8]
   - Suture with a 7-0 or 8-0 dural suture if accessible in a watertight fashion, using the Valsalva maneuver to confirm the closure.

■ Answers (*continued*)

- Cover with a dry piece of Gelfoam (Pfizer Pharmaceuticals, New York, NY) or collagen matrix.
- Cover with fibrin glue or hydrogel sealant.
- You may need to resect more bone to further the exposure and allow access to the whole tear.[9]
- Continue appropriate antibiotics.

8. *Why do you not remove the instrumentation of the previous fusion?*
   - The infection on the MRI does not extend to the previously treated levels.
   - The onset of symptoms is very recent as the surgery at the L3–L4 level was performed in the past 2 weeks. Therefore, the formation of the glycocalyx over the rod and other used material is improbable.[2,3]
   - Titanium materials have a porous surface that allows the penetration of antibiotics.[6]
   - Good results have been shown when leaving the instrumentation in place, even in cases where the infection was involving those instrumented levels, if thorough debridement is performed and antibiotic therapy is well managed.[10,11]

9. *Why is the piece of facet detached?*
   - The bone is likely detached due to erosion from osteomyelitis.

10. *What condition do you now worry about given the detached facet and how do you manage it?*
    - You worry about two entities:
      - Osteomyelitis and spread of the infection to bone
      - Instability and the possibility of spinal deformity
    - Your management should now involve placing the patient in a brace postoperatively and obtaining flexion-extension lumbar spine radiographs.
    - You may repeat radiographs in 2 to 4 weeks as osteomyelitic changes may become visible radiographically only after 2 to 3 weeks.[3]
    - He may need a lumbar instrumented fusion once the infection has healed if instability is then demonstrated.[12]
    - Treatment with antibiotics does differ in cases of osteomyelitis: he then needs 8–12 weeks of intravenous antibiotics instead of only 4–6 weeks (as in cases of simple epidural abscess with no bony involvement).[5]
    - Hyperbaric oxygenation can help to promote host immune defense response and stimulate vascularization of the injured tissues.[13]

■ References

1. Parkinson JF, Sekhon LH. Spinal epidural abscess: appearance on magnetic resonance imaging as a guide to surgical management. Report of five cases. Neurosurg Focus 2004;17(6):E12
2. Katonis P, Tzermiadianos M, Papagelopoulos P, Hadjipavlou A. Postoperative infections of the thoracic and lumbar spine: a review of 18 cases. Clin Orthop Relat Res 2007;454:114–119
3. Quiñones-Hinojosa A, Jun P, Jacobs R, Rosenberg WS, Weinstein PR. General principles in the medical and surgical management of spinal infections: a multidisciplinary approach. Neurosurg Focus 2004;17(6):E1
4. Darouiche RO. Spinal epidural abscess. N Engl J Med 2006;355(19):2012–2020
5. Sendi P, Bregenzer T, Zimmerli W. Spinal epidural abscess in clinical practice. QJM 2008;101(1):1–12
6. Hsieh PC, Wienecke RJ, O'Shaughnessy BA, Koski TR, Ondra SL. Surgical strategies for vertebral osteomyelitis and epidural abscess. Neurosurg Focus 2004;17(6):E4
7. Löhr M, Reithmeier T, Ernestus RI, Ebel H, Klug N. Spinal epidural abscess: prognostic factors and comparison of different surgical treatment strategies. Acta Neurochir (Wien) 2005;147(2):159–166
8. Wu AS, Griebel RW, Meguro K, Fourney DR. Spinal subdural empyema after a dural tear. Case report. Neurosurg Focus 2004;17(6):E10
9. Sassmannshausen GM, Ball PA, Abdu WA. Miscellaneous postoperative complications of spinal surgery. In: Bohlman HH, Boden SC, eds. The Failed Spine. Philadelphia: Lippincott Williams & Wilkins; 2003:290–302
10. Picada R, Winter RB, Lonstein JE, et al. Postoperative deep wound infection in adults after posterior lumbosacral spine fusion with instrumentation: incidence and management. J Spinal Disord 2000;13(1):42–45
11. Weinstein MA, McCabe JP, Cammisa FP Jr. Postoperative spinal wound infection: a review of 2,391 consecutive index procedures. J Spinal Disord 2000;13(5):422–426
12. Lee MC, Wang MY, Fessler RG, Liauw J, Kim DH. Instrumentation in patients with spinal infections. Neurosurg Focus 2004;17(6):E7
13. Chang WC, Tsou HK, Kao TH, Yang MY, Shen CC. Successful treatment of extended epidural abscess and long segment osteomyelitis: a case report and review of the literature. Surg Neurol 2008;69(2):117–120

Case 100 Chiari I Malformation

Mahmoud A. Al Yamany, Homoud Aldahash, and Abdulrahman J. Sabbagh

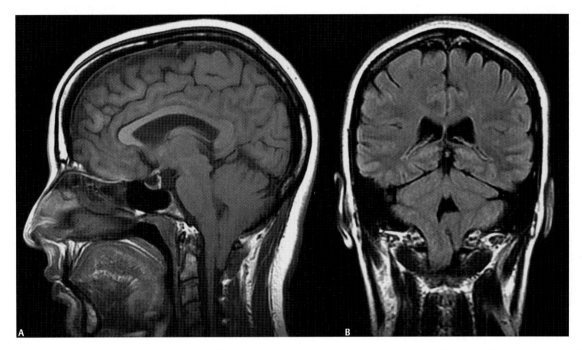

Fig. 100.1 **(A)** Sagittal and **(B)** coronal T2-weighted magnetic resonance images, demonstrating small posterior fossa, descended cerebellar tonsils down to the level of C1–C2 level posteriorly, and compression of the cranio–cervical junction and cervical spinal cord.

■ Clinical Presentation

- A 32-year-old woman presents with a long history of neck pain, intermittent bilateral shoulder pain, worsened with neck flexion and extension and during coughing and/or sneezing.
- She also complains of intermittent numbness in the tips of her fingers bilaterally.
- On physical examination, she has no neurologic deficits.

- Her past medical history is remarkable for an operation as a child for scoliosis, which was corrected at the age of 13 years. She did not have any further problem in that regard.
- Magnetic resonance imaging (MRI) is obtained and shown in **Fig. 100.1**.

■ Questions

1. What is the differential diagnosis?
2. What does the sagittal image of the MRI demonstrate?
3. Describe your management.
4. What is the expected outcome?
5. What are the possible complications of this procedure?

Assume this patient presented with progressive difficulty walking and spasticity. If she also presented with a spine MRI showing a syrinx in the upper thoracic and lower cervical cord, what would be your answers to the following questions?

6. What is the best management for the syrinx?
7. What are the pathogenesis theories of syringomyelia in Chiari I malformation?
8. Would you expect radiologic or clinical improvement to occur first?
9. How long would you wait before you expect the syrinx to start narrowing?
10. What are the different types of Chiari malformations?

■ Answers

1. *What is the differential diagnosis?*
   - Differential diagnosis includes
     - Hydrocephalus
     - Chiari malformation with cervical spinal cord syrinx
     - Isolated cervical spinal cord syrinx following scoliosis surgery
     - Cervical spine spondylosis
     - Tumors of the cervicomedullary junction or cervical spine

2. *What does the sagittal image of the MRI demonstrate?*
   - Sagittal MRI of the brain demonstrates
     - Small posterior fossa
     - Descended cerebellar tonsils, below the level of the craniocervical junction
     - Secondary myelomalacia of the cervical spinal cord

3. *Describe your management.*
   - Management consists of suboccipital craniotomy.
     - Removing the rim of the foramen magnum and the posterior arch of C1
     - This is followed by duraplasty, with or without arachnoid lyses and/or tonsillar resection.

4. *What is the expected outcome?*
   - The expected outcome would be a stabilization of symptoms or arrested symptom progression.
   - There is a chance of improvement in her neurologic condition and a good chance of improvement of the headache and neck and shoulder pain.[1–3]

5. *What are the possible complications of this procedure?*
   - Possible complications of the procedure include the following[4]:
     - Cerebrospinal fluid (CSF) leak
     - Subdural hygroma
     - Wound infection
     - Further herniation of the tonsils due to raised intracranial pressure
     - There is a small chance of intraoperative neural tissue injury.
     - Postoperative headache – causes include chemical meningitis from the patch or glue
     - Possibility of nocturnal respiratory depression following posterior fossa manipulation (more common in Chiari type II)

6. *What is the best management for the syrinx?*
   - First line of management is treating the Chiari malformation via a suboccipital decompression[1] (see answer of Question 3 for details).
   - Alternative options include adding a syringosubarachnoid shunt after the Chiari decompression in selected cases (presence of a large syrinx, with significant thinning of the spinal cord tissue and obliteration of the spinal subarachnoid space, especially when combined with syrinx-related symptoms),[5] or syringopleural shunt.

7. *What are the pathogenesis theories of syringomyelia in Chiari I malformation?*
   - Several theories exist:
     - Gardner's hydrodynamic theory[6]:
       - First to recognize the frequent association of syringomyelia with Chiari I malformation
       - Delay in the perforation of the roof of the rhombencephalon
       - Subarachnoid space does not fully open.
       - CSF becomes trapped in ventricular system.
       - The exaggerated pulsations are directed into the central canal causing hydromyelia.
     - Williams theory[7]
       - Postulated and later confirmed that such an obstruction could act as a valve, allowing CSF to cross the foramen magnum rostrally more effectively than caudally
       - Craniospinal dissociation is described where CSF may be "sucked" from the 4th ventricle into the central canal.
     - Ball and Dayan theory[8]
       - Activities that increase thoracic or abdominal pressure such as coughing and straining causes the spinal CSF to be diverted into the spinal cord parenchyma along dilated Virchow–Robin spaces.
     - Aboulker theory[9]
       - Spinal CSF enters into the cord by way of the dorsal root entry zone.
       - Absorption occurs either by
         - Blood vessels of the spinal gray matter
         - Rostral drainage through the central canal into the 4th ventricle
     - Oldfield theory[10,11]
       - The force that pushes spinal subarachnoid CSF into the cord parenchyma is the CSF pulsation pressure occurring during the cardiac cycle.
       - This pulsation will drive CSF into the cord along perivascular spaces.
     - Other theories such as Greitz[12] (intramedullary pulse pressure theory)
       - Suggests that syringomyelia is caused by increased pulse pressure in the spinal cord and that the syrinx consists of extracellular fluid rather than CSF

8. *Would you expect radiologic or clinical improvement to occur first?*
   - Expect to see improvement in clinical symptoms before radiologic improvement.

9. *How long would you wait before you expect the syrinx to start narrowing?*
   - The radiologic improvement in the width of the syrinx is expected within the first 3–6 months, but continued narrowing of the syrinx may take years.

■ Answers (*continued*)

- According to Wetjen et al.'s series of 29 patients with syringomyelia and Chiari I malformations, the average diameter of the syrinx preoperatively is ~6.9 mm (with a 2.1 mm standard deviation), whereas postoperatively it is less than 1.5 mm at last evaluation ($p < 0.0001$).
- The median time for the syrinx narrowing is 3.6 months after a Chiari decompression is completed.[11]

10. *What are different types of Chiari malformations?*
- There are four types of Chiari malformations.[13]
- See **Fig. 100.2** for details of each of the three main types.
- Note that Chiari type IV includes cerebella hypoplasia.[13]

Chiari Malformations

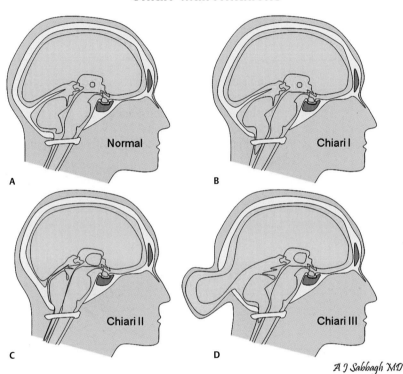

Fig. 100.2   Diagrams demonstrating normal posterior fossa appearance and variants of Chiari malformations on sagittal planes. **(A)** Normal posterior fossa anatomy. **(B)** Chiari malformation type I: shallow posterior fossa, tonsillar descent down to the level of C1–C2 junction, and posterior compression of the cervical spinal cord. **(C)** Chiari malformation type II: shallow posterior fossa, descent of the cerebellar hemispheres, vermis, and tonsils to the upper cervical spinal canal level, and posterior compression of the brainstem and the cervical spinal cord. **(D)** Chiari malformation type III: shallow posterior fossa, tonsillar herniation, brainstem and cervical spinal cord compression, and associate occipital encephalocele.

■ References

1. Attenello FJ, McGirt MJ, Gathinji M, et al. Outcome of Chiari-associated syringomyelia after hindbrain decompression in children: analysis of 49 consecutive cases. Neurosurgery 2008;62(6):1307–1313

2. Kumar R, Kalra SK, Vaid VK, Mahapatra AK. Chiari I malformation: surgical experience over a decade of management. Br J Neurosurg 2008;22(3):409–414

3. Hayhurst C, Richards O, Zaki H, Findlay G, Pigott TJ. Hindbrain decompression for Chiari-syringomyelia complex: an outcome analysis comparing surgical techniques. Br J Neurosurg 2008;22(1):86–91

4. Munshi I, Frim D, Stine-Reyes R, Weir BK, Hekmatpanah J, Brown F. Effects of posterior fossa decompression with and without duraplasty on Chiari malformation-associated hydromyelia. Neurosurgery 2000;46(6):1384–1389

5. Alzate JC, Kothbauer KF, Jallo GI, Epstein FJ. Treatment of Chiari I malformation in patients with and without syringomyelia: a consecutive series of 66 cases. Neurosurg Focus 2001;11(1):E3

6. Gardner WJ. Hydrodynamic mechanism of syringomyelia: its relationship to myelocele. J Neurol Neurosurg Psychiatry 1965;28:247–259

7. Williams B. The distending force in the production of "communicating syringomyelia." Lancet 1969;2(7613):189–193

8. Ball MJ, Dayan AD. Pathogenesis of syringomyelia. Lancet 1972;2(7781):799–801

9. Aboulker J. La syringomyelie et les liquides intra-rachidiens. Neurochirurgie 1979;25(Suppl):1–144

10. Oldfield EH, Muraszko K, Shawker TH, Patronas NJ. Pathophysiology of syringomyelia associated with Chiari I malformation of the cerebellar tonsils. J Neurosurg 1994;80(1):3–15

11. Wetjen NM, Heiss JD, Oldfield EH. Time course of syringomyelia resolution following decompression of Chiari malformation type 1. J Neurosurg Pediatr 2008;1(2):118–123

12. Greitz D. Unraveling the riddle of syringomyelia. Neurosurg Rev 2006;29(4):251–263

13. Oakes WJ. Chiari malformations, hydromyelia, syringomyelia. In: Rengashary SS, Wilkins RH, eds. Neurosurgery. 2nd ed. New York: McGraw-Hill; 1996: 3593–3616

Case 101   Median Nerve Entrapment at the Wrist

Gaetan Moise and Christopher J. Winfree

■ Clinical Presentation

- An 83-year-old right-handed woman without significant medical history presents with 3–4 weeks history of "tingling" in her first through third digits of the left hand.

- Episodes are transient, mildly painful, and typically occur at night awakening her from sleep.

■ Questions

1. What is the differential diagnosis?
2. What are possible locations of median nerve entrapment?
3. What is the most likely diagnosis?
4. What special physical exam findings and maneuvers would support this diagnosis?
5. What diagnostic tests should be ordered?
6. What nonsurgical measures can be attempted to ameliorate the patient's symptoms?
7. When should surgery be considered?
8. What are the surgical options?
9. What complications are associated with carpal tunnel release?

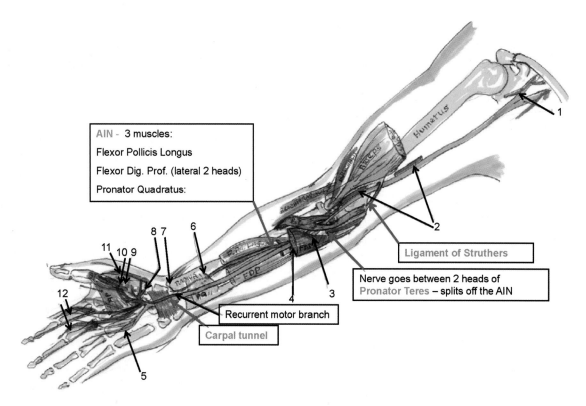

Fig. 101.1 Artist's rendering of median nerve anatomical course and locations of entrapment. Sites of entrapment are highlighted in pink. AIN, anterior interosseous nerve; FDP or Flexor Dig. Prof., flexor digitorum profundus; PQ, pronator quadrates; AP, adductor pollicis; PT, pronator teres; F. Pol. Longus, flexor pollicis longus; FDS, flexor digitorum superficialis. (1) Lateral and medial cords join to form the median nerve. (2) Median nerve descends along the medial edge of the brachial artery. (3) Median nerve passes under the flexor digitorum superficialis (arcade forms the Sublimis Bridge). (4) Median nerve descends between flexor digitorum superficialis and profundus. (5) Sensory branches of the median nerve. (6) Anterior interosseous nerve (AIN) reaches deep to the pronator quadrates. (7) AIN gives off the wrist articular branches. (8) Recurrent motor branch variation. (9) Abductor pollicis. (10) Flexor pollicis. (11) Opponens pollicis. (12) Lumbricals I and II.

■ Answers

1. *What is the differential diagnosis?*
   - Carpal tunnel syndrome (CTS)
   - Cervical radiculopathy
   - Brachial plexopathy
   - Supracondylar process syndrome (Struthers' ligament)
2. *What are possible locations of median nerve entrapment?*
   - **Figure 101.1** shows the anatomic localizations of median nerve compression sites.
3. *What is the most likely diagnosis?*
   - CTS results from median nerve compression at the carpal tunnel, a structure formed by several bones of the wrist and the transverse carpal ligament.[1]
   - The pathophysiology is thought to involve mechanical compression upon and ischemic changes within the median nerve.
   - Causes include repetitive hand movements, pregnancy, diabetes mellitus, acromegaly, hypothyroidism, multiple myeloma, amyloidosis, mucopolysaccharidosis, and rheumatoid arthritis.
   - It is the most common peripheral nerve compression syndrome and affects about 1–3% of adults.
   - Classic symptoms are restricted to a median nerve distribution distal to the carpal tunnel, but patients can present with proximal arm pain as well.
4. *What special physical exam findings/maneuvers would support this diagnosis?*
   - Phalen's test: patient rests elbows on exam table with forearms upright and allows wrist flexion with gravity assistance. Considered positive if median nerve distribution paresthesias commence or increase within 60 seconds.
   - Tinel sign: percussion of the median nerve at the wrist. Considered positive if reproduces paresthesias in a median nerve distribution.
   - Durkan's compression test: application of continuous pressure to the median nerve at the transverse carpal ligament produces median nerve paresthesias, which are relieved by release of pressure.
   - Sensory: for example, two-point discrimination, monofilament testing, vibration detection
5. *What diagnostic tests should be ordered?*
   - Electromyography and nerve conduction studies (EMG/NCS) are the standard diagnostic tests for CTS; conduction slowing of the median nerve across the wrist and denervational changes in the distal median-innervated muscles are commonly seen in CTS.
   - Cervical spinal imaging studies are unnecessary to make the diagnosis of CTS but are helpful to exclude other problems in the differential diagnosis such as cervical radiculopathy.
   - In this case, physical exam and NCS were consistent with the diagnosis of left-sided CTS; magnetic resonance imaging of the cervical spine was unremarkable.
6. *What nonsurgical measures can be attempted to ameliorate the patient's symptoms?*
   - Improve ergonomics associated with precipitating activities[2]
   - Avoid repetitive, stressful movements
   - Wrist splinting
   - Oral corticosteroids
   - Local injection of corticosteroids into carpal tunnel[3]
   - Nonsteroidal antiinflammatory medications, diuretics, vitamin supplements, and chiropractic manipulation are not thought to be helpful.
7. *When should surgery be considered?*
   - Persistence of symptoms that do not improve with a month or so conservative management.[3]
   - Evidence of conduction slowing along the median nerve at the wrist on NCS.
   - Weakness of median-innervated muscles need not be present, but prompt earlier surgical intervention if present.
   - Denervational changes on needle EMG of median-innervated muscles distal to the carpal tunnel need not be present, but prompt earlier surgical intervention if present.
8. *What are the surgical options?*
   - Mini-open carpal tunnel release involves decompressing the median nerve at the wrist through a 2-cm incision; although the patients may gently use the operated hand almost immediately, the incision requires a month or so of healing prior to aggressive work or rehabilitation activities (**Fig. 101.2 and Fig. 101.3**).[4]
   - Endoscopic carpal tunnel release involves decompressing the median nerve at the wrist through two 5-mm incisions; recovery times prior to return to work or aggressive physiotherapy are shorter after the endoscopic release compared with open release.[4]
   - Endoscopic carpal tunnel release is somewhat more expensive and has a higher risk of complications when performed by the inexperienced surgeon than open release.[4]
9. *What complications are associated with carpal tunnel release?*
   - Injury to the main trunk median nerve, the palmar cutaneous branch, or the recurrent motor branch[5]
   - Incomplete release
   - Painful scar
   - Injury to the superficial palmar arch
   - Infection
   - Complex regional pain syndrome

■ Answers (*continued*)

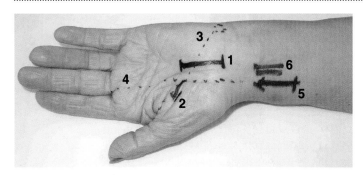

Fig. 101.2 Intraoperative photograph of the patient featured in this case, illustrating the superficial landmarks, incision, and surgical anatomy of the mini-open carpal tunnel release. The incision (1) is roughly 2 cm in length and begins 1–2 mm distal to the wrist crease and in line with the radial aspect of the 4th digit. The recurrent motor branch of the median nerve (2) is located at the intersection of Kaplan's line, (3) drawn from the pisiform bone to the angle of the thumb, and the line drawn in line with the radial aspect of the 3rd digit. (4) The palmar cutaneous branch of the median nerve (5) originates 5 cm proximal to the wrist crease along the radial aspect of the median nerve and generally traverses the wrist within its own fascial tunnel. The palmaris longus tendon (6) is sometimes seen proximal and just radial to the incision.

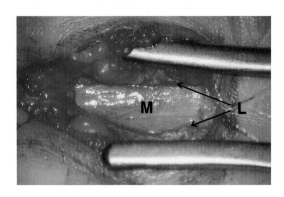

Fig. 101.3 Intraoperative photograph of the patient featured in this case, illustrating the median nerve (M) following division of the transverse carpal ligament (L). Elevation of the skin at each end of the incision by a small handheld retractor permits decompression of a total length of ~10 cm of median nerve through the 2 cm incision.

■ References

1. Katz JN, Simmons BP. Carpal tunnel syndrome. N Engl J Med 2002;346:1807–1812
2. Gerritsen AAM, de Crom MCTFM, Struijs MA, Scholten RJPM, de Vet HCW, Bouter LM. Conservative treatment options for carpal tunnel syndrome: a systematic review of randomized controlled trials. J Neurol 2002;249:272–280
3. Marshall S, Tardif G, Ashworth N. Local corticosteroid injection for carpal tunnel syndrome. Cochrane Database Syst Rev 2007; (2):CD001554
4. Scholten RJ, Mink van der Molen A, Uitdehaag BM, Bouter LM, de Vet HC. Surgical treatment options for carpal tunnel syndrome. Cochrane Database Syst Rev 2007;(4):CD003905
5. Russell SM, Kline DG. Complication avoidance in peripheral nerve surgery: injuries, entrapments, and tumors of the extremities–part 2. Neurosurgery 2006; 59(4, Suppl 2):ONS449–ONS456

Case 102   Brachial Plexus Injury and Horner Syndrome

Stephen M. Russell

■ Clinical Presentation

- A 35-year-old woman was an unrestrained driver in a car accident. She struck her shoulder against the steering wheel, which caused right-arm weakness and numbness.
- She is unable to raise the arm or flex at the elbow.
- Painful paresthesias and numbness in the thumb and index finger have also been present since the accident.
- Imaging revealed no fractures or rotator cuff tears. Despite physical therapy, she has had no evidence of recovery in the 3 months since the accident.

- On examination, she has atrophy of the deltoid, supraspinatus, infraspinatus, and biceps muscles. She cannot flex, abduct, or externally rotate the arm at the shoulder joint. She also cannot flex at the elbow or supinate the forearm.
- The rest of her arm and hand muscles are full strength.
- She has numbness along the radial forearm and hand, including the thumb and index finger.
- She has a positive Tinel's sign in the right supraclavicular space that radiates to the index finger.

■ Questions

1. What is your differential diagnosis for this woman?
2. What are sensory territories and muscles innervated by C5/C6 (i.e., the upper trunk)?
3. What diagnostic tests would you order for this patient?
4. Why wait 3 months prior to performing surgery?
5. What are the surgical outcomes of brachial plexus surgery?
6. Are there any surgical options if the injury was longer than 2 years ago?

7. If this patient had presented instead with numbness on the dorsum of his hand, weakness in the hand intrinsic muscles, as well as ptosis and myosis in one eye, where would the lesion then be localized?
8. What other anatomic site can give the same eye findings?
9. How do these eye findings affect prognosis?

■ Answers

1. *What is your differential diagnosis for this woman?*
   - She has a brachial plexus stretch injury involving C5/C6 and/or the upper trunk (Erb palsy).
   - Less likely diagnoses would include cerebral contusion or stroke, brachial neuritis, cervical spine fracture or herniated disc, and musculoskeletal injuries to the shoulder and arm.
2. *What are sensory territories and muscles innervated by C5/C6 (i.e., the upper trunk)?*
   - The location of combined C5/C6 and/or upper trunk sensory loss is depicted in **Fig. 102.1**.[1]
   - Patients with an upper trunk (Erb) palsy would be weak in the following muscles: rhomboids, deltoid, supraspinatus, infraspinatus, clavicular head of the pectoralis major, biceps, brachialis, brachioradialis, and possibly the latissimus dorsi.
   - In general, patients cannot abduct the shoulder or flex the elbow.[1]

3. *What diagnostic tests would you order for this patient?*
   - It is important to image (magnetic resonance imaging [MRI] or computed tomography [CT] myelogram) the cervical spine to exclude rootlet avulsion because if present, graft repair from avulsed spinal nerves would not be an option.
   - Electrodiagnostic evaluation must wait for 3–4 weeks so any signs of muscle denervation would be apparent after wallerian degeneration has occurred.
   - A repeat electrodiagnostic test 3 months later may reveal subclinical improvement.
   - A radiograph of the shoulder is important to exclude fractures and dislocations.
4. *Why wait 3 months prior to performing surgery?*
   - A 3-month waiting period is recommended because many patients with brachial plexus stretch injuries recover spontaneously within a few months (neurapraxic injuries), this initial observation period prevents them from undergoing surgery.

■ **Answers** (*continued*)

Upper Trunk Sensory Loss (C5/C6)

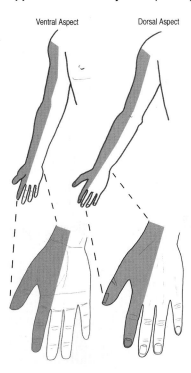

Ventral Aspect   Dorsal Aspect

Fig. 102.1   Location of upper trunk (combined C5/C6) sensory loss. Patients with an Erb's palsy (upper trunk) brachial plexus stretch injury can have numbness, paresthesias, and pain in this distribution. In practice, however, patients are usually most symptomatic in the affected portion of the hand. (From Russell SM. Examination of Peripheral Nerve Injury: An Anatomical Approach. New York: Thieme Medical Publishers; 2007. Adapted with permission.)

- Furthermore, for patients with axonotmetic injuries, providing adequate time for the axons to regenerate across the injury site one can then reliably conclude that an absence of an intraoperative nerve action potential across this injured segment would indicate that a spontaneous recovery would not occur.[2] Therefore, this segment of injured nerve is replaced with sural nerve grafts.

5. *What are the surgical outcomes of brachial plexus surgery?*
   - This depends on whether nerve grafts were used. If the upper trunk is scarred but has a positive nerve action potential recording across its injured segment, then only scar tissue is removed and no grafts are used (**Fig. 102.2A-C**).
   - These patients do well, with an 80–90% chance of achieving grade ⅗ or better muscle strength on the Medical Research Council scale.
   - Alternatively, when there is an absent nerve action potential recording across the injured segment of nerve, or if the nerve is obviously transected, sural grafts are used to reconstruct the nerve (**Fig. 102.2D-F**).
   - The chance of these patients achieving grade ⅗ or better muscle strength is ~50% (results depend on patient age, surgical delay, distance to recipient muscles, and graft length).[3,4]

6. *Are there any surgical options if the injury was longer than 2 years ago?*
   - Nerve repair rarely works if performed more than 2 years after the injury.
   - In these patients, and for those who did not improve much after a previous brachial plexus repair, other surgical options are available, including tendon transfers (e.g., Steindler procedure for arm flexion) and free muscle transfers (e.g., gracilis vascularized flap for elbow flexion).

7. *If this patient had presented instead with numbness on the dorsum of his hand, weakness in the hand intrinsic muscles, as well as ptosis and myosis in one eye, where would the lesion then be localized?*
   - The lesion described represents a preganglionic brachial plexus injury with Horner syndrome.
   - Nerve roots involved include C8 and T1 (and possibly C7).
   - Other clinical findings may also include anhidrosis, and serratus anterior paralysis (long thoracic nerve, innervation from C7 root).
   - A meningocele may be seen on imaging studies at the level of these cervical roots.
   - The sympathetic chain has also been damaged and avulsed; damage is proximal to the dorsal root ganglion.

■ **Answers (continued)**

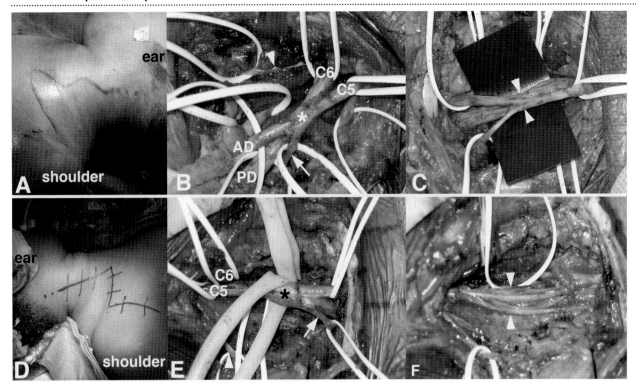

Fig. 102.2 Surgical exploration of the brachial plexus. Images **(A–C)** represents an 11-year-old boy who was struck by a car and sustained a left-sided brachial plexus injury with no return of function by 6 months. **(A)** An exploration was performed using a curvilinear supraclavicular incision (images **[B,C]** are in the same orientation as **[A]**). **(B)** The upper portion of the left brachial plexus was exposed, including the C5 and C6 nerve roots, anterior (AD) and posterior (PD) divisions of the upper trunk (*), suprascapular nerve (*white arrow*), and phrenic nerve (*arrowhead*). **(C)** The upper trunk was scarred, but had a positive nerve action potential across it; therefore, only a neurolysis (i.e., scar tissue removal) was performed (between the arrowheads). Images **(D–F)** represent a right-sided brachial plexus exposure (see presentation section for more information about this patient). **(D)** An exploration of the right brachial plexus was performed using a supraclavicular incision (images **[E,F]** are in the same orientation as **[C]**). **(E)** The right upper trunk was markedly neuromatous (*). C5, C6, as well as the suprascapular (*white arrow*) and spinal accessory (*arrowhead*) nerves were exposed. **(F)** There was no action potential recording across the injured upper trunk; therefore, six sural nerve cables grafts were used to reconstruct the upper trunk (between the arrowheads). (From Tender G, Kline D. Anterior supraclavicular approach to the brachial plexus. Neurosurgery 2006;58(S2):ONS 360–364.)

8. *What other anatomic site can give the same eye findings?*
   - Horner syndrome can be categorized in three types depending on the level of the injured neurons (**Fig. 102.3** for an anatomic illustration).[5–9]
   - First-order neuron lesions may present with hemisensory loss, dysarthria, dysphagia, ataxia, vertigo, and nystagmus. Anhidrosis affects the ipsilateral side of the body. Causes include the following:
     - Chiari malformations, syringomyelia[10]
     - Basal meningitis or skull-base tumors
     - Stroke with Wallenberg syndrome (lateral medullary syndrome)
     - Multiple sclerosis
     - Neck trauma and/or dissection of the vertebral artery
     - Pituitary tumors
   - Second-order neuron lesions (as in this case) may present with facial, neck, axillary, shoulder or arm pain, cough, hemoptysis, history of thoracic or neck procedures or trauma, anhidrosis of the ipsilateral face. Causes include the following:
     - Pancoast tumor or cervical rib
     - Birth trauma
     - Aortic dissection
     - Central venous line placement, chest tube placement[11]
     - Trauma or surgical injury to the neck or upper thorax
     - Hilar lymphadenopathy
     - Middle ear lesions[12]

■ **Answers (*continued*)**

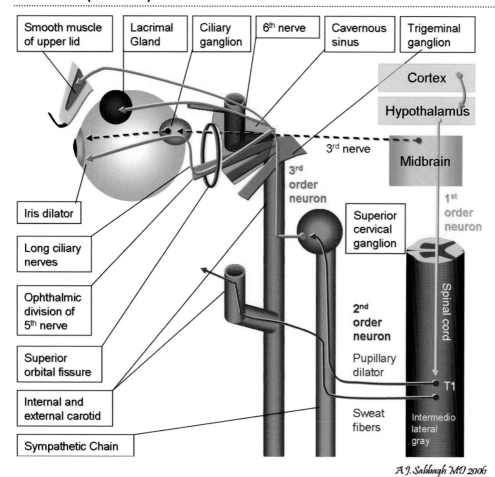

Fig. 102.3 Horner syndrome – anatomic depiction of the involved pathways. **(A)** First-order neurons (central sympathetic) start at the posterolateral hypothalamus, descend uncrossed via the midbrain and pons, and end in the intermediolateral gray at the level of C8 to T2. **(B)** Second-order preganglionic pupillomotor fibers leave the spinal cord at T1, join the cervical sympathetic chain, close to the pulmonary apex. These nerves ascend through the sympathetic chain and synapse in the superior cervical ganglion near the bifurcation of the common carotid artery (around C3 to C4 levels). **(C)** Third-order neurons: Pupillomotor fibers (postganglionics) leave the superior cervical ganglion and migrate along the internal carotid artery. Vasomotor and the sudomotor fibers branch off shortly after the postganglionic fibers leave the superior cervical ganglion. These fibers travel along the external carotid artery to innervate the blood vessels and sweat glands of the face. The pupillomotor fibers enter the cavernous sinus while traveling along the internal carotid artery. These fibers then join the abducens nerve (CN VI) in the cavernous sinus and enter through the superior orbital fissure into the orbit along with the ophthalmic branch of the trigeminal nerve (CN V1) via the long ciliary nerves. The long ciliary nerves innervate Müller muscle and the iris dilators. (From Patten JP. Neurological Differential Diagnosis. 2nd ed. Glasgow: Springer Verlag; 1996. Reede DL, Garcon E, Smoker WR, Kardon R. Horner's syndrome: clinical and radiographic evaluation. Neuroimaging Clin N Am 2008;18(2):369–385 xi. Bardorf CM. Horner syndrome. emedicine.com 2006. Available at: http://www.emedicine.com/OPH/topic336.htm. Accessed April 22, 2009.)

- Third-order neuron lesions may present with diplopia from sixth nerve palsy, numbness in the distribution of the first or second division of the trigeminal nerve, and pain. Anhidrosis is either absent or limited (fibers travel with the external carotid artery). Causes include the following:
  - Internal carotid artery dissection[13]
  - Raeder's paratrigeminal syndrome
  - Carotid cavernous fistula
  - Herpes zoster

9. *How do these eye findings affect prognosis?*
- Nerve damage proximal to the dorsal root ganglion (demonstrated by the presence of a Horner syndrome) usually cannot be directly surgically repaired.
- This often requires a neurotization procedure, which is more complex and has poorer outcomes.[14]
- In a retrospective study on 51 patients, outcomes of neurotization at the level of the brachial plexus show results of ~38% useful recovery.[15]

■ **References**

1. Russell SM. Examination of Peripheral Nerve Injury: An Anatomical Approach. New York: Thieme Medical Publishers; 2007

2. Tiel RL, Happel JT, Kline DG. Nerve action potential recordings method and equipment. Neurosurgery 1996;39(1):103–108

3. Kim DH, Cho Y, Tiel RL, Kline DG. Outcomes of surgery in 1019 brachial plexus lesions treated at Louisiana State University Health Sciences Center. J Neurosurg 2003;98(5):1005–1016

4. Kandenwein JA, Kretchmer T, Engelhardt M, Richter HP, Antoniadis G. Surgical interventions for traumatic lesions of the brachial plexus: a retrospective study of 134 cases. J Neurosurg 2005;103(4):614–621

5. Walton KA, Buono LM. Horner syndrome. Curr Opin Ophthalmol 2003;14(6):357–363

6. Patten JP. Neurological Differential Diagnosis. 2nd ed. Glasgow: Springer-Verlag; 1996

7. Haines DE. Fundamental Neuroscience for Basic and Clinical Applications. 3rd ed. Philadelphia: Churchill Livingstone Elsevier; 2006

8. Reede DL, Garcon E, Smoker WR, Kardon R. Horner's syndrome: clinical and radiographic evaluation. Neuroimaging Clin N Am 2008;18(2):369–385

9. Bardorf CM. Horner syndrome. emedicine.com 2006. Available at: http://www.emedicine.com/OPH/topic336.htm. Accessed April 22, 2009

10. Kerrison JB, Biousse V, Newman NJ. Isolated Horner's syndrome and syringomyelia. J Neurol Neurosurg Psychiatry 2000;69(1):131–132

11. Levy M, Newman-Toker D. Reversible chest tube Horner syndrome. J Neuroophthalmol 2008;28(3):212–213

12. Spector RH. Postganglionic Horner syndrome in three patients with coincident middle ear infection. J Neuroophthalmol 2008;28(3):182–185

13. Flaherty PM, Flynn JM. Horner syndrome due to carotid dissection. J Emerg Med 2008; Sep 12 Epub

14. Midha R, Zager E. Surgery of Peripheral Nerves. A Case-Based Approach. New York: Thieme Medical Publishers; 2007

15. Moiyadi AV, Devi BI, Nair KP. Brachial plexus injuries: outcome following neurotization with intercostal nerve. J Neurosurg 2007;107(2):308–313

Case 103   Neurogenic Thoracic Outlet Syndrome

Stephen M. Russell

■ Clinical Presentation

- A 32-year-old woman presents with a one-year history of left-hand weakness and incoordination, numbness in her medial left forearm, and paresthesias in her left fifth digit when she rotates her head to the right.
- Her weakness temporarily worsens with overhead arm activity, including combing her hair and reaching for items.
- She denies sensory symptoms in the thumb or first two fingers.

- She is a slim woman with a long neck and poor posture.
- On examination, she has mild atrophy and weakness in both the median and ulnar innervated hand intrinsic muscles compared with the opposite hand, hypesthesia along the medial left forearm, and a positive Tinel sign with gentle tapping in the left supraclavicular space.
- Her radial pulse disappears in either arm when the arm is raised above her head.

■ Questions

1. What is your differential diagnosis?
2. Describe the myotome and dermatome for C8, T1, and the lower trunk.
3. What diagnostic studies would you request to help confirm the diagnosis?
4. What are the different types of thoracic outlet syndrome?
5. What is the proposed pathophysiology of neurogenic thoracic outlet syndrome?
6. What are the treatment options?
7. What is the success rate of surgery for neurogenic thoracic outlet syndrome?

■ Answers

1. *What is your differential diagnosis?*
   - Considering that her neurologic examination localizes her pathology to the lower trunk, the working diagnosis would be neurogenic thoracic outlet syndrome.
   - The differential diagnosis for neurogenic thoracic outlet includes cervical radiculopathy, carpal tunnel syndrome, ulnar nerve entrapment at the elbow, motor neuron disease, and a Pancoast tumor.[1]
2. *Describe the myotome and dermatome for C8, T1, and the lower trunk.*
   - Together, C8 and T1 innervate all of the hand intrinsic musculature via both the ulnar and median nerves (they also provide contribution to some more proximal muscles).
   - **Figure 103.1** demonstrates the combined dermatome of C8 and T1, which represents the region of possible numbness or paresthesias in patients with neurogenic thoracic outlet syndrome.
   - Classically, these patients have paresthesias and numbness along the medial forearm.

3. *What diagnostic studies would you request to help confirm the diagnosis?*
   - An apical lordotic radiograph of the cervical spine should reveal any cervical ribs or "beaked" C7 transverse processes.
   - Magnetic resonance imaging (MRI) with and without contrast of the brachial plexus (which should include the cervical spine) is ordered to exclude a herniated disc, foraminal stenosis, and tumors.
   - Although frequently normal in mild cases, electrodiagnostic studies can reveal denervation in both ulnar and median innervated hand muscles (e.g., first dorsal interosseous and abductor pollicis brevis, respectively) and perhaps an absent nerve action potential from the medial antebrachial cutaneous nerve.
4. *What are the different types of thoracic outlet syndrome?*
   - Thoracic outlet is categorized as neurogenic, vascular, or disputed.[2]

■ **Answers (*continued*)**

Lower Trunk Sensory Loss (C8/T1)

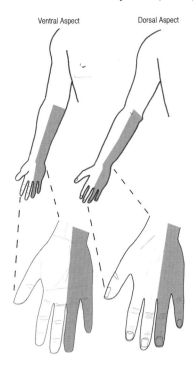

Ventral Aspect   Dorsal Aspect

Fig. 103.1 Location of lower trunk sensory loss (i.e., combined C8 and T1 sensory loss). Although variable, patients with neurogenic thoracic outlet syndrome often have sensory loss or paresthesias confined to the medial forearm (T1 dermatome), and less so in the small finger. (From Russell SM. Examination of Peripheral Nerve Injury: An Anatomical Approach. New York: Thieme Medical Publishers; 2007. Reprinted with permission.)

- Neurogenic and vascular thoracic outlet are both quite rare; the disputed type is much more common.
- Neurogenic thoracic outlet syndrome requires clear demonstration of objective neurologic finding on examination or diagnostic tests, including atrophy, electrodiagnostic testing abnormalities, a cervical rib, and/or focal nerve swelling on MRI.
  - If no objective findings are present, the patient should be observed for their subsequent development.
5. *What is the proposed pathophysiology of neurogenic thoracic outlet syndrome?*
  - Most experts believe that accessory ligaments and/or fascial bands related to a cervical rib or "beaked" C7 transverse process compress and distort the brachial plexus in patients with neurogenic thoracic outlet syndrome.[3]
  - It remains controversial whether the anterior scalene, per se, is responsible for nerve entrapment.
6. *What are the treatment options?*
  - For patients with mild symptoms and signs, posture training and a trial of physical therapy may lead to improvement.

- If atrophy and/or weakness are present, then surgical decompression of the brachial plexus is indicated.
- Once profound and chronic atrophy is present, however, the chance of surgical decompression causing a substantial improvement is unlikely.
- Therefore, early treatment is optimal.
- An anterior suprascapular exposure of the brachial plexus is the preferred approach by neurosurgeons in patients with neurogenic thoracic outlet syndrome (**Fig. 103.2**).[4]
7. *What is the success rate of surgery for neurogenic thoracic outlet syndrome?*
  - If preoperatively the patient only has provocative symptoms (e.g., with overhead arm use), and only minimal signs of weakness and atrophy (i.e., mild cases), then surgical decompression leads to improvement in 85–90% of patients.
  - When significant atrophy and weakness are present (moderate-to-severe cases), the chance of partial improvement is approximately two-thirds.[5]

■ Answers (*continued*)

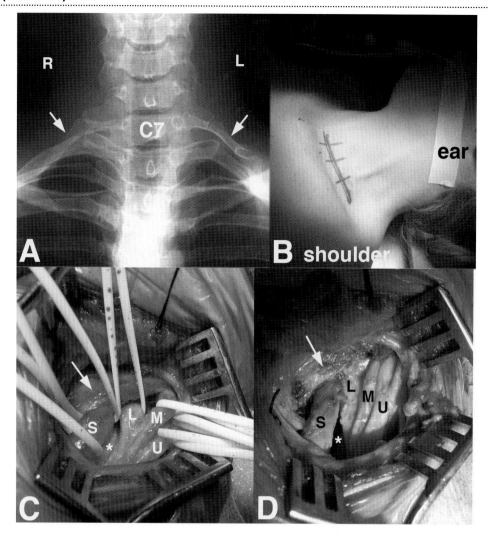

Fig. 103.2 Woman with left-sided neurogenic thoracic outlet syndrome. **(A)** Apical lordotic radiograph demonstrating bilateral cervical ribs (*white arrows*). **(B)** The transverse incision used to expose the left-sided brachial plexus. Care must be taken to preserve the supraclavicular sensory nerves, which are subcutaneous and often traverse the operative field. (Subsequent operative images are in the same orientation as depicted here). **(C)** The brachial plexus (upper [U], middle [M], and lower [L] trunks), subclavian artery (S), cervical rib (*), and anterior scalene (*white arrow*) are all exposed via an anterior supraclavicular approach. The clavicle is to the left of the operative exposure; therefore, the subclavian artery and lower trunk are significantly stretched over the top of the cervical rib and displaced in a cranial direction. **(D)** The cervical rib and its underlying attachments to the first rib have been removed (*). A portion of the scalene muscle has also been removed. The neurovascular structures are now under no tension.

■ References

1. Russell SM. Examination of Peripheral Nerve Injury: An Anatomical Approach. New York: Thieme Medical Publishers; 2007
2. Huang JH, Zager EL. Thoracic outlet syndrome. Neurosurgery 2004;55(4):897–902
3. Roos DB. Congenital anomalies associated with thoracic outlet syndrome. Anatomy, symptoms, diagnosis, and treatment. Am J Surg 1976;132(6):771–778
4. Tender GC, Kline D. Anterior supraclavicular approach to the brachial plexus. Neurosurgery 2006;58(4, Suppl 2):ONS-360–ONS-364
5. Tender GC, Thomas AJ, Thomas N, Kline DG. Gilliatt-Sumner hand revisited: a 25-year experience. Neurosurgery 2004;55(4):883–890

Case 104   Right Axillary Mass with Tinel Sign

Deepa Danan and Christopher J. Winfree

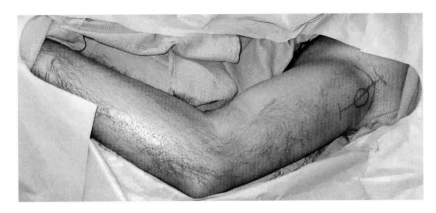

Fig. 104.1 Intraoperative photograph demonstrating location of the mass in the axilla of the right upper extremity (circle) and placement of the overlying incision. The arm is draped into the field to facilitate interpretation of intraoperative nerve stimulation. Specifically, the incision along the course of the nerve to permit tumor removal is located along a portion of the nerve that, when stimulated, does not produce muscle contractions, so that the risk of neurologic injury is reduced.

■ Clinical Presentation

- A 44-year-old right-handed man with no significant medical history, about one year ago noticed a palpable mass in his right axilla without any symptoms of pain, sensory loss, or weakness in the upper extremity.
- He has not noticed any change in size of the mass during this time.
- Detailed peripheral nerve examination showed 5/5 (Medical Research Council scoring system) strength bilaterally in shoulder girdle, upper arm, radial, median, and ulnar innervated muscles, and showed no sensory deficit to light touch or pinprick.
- Although palpation of the mass was not painful, tapping the mass generated a distinct Tinel sign radiating distally along the medial aspect of the arm, forearm, and the fourth and fifth digits (**Fig. 104.1**).

■ Questions

1. What is in this patient's differential diagnosis?
2. What components of the history and physical examination suggest a benign versus malignant diagnosis?
3. Are you going to order any tests? If so, which one(s)?
4. What is the appropriate course of treatment?
5. What is the typical outcome for benign lesions in this location?
6. What is the typical outcome for malignant lesions in this location?

■ Answers

1. *What is in this patient's differential diagnosis?*
   - An axillary mass that generates a prominent Tinel sign is most likely to be a benign peripheral nerve sheath tumor; schwannoma and neurofibroma are, by far, the most common types of nerve sheath tumors.[1]
   - Malignant peripheral nerve sheath tumor and other nerve sheath tumors, such as lipoma, hamartoma, and focal hypertrophic neuropathy, are also possibilities.
   - A connective tissue tumor not arising from the surrounding nerve(s) may, in certain cases, generate a Tinel sign due to extrinsic compression of the nerve and should be included in the differential diagnosis.
2. *What components of the history and physical examination suggest a benign versus malignant diagnosis?*
   - The clinical course is suggestive of a benign lesion.
   - Malignant peripheral nerve sheath tumors typically present as painful, rapidly enlarging lesions, sometimes accompanied by neurologic deficits.[1]

■ Answers (*continued*)

- A painless lesion with an unchanging size over the course of a year is most likely benign.

3. *Are you going to order any tests? If so, which one(s)?*
   - Electromyography and nerve conduction studies (EMG/NCS) may help localize the site of origin of the tumor, and document any neurologic injury caused by the tumor, but are not crucial in the workup of these patients.
   - Imaging studies are more important than EMG/NCS; magnetic resonance imaging (MRI) using T1-weighted, fat-saturated, gadolinium-enhanced images generally show peripheral nerve tumors in this location quite nicely.

4. *What is the appropriate course of treatment?*
   - Brachial plexus exploration for gross total excision of the lesion is performed to ascertain a diagnosis, establish prognosis, provide symptomatic relief, and prevent progression of disease.[1]
   - Benign lesions are generally easily removed from the parent nerve using microdissection techniques.
   - After appropriate identification and neurolysis of the involved neural element, a longitudinal incision over the length of the tumor is made; benign tumors are then easily separated from the nerve fascicles, and the attached nerve fascicles are divided (**Figs. 104.2, 104.3, and 104.4**).[1]
   - When dissection planes are difficult to obtain, or if the tumor is unusually adherent or grossly invad-

ing surrounding tissue planes, then malignancy is suspected and intraoperative frozen section is performed.
   - If malignancy is confirmed on biopsy, then attempts at resection are abandoned; once final pathology is confirmed in subsequent days, then adjuvant therapy, such as radiation, and/or chemotherapy may be indicated.[2]
   - When possible, limb-sparing oncologic resection is attempted; when limb-sparing techniques are not possible, the limb amputation is performed.[3]

5. *What is the typical outcome for benign lesions in this location?*
   - Benign schwannomas are associated with about a 7% risk of neurologic injury at the time of excision, and have a very low recurrence rate.
   - Benign neurofibromas have a higher risk of neurologic injury (20%) and may have a somewhat higher recurrence rate.[4]

6. *What is the typical outcome for malignant lesions in this location?*
   - Unfortunately, despite aggressive surgical and adjuvant therapies, malignant peripheral nerve sheath tumors remain quite lethal.
   - In one series, the recurrence rate was ~50% by 5 years.[3]
   - In another series, the mean survival was just over 2 years.[1]

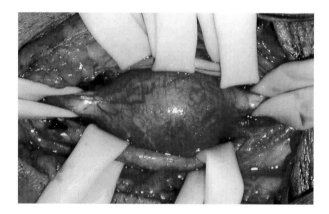

Fig. 104.2 Intraoperative photograph during infraclavicular brachial plexus exploration. Penrose drains have been used to isolate and retract neurovascular elements. The ulnar nerve, in the center of the field, has undergone fusiform enlargement by the tumor. The median nerve is seen in the upper portion of the exposure, while the basilic vein is seen below.

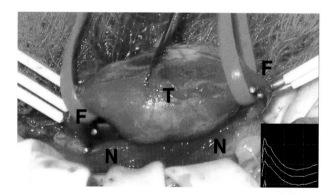

Fig. 104.3 Intraoperative photograph during excision of the tumor. The tumor (T) has been separated from the parent nerve (N), and remains attached by afferent and efferent fascicles (F). Intraoperative nerve action potential recordings (Inset, flat tracing) using special hook electrodes show that the attached tumor-associated fascicles are nonfunctional, and may be sacrificed without yielding a neurologic deficit.

■ Answers (*continued*)

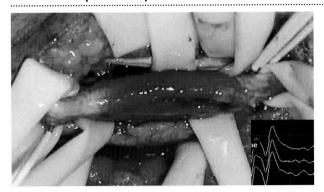

Fig. 104.4 Intraoperative photograph following gross total excision of the tumor. Intraoperative nerve action potential recordings (Inset, robust tracing) using special hook electrodes show that the ulnar nerve, though bruised, remains both anatomically and functionally intact.

■ References

1. Kim DH, Murovic JA, Tiel RL, Moes G, Kline DG. A series of 397 peripheral neural sheath tumors: 30-year experience at Louisiana State University Health Sciences Center. J Neurosurg 2005;102(2):246–255
2. Baehring JM, Betensky RA, Batchelor TT. Malignant peripheral nerve sheath tumor: the clinical spectrum and outcome of treatment. Neurology 2003;61(5):696–698
3. Wong WW, Hirose T, Scheithauer BW, Schild SE, Gunderson LL. Malignant peripheral nerve sheath tumor: analysis of treatment outcome. Int J Radiat Oncol Biol Phys 1998;42(2):351–360
4. Artico M, Cervoni L, Wierzbicki V, D'Andrea V, Nucci F. Benign neural sheath tumours of major nerves: characteristics in 119 surgical cases. Acta Neurochir (Wien) 1997;139(12):1108–1116

Case 105   Ulnar Nerve Compression at the Elbow

Stephen M. Russell

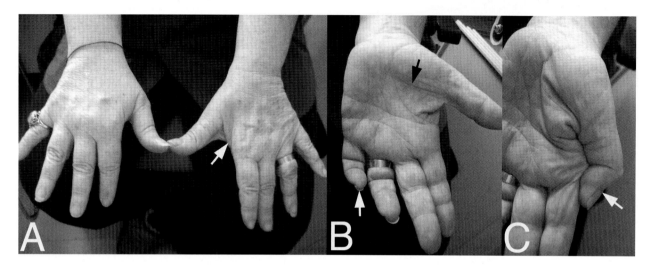

Fig. 105.1   A patient with severe left ulnar nerve entrapment at the elbow with clinical signs shown in **(A–C)**. See Answer section for further description.

■ Clinical Presentation

- A 50-year-old woman presents with 6 weeks of elbow pain localized to the left medial epicondyle.
- It began after a prolonged period of holding the telephone with the affected hand.
- A few days later she woke one morning with complete numbness in the small finger.
- Then over the ensuing weeks, she developed progressive hand atrophy, weakness, and incoordination.

- Her examination reveals dense numbness to light touch and pinprick on the hypothenar eminence (including the dorsum of the hand in this area), as well as the small finger and adjacent half of the ring finger.
- Severe atrophy of most hand intrinsic muscles is noted.
- Tapping in the retrocondylar groove causes paresthesias to occur in the small finger. **Figure 105.1** illustrates the patient's hands.
- She has no neck pain and no Spurling sign.

■ Questions

1. What is your differential diagnosis?
2. In **Fig. 105.1A**, what atrophic muscle is labeled with the white arrow?
3. In **Fig. 105.1B**, what atrophic muscle is labeled with the black arrow?
4. In **Fig. 105.1B**, the white arrow indicates an examination finding that is commonly encountered with her diagnosis, what is it?
5. In **Fig. 105.1C**, the white arrow indicates another examination finding that is commonly encountered with her diagnosis; what is it?

6. Describe the McGowan classification of ulnar nerve entrapment.
7. What are the nonoperative treatment options available?
8. What are the indications for surgery?
9. What are her surgical options for ulnar nerve decompression and/or transposition?
10. Describe the efficacy and common complications of ulnar nerve decompression and/or transposition.

■ Answers

1. *What is your differential diagnosis?*
   - Her history and examination are classic for an ulnar nerve entrapment at the elbow, including her reporting a period of prolonged flexion that may have instigated her somewhat rapid progression of symptoms, a clear sensory loss in an ulnar nerve distribution, and the evidence of ulnar innervated hand intrinsic atrophy.[1]
   - Other less likely diagnoses would include a C8 radiculopathy, an ulnar nerve entrapment at the wrist, and rarely, neurogenic thoracic outlet syndrome.

2. *In* **Fig. 105.1A**, *what atrophic muscle is labeled with the white arrow?*
   - There is marked atrophy of the first dorsal interosseous muscle.
   - Atrophy of this muscle is usually the most obvious with moderate to severe ulnar nerve injury/entrapment.

3. *In* **Fig. 105.1B**, *what atrophic muscle is labeled with the black arrow?*
   - Although most muscles of the thenar eminence are innervated by the median nerve, the largest one, the adductor pollicis, is innervated by the ulnar nerve; therefore, patients with ulnar neuropathy can also have atrophy of their thenar eminence.

4. *In* **Fig. 105.1B**, *the white arrow indicates an examination finding that is commonly encountered with her diagnosis; what is it?*
   - When the patient opens her affected hand, an "ulnar claw hand" is revealed. This consists of ring and small finger hyperextension at the knuckles (metacarpal-phalangeal joints) with superimposed interphalangeal joint flexion secondary to a tenodesis effect.

5. *In* **Fig. 105.1C**, *the white arrow indicates another examination finding that is commonly encountered with her diagnosis; what is it?*
   - A positive Froment sign
   - In patients with severe ulnar neuropathy, the adductor pollicis cannot adduct a straight thumb.
   - Instead, the patient flexes the distal interphalangeal joint (median innervated flexor pollicis longus) to oppose the thumb against the hand.

6. *Describe the McGowan classification of ulnar nerve entrapment.*
   - Dr. McGowan classified ulnar nerve entrapment at the elbow as follows[2]:
     - Grade 1: purely subjective symptoms with mild hypesthesia
     - Grade 2: sensory loss with slight wasting and weakness of the hand intrinsic muscles
     - Grade 3: severe sensorimotor deficits

7. *What are the nonoperative treatment options available?*
   - Very few nonoperative treatments are available.
   - Some include wearing an elbow pad or an elbow splint; however, compliance with these is poor.
   - Physical and occupational therapy may be effective in resolving mild cases.

8. *What are the indications for surgery?*
   - Surgery is usually recommended for McGowan grade 2 and 3 ulnar nerve entrapments.
   - As a general rule, if there are not periods during the day where the hand is normal, then nerve damage is likely occurring and surgery should be an option.
   - Some patients with McGowan grade 1 entrapments request surgery when other conservative measures have failed.

9. *What are her surgical options for ulnar nerve decompression and/or transposition?*
   - There are many surgical options for decompressing the ulnar nerve at the elbow (**Fig. 105.2**).
   - One should use a technique they have personal experience with because, in general, most techniques are equally efficacious.
   - Simple in situ decompression of the ulnar nerve has become more popular as of late because of a few recent randomized trials concluding that a simple decompression is as effective as a transposition.[3-5]

10. *Describe the efficacy and common complications of ulnar nerve decompression and/or transposition.*
    - The results of ulnar nerve decompression and/or transposition are that 60–80% of patients improve, while the rest are the same, or occasionally are worse over time.[3-5]
    - Complications include wound pain, elbow numbness, and neuroma formation from injury to the posterior division of the medial antebrachial cutaneous nerve (**Fig. 105.2A**).

■ **Answers (*continued*)**

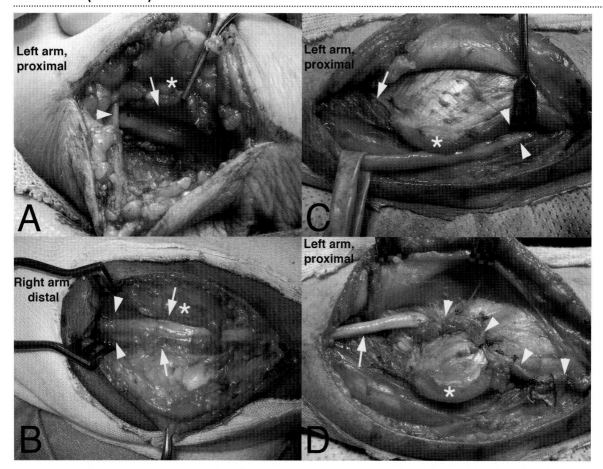

Fig. 105.2 Intraoperative photographs of decompression and/or transposition techniques for ulnar neuropathy localized to the elbow. Arm laterality, orientation, as well as location of the medial epicondyle (*) are provided for each photograph. **(A)** A simple, in situ decompression of the ulnar nerve (same patient as **Fig. 105.1**). Osborne's ligament has been transected and is held open by a forceps (*white arrow*). Although not visible, the ulnar nerve has been decompressed for 2–3 inches beyond both the proximal and distal exposures. The posterior branch of the medial antebrachial cutaneous nerve (*arrowhead*) often traverses the operative exposure and is at risk for iatrogenic injury. **(B)** Another simple decompression in a different patient. To release the cubital tunnel, both

the two heads of the flexor carpi ulnaris (*arrowheads*) as well as the Osborne's ligament (*arrows*) have been released to decompress the ulnar nerve. **(C)** Exposure of the ulnar nerve prior to a submuscular transposition in a patient with moderate ulnar neuropathy. The ulnar nerve is fully neurolysed and is isolated with a Penrose drain. The heads of the flexor carpi ulnaris have been separated (*arrowheads*), and the medial intermuscular septum has been removed (*arrow*). Failure to remove this septum may lead to iatrogenic nerve compression when the ulnar nerve is subsequently transposed under the flexor-pronator mass. **(D)** Same patient as in **C**. The ulnar nerve (*arrow*) has been placed under the flexor–pronator muscle mass, which has been sutured back together (*arrowheads*).

■ **References**

1. Russell SM. Examination of Peripheral Nerve Injury: An Anatomical Approach. New York: Thieme Medical Publishers; 2007
2. McGowan AJ. The results of transposition of the ulnar nerve for traumatic ulnar neuritis. J Bone Joint Surg Br 1950;32:293–301
3. Bartels RH, Vehagen WI, van der Wilt GJ, Meulstee J, van Rossum LG, Grotenhuis JA. Prospective randomized controlled study comparing simple decompression versus anterior subcutaneous transposition for idiopathic neuropathy of the ulnar nerve at the elbow: Part 1. Neurosurgery 2005;56(3):522–530
4. Gervasio O, Gambardella G, Zaccone C, Branca D. Simple decompression versus anterior submuscular transposition of the ulnar nerve in severe cubital tunnel syndrome: a prospective randomized study. Neurosurgery 2005;56(1):108–117
5. Biggs M, Curtis J. Randomized, prospective study comparing ulnar neurolysis in situ with submuscular transposition. Neurosurgery 2006;58(2):296–304

Case 106   Lower Extremity Peripheral Nerve Sheath Tumor

Robert L. Tiel

■ Clinical Presentation

- A 15-year-old right-handed boy presented with a lump on the posterior lateral aspect of his right leg, just above the popliteal crease.
- Although the lump is usually painless, if knocked or manipulated he experiences a shooting sensation down his leg into the side and top of his foot.
- The frequent pains thus generated have forced him to abandon playing soccer.
- His neurologic examination is normal.
- When the lump is palpated it seems to have the dimensions of a large olive-sized (2 × 2 × 2-cm) mass. It moves from right to left, but not vertically. When lightly percussed, a sharp sensation is elicited, which goes into the dorsum of the right foot.
- Other physicians had previously seen the patient. After a magnetic resonance imaging (MRI) scan had been obtained (**Fig. 106.1**), they advised him to have the lump monitored, to limit his activities, and to "live with" the condition.

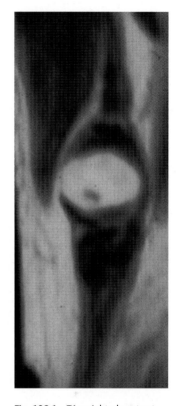

Fig. 106.1   T1-weighted contrast-enhanced magnetic resonance image of a schwannoma. Note widening of the nerve.

■ Questions

1. What is your working diagnosis?
2. Provide a detailed differential diagnosis.
3. What are the ancillary diagnoses for which he should be evaluated?
4. What are the clinical findings associated with these diagnoses?
5. The mother has a friend in whom neurofibromatosis was suspected; she states that this friend was sent to an ophthalmologist for diagnosis. Why?
6. She asks you if this tumor could be malignant. What is your answer?
7. The other physicians recommended "living with" the condition. What are this patient's options? What are the risks to the patient?
8. Should surgical excision be advised?
9. Should a needle biopsy be performed first?
10. Which incision should be used for general exposure?
11. Describe the steps in removing the tumor.
12. Should a frozen section be requested?
13. The tumor is removed; final sections are available for review 3 days later. Representative samples are shown in **Figs. 106.2, 106.3, 106.4, and 106.5**. What is your diagnosis?
14. Which immunohistochemical stains are useful in diagnosing peripheral nerve sheath tumors?

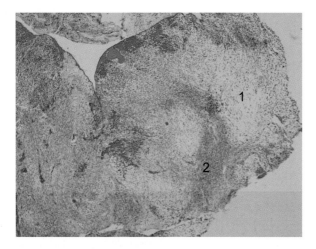

Fig. 106.2 Low magnification (40×) of tumor with two areas of interest (hematoxylin and eosin [H&E] stained).

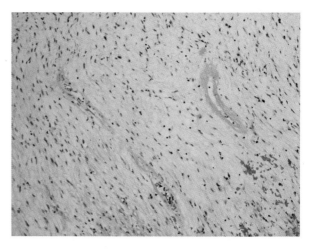

Fig. 106.3 High magnification (200×) of area 1 (H&E) stained).

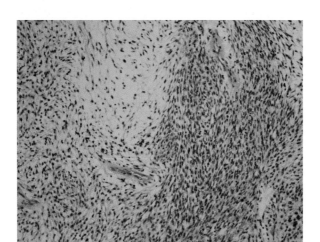

Fig. 106.4 High magnification (200×) of area 2 (H&E stained).

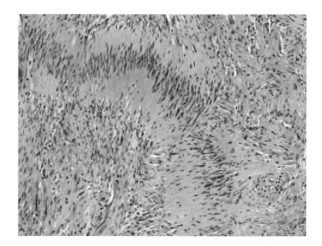

Fig. 106.5 High magnification (200×) of tumor pathology (H&E stained).

■ Answers

1. *What is your working diagnosis?*
   - The working diagnosis is that of peripheral nerve sheath tumor.
   - The lump suggests tumor pathology. The MRI (**Fig. 106.1**) shows a contrast-enhancing intraneural mass widening the nerve.
   - The lateral mobility is evident, but vertical mobility strongly suggests a lesion within a movable peripheral nerve.
   - Finally, the paresthesias associated with manipulation point toward primary neural involvement in a specific peripheral nerve distribution (in this case the common peroneal nerve).
2. *Provide a detailed differential diagnosis.*

- The differential diagnosis of nerve sheath tumor includes the following[1]:
- Benign tumors
  - Schwannoma
    - Cellular schwannoma
    - Plexiform schwannoma
    - Melanotic schwannoma
  - Neurofibroma
    - Diffuse (cutaneous)
    - Localized
    - Plexiform
  - Perineurioma
  - Nerve sheath myxoma
  - Granular cell tumor
  - Ganglioneuroma

■ Answers (*continued*)

- Malignant tumors
  - Malignant peripheral nerve sheath tumors (MPNST)
  - Variants of above
  - Secondary neoplasms
- Tumor-like lesions
  - Reactive lesions
    - Traumatic neuroma
    - Inflammatory pseudotumor
  - Inflammatory and infectious lesions
  - Intraneural ganglion cysts
  - Hyperplastic lesions
    - Localized hypertrophic neuropathy
  - Hamartomas
    - Fibrolipomatous hamartoma

3. *What are the ancillary diagnoses for which he should be evaluated?*
   - The presence of a peripheral nerve sheath tumor warrants evaluation for neurofibromatosis types 1 (NF-1) and 2 (NF-2) and for schwannomatosis.

4. *What are the clinical findings associated with these diagnoses?*
   - Diagnostic criteria for NF-1[2] (two or more of the following):
     - Six or more café-au-lait spots
       - Greater than 1.5 cm or larger in postpubertal individuals
       - Greater than 0.5 cm or larger in prepubertal individuals
     - Two or more neurofibromas of any type
     - One or more plexiform neurofibromas
     - Axillary or groin freckling, an optic pathway glioma, two or more Lisch nodules
     - A first-degree relative with NF-1 (as defined by the preceding criteria)
     - Characteristic osseous lesions, such as sphenoid dysplasia
   - Diagnostic criteria for NF-2[3]
     - The main characteristic of NF-2 is the presence of bilateral vestibular schwannomas – tumors arising from the vestibular branch of the eighth cranial nerve (CN VIII).
     - Other diagnostic features consistent with NF-2
       - A first-degree relative with NF-2
       - A unilateral vestibular schwannoma in a patient younger than age 30 years
     - Or any two of the following:
       - Meningioma
       - Glioma
       - Schwannoma
       - Juvenile posterior subcapsular lenticular opacities
       - Juvenile cortical cataracts

- Diagnostic criteria for schwannomatosis[3,4]
  - Individuals should not fulfill the diagnostic criteria for NF-2 or have any of the following:
    - A vestibular schwannomas of CN VIII
    - Constitutional NF-2 mutation
    - First-degree relative with NF-2
  - Definite schwannomatosis
    - Older than 30 years and two or more nonintradermal schwannomas (at least one confirmed by histology)
    - One schwannoma confirmed with histology and a first-degree relative who meets the above requirements.
    - Lack of radiographic evidence of CN VIII tumor on an imaging study performed after age 18 years.
  - Possible schwannomatosis
    - Older than 30 and two or more nonintradermal schwannomas (at least one confirmed by histology)
    - Older than 45 years and no symptoms of CN VIII dysfunction and two or more nonintradermal schwannomas (at least one confirmed by histology)
    - Radiographic evidence of a schwannoma and a first-degree relative who meets the criteria for definite schwannomatosis

5. *The mother has a friend in whom neurofibromatosis was suspected; she states that this friend was sent to an ophthalmologist for diagnosis. Why?*
   - The ophthalmologists would be conducting a slit-lamp evaluation to identify Lisch nodules or posterior subcapsular lenticular opacities.
   - A Lisch nodule is a melanocytic hamartoma of the iris.
     - They appear after age 3.
     - They are present in 90% of NF-1 patients.
     - They are specific for NF-1.
     - They are usually clear yellow to brown.
     - A slit-lamp examination may be necessary to differentiate them from nevi on the iris, where they present as flat or minimally elevated, densely pigmented lesions with blurred margins.
   - Juvenile posterior subcapsular lenticular opacities
     - Usually asymptomatic
     - Occur in NF-2

6. *She asks you whether this tumor could be malignant. What is your answer?*
   - The possibility of malignancy is always present until the permanent histologic sections are evaluated.
   - Incidence in the general population is 0.0001%.[5]
   - Although the likelihood of malignant transformation is higher in NF-1 patients, only half of malignant nerve sheath tumors arise from NF-1 patients; the other half arise de novo from people without neurofibromatosis.

■ **Answers (***continued***)**

- From the clinical perspective the tumor size and the presence of a more constant pain suggest the diagnosis of malignancy.
  - Loss of function in the distribution of the nerve suggests malignancy. Although benign nerve sheath tumors may attain a large size, they usually displace the fascicles aside and involve the fascicles minimally.
  - A Tinel sign or mechanical irritability should not be confused with the pain of malignancy, which is more constant and often throbs "at night".

7. *The other physicians recommended living with the condition. What are this patient's options? What are the risks to the patient?*
   - The patient with a nerve sheath tumor has the following options:
   - Live with the tumor (observation)
     - Have its growth monitored
     - If it grows, have it operated upon.
   - Have the tumor resected
     - Resection of the tumor causes little morbidity.
       ▪ The risk of schwannoma together with a normal examination
         • Will lead to no postoperative motor deficit in 90% of operated cases
         • Resolves nerve irritability and pain in 75% of operated cases
       ▪ The risk of solitary neurofibroma without motor deficit
         • Allows 78% to have no postoperative motor deficit
         • Allows pain to be resolved or improved in 88% of cases[6]

8. *Should surgical excision be advised?*
   - Given the relatively low risks of resection combined with the uncertainty of diagnosis, resection represents the single best option unless age or associated medical morbidity precludes surgery.
   - The lifetime focal cure rate for schwannomas is 95%.
   - The histologic diagnosis is determined and the tumor definitively treated.

9. *Should a needle biopsy be performed first?*
   - No, needle biopsy should not be advised for most nerve sheath tumors.[6]
   - In contradistinction to other soft tissue tumors, biopsy of nerve sheath tumors increases the morbidity of management.
   - The biopsy needle must first blindly traverse the nerve sheath tumor, piercing the outside capsule and displaced fascicles, risking nerve damage to a functioning nerve.
   - Intraneural tissue planes that aid in tumor removal might be lost by biopsy-related hemorrhage or scarring.
   - An exception may be large painful tumors that show increased activity on positron emission tomography scanning because a targeted biopsy might allow determination of malignancy prior to operation.

10. *Which incision should be used for general exposure?*
    - An extensile incision should be located over the tumor and along the course of the nerve.
    - For the peroneal nerve above the popliteal fossa a "Lazy S" incision would be appropriate (**Fig. 106.6**).

11. *Describe the steps in removing the tumor.*
    - The steps in tumor removal proximal to an entrapment site (for the peroneal nerve, the fibular head) include the following[7]:
      - The skin incision is made and the peroneal nerve and tumor are freed from all surrounding tissue.
      - In the location where the peroneal nerve can be entrapped by the fascial tissue at the head of the fibula, the nerve is "released" past the fibular head, well into the peroneus longus muscle.
      - Nerve action potential (NAP) recording (if available) is performed along the entire nerve. A NAP should be easily recordable (**Fig. 106.7**).
      - Attention is turned to the tumor once the nerve and its branches have been completely neurolysed.
      - A fascicle-free area of the is tumor is determined
        ▪ By inspection (**Fig. 106.8**)
        ▪ By cautious nerve stimulation (**Fig. 106.9**)
      - Attempting to discover the dissection plane of the tumor, the surgeon makes an incision into the tumor and its primary fascicle and gentle dissection is used to develop this plane between tumor and fascicles (**Fig. 106.10**).
      - The tumor and its primary entry and exit fascicle are dissected out (**Fig. 106.11**).
      - A NAP recording is done of the entering fascicle (**Fig. 106.12**). A flat trace is elicited, thereby insuring that the fascicle from which the tumor arose is nonfunctioning or solely sensory.
      - The tumor is removed well into the originating and exiting fascicle to ensure complete tumor excision (**Fig. 106.13**).
      - A whole nerve NAP is recorded after resection to insure a functioning nerve.
      - The meticulous hemostasis of the tumor bed is achieved prior to closure.
      - The incision is closed.

12. *Should a frozen section be requested?*
    - A frozen section is usually unnecessary if the tumor dissection proceeds easily.
    - If dissection planes are not found:
      - The nerve adheres to soft tissue structures, and a frozen section may be warranted to evaluate the suspected tissue for malignancy or alternative diagnosis.
    - If the nerve seems unusually hard or fibrotic:
      - The diagnosis of peripheral nerve pseudotumor is now being considered, and a representative sample is usually warranted to determine whether dissection should proceed.

■ Answers (*continued*)

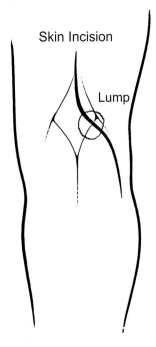

Fig. 106.6   Incision for exposing the right common peroneal nerve to expose the nerve sheath tumor.

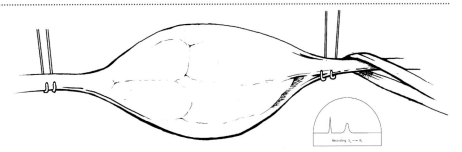

Fig. 106.7   The tumor and nerve are dissected free from surrounding connective tissue and a positive nerve action potential is recorded.

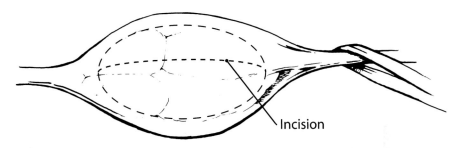

Fig. 106.8   A fascicle-free area is determined from inspection.

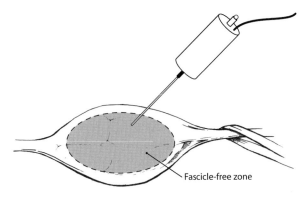

Fig. 106.9   An area of no stimulation is mapped out using a disposable hand held stimulator set on 2 mA.

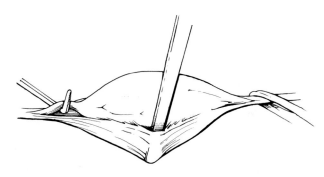

Fig. 106.10   An incision is made into the nerve and a plane of dissection between the tumor and the nerve is developed.

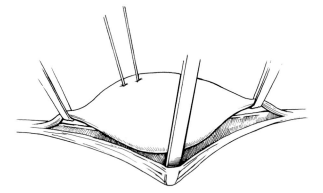

Fig. 106.11   Stitch retraction is sometimes useful in manipulating the tumor to aid in the intraneural dissection of the tumor from the surrounding nerve.

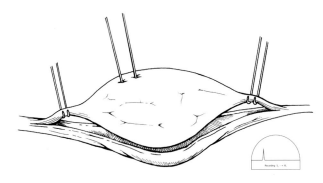

Fig. 106.12   A nerve action potential cannot be recorded across the involved fascicle indicating that the fascicle is either pure sensory or contains no useful motor fibers.

■ **Answers (continued)**

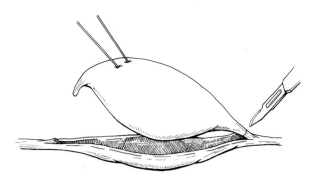

Fig. 106.13 The tumor is sharply cut at both ends where the fascicle of origin is of normal caliber.

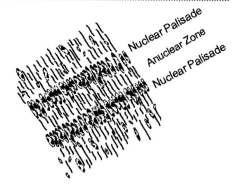

Fig. 106.14 Diagram of a Verocay body.

13. *The tumor is removed; final sections are available for review 3 days later. Representative samples are shown in* **Figs. 106.2, 106.3, 106.4, and 106.5**. *What is your diagnosis?*
   • The diagnosis is benign schwannoma.[8]
   • Antoni A pattern (**Fig. 106.4**)
      – Compact elongated cells with tapered spindle-shaped nuclei
      – Variable chromasia
      – Ample pink cytoplasm
   • Antoni B pattern (**Fig. 106.3**)
      – Loose texture "cobweb like meshwork"
      – Multipolar processes
      – Round and oval nuclei
      – Occasional microcysts

   • Verocay bodies (**Fig. 106.5**)
      – Nuclear clusters in a palisading arrangement
      – Double rows of nuclei separated by aligned eosinophilic cell processes (**Fig. 106.14**)
14. *Which immunohistochemical stains are useful in diagnosing peripheral nerve sheath tumors?*
   • The immunohistologic stains useful in identifying peripheral nerve tumors are summarized in **Table 106.1**.[9-14]
   • They include
      – S-100 (so called because of its solubility in 100% saturated ammonium sulfate)
      – CD-34 (cluster of differentiation molecule)
      – EMA (epithelial membrane antigen)
      – Nestin

■ Answers (*continued*)

Table 106.1   Immunohistochemistry of Peripheral Nerve Sheath Tumors

Marker	Function	Specificity	Schwannoma	Neurofibroma	Perinerinoma [9,10,11]	MPNST
S-100	Described initially by Moore,[12] constitutes a large family of at least 20 proteins with calcium binding ability	Present in the cytosol of glial and Schwann cells, and also, in adipocytes and chondrocytes, although in very low concentrations in the latter two	Strongly positive ++++	Variable ++ to ++++	Less than 5% positive - to +	Variable 50% positive - to ++
CD-34 (human progenitor cell antigen)[13]		Immunoreactive to endoneurial fibroblasts	Negative Antoni A positive Antoni B - to +	Positive +++	Variable - to ++	Variable - to +
EMA[10,14]	A large, highly glycosylated protein (MUC1)	Expressed on the apical membrane of many epithelial cells	Negative -	Variable - to +	Positive ++++	Variable - to +
Nestin[11]	Intermediate filament protein	Expressed in neuroectodermal stem cells	Variable - to ++	Variable - to +		Positive +++

Abbreviations: MPNST, malignant peripheral nerve sheath tumor; +, positive expressivity; -, negative expressivity; EMA, epithelial membrane antigen.

■ References

1. Scheithauer BW. Tumors of the Peripheral Nervous System. 3rd ed. [Fascicle 23]. In Rosai J, Sobin LH, eds.. Atlas of Tumor Pathology. Washington DC: Armed Forces Institute of Pathology; 2007
2. Ferner RE, Huson SM, Thomas N, et al. Guidelines for the diagnosis and management of individuals with neurofibromatosis 1. J Med Genet 2007;44(2):81–88
3. Ferner RE. Neurofibromatosis 1 and neurofibromatosis 2: a twenty first century perspective. Lancet Neurol 2007;6(4):340–351
4. MacCollin M, Chiocca EA, Evans DG, et al. Diagnostic criteria for schwannomatosis. Neurology 2005;64(11):1838–1845
5. Ducatman BS, Scheithauer BW, Piepgras DG, Reiman HM, Ilstrup DM. Malignant peripheral nerve sheath tumors. A clinicopathologic study of 120 cases. Cancer 1986;57(10):2006–2021
6. Kline DG, Hudson AR. Nerve Injuries: Operative Results of Major Nerve Injuries, Entrapments, and Tumors. Philadelphia: W.B. Saunders; 1995
7. Kline DJ, Hudson AR, Kim DH. Atlas of Peripheral Nerve Surgery. Philadelphia: Saunders; 2001
8. Ellison D, Love S, Chimell L, Harding B, Lowe JS, Vinters HV. Neuropathology — A Reference Text to CNS Pathology. St. Louis: Mosby; 2004
9. Hornick JL, Fletcher CD. Soft tissue perineurioma: clinicopathologic analysis of 81 cases including those with atypical histologic features. Am J Surg Pathol 2005;29(7):845–858
10. Limacher JM, Acres B. MUC1, a therapeutic target in oncology. Bull Cancer 2007;94(3):253–257
11. Shimada S, Tsuzuki T, Kuroda M, et al. Nestin expression as a new marker in malignant peripheral nerve sheath tumors. Pathol Int 2007;57(2):60–67
12. Moore BW. A soluble protein characteristic of nervous system. Biochem Biophys Res Commun 1965;19:739–744
13. Weiss SW, Nickoloff BJ. CD-34 is expressed by a distinctive cell population in peripheral nerve, nerve sheath tumors, and related lesions. Am J Surg Pathol 1993;17(10):1039–1045
14. Hirose T, Tani T, Shimada T, Ishizawa K, Shimada S, Sano T. Immunohistochemical demonstration of EMA/Glut1-positive perineurial cells and CD34-positive fibroblastic cells in peripheral nerve sheath tumors. Mod Pathol 2003;16(4):293–298

Case 107   Foot Drop and Peroneal Nerve Injury

Robert L. Tiel

■ Clinical Presentation

- An 18-year-old college freshman suffers a right knee dislocation during fall football practice.
- He has immediate loss of dorsiflexion of the right foot on the field.
- He is discovered to have an anterior and posterior cruciate ligament (ACL; PCL) and lateral collateral ligament tears.
- He is scheduled for orthopedic knee surgery and his ligaments are repaired.
- The peroneal nerve, which was seen in surgery, was believed to be "intact" but slightly bruised.
- He is seen 4 months later in consultation with the following physical examination of his right leg.
- Motor examination right lower extremity (Medical Research Council scale)
  - Iliopsoas: 5/5
  - Quadriceps femoris: 5/5
  - Tibialis anterior: 0/5
  - Extensor hallicis longus: 0/5
  - Extensor digitorum communis: 0/5
  - Peroneus longus/brevis: 3/5
  - Posterior tibialis: 4+/5
  - Plantar flexion (soleus/gastrocnemius): 4+/5
  - Toe flexion: 4+/5

- Sensory examination of the right lower extremity
  - Web space between first and second toes numb to pin
  - Dorsum of foot numb to pin
  - Lateral border of foot slightly decreased compared with left foot
  - Sole of foot same compared with the left foot
- Deep tendon reflexes (DTRs)
  - Right 2+ knee jerk (KJ) 1+ ankle jerk (AJ) (with reinforcement)
  - Left 2+ KJ 2+ AJ

■ Questions

1. What physical finding must be checked on the football field and in the emergency room?
2. Is the nerve injured?
3. What is the Seddon or Sunderland grade?
4. Where is the nerve(s) injured?
5. Does the patient need any orthosis? If so what type?
6. Which plan of care should be arranged?
7. Which electrodiagnostic tests should be ordered and when? Which muscles should be examined?
8. When, if ever, should this nerve injury be explored?
9. What incision should be used? How do you find the peroneal nerve when all you see is fat? What is the relation of the common peroneal nerve to the fibular head?
10. When, if ever, should the nerve(s) be repaired?
11. What are the results of operative repair at this level for foot drop?
12. What are patient's alternatives to nerve repair?

Table 107.1 Correlation between Seddon and Sunderland Nerve Injury Grading

Clinical State of the Nerve	Demyelination, conduction block	Disruption of the nerve fibers, endoneurium intact	Disruption of the endoneurium, perineurium intact	Disruption of the perineurium, epineurium intact	Complete disruption of the epineurium, nerve severed
Seddon	Neuropraxia	Axonotmesis	Neurotmesis	Neurotmesis	Neurotmesis
Sunderland	Grade 1	Grade 2	Grade 3	Grade 4	Grade 5

Source: Seddon H. Surgical Disorders of the Peripheral Nerves. Edinburgh: Churchill Livingstone; 1972; Sunderland S. Nerve and Nerve Injuries. New York: Churchill Livingston; 1978.

■ Answers

1. *What physical finding must be checked on the football field and in the emergency room?*
   - The most important physical finding in this case was the presence of a palpable distal pulse.
   - Unrecognized ischemia can lead to loss of limb and even death.
   - Using the Doppler ultrasound and/or angiography to assess the vasculature can further insure that the leg is viable.
2. *Is the nerve injured?*
   - Yes, there is no function of the muscles of dorsiflexion and no mention of direct injury to the muscles; so therefore the nerve is injured and not working properly after injury.
3. *What is the Seddon or Sunderland grade?*
   - The injury is either axonotmetic or neurotmetic by the Seddon classification or Sunderland grade 2–4 (**Table 107.1**).
   - Determining either the Seddon or Sunderland grade acutely is impossible upon initial presentation.
   - Because after 4 months, there has been no recovery of function, then this is not a neurapraxic injury – not a (Seddon) or a Sunderland grade 1 injury.
   - The Sunderland grade cannot be 5 as the nerve was inspected and appears to be in continuity.
4. *Where is the nerve injured?*
   - Localization of the nerve injury is at the level of the peroneal division from the sciatic nerve.
   - There is mild injury of the tibial division and complete injury of the peroneal.

- The peroneal nerve is tethered at this bifurcation and some damaging energy has been transmitted to the tibial nerve.
- The normal cross-sectional diameter of the sciatic nerve just proximal to the split is 11–12 mm, the tibial nerve is usually 6 mm and the peroneal nerve 5 mm at its origin.
- After a stretch injury these measurements increase and the peroneal nerve might be 11–12 mm and the tibial nerve 7 mm demonstrating the internal fibrosis and injury which accompanied the dislocation (**Fig. 107.1**).

5. *Does the patient need any orthosis? If so what type?*
   - Almost all patients will benefit from a well-fitting orthosis.
   - The most common is the in the shoe ankle-foot orthosis (AFO), but there exist many variations on this model. The specific purpose of an AFO is to provide toe dorsiflexion during the swing phase, medial and/or lateral stability at the ankle while standing, and, if necessary, push-off stimulation during the late stance phase.
   - The goal of bracing is to prevent toe and foot drop while walking, which would contribute to tripping.
   - Additionally, the ankle also needs the lateral support to avoid spontaneous inversion and twisting of the ankle joint.
   - For those so inclined, a stiff lace-up work boot or a cowboy boot can reasonably serve these dual purposes.

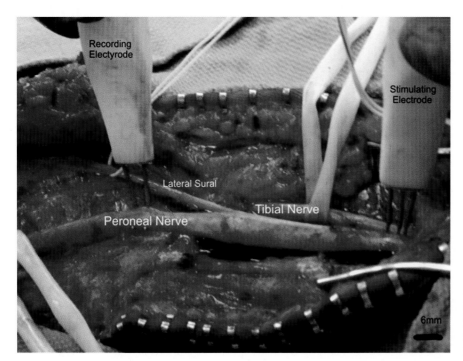

Fig. 107.1   Nerve action potential recording of a stretched peroneal nerve showing increased diameter well into the sciatic nerve at the sciatic bifurcation into the common peroneal nerve and the tibial nerve.

■ Answers (*continued*)

6. *Which plan of care should be arranged?*
   - The essential question with all nerve injuries and this one in particular is whether the nerve will recover spontaneously or not.
   - Waiting 3–4 months is recommended unless evidence exists that the nerve is divided.
   - Fitting for an orthosis and treating symptomatically for pain are both interventions usually warranted.
7. *Which electrodiagnostic tests should be ordered and when? Which muscles should be examined?*
   - Waiting 4 months, all hope of a neurapraxic recovery has disappeared.
   - An electromyographic study is to determine whether any nerve fibers have returned to their respective muscles through the injury.
   - An axonotmetic injury (Sunderland 2) will usually recover on its own.
   - The pattern of injury indicates that both the tibial and peroneal divisions of the sciatic nerve have been involved.

- The goal of electromyography (EMG) is to determine the range of involvement. The short head of biceps is supplied by the lateral peroneal division of the sciatic nerve. A normal pattern here ensures that the injury is lower on the sciatic nerve.
- Muscles innervated by the peroneal nerve should be examined. Because the peroneal nerve divides into the superficial peroneal nerve and the deep peroneal nerve, representative muscles from both peroneal divisions should be examined.
- These muscles include the tibialis anterior from the deep peroneal nerve and peroneus longus from the superficial peroneal nerve.
- Tibial nerve innervated muscles should also be evaluated, such as the gastrocnemius muscle and the posterior tibial muscle.
- EMG involvement of the posterior tibial muscle in cases of foot drop will localize the injury to a level at or above the sciatic nerve bifurcation.

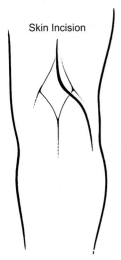

Fig. 107.2 The "lazy S" incision used for peroneal nerve exposure of the right peroneal nerve, posterior view.

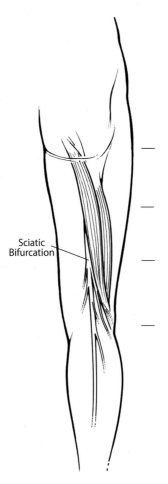

Fig. 107.3 The thigh can be divided into thirds. The bifurcation of the sciatic is at the junction of the lower and middle third of the thigh.

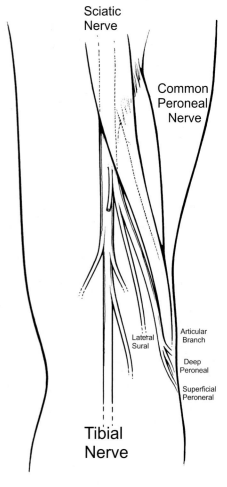

Fig. 107.4 The peroneal nerve is to be found on the medial side of the junction of the short head of biceps and the long head of the biceps femoris tendon.

■ Answers *(continued)*

- An isolated peroneal injury will not show involvement of the posterior tibial muscle.

8. *When, if ever, should this nerve injury be explored?*
   - The nerve should be explored 3–4 months after injury if no recovery is observed and none demonstrated on EMG.[1]
   - If EMG shows some recovery, it is worth waiting 8 weeks and repeating the clinical and if necessary electrical examination.
   - When EMG recovery is not enough to power useful regeneration then operative repair is required.

9. *What incision should be used? How do you find the peroneal nerve when all you see is fat? What is the relation of the common peroneal nerve to the fibular head?*
   - A "lazy S" incision on the back of the leg provides adequate "extensile" exposure and avoids going perpendicular to the knee flexion crease (**Fig. 107.2**).
   - The tibial and peroneal nerves split from the sciatic at the lower third of the thigh (**Fig. 107.3**).
   - The peroneal nerve lies along the medial edge of the short head and medial edge of the tendon of the biceps femoris, which is easily differentiated from the surrounding fat (**Fig. 107.4**).
   - The peroneal nerve can be palpated at the fibular head.
   - This is a point of fixation where the common peroneal nerve dives under the peroneus longus muscle.[2]

10. *When, if ever, should the nerve(s) be repaired?*
    - The nerve should be repaired when no clinical or electromyographic evidence of recovery exists.
    - Nerve action potential (NAP) recording can be done over the affected segment (**Fig. 107.1**).
    - If a regenerative response is noted, then spontaneous recovery to M3 or greater will occur 90% of the time.

- If no recording is elicited, the damaged segment will be resected back to healthy, bleeding, and pouting fascicles and the gap repaired with sural nerve grafts.
- If the damaged segment is greater than 10 cm, orthopedic procedures of recovery with graft repair are so poor that closure may be all that is indicated at this time. An orthopedic procedure such as tendon transfer may then be contemplated at a later time.

11. *What are the results of operative repair at this level for foot drop?*
    - The results of operative repair for peroneal nerve injury are very much distance dependent.
    - Pooled literature shows a 29–50% recovery to M3 or greater with graft repair and a 39–100% recovery with primary suture repair.[3]
    - Graft length is a determinate with 70% recovery for grafts <5 cm, 35% for grafts 6–12 cm and 18% for grafts over 12 cm.[4]
    - Most knee dislocations injure the nerve from its fibular fixation into the sciatic bifurcation thereby requiring long grafts, usually greater than 12 cm, thus predicting poor results.

12. *What are patient's alternatives to nerve repair?*
    - Currently, no acceptable nerve transfers for this nerve injury exist.
    - After a year without neurologic recovery, orthopedic solutions become necessary.
    - The posterior tibialis tendon provides the energy of dorsiflexion.
    - Depending upon the completeness of injury, different variations of tendon transfer are employed.[5]
    - After minor recovery in the evertor muscles (M2), tibialis posterior transfer appears to be more effective.

■ References

1. Kline DG, Hudson AR. Nerve Injuries: Operative Results of Major Nerve Injuries, Entrapments, and Tumors. Philadelphia: W.B. Saunders; 1995
2. Kline DJ, Hudson AR, Kim DH. Atlas of Peripheral Nerve Surgery. Philadelphia: Saunders; 2001
3. Tiel RL, Kline DG. Peripheral nerve injury. In Reiling RB, Eiusman B, McKellar DP, eds. Prognosis and Outcomes in Surgical Diseases. St. Louis, MO: Quality Medical Publishing; 1999: 392–395
4. Kim DH, Kline DG. Management and results of peroneal nerve lesions. Neurosurgery 1996;39:312–320
5. Gould JS, Curry EE. Tendon Transfers as Reconstructive Procedures in the Leg and Foot Following Peripheral Nerve Injuries. In: Van Beek AL, Omer GE SM, eds. Management of Peripheral Nerve Problems. Philadelphia: W.B. Saunders; 1998: 717–730

Section III Neurology

Case 108   Temporal Lobe Epilepsy

Abdulrahman J. Sabbagh, Lahbib B. Soualmi, Fawziah A. Bamogaddam, Khurram A. Siddiqui, and Shobhit Sinha

■ Clinical Presentation

- A 28-year-old left-handed woman presents with the diagnosis of epilepsy since childhood.
- She suffers from two types of seizures.
  - The first type is described as a diurnal episode preceded by an aura of a rising abdominal sensation and fear followed by loss of awareness associated with lip smacking and fine hand-motor automatisms. This is followed by postictal tiredness (2 to 3 per day).
  - The second type consists of nocturnal convulsions (2 to 3 per week).
- She was tried on several antiepileptics, and currently her epilepsy is refractory to triple medications.

■ Questions

1. How do you classify her seizures?
2. Where would you localize her first type of seizures?
3. What would be your presurgical management steps?

She had video electroencephalography (EEG) monitoring that showed ictal and interictal evidence of a right temporal focus.

A magnetic resonance imaging (MRI) scan of the brain is performed (**Fig. 108.1**).

Neuropsychological evaluation reveals normal intelligence, verbal and visuospatial memory. She was shown to be strongly left hemisphere dominant, and Wada test lateralized her verbal functions, memory, and speech to the left side.

4. Describe the finding shown on the MRI.
5. What surgical options are available for this patient?
6. According to current evidence-based studies, what is the expected seizure outcome after temporal lobe surgery compared with best medical management?
7. What is the chance of her becoming completely seizure free (Engel class Ia) after successful surgery? What are the chances of being on monotherapy after surgery? What are the chances of antiepileptic drug freedom after surgery?
8. What are the possible complications associated with temporal lobe epilepsy surgery?
9. Describe the surgical principles in temporal lobe epilepsy surgery.
10. What is the central point? How does it help you during temporal lobe resection?
11. What is Meyer's loop and how can it be avoided during temporal lobe surgery?

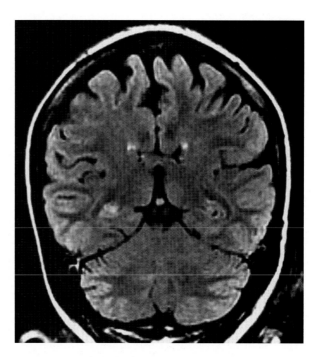

Fig. 108.1 Fluid-attenuated inversion-recovery coronal magnetic resonance image of the brain.

■ Answers

1. *How do you classify her seizures?*
   - The first type is a complex partial seizure.
   - The second type is probable secondary generalized tonic-clonic seizure.
2. *Where would you localize her first type of seizures?*
   - The semiology localizes these seizures to the temporal lobe.
3. *What would be your presurgical management steps?*
   - Management steps include the following:
     - Obtaining a full history and clinical examination
     - Verifying antiepileptic medication serum levels
     - Obtain EEG followed by video EEG telemetry if the EEG was not conclusive.
     - Obtain MRI of the brain
     - Neuropsychological evaluation
     - Wada testing (Dr. Juhn Wada's intracarotid sodium amobarbital procedure to lateralize speech and memory functions[1])
4. *Describe the finding shown on the MRI.*
   - **Figure 108.1** showing a hyperintense signal demonstrates atrophy in the right hippocampus greater than on the left side.
   - These are characteristic features of mesial temporal sclerosis (MTS).
5. *What surgical options are available for this patient?*
   - As all seizures are coming from the right nondominant temporal lobe along with evidence of right-sided MTS the surgical options are as follows:
     - Corticoamygdalohippocampectomy (temporal lobectomy)
     - Selective amygdalohippocampectomy
       - Transsylvian (Yaşargil technique)[2]
       - Transcortical (Olivier technique)[3]
6. *According to current evidence-based studies, what is the expected seizure outcome after temporal lobe surgery compared with best medical management?*
   - According to Wiebe et al.[4] (the only randomized controlled trial assessing temporal lobe epilepsy surgery as of 2008), the number of patients needed to treat for one patient to become free of disabling seizures is two.

- 58% of surgical cases compared with 8% of best medical management cases will be free of disabling seizures.[4]
- Long-term favorable seizure outcome (Engel class I and II) ranges between 50–90%.[5,6]
7. *What is the chance of her becoming completely seizure-free (Engel class Ia) after successful surgery? What are the chances of being on monotherapy after surgery? What are the chances of antiepileptic drug freedom after surgery?*
   - According to the McGill group, 40–58% of patients undergoing temporal lobe epilepsy surgery end up in the Engel Ia class — seizure free.[6]
   - The chance of becoming antiepileptic drug free according to Téllez-Zenteno et al. is 20%.[7]
   - Based on the same study 41% will be on monotherapy.[7]
8. *What are the possible complications associated with temporal lobe epilepsy surgery?*
   - Complications vary among centers and range between 5–10%.[4] They include
     - Infections
     - Hematoma
     - Hemiparesis
     - Memory and language deficits
     - Contralateral upper quadrantanopia — pie-in-the-sky deficit (Some consider it to be an expected finding rather than a complication.)
9. Describe the surgical principles in temporal lobe epilepsy surgery.
   - The following summarizes the steps in the temporal lobe surgery and corticoamygdalohippocampectomy[2,3,8]:
     - Positioning:
       - The aim here is to have the operative field (frontotemporal area) almost horizontal
       - Patient is supine, head in pins, roll under the shoulder.
       - The head is kept higher than the heart and turned 60 degrees, slightly extended, and exposing the temple.
       - Make sure the neck veins are not compressed or over stretched to avoid compressing the neck veins.

■ Answers (*continued*)

- Neuronavigation is used to tailor the skin incision and bony opening.
- Craniotomy:
  - Question mark skin incision from the zygoma just anterior to the ear going back around the pinna and up and parallel to the temporalis line to the hairline
  - Then temporalis fascia incision and muscle opening are done.
  - Exposure of the pterion, the zygomatic root is performed.
  - The craniotomy should reach the anteroinferior-most of the temporal base and then taken to the limits of the skin incision, making sure exposure comprises at least 6.5 cm behind the temporal tip.
  - This is followed by controlling the middle meningeal artery and durotomy.
- Temporal neocorticectomy:
  - The sylvian vein and especially the vein of Labbé (located 5 to 6 cm behind the temporal tip) need to be protected.
  - The middle cerebral artery branches must be avoided.
  - This is achieved via a subpial resection of the first temporal gyrus on the nondominant hemisphere and following the pia of the sylvian fissure.

- Posteriorly, the dissection is performed up to the central point or as tailored by functional imaging if the speech area is close by.
- More medially the temporal resection should not reach or cross the petrous ridge and the temporal horn roof (Meyer's loop) should be avoided.
- Amygdalohippocampectomy and parahippocampal gyrectomy:
  - After opening the lateral wall and the lateral part of the roof of the temporal horn one should identify the collateral eminence and the lateral ventricular sulcus.
  - Medial to the sulcus is the hippocampus (**Fig. 108.2**). The fimbria is identified by moving the choroid plexus superiorly and posteriorly (**Fig. 108.2**).[3]
  - The fimbria and the stria terminalis join, making the anterior border of the choroid fissure (**Fig. 108.2**).[3]
  - The amygdale should be identified anterior and medial through the temporal horn.
  - Using the ultrasonic aspirator the parahippocampus and then the rest of the hippocampal formation is emptied above and below the hippocampal sulcus while holding it with forceps.

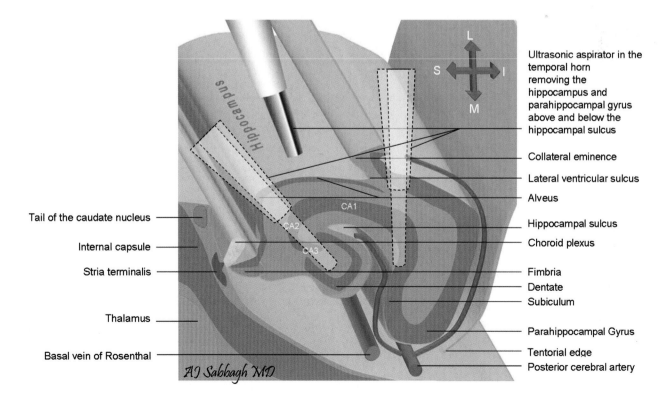

Fig. 108.2   Artist's rendering of hippocampal resection. L, lateral; M, medial; S, superior; I, inferior; CA, cornu ammonis.

■ Answers *(continued)*

- The posterior limit of the hippocampal removal should be at the tectal cistern.
- Care should be taken not to injure the posterior cerebral artery, the basal vein, or the third cranial nerve and cross cerebri medially.
- The dorsomedial limit of removal of the amygdala corresponds to the entorhinal sulcus.
- Intraoperative imaging (if available, such as iMRI or iCT) is particularly helpful to confirm completeness of resection or for reregistration after brain shifts.
- Microscope magnification is very helpful at this stage.

10. *What is the central point? How does it help you during temporal lobe resection?*
- The central point is the meeting point between the motor (M) and sensory (S) strips (there may be a connecting sulcus in the hand area of the homunculus at that level referred to as "pli de passage fronto-pariétal moyen" of Broca[9]).
- The dotted line indicates extent of resection (**Fig. 108.2**).

11. *What is Meyer's loop and how can it be avoided during temporal lobe surgery?*
- It represents the part of optic radiation that projects from the relay neurons in the lateral geniculate body (thalamus) forward and lateral.
- These projections loop on the roof of the temporal horns all the way just beyond them, anterosuperiorly, then backward toward the occipital visual cortex along the calcarine fissure (**Fig. 108.3**).[10,11]
- The loop should be protected during surgery by avoiding the roof of the temporal horns.
- For selective amygdalohippocampectomy:
  - Transcortical: through the middle temporal gyrus onto the lateral wall of the temporal horn would be a safe pathway.
  - Transsylvian: incisions at the level of the limen insulae, or the adjacent 5 mm of the inferior insular sulcus should be a safe pathway.

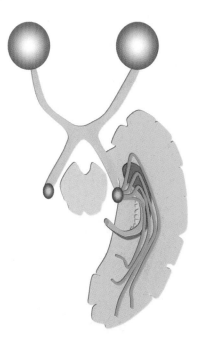

Fig. 108.3 Artist's rendering of Meyer's loop and the visual system. Meyer's loop is illustrated as the structure in turquoise blue. The optic nerve and chiasm are in bright yellow; the lateral geniculate body is the small darker yellow sphere; the temporal horn and contents are in red and orange.

■ References

1. Wada J, Rasmussen T. Intracarotid injection of sodium amytal for the lateralization of cerebral speech dominance. 1960. J Neurosurg 2007;106(6):1117–1133

2. Wieser HG, Yaşargil MG. Selective amygdalohippocampectomy as a surgical treatment of mesiobasal limbic epilepsy. Surg Neurol 1982;17(6):445–457

3. Olivier A. Transcortical selective amygdalohippocampectomy in temporal lobe epilepsy. Can J Neurol Sci 2000;271(1, Suppl):S68–S76

4. Wiebe S, Blume WT, Girvin JP, Eliasziw M. Effectiveness and efficiency of surgery for Temporal Lobe Epilepsy Study Group. A randomized, controlled trial of surgery for temporal-lobe epilepsy. N Engl J Med 2001;345(5):311–318

5. Téllez-Zenteno JF, Dhar R, Wiebe S. Long-term seizure outcomes following epilepsy surgery: a systematic review and meta-analysis. Brain 2005;128(Pt 5):1188–1198

6. Tanriverdi T, Olivier A, Poulin N, Andermann F, Dubeau F. Long-term seizure outcome after mesial temporal lobe epilepsy surgery: corticalamygdalohippocampectomy versus selective amygdalohippocampectomy. J Neurosurg 2008;108(3):517–524

7. Téllez-Zenteno JF, Wiebe S. Long-term seizure and psychosocial outcomes of epilepsy surgery. Curr Treat Options Neurol 2008;10(4):253–259

8. Yoshor D, Hamilton WJ, Grossman RG. Temporal lobe operations for drug resistant epilepsy. In: Roberts DW, Schmidek HH, eds. Schmidek and Sweet's Operative Neurosurgical Techniques: Indications, Methods and Results. Philadelphia: Saunders Elsevier; 2006

9. Broca P. Description Elementaires des Circonvolutions Cerebrales. Paris: Memoires d'Anthropologie;1888:707–804

10. Choi C, Rubino PA, Fernandez-Miranda JC, Abe H, Rhoton AL Jr. Meyer's loop and the optic radiations in the transsylvian approach to the mediobasal temporal lobe. Neurosurgery 2006; 59(4, Suppl 2):ONS228–ONS235

11. Gonzalez LF, Smith K. Meyer's loop. Barrow Quarterly 2002;18(1):4–7

Case 109 Corpus Callosotomy for Drop Attacks

Abdulrahman J. Sabbagh, Jeffrey Atkinson, Jean-Pierre Farmer, and José Luis Montes

■ Clinical Presentation

- A 14-year-old right-handed girl was diagnosed with multifocal epilepsy since the age of 4 years.
- Her epilepsy has become progressive with time and has been intractable for the past 3 years.
- Her seizures are described as staring events that occur 2–4 times a day and atonic drop attack that occur once or twice daily despite compliance with triple therapy.

- She is on three antiepileptic medications, without which she has frequent generalized tonic clonic seizures.
- On examination she is somewhat cognitively subnormal. She has multiple scalp scars of different ages from repeated falls.

■ Questions

1. How would you investigate this case?

Magnetic resonance imaging (MRI) of the brain was essentially normal. Electroencephalography (EEG) showed bilateral multifocal epilepsy.

2. What are the surgical options?
3. What would you tell the parents regarding expected seizure outcome after surgery?
4. What are the predictors of a better outcome?

You operate on her and perform an anterior two-thirds corpus callosotomy. Postoperatively she is well and awake but would not interact or speak for the first few days. She returns to her normal self by the end of the week.

5. The parents were concerned; what do you tell them happened?
6. What are the possible complications related to corpus callosotomy?
7. What are the indications for corpus callosotomy?
8. Describe the parts of the corpus callosum.
9. Compare the callosotomy procedure with vagal nerve stimulation.
10. What are the approaches for corpus callosotomy?

■ Answers

1. *How would you investigate this case?*
   - Investigations include the following:
     - Drug levels to check compliance
     - Single photon emission tomography (SPECT) scans
       - Ictal mode
       - Interictal mode
     - MRI brain
     - Video electroencephalogram telemetry
2. *What are the surgical options?*
   - Surgical options for intractable multifocal epilepsy include[1-3]
     - Corpus callosotomy
       - Anterior two-thirds callosotomy
       - Complete callosotomy (not recommended for almost normal children)
     - Vagal nerve stimulator

3. *What would you tell the parents regarding expected seizure outcome after surgery?*
   - This surgery is palliative.
   - It is more effective in treating atonic or drop attacks compared with other epilepsy types.[1,2]
   - A meta-analysis/systematic review of the literature showed that the long term seizure outcome is 35% of patients with callostomy become free of most disabling seizures.[4]
4. *What are the predictors of a better outcome?*
   - Factors predicting better chance of improvement include the following:
     - Lateralization
     - Frontal origin of seizures
     - Extent of corpus callosum resection[1,5,6]

■ Answers (*continued*)

5. *The parents were concerned; what do you tell them happened?*
   - She has developed the expected postcallosotomy transient mutism.[7]
6. *What are the possible complications related to corpus callosotomy?*
   - Postoperative complications are as follows:
     - Mortality risk is less than 1% and morbidity rates are 6–30%.[6,8,9]
     - The callosal syndrome includes[8,10,11]
       - Inability to name objects presented briefly to the left visual hemifield
       - Left hemialexia
       - Left hemianomia
       - Difficulty imitating the hidden other hand
       - Unilateral tactile anomia
       - Unilateral left agraphia
       - Right-hand constructional apraxia (inability to copy a complex design with the right hand, but ability to outperform this by using the left hand)
     - Interhemispheric retraction
       - Supplementary motor area injury
       - Cingulate gyrus injury
     - Vascular compromise or injury to the following:
       - Superior sagittal sinus hemorrhage or occlusion
       - Pericallosal and supramarginal artery injury
     - Disconnection syndrome[7]
7. *What are the indications for corpus callosotomy?*
   - Callosotomy is a palliative treatment aimed at seizure reduction rather than seizure cure.
   - It is indicated for intractable multifocal epilepsy that is not amenable to resection of an epileptic focus and that is associated with drop attacks.[1,2]
   - Such examples include patients with severe Lennox–Gastaut syndrome.
8. *Describe the parts of the corpus callosum.*
   - Parts of the corpus callosum are described below (**Fig. 109.1**).
     - Rostrum
     - Genu
     - Body
     - Isthmus
     - Splenium
     - Forceps minor and major
   - **Figure 109.1** also shows the approximate locations of connecting fibers of major cortical brain regions.[12]
9. *Compare the callosotomy procedure with vagal nerve stimulation.*
   - Better seizure control can be achieved by callosotomy, especially drop attacks.[3]
   - Vagal nerve stimulation is less invasive.
   - Vagal nerve stimulation is reversible unlike callosotomy.
   - Vagal nerve stimulation has less morbidity.
   - Vagal nerve stimulation requires battery changes and a closer follow-up.[3]

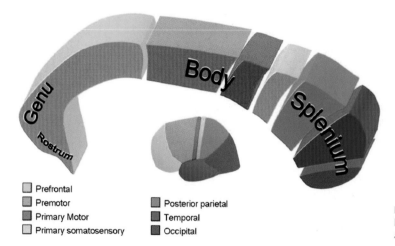

Prefrontal
Premotor
Primary Motor
Primary somatosensory
Posterior parietal
Temporal
Occipital

Fig. 109.1 Parts of the corpus callosum. The approximate locations of connecting fibers of major cortical brain regions are highlighted in the smaller unlabeled image.

■ Answers *(continued)*

10. *What are the approaches for corpus callosotomy?*
    - Standard anterior two-thirds callosotomy[1] or complete callosotomy[2]
      - Supine position
        - Slight flexion with placement of the midline of the cranium at a right angle to the floor
        - Single or double skin openings (anterior and posterior)
        - Interhemispheric approach by entering the cranium at the nondominant hemisphere and/or the side with the least crossing superior sagittal sinus tributaries obstructing the way (neuronavigation is very helpful in outlining those vessels preoperatively).[13]
      - Lateral position (Olivier technique[1])
        - Letting the side of entry inferior, so the brain will sag with gravity to help open the interhemispheric fissure without retraction (**Fig. 109.2**)

- Two-stage approach[13]
  - Starting with the two-thirds callosotomy approach and planning for the remaining one-third at a second stage if seizures need better control despite improvement.
- Other techniques
  - Endoscopic approach[14]
  - Gamma knife or other forms of radiosurgery[15]

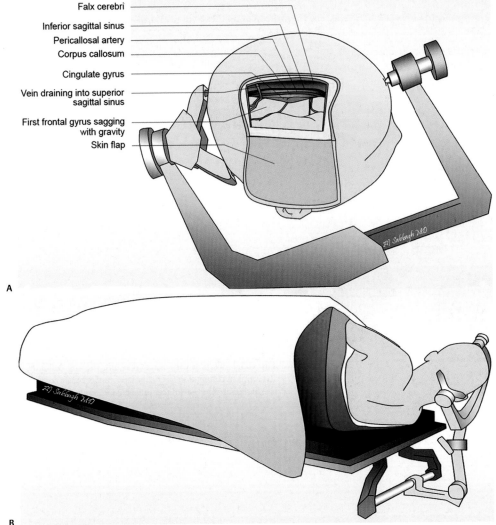

Falx cerebri
Inferior sagittal sinus
Pericallosal artery
Corpus callosum
Cingulate gyrus
Vein draining into superior sagittal sinus
First frontal gyrus sagging with gravity
Skin flap

A

B

Fig. 109.2 Corpus callosotomy via lateral positioning. **(A)** Shows head positioning with respect to the floor, bone flap opening, and exposure. Note that the side of entry is inferior so the brain sags with gravity to help open the interhemispheric fissure without the need for retraction. **(B)** Patient positioning on the bed with Mayfield three-point fixation head holder.

■ References

1. Oguni H, Olivier A, Andermann F, Comair J. Anterior callosotomy in the treatment of medically intractable epilepsies: a study of 43 patients with a mean follow-up of 39 months. Ann Neurol 1991;30(3):357–364

2. Shimizu H. Our experience with pediatric epilepsy surgery focusing on corpus callosotomy and hemispherotomy. Epilepsia 2005;46(Suppl 1):30–31

3. Nei M, O'Connor M, Liporace J, Sperling MR. Refractory generalized seizures: response to corpus callosotomy and vagal nerve stimulation. Epilepsia 2006;47(1):115–122

4. Téllez-Zenteno JF, Dhar R, Wiebe S. Long-term seizure outcomes following epilepsy surgery: a systematic review and meta-analysis. Brain 2005;128(Pt 5):1188–1198

5. Sunaga S, Shimizu H, Sugano H. Long-term follow-up of seizure outcomes after corpus callosotomy. Seizure 2009;18(2):124–128. Sep 15. Epub

6. Maehara T, Shimizu H. Surgical outcome of corpus callosotomy in patients with drop attacks. Epilepsia 2001;42(1):67–71

7. Quattrini A, Del Pesce M, Provinciali L, et al. Mutism in 36 patients who underwent callosotomy for drug-resistant epilepsy. J Neurosurg Sci 1997;41(1):93–96

8. Jea A, Vachhrajani S, Widjaja E, et al. Corpus callosotomy in children and the disconnection syndromes: a review. Childs Nerv Syst 2008;24(6):685–692

9. Sakas DE, Phillips J. Anterior callosotomy in the management of intractable epileptic seizures: significance of the extent of resection. Acta Neurochir (Wien) 1996;138(6):700–707

10. Balsamo M, Trojano L, Giamundo A, Grossi D. Left hand tactile agnosia after posterior callosal lesion. Cortex 2008;44(8):1030–1036

11. Moroni C, Belin C, Haguenau M, Salama J. Clinical callosum syndrome in a case of multiple sclerosis. Eur J Neurol 2004;11(3):209–212

12. Hofer S, Frahm J. Topography of the human corpus callosum revisited–comprehensive fiber tractography using diffusion tensor magnetic resonance imaging. Neuroimage 2006;32(3):989–994

13. Hodaie M, Musharbash A, Otsubo H, et al. Image-guided, frameless stereotactic sectioning of the corpus callosum in children with intractable epilepsy. Pediatr Neurosurg 2001;34(6):286–294

14. Guerrero MH, Cohen AR. Endoscope-assisted microsurgery of the corpus callosum. Minim Invasive Neurosurg 2003;46(1):54–56

15. Smyth MD, Klein EE, Dodson WE, Mansur DB. Radiosurgical posterior corpus callosotomy in a child with Lennox-Gastaut syndrome. Case report. J Neurosurg 2007;106(4, Suppl):312–315

Case 110   Vagal Nerve Stimulator

Nazer H. Qureshi

■ Clinical Presentation

- A 16-year-old boy with cerebral palsy and a long history of seizures is referred to you for a vagal nerve stimulator (VNS) placement.

- The mother wishes the generator to be placed on the right side because of flexion contractures in the left upper extremity.

■ Questions

1. What is the mechanism of action of VNS?
2. What is the United States Food and Drug Administration (FDA-) approved indication for VNS in the treatment of epilepsy?
3. How do you identify the vagal nerve in the neck for implantation?
4. Where on the vagal nerve should the lead wires be ideally placed and is there any concern regarding VNS placement on the right side?
5. What are the reported results for VNS use in epilepsy?
6. What are the usual initial VNS settings for use?
7. What are the usual side effects of VNS placement?
8. The patient returns to you a month later with pus draining out from the battery site. What are your options?
9. Antibiotics and your debridement cleared the infection. What are you going to do next?
10. A few weeks after reimplantation of the battery at the new site, the patient presents with infection along the leads extending into the neck. What are your options now?
11. Nine months after all the infection is cleared, the patient is referred to you once more for reimplantation of VNS. What are your options now?
12. Other than the treatment of seizures, is there any other indication for VNS placement?

■ Answers

1. *What is the mechanism of action of VNS?*
   - The precise mechanism of action of VNS is unknown.
   - It has been suggested that VNS has action on various regions of the brain including the locus ceruleus, amygdala, hippocampus, and contralateral somatosensory cortex.
   - Another proposed mechanism of action is the possibility that VNS increases γ-aminobutyric acid (GABA) and glycine levels in the brain.
   - Ben-Menachem et al.[1] measured amino acid and neurotransmitter metabolite concentrations in cerebrospinal fluid (CSF) samples of patients on clinical trials of VNS before and 3 months after VNS placement.
   - Their results showed an increase in GABA level among patients that failed to respond to VNS stimulation, those with a lower setting of stimulation, as well as patients who had undergone a long-term VNS stimulation.

- Yet others have indicated that VNS decreases cortical epileptiform activity directly and possibly also affects blood flow through different regions of the brain.[2,3]

2. *What is the FDA-approved indication for VNS in the treatment of epilepsy?*
   - In 1997, the FDA approved implantation of VNS as an adjunctive therapeutic modality in reducing the frequency of seizures in adults and adolescents over 12 years of age with partial onset seizure that are refractory to antiepileptic medications.[4]
   - Although the FDA indication for VNS excludes other types of epilepsies, most epileptologists and neurosurgeons believe the indications for placement of VNS to be more widespread.[5,6]

3. *How do you identify the vagal nerve in the neck for implantation?*

■ Answers (*continued*)

- The vagal nerve is in the posterior part of carotid sheath between the carotid artery and internal jugular vein.
- Caution is advised to differentiate the vagus from the phrenic nerve, which traverses in the anterior part of the sheath.

4. *Where on the vagal nerve should the lead wires be ideally placed, and is there any concern regarding VNS placement on the right side?*
   - The right vagal nerve innervates the sinoatrial (SA) node more than 60%, whereas the left vagal nerve mostly innervates the atrioventricular (AV) node of the heart.
   - Placement of the leads on the right vagal nerve is contraindicated, as the stimulation will result in asystole.
   - The risk of bradycardia exists even when the electrodes are placed on the left vagal nerve.
   - What the mother wished was for the battery pocket to be placed on the right side secondary to flexion contractures of the left upper extremity. This can be done and should be considered given the contractures.[7]
   - The ideal place for implantation of leads on vagus is in the middle part of the neck proximal to the branches to the cardiac plexus.
   - The three lead wires are placed from proximal to distal along the nerve.

5. *What are the reported results for VNS use in epilepsy?*
   - In the Vagus Nerve Stimulation Study Group E05 trial, the median reduction in seizure frequency at 12 months after completion of the initial double-blind study was 45%.[8]
   - Overall, 35% of the patients had a reduction in seizures of at least 50%; 20% of the patients demonstrated a 75% reduction in their seizure frequency.[8]
   - Similar results have also been reported in the XE5 trial.[9]
   - A 12-year retrospective review of the effectiveness of VNS in 48 patients with intractable partial epilepsy reported a mean decrease in seizure frequency by 26% after 1 year, 30% after 5 years, and 52% after 12 years.[10]

6. *What are the usual initial VNS settings for use?*
   - Although some centers initiate stimulation the day after implantation, usually the generator is kept turned off and an increase in output is advanced by the neurologists after a 2-week postoperative period.
   - Typically, the output is adjusted to tolerance, using a 30-Hz signal frequency, with a 500-microsecond pulse width for 30 seconds of "on" time and 5 minutes of "off" time.
   - This is not standard and multiple variations exist depending on the clinical situation.

7. *What are the usual side effects of VNS placement?*
   - The most common side effects of VNS are cough, hoarseness, and throat pain.
   - Unlike antiepileptic drugs, VNS has not been associated with adverse effects such as depression, fatigue, confusion or cognitive impairment, etc.

8. *The patient returns to you a month later with pus draining out from the battery site. What are your options?*
   - Infection at the site of battery would necessitate removal of the battery and treatment with debridement and antibiotics.[11]
   - The lead wire could be left in place and moved away from the infected site.

9. *Antibiotics and your debridement cleared the infection. What are you going to do next?*
   - Once the infection is cleared, a new battery should be implanted at another site in the anterior chest wall and reconnected to the lead wires.

10. *A few weeks after reimplantation of the battery at the new site, the patient presents with infection along the leads extending into the neck. What are your options now?*
    - If there is suspicion of infection along the lead wires, then the neck incision should be opened and explored.[12]
    - The wires should be cut close to the vagus nerve's lead implantation site and the leads should be left in situ.
    - Attempting to remove the leads from the vagus nerve will result in injury to the nerve.

11. *Nine months after all the infection is cleared, the patient is referred to you once more for reimplantation of VNS. What are your options now?*
    - The vagus nerve can be explored proximally in the neck and if it is possible to implant another set of leads on the vagus nerve, it should be done proximal to its cardiac branches.

12. *Other than the treatment of seizures, is there any other indication for VNS placement?*
    - Other indications for use of VNS include refractory depression, and research is being conducted for its use in the treatment of such varied diseases as anxiety disorders, Alzheimer disease, migraines, and fibromyalgia.[13,14]

■ References

1. Ben-Menachem E, Hamberger A, Hedner T, et al. Effects of vagus nerve stimulation on amino acids and other metabolites in the CSF of patients with partial seizures. Epilepsy Res 1995;20(3):221–227

2. McLachlan RS. Suppression of interictal spikes and seizures by stimulation of the vagus nerve. Epilepsia 1993;34(5):918–923

3. Henry TR, Bakay RA, Votaw JR, et al. Brain blood flow alterations induced by therapeutic vagus nerve stimulation in partial epilepsy: I. Acute effects at high and low levels of stimulation. Epilepsia 1998;39(9):983–990

4. Schachter SC. Vagus nerve stimulation therapy summary: five years after FDA approval. Neurology 2002;59(6, Suppl 4):S15–S20

5. Nierenberg AA, Alpert JE, Gardner-Schuster EE, Seay S, Mischoulon D. Vagus nerve stimulation: 2-year outcomes for bipolar versus unipolar treatment-resistant depression. Biol Psychiatry 2008;64(6):455–460

6. Ansari S, Chaudhri K, Al Moutaery KA. Vagus nerve stimulation: indications and limitations. Acta Neurochir Suppl (Wien) 2007;97(Pt 2):281–286

7. Spuck S, Nowak G, Renneberg A, Tronnier V, Sperner J. Right-sided vagus nerve stimulation in humans: an effective therapy. Epilepsy Res 2008;82(2-3):232–234

8. Morris GL III, Mueller WM. Long-term treatment with vagus nerve stimulation in patients with refractory epilepsy. The Vagus Nerve Stimulation Study Group E01–E05. Neurology 1999;53(8):1731–1735

9. Amar AP, DeGiorgio CM, Tarver WB, Apuzzo ML. Long-term multicenter experience with vagus nerve stimulation for intractable partial seizures: results of the XE5 trial. Stereotact Funct Neurosurg 1999;73(1–4):104–108

10. Uthman BM, Reichl AM, Dean JC, et al. Effectiveness of vagus nerve stimulation in epilepsy patients: a 12-year observation. Neurology 2004;63(6):1124–1126

11. Smyth MD, Tubbs RS, Bebin EM, Grabb PA, Blount JP. Complications of chronic vagus nerve stimulation for epilepsy in children. J Neurosurg 2003;99(3):500–503

12. Ortler M, Luef G, Kofler A, Bauer G, Twerdy K. Deep wound infection after vagus nerve stimulator implantation: treatment without removal of the device. Epilepsia 2001;42(1):133–135

Case 111   Progressive Multifocal Leukoencephalopathy

Ravi Pande, Maya Nader, and Remi Nader

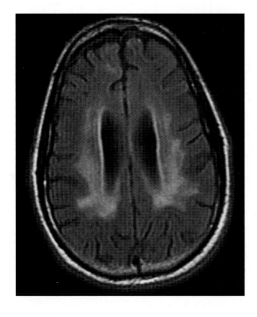

Fig. 111.1   Axial fluid-attenuated inversion-recovery magnetic resonance image of the brain.

■ Clinical Presentation

- A 30-year-old African American man who is deaf presented to your clinic with balance problems and frequent falls. His mother has noticed these symptoms over the past 4–6 months.
- The symptoms are progressively getting worse; now he has to use a walker to ambulate.

- Clinical examination reveals intact cranial nerves, except for deafness. Upper extremity strength is 5/5, lower extremity strength is 4+/5, and he is significantly ataxic while ambulating.

■ Questions

1. What is your next step in the workup of this patient?
2. Describe the magnetic resonance imaging (MRI) findings seen on **Fig. 111.1**.
3. What is your differential diagnosis?
4. What more of the history would you need after reviewing this MRI?

In this case, his aunt did provide the information that he was in multiple same-sex sexual relationships.

5. What further tests would you order?
6. What surgical options would you consider? Under what circumstance?

Test results obtained are as follows. The patient is human immunodeficiency virus (HIV)-positive with a viral load of 750,000 and a cluster of differentiation 4 (CD4) count of 61. Cerebrospinal fluid (CSF) analysis yielded protein level of 105. Polymerase chain reaction (PCR) for JC-virus was negative. CSF immunoglobulin G (IgG) index was high with nine oligoclonal bands (probable markers of demyelination and blood–brain barrier leakage).

7. What are the yields of a brain biopsy in a patient with acquired immunodeficiency syndrome (AIDS)?
8. Discuss your diagnosis after reviewing the test results.
9. What is your management?
10. What is the prognosis?

■ Answers

1. *What is your next step in the workup of this patient?*
   - Obtain an MRI of the brain.
   - Obtain a neurology consultation.
   - May also consider obtaining MRI of the cervical and thoracic spine to rule out causes of myelopathy
2. *Describe the MRI findings seen in* **Fig. 111.1**.
   - MRI of the brain shows extensive periventricular demyelination with some degree of atrophy. On the contrast images (not shown), there was no enhancement.
3. *What is your differential diagnosis?*
   - Differential diagnosis is broad and includes the following[1]:
     - Multiple sclerosis (lesions should typically enhance with contrast)
     - Acute disseminated encephalomyelitis (ADEM)
     - Progressive multifocal leukoencephalopathy (PML)
   - Other less likely diagnosis include
     - Neoplasms (primary or metastatic — atypical as there is no enhancement, no mass effect, and lesions are diffuse)
     - Infectious causes (herpes encephalitis — atypical location)
     - Vascular (small vessel disease — also atypical location)
     - Medication or vitamin deficiencies (vitamin B6 [pyridoxine] deficiency)
4. *What more of the history would you need after reviewing this MRI?*
   - Important history facts to seek include
     - Medical and surgical history
     - Medications taken
     - Family history
     - Other social history
       - Drugs, alcohol, smoking
       - Diet history
       - Sexual contacts and relationships
5. *What further tests would you order?*
   - Toxicology screen
   - HIV panel

   - CSF analysis, including
     - Usual tests (cell count, cytology, cultures, glucose, protein)
     - Viral analysis — particularly PCR for JC-virus[2]
     - CSF immunoglobulin G index
     - Toxoplasmosis titers
6. *What surgical options would you consider? Under what circumstance?*
   - A brain biopsy may be considered if the tests remain inconclusive.
     - This is particularly useful in patients with AIDS who have intracerebral lesions and negative toxoplasmosis titers.[3]
   - There is no focal lesion or mass effect. Therefore, there are no further indications for surgical intervention (aside from obtaining a diagnostic biopsy).[4]
7. *What are the yields of a brain biopsy in a patient with AIDS?*
   - Overall yields range from 67–92%.[3,5–7]
   - In a study on 246 patients with AIDS, a definitive diagnosis was obtained in 92.3% of patients who underwent a biopsy.[3]
     - Lymphoma was the most frequent diagnosis (52.9% of patients).
     - This was followed by progressive multifocal leukoencephalopathy (18.9% of patients).
     - After lymphoma, toxoplasmosis (8.1% of patients) was the most frequently diagnosed.
   - Of note, however, is that a contrast-enhancing lesion will yield a diagnosis more frequently than a non-contrast-enhancing lesion.
     - In a study on 25 AIDS patients, the proportion of biopsies of contrast-enhancing lesions that were diagnostic and contributing to the patients' therapeutic management was 87.5%. However, only 67% of the biopsies of nonenhancing lesions were diagnostic, and none of these lesions were treatable.[5]
8. *Discuss your diagnosis after reviewing the test results.*
   - HIV with AIDS

■ Answers *(continued)*

- Probable PML[8]
  - PML is a rare subacute demyelinating disease caused by an opportunistic papovavirus called JC-virus (JCV) or in some cases by the SV-40 strain.
  - It occurs in patients with defective cell-mediated immunity (2–5% of patients with AIDS),[9] in 1 in 1000 patients treated with Tysabri (Natalizumab; biogen idec, Cambridge, MA; immunosuppressant used in the treatment of multiple sclerosis),[10] in patients with carcinoma and sarcoidosis, and in therapeutically immunosuppressed patients (e.g., transplant patients).
  - A few cases have been reported in the absence of underlying disease.
  - Pathology reveals eosinophilic intranuclear inclusions of papovavirus causing destruction of the oligodendroglia with relative sparing of axons.
  - Demyelination is most prominent in the subcortical white matter, with involvement of cerebellum, brainstem, or spinal cord white matter being less common.
  - With disease progression, the demyelinated areas coalesce to form large lesions.
  - Clinical manifestations are diverse and related to the location and number of lesions.[9]
    - Onset is subacute to chronic with focal or multifocal signs (hemiplegia, sensory abnormalities, visual field cuts, and other focal signs of lesion in the cerebral hemisphere).
    - Cranial nerve lesions, ataxia, and spinal cord involvement are less common.
    - Dementia ensues as the number of lesions increase.
  - A definitive diagnosis of PML can be made by brain biopsy.
  - CSF is usually normal.
  - JC virus DNA can be detected in CSF by nested PCR (n-PCR).[11]

9. *What is your management?*
   - There is no definitive treatment available for PML.
   - Highly active antiretroviral therapy should be initiated with the goals as follows:[12]
     - Improvement of CD4 count
     - Normalization of viral load
     - Neurologic stabilization of PML symptoms

10. *What is the prognosis?*
    - The diagnosis of PML has an overall grim outlook.[11]
    - The course of PML usually lasts months with 80% of patients dying within 9 months.
    - Rarely, survival may be several years, with the longest verified course being 6 years.

■ References

1. Osborn AG. Diagnostic Neuroradiology. St. Louis, MO: Mosby; 1994

2. Ferrante P, Omodeo-Zorini E, Caldarelli-Stefano R, et al. Detection of JC virus DNA in cerebrospinal fluid from multiple sclerosis patients. Mult Scler 1998;4(2):49–54

3. Rosenow JM, Hirschfeld A. Utility of brain biopsy in patients with acquired immunodeficiency syndrome before and after introduction of highly active antiretroviral therapy. Neurosurgery 2007;61(1):130–140

4. Hall WA, Truwit CL. The surgical management of infections involving the cerebrum. Neurosurgery 2008;62(2, Suppl):519–530

5. Chappell ET, Guthrie BL, Orenstein J. The role of stereotactic biopsy in the management of HIV-related focal brain lesions. Neurosurgery 1992;30(6):825–829

6. Iacoangeli M, Roselli R, Antinori A, et al. Experience with brain biopsy in acquired immune deficiency syndrome-related focal lesions of the central nervous system. Br J Surg 1994;81(10): 1508–1511

7. Luzzati R, Ferrari S, Nicolato A, et al. Stereotactic brain biopsy in human immunodeficiency virus-infected patients. Arch Intern Med 1996;156(5):565–568

8. Weber T. Progressive multifocal leukoencephalopathy. Neurol Clin 2008;26(3):833–854 x–xi

9. Vidal JE, Penalva de Oliveira AC, Fink MC, Pannuti CS, Trujillo JR. Aids-related progressive multifocal leukoencephalopathy: a retrospective study in a referral center in São Paulo, Brazil. Rev Inst Med Trop Sao Paulo 2008;50(4):209–212

10. Goodin DS, Cohen BA, O'Connor P, et al. Assessment: the use of natalizumab (Tysabri) for the treatment of multiple sclerosis (an evidence-based review): Report of the Therapeutics and Technology Assessment Subcommittee of the American Academy of Neurology. Neurology 2008;71(10):766–773

11. Sadler M, Nelson MR. Progressive multifocal leukoencephalopathy in HIV. Int J STD AIDS 1997;8(6):351–357

12. Aksamit AJ. Progressive multifocal leukoencephalopathy. Curr Treat Options Neurol 2008;10(3):178–185

Case 112   Neuromyelitis Optica

Xiaohong Si and Robert Herndon

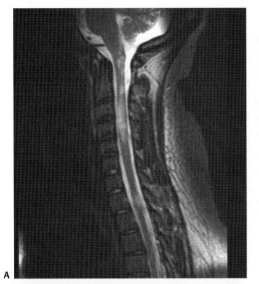

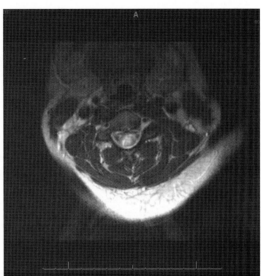

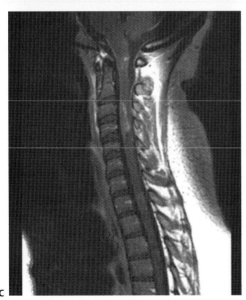

Fig. 112.1 Magnetic resonance imaging of spine with findings of multilevel increase signal and suggest edema on T2-weighted images within the spinal cord. **(A)** Sagittal and **(B)** axial T2-weighted images are demonstrated. The longest extends just below obex to the C5 level. There is second region of increased signal extending from the superior to the inferior margin of the T2 vertebra. **(C)** Sagittal T1-weighted MRI with contrast: this is a postcontrast view of the same lesion in **(A)**. Note the contrast enhancement at level of C3–C4.

■ Clinical Presentation

- A 20-year-old African American woman presented with blurred vision and headaches a few years ago.
- She was then diagnosed with optic neuritis and had a suspected diagnosis of multiple sclerosis (MS).
- At this time, magnetic resonance imaging (MRI) of the brain showed two small periventricular lesions on T2-weighted images.
- She was treated with interferon β-1a (Avonex, Biogen Idec, Cambridge, MA) without significant improvement.

- At the age of 25, she presents now with muscle weakness and numbness in her legs.
- MRI of cervical spine demonstrates multilevel increase signal suggesting edema on T2-weighted images within the spinal cord (**Fig. 112.1**). This abnormal signal within the cervical cord was more prominent with contrast enhancement.

■ Questions

1. What is the differential diagnosis?

Her condition declined steadily over the last decade to the extent that she lost the ability to communicate and ambulate.

2. What is the next step in your assessment?

Her medical history is remarkable for systemic lupus erythematosus. Physical examination reveals some disorientation, unintelligible speech, with some limitations, as she was not following commands. Her reflexes were increased with ankle clonus.

3. What imaging and other diagnostic studies would you like to obtain?

MRI of the brain showed mild cerebral atrophy with two small nonspecific periventricular lesions on T2-weighted images. Electromyography and nerve conduction studies (EMG/NCS) performed on proximal and distal muscles in the upper and lower extremity show myopathic motor units with poor and irregular recruitment. The changes in muscles were interpreted as most likely from disuse and upper motor neuron disorder. Visual evoked potentials show anterior visual pathway dysfunction from the right eye. Findings are normal from the left eye.

4. What are the diagnostic criteria of neuromyelitis optica (NMO)?
5. What specific laboratory tests can be used as evidence to support the diagnosis of NMO?

Laboratory testing results were as follows: urine mucopolysaccharides and oligosaccharides were normal. NMO antibody level was 1:30,720 (normal range is 1:120). Pyruvate level was 0.049–0.183 (normal range is 0.030–0.080). Lactic acid level was 1.1–2.9 (normal range is 0.7–2.1). Antinuclear antibodies (ANA) were 359 U, anti-Smith antibody was 495 U, anti-double-stranded DNA (DS-DNA) was 353 U (all of which are elevated above normal range). Cerebrospinal fluid (CSF) studies are summarized in **Table 112.1**. DNA analysis revealed normal mitochondrial DNA.

6. What is the relation between NMO and MS?
7. What is the most common mistake a neurosurgeon can make when encountering a patient with myelitis coinciding with spondylotic change in the spinal cord?

Table 112.1   Summary of Cerebrospinal Fluid (CSF) Studies

CSF Study	Patient Value	Normal Range
Protein	67	40–70 mg/dL
Glucose	28	12–60 mg/dL
WBC	4	0–5 WBC/cmm
RBC*	7558	0 RBC/cmm
MS Panel	No oligoclonal bands	Not present

Abbreviations: RBC, red blood cell; WBC, white blood cell.

*The RBC in this case represents a bloody spinal tap.

■ Answers

1. *What is the differential diagnosis?*
   - Differential diagnosis included cervical disks myelopathy, systemic lupus erythematosus (SLE), transverse myelitis, vasculitis, spinal cord tumor, infectious or postinfectious processes.

2. *What is the next step in your assessment?*
   - Obtain a detailed history including past medical history, medications, allergies, social history, etc.
   - Obtain a detailed physical and neurologic examination.
   - Obtain laboratory panel, including CSF studies and other demyelinating panel.

3. *What imaging and other diagnostic studies would you like to obtain?*
   - MRI of the brain
   - EMG/NCS
   - Visual evoked potentials

4. *What are the diagnostic criteria of neuromyelitis optica (NMO)?*
   - Neuromyelitis optica was originally defined as an idiopathic inflammatory and demyelinating disease of the central nervous system.
   - It is characterized by optic neuritis and myelitis.
   - It was described by Eugene Devic in 1894 and is also known as Devic disease.
   - The diagnostic criteria of NMO[1–3] includes the following:
     – Optic neuritis
     – Acute myelitis
     – No clinical or neurologic disease outside the optic nerve and spinal cord
     – Serology testing (see question below)

5. *What specific laboratory tests can be used as evidence to support the diagnosis of NMO?*
   - NMO antibody (NMO immunoglobulin G[IgG]) is targeted to aquaporin-4, which is a water channel located on the astrocyte foot processes associated with endothelial tight junctions and cerebral microvessels.[4]
   - NMO-IgG was present in the serum of 91% of patients with NMO, whereas this antibody is present in only 9% of MS patients.[5]

6. *What is the relation between NMO and MS?*
   - NMO is now considered as a distinct entity, separate from MS.
   - The clinical course of NMO was initially thought to be monophasic.
   - It was found to occur as a monophasic illness, that is, either fulminant and fatal or associated with varying degrees of recovery.
   - Its course can be variable. Polyphasic courses characterized by relapses and remissions also occur.
   - Although the clinical course of NMO is similar to a certain type of MS (progressive relapsing MS), NMO patients respond poorly to traditional MS treatments.[6]
   - In addition, the diverse sources of evidence support the hypothesis that NMO is dominated by humoral mechanisms; this is distinct from classic MS.[7]
   - The understanding of the pathogenesis of NMO leads to more effective treatments as well as further explorations into new treatments.[8]

7. *What is the most common mistake a neurosurgeon can make when encountering a patient with myelitis coinciding with spondylotic change in the spinal cord?*
   - Spinal surgery may be mistakenly performed to decompress a case of myelitis with associated mild spondylosis.
   - Neurosurgeons must always be aware of the other causes of myelopathy. These conditions include parainfections or postinfections, systemic autoimmune disease, paraneoplastic syndromes, MS, Devic disease, as well as vascular causes.
   - Therefore, it is necessary to have a more thoughtful workup on these patients.

■ References

1. Wingerchuk DM. Neuromyelitis optica: current concepts. Front Biosci 2004;9:834–840
2. Wingerchuk DM. Neuromyelitis optica. Int MS J 2006;13(2):42–50
3. Wingerchuk DM, Lennon VA, Pittock SJ, Lucchinetti CF, Weinshenker BG. Revised diagnostic criteria for neuromyelitis optica. Neurology 2006;66(10):1485–1489
4. Takahashi T, Fujihara K, Nakashima I, et al. Anti-aquaporin-4 antibody is involved in the pathogenesis of NMO: a study on antibody titre. Brain 2007;130(Pt 5):1235–1243
5. MacReady N. Autoantibody discovery sheds light on NMO, MS differentiation. Psychiatric Times 2006; Sep 1
6. Lalive PH, Perrin L, Chofflon M. Neuromyelitis optica/Devic's syndrome: new perspectives. Rev Med Suisse 2007;3(106):950–955
7. Wingerchuk DM. Neuromyelitis optica: new findings on pathogenesis. Int Rev Neurobiol 2007;79:665–688
8. Matiello M, Jacob A, Wingerchuk DM, Weinshenker BG. Neuromyelitis optica. Curr Opin Neurol 2007;20(3):255–260

Case 113 Normal Pressure Hydrocephalus

Remi Nader

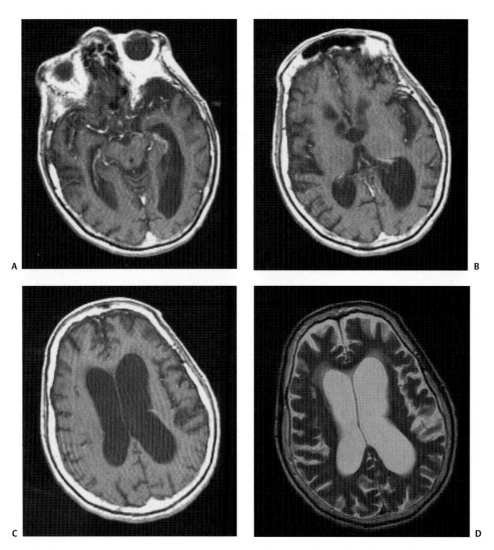

Fig. 113.1 **(A–C)** Sequential axial T1-weighted magnetic resonance images of the brain with infusion of intravenous contrast. **(D)** A T2-weighted axial image at the level of the lateral ventricles is shown.

■ Clinical Presentation

- A 64-year-old woman with dementia and a history of previous head injury ~30 years ago presents with progressive deterioration in her mental status with further dementia as well as incontinence over the past year.
- Over the past 2 months, she has been having some increased drowsiness as well as decreased appetite and some weight loss. She is becoming more agitated.

- She has had some decreased vocalization in the past year.
- The patient has been nonambulatory for ~6 months.
- The remainder of her neurologic examination is within normal limits.
- Magnetic resonance imaging (MRI) is obtained and pertinent images are shown in **Fig. 113.1**.

■ Questions

1. Interpret the MRI.
2. Provide a differential diagnosis and the most likely diagnosis.
3. What are the main clinical criteria for the most likely diagnosis?
4. What is Evans' ratio?
5. What other conditions predispose to this diagnosis?
6. What diagnostic studies can confirm this diagnosis?
7. What are the limitations of these studies?
8. What treatment measures are available for this condition?
9. What are the main complications of these treatment measures?
10. Name some prognostic factors for the treatment of this condition.

■ Answers

1. *Interpret the MRI.*
   - MRI shows diffuse brain atrophy and ventriculomegaly.
   - The degree of ventriculomegaly appears to be disproportionately elevated compared with the amount of atrophy.
   - There appears to be some transependymal cerebrospinal fluid (CSF) transudation in the form of periventricular high signal on T2-weighted images.
2. *Provide a differential diagnosis and the most likely diagnosis.*
   - Normal pressure hydrocephalus (NPH) — most likely
   - Differential diagnosis of dementia includes (mnemonic is "CITTEN DIVA," more common conditions are in boldface)[1,2]
     - Congenital/developmental: Huntington disease
     - Infectious: syphilis, human immunodeficiency virus (HIV), meningitis, herpes encephalitis
     - Traumatic: **posttraumatic dementia**, concussion, chronic subdural hematoma, hypoxia
     - Tumor: metastatic disease, carcinomatosis
     - Endocrine: Addison disease, Cushing syndrome, diabetes mellitus, thyroid and parathyroid disease, renal failure
     - Neurologic: **Alzheimer disease**, Parkinson, Pick dementia
     - Drugs/medications: alcohol induced, vitamin B12 or folate deficiency, pellagra, vitamin B1 deficiency
     - Inflammatory: multiple sclerosis, prion disease
     - Vascular: diffuse small vessel disease, stroke
     - Acquired and other: depression, psychosis
3. *What are the main clinical criteria for the most likely diagnosis?*
   - The Adams triad includes[3]
     - Ataxia: precedes other symptoms, wide based, "glued to the floor," difficult initiation of gait
     - Dementia: memory, bradyphrenia, bradykinesia
     - Urine incontinence
   - Other criteria include male sex, age greater than 60 years, communicating hydrocephalus, normal pressure on lumbar puncture

4. *What is Evans' ratio?*
   - The ratio of the maximum width of the frontal horns to the maximum width of the inner table of the cranial vault[4]
   - If the ratio is greater than 0.3, then there is a greater likelihood of hydrocephalus.[2]
5. *What other conditions predispose to this diagnosis?*
   - Postsubarachnoid hemorrhage
   - Posttrauma
   - Postmeningitis
   - After posterior-fossa surgery
   - Tumor, carcinomatous meningitis
   - Alzheimer disease
   - Aqueductal stenosis
6. *What diagnostic studies can confirm this diagnosis?*
   - Diagnostic studies are outlined below[2,3,5]:
     - CSF "tap" test by performing a lumbar puncture (LP) with removal of 40 to 50 cc of CSF followed by assessment of improvement of cognitive abilities
     - Serial LP
     - Continuous intracranial pressure (ICP) monitoring
     - Lumbar drain placement
     - Radionucleotide cisternography
7. *What are the limitations of these studies?*
   - Limitations of the studies include the following[2,3]:
     - CSF "tap" test has a poor sensitivity (26–62%).[3]
     - LP: An opening pressure (OP) greater than 10 (but less than 18 mm H_2O) is associated with a higher response rate to shunting.
     - Continuous ICP monitoring: Normal OP, but pressure peaks greater than 270 mm H_2O or recurrent B waves are predictors of better prognosis with shunting.
     - Radionucleotide cisternography: Persistence of ventricular activity in a late scan (after 48–72 hours) is associated with a 75% chance of improving with shunting (this is also the case if the ratio of ventricular to total intracranial activity (V/T) is greater than 32%).

■ Answers (*continued*)

8. *What treatment measures are available for this condition?*
   - Ventriculoperitoneal shunt
     - Medium-pressure valve shunt
     - Programmable shunt
   - Other shunt types: ventriculopleural or ventriculoatrial
   - Third ventriculostomy (only in cases of obstructive hydrocephalus)[3,6]

9. *What are the main complications of these treatment measures?*
   - Complication rate of shunting in NPH is 30–40%. These include[3]
     - Subdural hematoma 8–17%
       - Higher rate if the patient is older or if a low pressure valve is used
       - Two thirds resolve spontaneously; one third needs evacuation and shunt tying.
     - Shunt infection, obstruction, or disconnection (10–31%)
     - Intraparenchymal hemorrhage
     - Seizure (4%)

10. *Name some prognostic factors for the treatment of this condition.*
   - The most likely symptom to improve is incontinence, then ataxia, and lastly dementia.
   - There is a better response rate if the gait impairment is the primary symptom.[4,5]
   - Long-term response rate is as high as 75%.[4]
   - The response is better if the symptoms are present for a shorter time.[4]
   - Some patients (e.g., with Alzheimer disease) will improve for a brief period and then worsen again.

■ References

1. Davidson S, Haslett C. Davidson's Principles and Practice of Medicine. Oxford: Churchill Livingstone; 1999
2. Relkin N, Marmarou A, Klinge P, Bergsneider M, Black PM. Diagnosing idiopathic normal-pressure hydrocephalus. Neurosurgery 2005;57(3, Suppl):S4–S16
3. Factora R, Luciano M. Normal pressure hydrocephalus: diagnosis and new approaches to treatment. Clin Geriatr Med 2006;22(3):645–657
4. McGirt MJ, Woodworth G, Coon AL, Thomas G, Williams MA, Rigamonti D. Diagnosis, treatment, and analysis of long-term outcomes in idiopathic normal-pressure hydrocephalus. Neurosurgery 2005;57(4):699–705
5. Marmarou A, Young HF, Aygok GA, et al. Diagnosis and management of idiopathic normal-pressure hydrocephalus: a prospective study in 151 patients. J Neurosurg 2005;102(6):987–997
6. Klinge P, Marmarou A, Bergsneider M, Relkin N, Black PM. Outcome of shunting in idiopathic normal-pressure hydrocephalus and the value of outcome assessment in shunted patients. Neurosurgery 2005;57(3, Suppl):S40–S52

Index

Note: Page numbers followed by *f* and *t* indicate figures and tables, respectively.